A Guide to
Dermatohistopathology

A Guide to Dermatohistopathology

THIRD EDITION

Hermann Pinkus, M.D., M.S.

Professor Emeritus and Former Chairman
Department of Dermatology and Syphilology
Wayne State University School of Medicine
Detroit, Michigan

Amir H. Mehregan, M.D.

Clinical Professor
Department of Dermatology and Syphilology
Associate, Department of Pathology
Wayne State University School of Medicine
Detroit, Michigan

APPLETON-CENTURY-CROFTS/New York

81 82 83 84 85 / 10 9 8 7 6 5 4 3 2 1

Prentice-Hall International, Inc., London
Prentice-Hall of Australia, Pty. Ltd., Sydney
Prentice-Hall of India Private Limited, New Delhi
Prentice-Hall of Japan, Inc., Tokyo
Prentice-Hall of Southeast Asia (Pte.) Ltd., Singapore
Whitehall Books Ltd., Wellington, New Zealand

Library of Congress Cataloging in Publication Data
Pinkus, Hermann.
  A guide to dermatohistopathology.

  Includes bibliographies and index.
  1. Skin—Diseases—Diagnosis. 2. Histology, Path-
ological. I. Mehregan, Amir H., joint author.
II. Title.
RL95.P56 1981   616.5′075   80–17968
ISBN 0–8385–3151–2

Text design: Judith F. Warm

Cover design: Gloria J. Moyer

PRINTED IN THE UNITED STATES OF AMERICA

cells, but it remains present in prickle cells until postnatal life.[4] In the adult, basal cells contain glycogen only in the exceptional circumstances of preparation for rapid proliferation after tape stripping or similar situations (Chap. 7, Fig. 7-2). Prickle cells may contain glycogen in any acanthotic epidermis (Figs. 5-4 and 27-5). Psoriatic epidermis contains it regularly.

The cells of the granular layer appear fusiform (Fig. 2-8A) in vertical sections of skin. Their true shape resembles that of a fried egg. It may be recognized in tangential sections of thick epidermis (Fig. 2-8B). The remnants of the nucleus produce a central bulge in the flattened cell body. The granular layer is a conspicuous feature in vertical sections stained with hematoxylin because keratohyalin has a strong affinity for this dye, a property it shares with chromatin and calcium salts without being related to either. Keratohyalin granules are colorless in the living tissue, but their close arrangement and refractivity have an effect similar to that of glass beads on a projection screen, making the skin surface look white. They also diffuse all colors below them, so that black or brown material in the dermis appears gray. A blue tinge is added by the opaqueness of the white dermal collagen.[11] These effects assume clinical significance in several dermatoses, e.g., lichen planus (Chap. 9), leukoplakia (Chap. 45), and certain pigmentary disorders (Chap. 30).

Another organelle, first described by Selby and by Odland, is present in the uppermost layers of prickle cells.[3] It is visible only under the electron microscope and has been given a variety of names: lamellar body, membrane coating granule, keratinosome, cementosome, or just Odland body. This granule seems to have important physiologic functions in the keratinization process and barrier function of the skin and is abnormal in certain skin diseases. It is probably related to lysosomes, containing acid phosphatase, and is 100 to 300 nm in diameter with a laminated internal structure. It also contains phospholipids. These granules migrate from the Golgi region to the cell membrane and, after being discharged from the cell, spread their contents in the intercellular spaces of the lower horny layer.

Keratinized Cells. The intimate processes of keratinization have become accessible to morphologic investigation only with the advent of electron microscopic and electron histochemical techniques. For our purposes, it suffices to say that normal epidermal keratinization requires tonofilaments and keratohyalin, and perhaps other cell constituents. Above the granular layer, the nuclei disappear. The cells assume the shape of pancakes and have dense membranes and poorly staining centers. Close apposition of the membranes of neighboring cells produces the so-called basketweave appearance of the stratum corneum. The apparently empty spaces are the cell bodies. The true shape of the corneocytes is best seen in scrapings or on tape strips from the skin surface where the cells appear as symmetrical or elongated polygonal flakes with diameters varying from 30 μ to more than 40 μ.[12] This type of examination reveals regional differences and shows characteristic alterations of horny cells in some dermatoses.[13,14] The transition zone between stratum granulosum and stratum corneum, if it is thick, can be recognized as stratum lucidum (Fig. 2-8A), the cells of which appear homogeneous under the light microscope.

Epidermal Biology

The diagram in Figure 2-9 relates the changes of cell size and shape with epidermal biology. Nature's economy requires only 4 broad and flat ker-

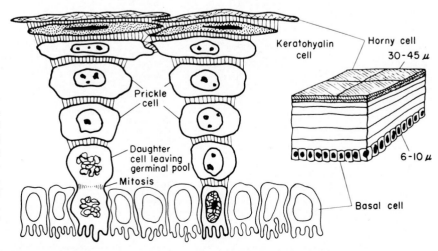

FIGURE 2–9.
Diagram of epidermal biology emphasizes changes in size and shape of keratinocytes from basal layer to horny layer. Insert shows 10 × 10 = 100 basal cells covering the same area as 2 × 2 = 4 keratinized cells. Mitotic division takes place in basal layer. (Adapted from Pinkus. In Handbuch der Haut-und Geschlechtskrankheiten, Ergänzungswerk, 1, 2, 1965. Courtesy of Springer-Verlag.)

atinized cells on the epidermal surface to cover the same area that is occupied by 100 columnar cells at the base. Thus, relatively infrequent mitoses in the basal germinal layer suffice to replace exfoliating surface layers, even if both surfaces are flat. Ordinarily, the presence of rete ridges makes the proportion of basal cells to keratinized cells much more favorable. Mitotic indices of 0.1 to 1 per 1000, as determined by various investigators, are quite sufficient for average epidermal turnover in which the total lifespan of a keratinocyte is about 40 to 56 days.[15,16] This slow renewal of the epidermis can be sped up tremendously in emergencies, such as removal of the stratum corneum by tape stripping (Fig. 7-2) or accidental trauma, and in disease, such as psoriasis.[17] The mitotic index may rise as high as 50 per 1000 viable cells. Under the reasonable assumption of 1 hour for mitotic duration, this makes complete renewal of the epidermis possible in 20 hours. It has been shown that in keeping with general biologic rules,[18] the epidermis needs 36 to 48 hours to retool for this speedup. (For further details see Chap. 5.)

The direction of renewal ("growth") in the human epidermis is outward under most circumstances that do not involve neoplasia or pseudoepitheliomatous proliferation.[19] The true biologic baseline for epidermal growth process is the epidermal–dermal interface. When the interlocking rete ridges and papillae elongate in psoriasis or lichen simplex, the suprapapillary portions of the epidermis are lifted up and moved farther away from this baseline. "Downgrowth" of the rete ridges does not exist in the sense that long ridges extend into a deeper level of the dermis. These points will be taken up in Chapters 5, 7, 8, 20, and 27).

Epidermal Architecture

The epidermis, a tissue consisting of living fragile cells in a state of steady biologic flux, forms a surprisingly tough outer coat without the benefit of extracellular skeletal substances. It is enabled to do so by myriads of intercellular connections, by a mechanically resistant outer covering consisting of its own dead elements which are produced by a complicated process of maturation, and by only partially understood physicochemical barriers formed by polar and nonpolar constitutents in the prekeratin and keratin layers. We have already referred to dermal–epidermal cohesion by means of rootlets of basal cells and dermal fibrils of the basement zone. We will now consider the grosser three-dimensional configuration of the outer and deep surfaces of the epidermis because their changes have significance in many dermatoses.

Inspection at low magnification[20,21] shows the surface of normal skin to be crisscrossed by coarser and finer wrinkles which assume special configurations in the ridged skin of palms and soles (dermatoglyphics). In histopathologic examination, most surface wrinkles appear as relatively minor depressions between fairly straight or slightly rounded stretches. More pronounced serrations of the outer contour are pathologic (papillomatosis, Chap. 5). The deep epidermal surface or epidermal–dermal interface is straight only in atrophic skin, except on the face. It carries a system of ridges between which the vascular papillae of the dermis are inserted. One might say that the epidermis fills all the interstices between the fingerlike papillae like a plastic mass and also provides a suprapapillary plate. This is illustrated in Figure 2-10, showing in

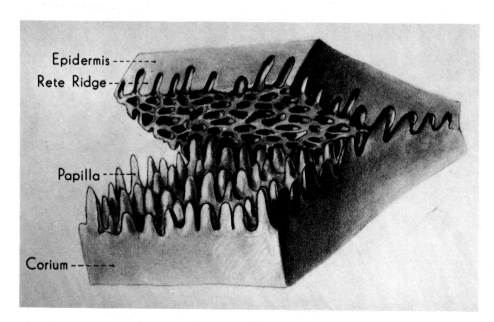

Epidermis

Rete Ridge

Papilla

Corium

FIGURE 2–10.
Artist's drawing of dermoepidermal interface. This three-dimensional view illustrates the effect that would result if epidermis were lifted after pretreatment of fresh skin with dilute acetic acid or other agents. Dermal papillae are pulled out of reciprocating depressions between epidermal ridges. Front of tissue block shows peglike cross sections of rete ridges as seen in paraffin sections, as in Figure 2-4.

Dedicated to
HILDA and VIRGINIA,
our patient and understanding wives,
and to the memory of FELIX PINKUS,
a master of cutaneous anatomy and pathology

Contents

VIII / Mucous Membranes, Hair, and Nail

Preface

To revise our book for a third edition, five years after the second one, presented more problems than anticipated. The second edition had been a careful overhaul of the first to correct details and to add new data. Collection of material during the last five years forced us to make more changes in format, which have been accomplished by a larger page size, printing in two columns, and the addition of about 100 new photomicrographs. In particular, we found it necessary to add a new chapter on immunofluorescence and illustrations of transmission and scanning electron microscopy. These are meant to provide a guide for further study rather than to cover the results of these new and valuable methods.

Another question was the selection of bibliographic references. We felt we should not confront the reader with our personal knowledge and opinions without offering the opportunity to consult other authors. We chose fairly lengthy lists of papers, most of them published in the last six years and either containing new work or more or less comprehensive lists of citations. We had to omit many valuable older references and much that is just as good as the papers cited.

Our general approach has remained the same. We collect those diseases and tumors in one spot that resemble each other and must be differentiated under the microscope, rather than pay attention to any clinical system of organization. We hope the book is complete enough to serve as a textbook of dermatohistopathology, but that it also continues to offer a guide for further individual study.

Again, we had the help of many friends who offered constructive criticism and advice, we received material of slides and photographs from colleagues, and we thank our publishers for their cooperation. Miss Elaine Krobock did a tremendous work in retyping and incorporating new material, and we are duly grateful.

SECTION

I

GENERAL PART

CHAPTER

1

Introduction and Aims

This book aims to be a guide to the interpretation of cutaneous biopsy sections and, therefore, is arranged according to histopathologic similarities and differences rather than in conformity with any clinical system of skin diseases. The book has grown out of the teaching experience of the authors and represents a modification of the instructional course given periodically to residents in the dermatologic and pathologic training programs in Detroit.

It has been our experience that dermatologic residents need a guide beyond the information offered in textbooks. They have to be shown how to look at a section, how to analyze it, and how to tell important pathologic changes from insignificant and coincidental abnormalities. Even before that, they have to be taught normal skin structure and how it appears in haphazard and not always ideally prepared sections. They have to learn to recognize the pitfalls of technical artifacts. In addition, and actually foremost, they have to be taught to think. Histologic diagnosis of skin diseases usually does not result from looking for individual features and adding them up mechanically. Students must realize that they see one fleeting moment in the pathologic process fixed and that each stained section is a random, two-dimensional sample of a three-dimensional organ and may not be representative of all the changes present in the biopsy specimen. They must examine multiple sections and learn to interpret what they see in the three dimensions of space and the fourth dimension of time.[1]

Some very good pathologists frown on too much interpretation: "Describe and diagnose on the basis of objective data" is the motto of many. However, all histopathologic examination includes interpretation, or we would be restricted to describing blue and red blotches rather than calling them epidermal cells, smooth muscle, or eosinophilic leukocytes. It is impossible to draw a distinct line between just enough and too much interpretation. What is called for is constant awareness of the distinction between observation and interpretation. One should not apply time-honored and worn expressions to histologic pictures but interpret them anew, when necessary, on the basis of lessons learned in many different fields: anatomy, experimental embryology, hematology, experimental pathology, biochemistry, and many others. The most profitable course is to observe first, then *consciously* to inject interpretation, and to point out to students as well as to readers of published articles why the interpretation is considered justified. Only then will we stimulate independent thinking and avoid being trapped in dogmatic statements.

All authors have personal opinions based on their education and training and the trend of their mental processes. This book, we feel sure, will be an outstanding example of such bias. We do not apologize, because all statements and interpretations are aimed at helping the student to make diagnoses by understanding what is going on in the tissue—or at least, what might be a reasonable explanation of the pathologic data in biologic terms.

In this respect, the authors continue on a path blazed by researchers like Jesionek,[2] when he called his book *Biology of Healthy and Diseased Skin*, and Kyrle,[3] when he wrote his *Lectures on Histobiology of Skin Diseases*. We hope that modern research on cutaneous biology in all its phases will enable us to come a little closer to the goal envisioned by the older authors.

We advise readers to consult frequently other available texts and to be eclectic in forming their own concepts. We hope that our specific aim in this book of showing students how to analyze their sections will be helpful for that purpose. Since publication of the first and second editions of this book, several new books have become available (Helwig and Mostofi;[4] Graham, Johnson, and Helwig;[5] Milne;[6] Okun and Edelstein;[7] Lever and Schaumburg-Lever;[8] Ackerman[9]), each with its own particular merits. In addition, the encyclopedic treatises of Allen[10] and Montgomery[11] are a must for the serious student. For those who read other languages, the two volumes of Gans and Steigleder,[12] the recent treatise edited by Schnyder,[13] and the concise text of Civatte[14] are recommended. The monumental German *Handbuch* edited by Jadassohn[15] and the supplementary volumes edited by Marchionini[16] remain the most complete source of information for the years before their publication. The annual *Year Books of Dermatology*[17] provide abstracts of and comments on current publications.

The first edition of the *Guide* restricted bibliographic references mainly to personal publications and to those of other authors that supported specific points in the text. We did not think it necessary to duplicate lengthy bibliographies available in other works. The second edition provided more references, which were chosen mainly from recent publications in order to give the reader a starting point for literary search. We have revised the bibliography by the inclusion of newer articles and the omission of others in this third edition. Omission of many excellent publications was painful, but the *Guide* is meant to inform and teach not to give balanced credit to published work. Another omission, which was called to our attention by several pathologists, is clinical description. Although we are aware that dermatopathology includes both macroscopic and microscopic examination of skin diseases, we decided to abide by our original purpose of being a guide to dermatohistopathology and not to lengthen the text by including material that is available in many books on clinical dermatology. An even more difficult decision was inclusion or omission of many new data acquired by histochemical, immunofluorescent, and electron microscopic techniques. Most of these techniques are performed in special laboratories, and many are not yet routine procedures in day-to-day diagnosis. We chose to refer to their results, wherever they enhance our insight into events recognizable by light microscopy. Details are discussed occasionally, and the normal structure of the skin has been illustrated by electron microscopic pictures contributed by Dr. Aurel Lupulescu of the Department of Dermatology and Syphilology of Wayne State University and by Dr. Walter H. Wilborn of the Department of Anatomy, University of South Alabama, Mobile. Dr. Thomas F. Downham II of Wayne State University contributed a chapter on immunofluorescent tests.

REFERENCES

1. Pinkus H: Four-dimensional histopathology. Arch Dermatol 82:681, 1960
2. Jesionek A: Biologie der Gesunden und Kranken Haut. Leipzig, Vogel, 1916
3. Kyrle J: Vorlesungen über Histo-Biologie der Menschlichen Haut und Ihrer Erkrankungen. Berlin and Vienna, Springer-Verlag, 1925
4. Helwig EB, Mostofi FK: The Skin. Baltimore, Williams & Wilkins, 1971
5. Graham J, Johnson W, Helwig EB: Dermal Pathology. Hagerstown, Md., Harper, 1972
6. Milne JA: An Introduction to the Diagnostic Histopathology of the Skin. London, Arnold, 1972
7. Okun MR, Edelstein LM: Gross and Microscopic Pathology of the Skin. Boston, Dermatopathology Foundation Press, 1976
8. Lever WF, Schaumburg-Lever G: Histopathology of the Skin; 5th ed. Philadelphia, Lippincott, 1975
9. Ackerman AB: Histologic Diagnosis of Inflammatory Skin Diseases. A Method by Pattern Analysis. Philadelphia, Lea & Febiger, 1978
10. Allen AC: The Skin, A Clinicopathological Treatise, 2nd ed. New York, Grune & Stratton, 1967
11. Montgomery H: Dermatopathology. New York, Harper & Row, Hoeber Medical Division, 1967
12. Gans, O, Steigleder GK: Histologie der Hautkrankheiten, 2nd ed. Berlin, Springer-Verlag, 1955
13. Schnyder UW (ed): Haut und Anhangsgebilde; Histopathologie der Haut, 1 and 2; 2nd ed. Doerr-Seifert-Uehlinger: Spezielle Pathologische Anatomie, Vol. 7. Berlin, New York, Springer-Verlag, 1978–1979
14. Civatte J: Histopathologie Cutanée. Paris, Editions Medicales Flammarion, 1967
15. Jadassohn J (ed): Handbuch der Haut-und Geschlechtskrankheiten. 23 vols. Berlin, Julius Springer, 1927–1937
16. Marchionini A (ed): Jadassohn's Handbuch der Haut und Geschlechtskrankheiten, Ergänzungswerk. 8 vols. Berlin, New York, Springer-Verlag, 1959-1980
17. Year Books of Dermatology. Chicago, Year Book, 1969–1979

CHAPTER

2

Normal Structure of Skin

The skin is a vitally important organ, has a complicated structure, and serves many functions.[1-3] "Normal skin," however, is an abstraction. Topography and differences of age, sex, and genetic constitution introduce so many variations that few general statements can be made. One has to have exact clinical information in order to adjudge a given section of skin normal or abnormal. Figure 2-1 illustrates four regions of skin photographed at identical magnification. Differences are obvious in the total dimensions of the organ, the absolute and relative thickness of epidermis and dermis, their architecture and structure, number and size of hair follicles and glands, and many other details.

It is of fundamental importance for the dermatopathologist to study the normal features of skin and their variations. He should also inform himself about embryologic development and the biology of the entire organ and its components. Some major misconceptions and misnomers in dermatology have resulted from inadequate knowledge of normal development, structure, and function. We will name only a few: the fibrovascular tumors of the central face in the tuberous sclerosis syndrome are to this day known by the misnomer "adenoma sebaceum" because Pringle did not realize in the nineteenth century how large normal sebaceous glands can be in this region. The now obsolete name "rete pegs" for the projections of the lower surface of the epidermis was based on failure to view the structure of the skin in three dimensions. Darier's division of skin cancers into "basal cell,"

"prickle cell," and "mixed" types was based on incomplete knowledge of epidermal biology and led to the strange misinterpretation that basal cells and prickle cells proliferate independently of each other, a concept that was corrected only many years later. Finally, use of the oversimplifying term "primary epithelial germ" for the mesodermal–ectodermal anlage of the pilar apparatus has held back for many years the recognition and investigation of epithelial–mesenchymal interaction in cutaneous neoplasia (Sec. VII).

The study of normal skin structure does not require an elaborate program of obtaining and preparing specimens of healthy skin. Many biopsy specimens submitted to the laboratory for diagnosis show normal features of some skin constituents. The student should establish a habit of examining all features of a skin section, not only those which are important for making a diagnosis. In many cases, one should spend more time and look at more sections studying the normal than interpreting the abnormal. Effort thus expended will be repaid manyfold by the experience gained whenever a difficult point of interpretation arises. The better anatomist and biologist becomes, in due time, the better dermatopathologist.

DEVELOPMENT

The skin of the fetus[2,4,5] is derived from ectoderm and mesoderm. From the simple epithelial layer

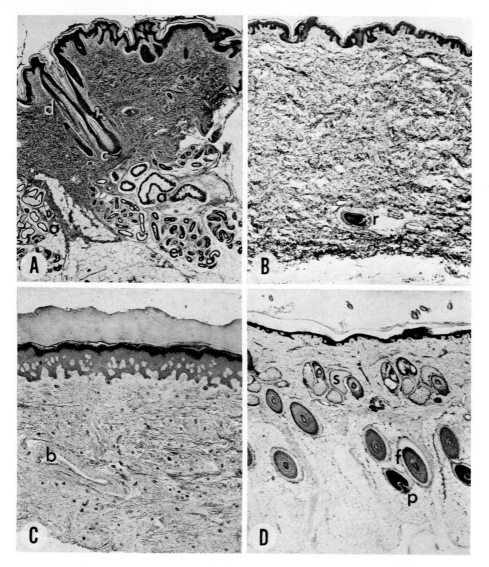

FIGURE 2–1.
Normal skin from four different body areas stained with H&E. ×21. **A.** *Axilla.* **B.** *Back of trunk.* **C.** *Sole.* **D.** *Scalp, a, apocrine coil; b, artery; c, catagen hair; d, apocrine duct; e, eccrine coil; f, fibrous root sheath; p, hair papilla; r, hair root; s, sebaceous gland.*

covering the surface of the embryo, the neuroectoderm is split off when the neural groove closes to form the neural tube. Material in the thickened rims of the groove (neural crest) contributes to the skin by forming the sympathetic nervous system and furnishing melanoblasts. The secondary ectoderm (Fig 2-2) soon becomes two-layered and later stratified (Fig. 2-3A) through mitotic activity greater than that needed to keep pace with general body growth. Ectoderm, in contrast to entoderm, has an inherent tendency toward stratification and expresses it even in tissue culture.[6] Glands derived from ectoderm are lined by at least two layers of epithelium.

While mitotic activity occurs in both layers of the primitive epidermis, it soon is restricted to the basal layer, which thus becomes the germinal layer (stratum germinativum) from which cells move outward to become mature and exfoliated. The outer layer of embryonic epidermis is called the *periderm* (the term "epitrichium" has no founda-

tion in human anatomy and is obsolete) and seems to fulfill a function of exchange between body and amniotic fluid. Electron microscopic studies have shown that the outer surfaces of periderm cells carry microvilli and fuzz, like those seen in ex-

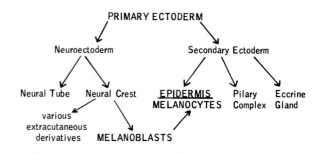

FIGURE 2–2.
Ectodermal derivatives. Note that the epidermis is but one of several ectodermal structures in the skin and that melanocytes reenter the skin secondarily as neuroectodermal derivatives and find their final location at the dermoepidermal junction.

change-active epithelia (Fig. 2-3B). After the sixteenth week, periderm is replaced by keratinizing cells, and the epidermis gradually assumes the characteristics of the stratified adult tissue.

The dermis (cutis and corium are synonyms) is furnished by embryonic mesoderm.[7] Portions of it are temporarily organized into somites and, thus, have metameral structure. Segmental organization, however, is soon obliterated in the skin, and major portions of it on head, neck, and extremities are not derived from somites. So-called dermatomes are established secondarily by the distribution of segmental nerves. Similarly, while some blood vessels are derived from segmental arteries, many form as plexus in the local mesenchyme. At certain periods, the embryonic skin is a blood cell-forming organ, a function that may be revived under pathologic conditions.[8] Connective tissue fibers are laid down gradually, reticulum and collagen earlier than elastin.[9]

The two types of cutaneous adnexa, pilar complexes and eccrine glands, are derived from the epidermal basal layer through individual acts of differentiation in which ectoderm and mesoderm interact. There is no invagination of epidermis, and the cells of each hair germ and eccrine germ form a new biologic unit. They grow by mitotic division of their own elements and penetrate downward

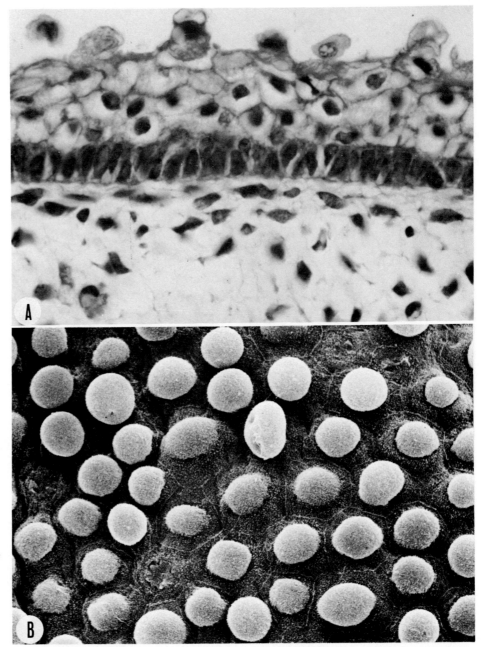

FIGURE 2–3.
Skin of fetal foot showing stratified epidermis, with columnar basal cells, pale (glycogen-rich) prickle cells, and exfoliating periderm cells. Not all areas of body achieve this high degree of fetal differentiation. Dermis is relatively unstructured, consisting of stellate cells and few thin collagen fibers suspended in mucinous ground substance. H&E. ×600. **B.** *Scanning electron micrograph of surface of similar skin. Polygonal outline of uppermost prickle cells. Protruding periderm cells showing microvilli, some of which have exfoliated. X840. (Courtesy of Dr. W. H. Wilborn.)*

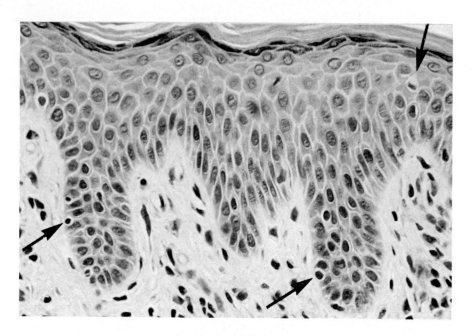

FIGURE 2–4.
Vertical section of adult epidermis. Well-developed ridges and papillae, thick stratum spinosum, and multiple stratum granulosum under the nonnucleated stratum corneum. Basal cells are more or less columnar. Two arrows point to junctional melanocytes. Arrow at right points to a high-level dendritic cell that may be a Langerhans cell. Papillae contain fixed tissue-type cells embedded in fibrillar connective tissue. H&E. X370.

through the dermis and upward through the epidermis to the surface.[2] While the eccrine apparatus remains a simple tubular unit throughout life, the pilar germ becomes a complex miniature organ consisting of hair root, sebaceous gland, apocrine gland, arrector muscle, and haarscheibe. In its growth and function, ectodermal and mesodermal components continuously interact, and the term "primary epithelial germ" should be abandoned in favor of either the older *hair germ* or the more inclusive *hair apparatus germ*. Many ultrastructural data on the embryology of human skin have been contributed by Hashimoto (reviewed by Holbrook[5]).

EPIDERMIS

The epidermis is a stratified epithelial tissue (Fig. 2-4) which renews itself continually through mitotic division of its basal cells. Daughter cells achieve suprabasal position and undergo a slow pro-

cess of maturation during which they are described as "prickle (spinous) cells," "granular (keratohyalin) cells," and "horny cells" or "corneocytes." All these phases of the epidermal keratinocyte (Table 2-1) are comparable to the maturing stages of the erythropoietic series, from stem cell through erythroblast and normoblast to erythrocyte. The mature keratinized cell is the functional end product of keratinopoiesis, just as the nonnucleated red cell is the all-important end product of hematopoiesis. Both are functionally active and biologically dead.

Epidermal Layers

Precise terminology is a prerequisite for clear thinking and scientific communication. We therefore list various definitions in Table 2-2. The term *basal cell* means cell at the base in contact with mesoderm. Basal cells anywhere in the skin are the principal germinal cells for epidermis and adnexa,

TABLE 2–1.
Biology of the Keratinocyte

Common Name	Biologic Function	Hematologic Analog
Basal cell	Principal matrix (epidermal germinative cell) adhesion to dermis	Medullary stem cell
Prickle (malpighian) cell	Auxiliary matrix, early stage of keratinization, mechanical stability	Erythroblast
Granular (keratohyalin) cell	Progressing keratinization, part of physiologic barrier	Normoblast
Keratinized (horny) cell (corneocyte)	Functionally mature, biologically dead, mechanical and chemical barrier	Erythrocyte

TABLE 2–2.
Definitions and Recommended Terms in Epidermal and Adnexal Histology

Epidermis

Definition

Epithelial tissue derived from embryonic ectoderm and covering the outer surface of the skin. See Figure 2-2. (Sometimes inappropriately used in a wider sense for all ectodermal epithelia in the skin.)

Recommended Terms

1. *Epidermis* for surface epithelium of skin
2. *Mucosal epithelium* for surface epithelium of oral and other mucous membranes
3. *Adnexal epithelium* (follicular, sebaceous, eccrine, and apocrine) for epithelial parts of hair follicles and cutaneous glands
4. *Ectodermal epithelium* when two or all of the above are meant
5. *Ectodermal modulated cell* for quasi-embryonic cell in wound healing or other emergency situations (see Fig. 2-13)
6. *Stratified* for any multilayered epithelium whether of ectodermal or entodermal origin
7. *Squamous* for any multilayered epithelium in which cells flatten and usually keratinize toward the surface
8. *Epidermoid* for any epithelium keratinizing in the epidermal (orthokeratotic) manner with keratohyalin formation

The Ubiquitous and Confusing Basal Cell

Anatomic Definition

1. Lowest cell in epidermis in contact with dermis
2. Outermost cell of cutaneous adnexa in contact with dermis

Recommended Terms

1. *Epidermal basal cell*
2. *Adnexal basal cell*

Physiologic Definition

1. Immature matrix cell of epidermis
2. Immature matrix cell of adnexa

Recommended Terms

1. *Epidermal matrix* (or *germinal*) *cell*
2. *Adnexal matrix cell*

Pathologic Definition

1. Immature cell of benign tumors
2. Specific cell of basal cell epitheliomas (basal cell carcinomas)

Recommended Terms

1. *Basaloid cell*
2. *Basalioma cell*

Keratinocyte

Definition

Any epithelial cell that is part of a keratinizing tissue

Recommended Terms:

1. *Epidermal keratinocyte* (Table 2-1)
2. *Adnexal keratinocytes* compose all parts of the hair and hair follicle, the sebaceous duct, and the intra-epidermal sweat duct (acrosyringium).

TABLE 2–2 (Continued).

3. *Prickle cell*, although actually a misnomer, remains the accepted term for cells between the basal and the granular or keratinized layers. *Spinous cell*, which has the same meaning, is less commonly used. *Squamous cell* implies that the cell either is or is expected to become a squame or flake. The term is applied mainly to the cells of epidermoid carcinomas.
4. *Keratinized cell* (*horny cell, corneocyte*) applies mainly to nonnucleated cells above the granular layer (orthokeratotic cells) but is also used for nucleated parakeratotic cells once they have reached the final stage of their development.

Nonkeratinocytes

Definition

Cells found in the epidermis which do not undergo keratinization

Recommended Terms

1. *Dendritic cells* comprising *melanocytes, Langerhans cells,* and *Merkel cells* all of which live in the epidermis as symbionts.
2. *Mesodermal cells* which have entered the epidermis by the process of exocytosis might be included in a wider sense but are better identified as small round cells, granulocytes, mast cells, and so on.
3. *Nonkeratinizing tumor cells* should be designated as nevus cells, malignant melanoma cells, Paget cells, and so on.

but under pathologic conditions, e.g., in psoriatic epidermis, the anatomic basal cells are not synonymous with physiologic germinal cells. In psoriasis and in other conditions of rapid epidermal proliferation, one or more suprabasal layers may be part of the stratum germinativum. When Krompecher introduced the term "basal cell carcinoma," he stretched the meaning of the phrase *basal cell* to a degree that became highly confusing and led thinking and investigation astray for decades. The small, dark-staining cells that form a large portion of the substance of benign epidermoid and adnexoid tumors, and the tumor cells of basal cell epitheliomas (basal cell carcinomas, basaliomas) bear only a very superficial resemblance to normal basal cells. They are basaloid cells, and in the case of basal cell epithelioma, we may call them *basalioma cells* (Sec. VII, Chaps. 33 to 39).

Basal Cells. Epidermal basal cells may be flat, cuboidal, or columnar. In conformity with their shape, they contain a round or ovoid nucleus which stains dark with hematoxylin and basic aniline dyes and has a coarse chromatin network, usually without a prominent nucleolus. In addition to their role as germinal cells, basal cells have the vitally important function of maintaining the connection

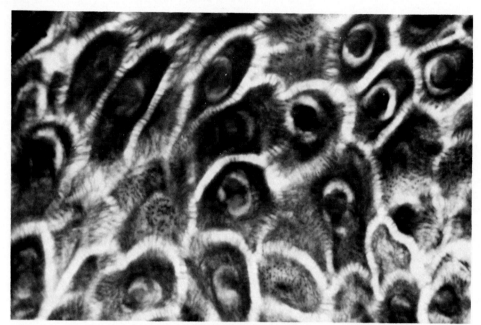

FIGURE 2–5.
Prickle cells in chronic ecze-matous dermatitis. Intercellular bridges are stretched across widened intercellular spaces. Bridges appear as dark dots where cut transversely, no free prickles. Slight thickening in center of some bridges repre-sents Bizzozero's nodule (des-mosome). Hematoxylin-Pon-ceau S-picric acid. X900.

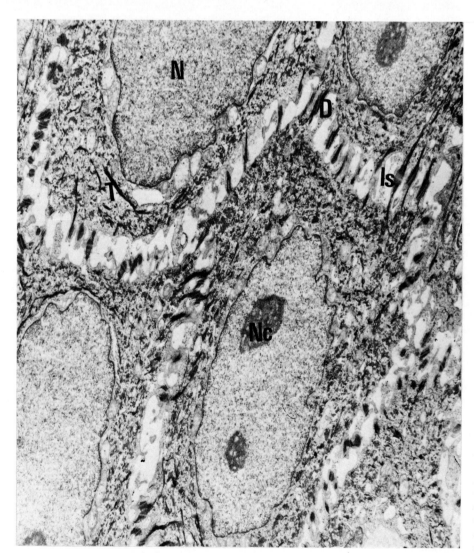

FIGURE 2–6.
Four prickle cells conntected by stretched intercellular bridges in slightly edematous skin. Dark tonofilaments (T) in the cytoplasm extend into the bridges and are connected to desmosomes (D). IS, intercel-lular space; N, nuclei, Nc, nu-cleoli. Electron micrograph. X11,200. (Courtesy of Dr. A.P. Lupulescu.)

between dermis and epidermis, which is insured by several mechanisms (p. 16–18). Basal cells possess numerous pedicles or rootlets which greatly increase the contact surface and are inserted between the felt of superficial dermal fibrils.

Other surfaces of the basal cell are connected with neighboring basal cells and prickle cells by means of desmosomes on which intracellular tonofibrils attach. Thick bundles of the latter are known as "Herxheimer spirals." Old disputes between light microscopists concerning the existence of tonofibrils and the nature of intercellular bridges have been laid to rest by the higher resolution of the electron microscope. Basal cells and prickle cells are much alike in their constituents and structure. The prickle cell differs from the basal keratinocyte due to its detachment from contact with mesoderm and its starting on the road to maturation and death (Chap. 5).

Prickle Cells and Granular Cells. The multiple layers of prickle cells (spinous cells) constitute what we call the *rete malpighi,* an old term which remains useful. *Prickle cell* itself is a misnomer inasmuch as the cells are not beset with free-ending prickles or spines. If a prickle cell becomes separated from its neighbors, as in pemphigus or other acantholytic dermatoses, its contour appears smooth under the light microscope. Only when keratinocytes are in contact with others do they develop intercellular connections (desmosomes). In not too well fixed preparations, these are drawn out into bridges and, in transverse section, give the appearance of prickles. When the pioneers wanted to study prickle cells, they chose condyloma acuminatum, the hyperplastic and edematous epidermis of which shows cellular detail much better than does normal tissue. Figure 2-5 represents hyperplastic epidermis of chronic eczematous dermatitis. Electron microscopy has shown that intercellular spaces normally are very narrow, that cell contours are convoluted and interlocking, and that desmosomes as circumscribed areas of attachment of the cell membranes are usually situated at the slants and not at the tips of the dovetailing pattern. With intercellular edema or in specimens in which fixation caused some shrinkage (Fig. 2-6), cells pull away from each other but remain connected by the desmosomes, which now seem to sit as bridge nodules (Bizzozero) at the center of cytoplasmic bridges. In spite of their complicated structure (Fig. 2-7), desmosomes break and re-form with relative ease,

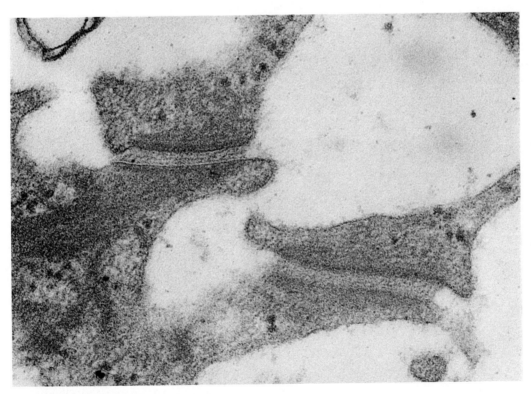

FIGURE 2–7.
High magnification of two desmosomes sitting at the center of stretched cytoplasmic bridges which contain dark tonofilaments. The desmosomes have several electron-dense and electron-lucent layers and a thickened plasma membrane at either side. (Courtesy of Dr. A.P. Lupulescu.)

probably within hours,[10] whenever keratinocytes move against each other or leukocytes migrate between them. The separated cell surfaces then have microvilli like numerous other cell types, but these are submicroscopic and are not to be confused with prickles.

The light microscopic image of prickles is due to tonofibrils, actually bundles of tonofilaments, which sweep from the interior of the cell to the desmosomes. Tonofibrils are largely responsible for the dense, somewhat bluish appearance of prickle cell cytoplasm in H&E sections. Tonofibrils are demonstrable with Unna's and other stains. They seem to be absent in cells of the intraepidermal sweat duct and in tumor cells of basaloid type. These cells possess ultramicroscopic tonofilaments, which are not arranged into bundles. Under the light microscope, such cells may be connected by thin cytoplasmic

bridges, but lack the intracytoplasmic component, the tonofibrils, which make the bridge a solid-appearing, ropelike structure. These points are discussed in Chapters 33 to 39.

Prickle cells are bulkier than basal cells, have vesicular nuclei with distinct membrane, and have one or several angular nucleoli (Fig. 2-6). Cells in the higher layers become flat and broad and eventually acquire keratohyalin granules, while the nucleus becomes pyknotic and then disappears. Normally, a cell may go through these stages in about two weeks, although individual variations exist.

The prickle cells are apt to contain glycogen. This substance, essential in carbohydrate metabolism, fills all layers of the embryonic epidermis. It is first absent in the early hair germ and later is distributed in a characteristic pattern (see Fig. 2-24). In the epidermis, glycogen disappears from basal

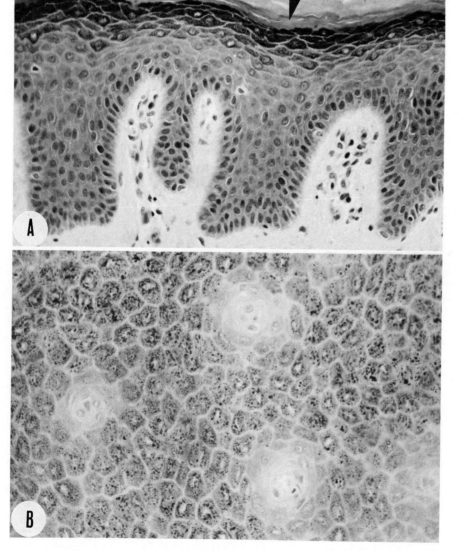

FIGURE 2–8.
A. *Vertical section of thick epidermis of volar skin showing a thick stratum granulosum and stratum lucidum (arrow) that appears darker than the stratum corneum. Two cells in stratum spinosum, consisting of dark nucleus and light halo, may be Langerhans cells. H&E. X370.* **B.** *Tangential section through stratum granulosum with cross sections of three eccrine sweat ducts. The polygonal shape of granular cells is well depicted. H&E. X370.*

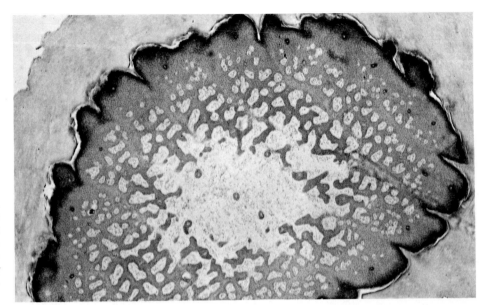

FIGURE 2–11.
Oblique section of finger skin. H&E. Pictures of this type, while confusing in histopathologic specimens (see Fig. 3-15), reveal three-dimensional architecture of epidermis and show regular spacing of cross-sectioned eccrine ducts.

diagrammatic form that rete pegs do not exist but are a misinterpretation of transverse section of rete ridges. Oblique sections of thick normal skin (Fig. 2-11) furnish surprising but highly instructive pictures which should be kept in mind in the interpretation of pathologic specimens, not all of which are embedded and cut in the ideal manner (Chap. 3).

Epidermal Symbiosis

The epidermis consists not only of the epidermal keratinocytes but of three other components. Two of these are the intraepidermal portions of pilar complex (acrotrichium) and eccrine apparatus (acrosyringium), and the third one consists of dendritic cells (melanocytes and Langerhans cells). To speak of the epidermis as a symbiosis appears justified if we consider that all four components maintain themselves in balance by mitotic division of their own germinal cells, that their interdependent life processes give various types of healthy epidermis its specific characteristics, and that they may act and react quite independently under pathologic conditions.

A description of the nonkeratinocytes (melanocytes and Langerhans cells) will be given at the end of the chapter. The adnexal keratinocytes of pilar and eccrine origin have a peculiarly ambivalent role. In fetal life (see below), these poral portions grow from their specific adnexal germs in the basal layer upward through the epidermis, while the main portion of the germ forms the intradermal structures. In adult life, acrosyringeal cells have several features by which one can distinguish them from epidermal keratinocytes with fair ease.[22] They

never contain melanin, even in the darkest Negro epidermis (Fig. 2-12), and do not contain microscopically visible tonofibrils (although electron microscopy reveals tonofilaments). These cells often have roundish nuclei with several small chromatin

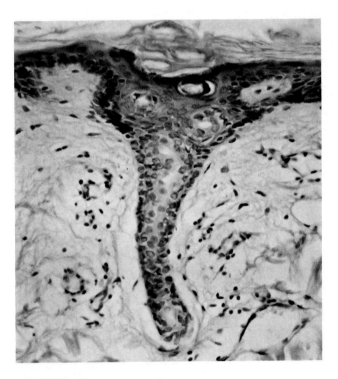

FIGURE 2–12.
Acrosyringium. Nonpigmented eccrine duct coils in relatively thin pigmented epidermis and is cut transversely six times in stratum malpighi and stratum corneum. Cells of intraepidermal eccrine unit contain keratohyalin in second and third turn and are fully keratinized in three upper turns. H&E. X180.

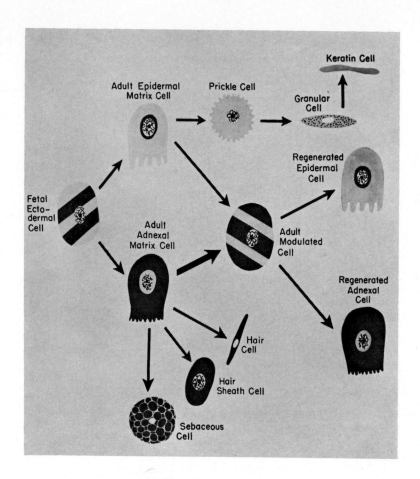

FIGURE 2–13.
Diagram of ectodermal pluripotentiality and modulation. Fetal ectodermal cell (left) has epidermal (light gray) and adnexal (dark) potential. Adult ectodermal cell, whether epidermal or adnexal matrix cell, preserves in latent form opposite potential (indicated by ring around nucleus), which becomes manifest in quasi-fetal modulated cell of healing wound. Modulated cells derived mainly from adnexal matrix cells redifferentiate in epidermal or adnexal direction.

masses and begin to form keratohyalin and keratinize at a deeper level in the epidermis than the epidermal keratinocytes. Their keratin tends to stain red in O&G sections (Chap. 3).

Acrotrichial keratinocytes, on the other hand, are practically indistinguishable from the epidermis that surrounds them. This has been the reason for the often repeated but incorrect statement that the follicular infundibulum is an invagination of the epidermal layers. It would lead too far to repeat at this point all the evidence for the existence of the intraepidermal follicular wall.[23] However, once we accept the concept, many features of skin pathology and especially of epidermal and adnexal neoplasia (Chaps. 33 to 38) assume biologic significance, and diagnostic acumen is enhanced.

Thus, acrosyringium and acrotrichium are biologically separate symbionts in the epidermis under normal and many abnormal conditions. However, in certain emergency situations, especially in wound healing, adnexal keratinocytes become modulated (Fig. 2-13), return to a quasi-embryonic state, and redifferentiate into epidermis indistinguishable from the one they replace. This ambivalence of adnexal cells must be kept in mind and will be referred to in later chapters.

JUNCTION

The line at which epidermis and dermis meet in vertical sections through the skin is in three-dimensional view an interface of complicated configuration (Figs. 2-11 and 2-12). PAS stain (Fig. 2-14) reveals a sharply defined thin zone of neutral mucopolysaccharides which is similarly prominent in immunofluorescent examinations in a number of diseases (Chap. 4). Electron microscopy (Fig. 2-15) has shown[22] that the cell membrane of the basal cell rootlets is paralleled in all its convolutions by a thin (300 nm), electron-dense basal lamina, which is separated from the cell membrane by an electron-lucent gap (lamina lucida). The cell membrane carries hemidesmosomes to which intracellular tonofilaments attach. The dense basal lamina is connected to underlying collagen fibrils by special anchoring fibrils. Details are illustrated diagrammatically in Figure 2-16 at three increasing magnifications.

This basement zone is what the term *junction* implies. It is a zone consisting of different materials, ordinarily insuring a firm cohesion between epidermis and dermis. How it is disrupted under pathologic conditions will be seen in the discussion

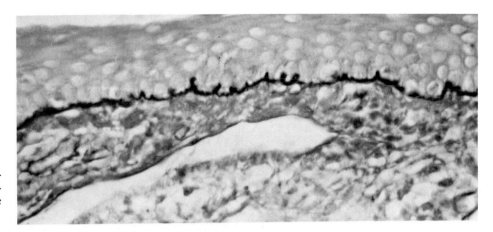

FIGURE 2–14.
PAS-positive basement membrane at dermoepidermal interface. Alcian blue-PAS-picric acid stain. X460.

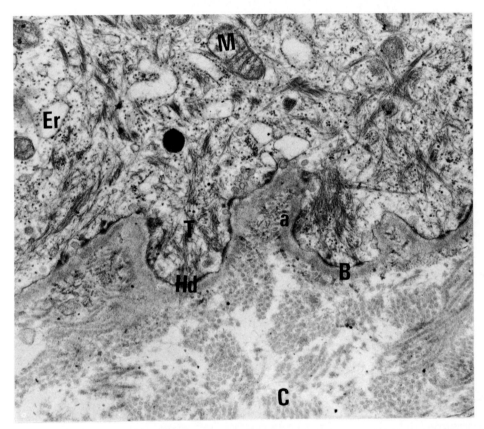

FIGURE 2–15.
Electron micrograph of dermoepidermal junction. Basal lamina (B) with anchoring fibrils (a) and hemidesmosomes (Hd) to which tonofilaments (T) extend. Mitochondrion (M) and rough endoplasmic reticulum (Er) in basal cell. Collagen fibrils (E) in dermis. X36,000. (Courtesy of Dr. A.P. Lupulescu.)

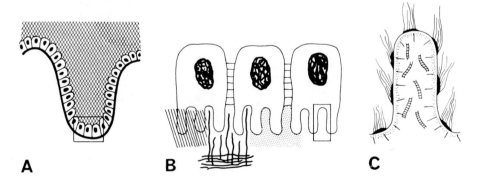

FIGURE 2–16.
*Diagrammatic representation of dermoepidermal junction as seen at different magnifications by different techniques. **A.** Low power shows rete ridge with basal cells. **B.** Three basal cells with rootlets. Reticulum fibers (at left), elastic fibers (center), and ground substance (right) demonstrated in basement zone by appropriate staining. **C.** Electron microscopy shows basal lamina with anchoring fibrils, basal cell membrane with half-desmosomes, tonofibrils in basal cells, and collagen in dermis.*

17

of subepidermal bullae (Chap. 11). The basement zone is not a line of division, an immovable structure, disrupted only in malignancy. It is very likely that some of its constituents are contributed by the epidermis, others by the dermis, and that basement membrane formation is the result of combined effort of the two tissues. Therefore, presence of basement membrane in a benign tumor or in basal cell epithelioma indicates that epithelium and mesenchyme are compatible and collaborating. Absence of basement membrane in a true carcinoma does not mean that it has been broken through and destroyed, but its formation has ceased because of the malignant character of the epithelial cells. When epidermis undergoes pseudocarcinomatous proliferation (Chap. 34), the benign but rapidly proliferating or migrating epithelium does not form a basement membrane until it returns to more normal conditions.

Basement membrane is also no physiologic barrier. Most substances injected into the dermis penetrate it easily. Neutrophils, lymphocytes, and Langerhans cells go through it from the dermis. Immunoglobulins collect on the membrane in many diseases, while the antibodies of pemphigus travel through it to bind to cell membranes. Electron microscopic and immunofluorescent methods have brought many new data, which are helpful in diagnosis and will be referred to in many of the later chapters.

DERMIS

The mesodermal component of the skin is conveniently divided into pars papillaris consisting of papillae and subpapillary layer, pars reticularis, and subcutaneous fat tissue or hypoderm. In all layers we encounter cells, fibers, and ground substance, plus the more highly structured vessels and nerves. Embedded in the dermis are pilar and eccrine apparatuses, which will be discussed later in this chapter.

Pars Papillaris

The pars papillaris contains relatively more cells and vessels than does the pars reticularis. It is structurally and functionally associated with the epidermis, with which it forms the *active skin*, an organ weighing close to 900 gm in the average adult. This estimate is based on the generally accepted value of 1.8 sq m for skin surface and 500 μ for combined thickness of epidermis and pars

papillaris. It is this part, about one tenth of the entire skin, which alone is involved in most of the common inflammatory dermatoses (Sec. II). Sweet[23] recently used "epidermal unit" with similar connotation, while Reed and Ackerman[24] unite papillary and periadnexal dermis under the term "adventitial dermis."

The frame of the pars papillaris is made of collagen fibers and thin bundles. Reticulum fibers are present in dense array just below the epidermis and are arranged vertical to the interface. Elastic fibers have a highly characteristic appearance and distribution. Thin fibers (Fig. 2-17) form a felt at a variable but topographically characteristic distance from the epidermis. From this base, even finer fibers rise vertically toward the epidermis without quite reaching it.[25] This brushwork of fine elastic fibers and its baseline are valuable landmarks by which to judge the distribution in depth of inflammatory infiltrate and tumor cells (Chap. 5). A special feature of face and extremities is the occurrence of elastic globes at the level of the basic felt.[26] It is generally accepted that all fibers of the dermis and the ground substance are manufactured by one race of fibroblasts, but the regulation of this process is poorly understood.[27]

Blood vessels form a subpapillary plexus from which capillary loops[28] enter the papillae. Lymph vessels are always present but are not easily identified. Somewhat larger lymph channels, especially on the lower extremities, may have a prominent elastic fiber basket (Fig. 25-3) surrounding the simple endothelium. Nerve fibers are not visible in routine stains, but Meissner's corpuscles (see Figs. 2-22 and 32-18) are identifiable in those regions where they occur.

The pars papillaris contains, in addition to endothelial cells, fibrocytes, histiocytes, and some small round cells, presumably lymphocytes (Chap. 5). It is impossible to separate fibrocytes from histiocytes (Chap. 5) in routinely stained normal skin. Only when histiocytes become macrophages and contain melanin or other substances can they be identified. We, therefore, use the noncommittal term *fixed-tissue-type cells* in our descriptions. Small numbers of mast cells (Fig. 44-11) are a normal constituent of all portions of the dermis. Ground substance is present in the form of neutral and acid mucin substances. The former are represented by the PAS-positive basement membrane below the epidermis (Fig. 2-15) and by similar membranes around blood vessels. Alcian blue usually reveals small amounts of hyaluronic acid, but metachromatic mucopolysaccharides are not normally found in the pars papillaris.

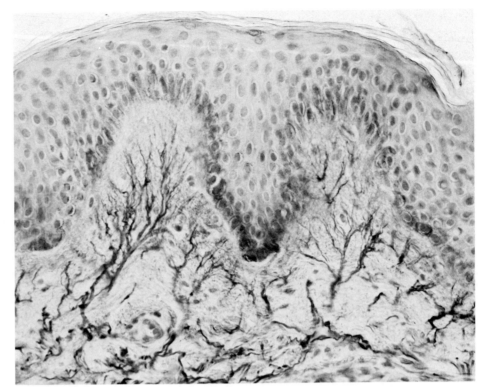

FIGURE 2–17.
Superficial elastic fibers of papillae and subpapillary layer. Brushlike thin fibrils ascend toward epidermis without quite reaching it. Slightly thicker fibers surround subpapillary vessels. O&G. X370.

Pars Reticularis

This portion constitutes the leather of hides and consists of a three-dimensional meshwork of collagen bundles which are accompanied by thick interconnected elastic fibers (Fig. 5-18, 26-6A) and ribbons in similar three-dimensional arrangement. The orientation of collagen bundles is strikingly demonstrated by polarized light (Fig. 2-18) because they are birefringent. They have preferential direction in any particular region of the body surface. This is the basis of Langer's lines of cleavage,

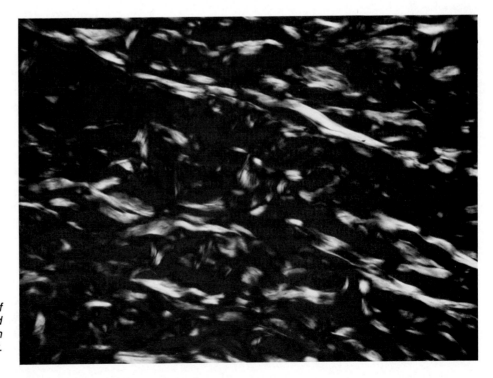

FIGURE 2–18.
Three-dimensional weave of collagen bundles is illustrated in this H&E-stained section photographed in polarized light. X180.

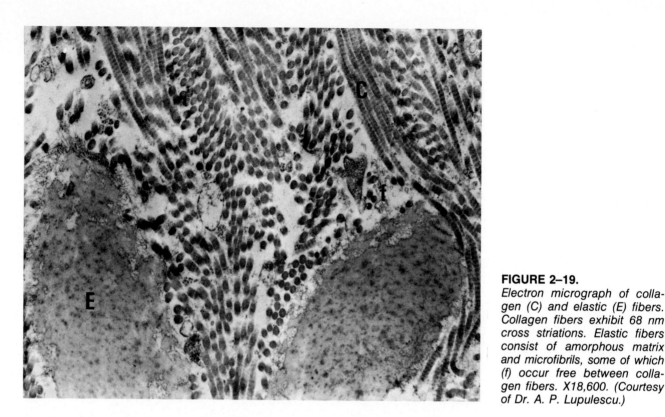

FIGURE 2–19.
Electron micrograph of collagen (C) and elastic (E) fibers. Collagen fibers exhibit 68 nm cross striations. Elastic fibers consist of amorphous matrix and microfibrils, some of which (f) occur free between collagen fibers. X18,600. (Courtesy of Dr. A. P. Lupulescu.)

which guide the direction of surgical incisions. It also explains why randomly oriented sections may show many long bundles in some cases or many roundish blocks in others. The latter should not be interpreted as fragmented bundles, and, similarly, cross sections of elastic fibers should not be mistaken for fragmented fibers. Electron microscopy shows longitudinal and transverse sections of collagen fibrils, approximately 100 nm thick, which are rhythmically banded, and much wider sections of elastic fibers which consist of microfibrils embedded in an amorphous matrix of elastin. Elastic microfibrils also occur free between the collagen fibrils (Fig. 2-19). The proportion of elastin and collagen varies with age. Relative quantity of collagen is highest in the third decade.[29] Ground substance is represented by vascular PAS-positive basement membranes and relatively weak and diffuse reaction to alcian blue. Any more pronounced reaction is pathologic.

Fibrocytes, histiocytes, mast cells, and blood vessels are present in relatively small number, but no norms have been established. Veins, arteries, and nerves usually are found together in triads as in most other organs, a fact that makes it easier to identify nerves which are sizable only in the deep dermis and become tiny in higher strata (Chap. 7). While arteriovenous anastomoses probably exist in all areas, the neuromyoarterial glomus of Masson is found most commonly on the volar surfaces of the hands and feet (Fig. 2-20).

Subcutaneous Tissue

Although it is an anatomic controversy whether fat tissue should be considered part of the skin, some of its histologic features need discussion. Not a few skin diseases affect the hypoderm, and various forms of panniculitis are definitely in the realm of the dermatopathologist. The border between dermis and subcutis is never sharp. Individual fat lobes protrude higher, and connective tissue septa, very similar to dermis, are a regular constituent of the hypoderm, often forming retinacula between skin and fascia. Eccrine coils and the lower portions of hair follicles may be embedded in fat tissue in the midst of dermis as a reminder that in fetal life every hair root and sweat gland penetrates into the subcutaneous fat. Fetal fat tissue develops in the form of individual fat organs around small blood vessels, and adult tissue retains a lobular structure and rich vascularity. Each fat lobule is supplied by only one arteriole, a fact that explains why transplanted tissue often necrotizes or becomes atrophic.[30] Fat cells, which have an average diameter of 94 μ,[31] have one feature worth looking for if there is doubt whether one deals with fat tissue or some form of vacuoles. The flat and ovoid nucleus often possesses a sharply defined central hole (Fig. 2-21).

The largest nervous end organs found anywhere in the body are present in subcutaneous tissue of the acral parts of the extremities. These Vater–Pa-

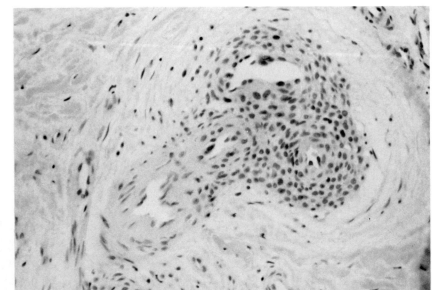

FIGURE 2–20.
Part of a neuromyoarterial glomus of Masson. Artery at left joins the Suquet-Hoyer canal, which is surrounded by multiple layers of glomus cells and thins out into a venous vessel at top. H&E. X400.

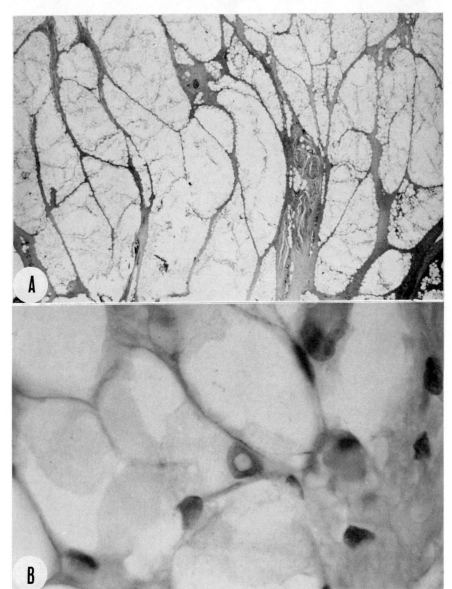

FIGURE 2–21.
*Subcutaneous fat tissue. **A.** Low power shows fat lobules separated by thin and thicker fibrous septa carrying blood vessels. X14. **B.** High power shows several fat cells with thin cross sections of peripheral nuclei. One nucleus is shown in frontal view with the characteristic hole (or thin spot). X1100.*

cini corpuscles consist of a central axon surrounded by multiple laminae of connective tissue which hold fluid ground substance between them to produce a hydrostatic balloonlike structure highly adapted to the perception of pressure changes in its surroundings (Fig. 2-22).

THE PILAR APPARATUS

The hair follicle is the most conspicuous part of most pilar complexes (Fig. 2-23), which also include sebaceous gland, hair muscle, and, in certain cases, apocrine gland. Moreover, pilar apparatuses often occur in groups of three (less commonly two, five, or more), and the biologic hairfield includes the haarscheibe and associated eccrine glands. Thus, the skin may be thought of as being organized into many tiny districts, an intriguing idea discussed by dermatologists at various times.[32] The grouped arrangement of hairs is most obvious in the neck area of many women, where the relatively large sebaceous glands produce visible papules.[33] It is also visible in many sections of children's skin,

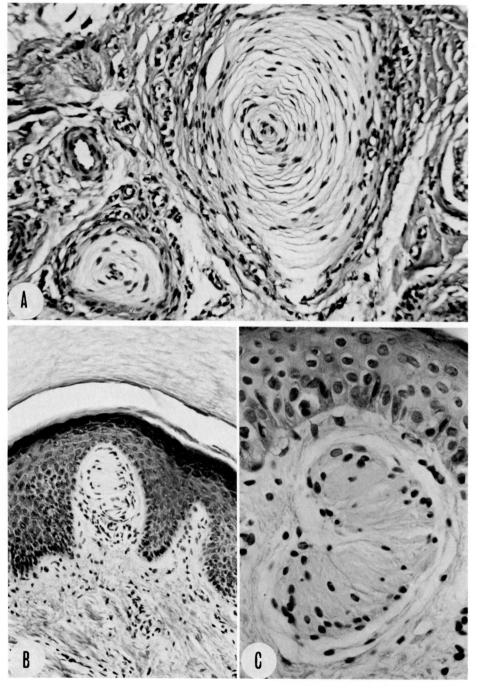

FIGURE 2–22.
Cutaneous nerve corpuscles. **A.** *Vater-Pacini corpuscle in subcutaneous tissue of palm. H&E. X180.* **B.** *Meissner corpuscle in papilla of finger. H&E. X400.* **C.** *Genital touch corpuscle from glans penis. H&E. X600.*

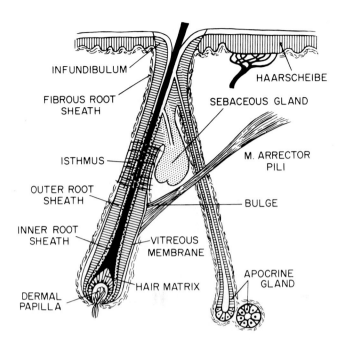

FIGURE 2–23.
Diagrammatic representation of pilar apparatus comprising hair follicle, sebaceous gland, apocrine gland, arrector muscle, and haarscheibe (hair disk). (From Pinkus. In Baccaredda-Boy, Moretti, and Frey (eds). Biopathology of Pattern Alopecia, 1968. Courtesy of S. Karger.)

and this should be kept in mind in many dermatoses affecting follicles. The previous presence of hair follicles can be deduced from the existence of an arrector muscle, which often is the sole remnant of an atrophic pilar complex.

Development

As pointed out above, each pilar apparatus comes into existence through a true act of embryonic differentiation[34] by which small groups of epidermal basal cells are converted into prospective hair germ cells. They become associated with mesenchymal elements, the precursors of fibrous root sheath and dermal papilla. The hair germ (Fig. 2-24) has bilateral symmetry and grows slantingly down through the developing dermis into the subcutaneous fat tissue. Follicles of genetically curled hairs acquire a curve during this process which may bring the hair matrix back under the site where the germ originated in the epidermis. At the same time, follicular cells grow slantingly upward through the epidermis to the surface (Fig. 2-24D) and form the hair canal, the earliest site of keratinization in the fetal skin.[35] Because of its bilateral symmetry, we can distinguish an anterior and posterior surface of the follicle, the latter corresponding to the side that forms an open angle with the lower

surface of the epidermis. Terminology is derived from the fact that most hairs of animals and humans are directed toward the tail end of the body.

While the hair germ's anterior surface remains smooth, its posterior surface soon develops two or three buds. The two constant ones (Fig. 2-24C) develop into the bulge and the sebaceous gland, the inconstant one into the apocrine gland. Their arrangement never varies: the bulge is lowest; the sebaceous bud, above it; and the apocrine bud, highest. The arrector muscle differentiates within a field of metachromatic mesenchyme, obviously under the influence of the hair follicle but not in di-

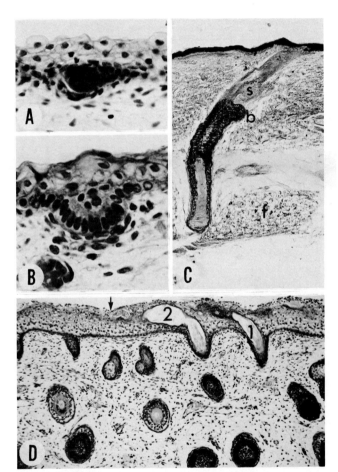

FIGURE 2–24.
Fetal hair follicles. A. Sagittal. B. Frontal view of early hair germ showing bilateral symmetry. There is no invagination of the epidermis; ectodermal and mesodermal components are well shown. H&E. C. Curved follicle of Negro fetus. b, bulge; s, sebaceous gland; f, fat tissue lobe. Glycogen is absent from hair matrix and its products and from the upper follicle above the bulge. PAS-light green. D. Fetal eyebrow showing well-differentiated hair roots in dermis and curved, slanting, and keratinized hair canals (1 and 2) in nonkeratinized epidermis. Arrow indicates distal end of hair canal 2. H&E. (From Pinkus. In Montagna and Ellis (eds). The Biology of Hair Growth, 1958. Courtesy of Academic Press.)

rect contact with it. The slender muscle fibers grow upward toward the epidermis and downward toward the bulge. The mesenchymal cells of the hair germ envelop the growing epithelial follicle in a fibrous sheath and form a terminal pad, part of which becomes enclosed in the hollow center of the hair matrix and develops into the dermal papilla.

Once matrix and papilla are united to form the bulbous lower end of the follicle, differentiation of the hair and its inner root sheath begins. Through intricate inductive processes, evidently originating in the dermal papilla, morphologically identical epithelial matrix cells begin to undergo maturation along five different pathways and form the distinct end products of Henle's layer, Huxley's layer, root sheath cuticle, hair cuticle, and hair cortex. A sixth product of adult hair matrix, the medulla, is absent in fetal hairs. Inner root sheath is made first and forms a protective cap over the fine tip of the hair, similar to the enveloping bracts of a plant shoot piercing the ground. However, the simile is not

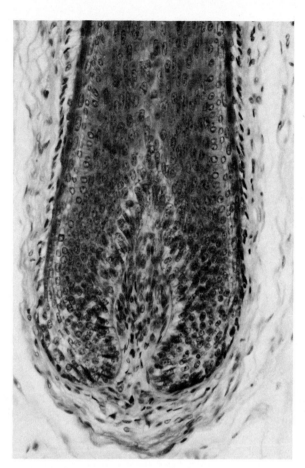

FIGURE 2–26.
Matrix region (bulb) of strong hair follicle. The fibrous root sheath surrounds the epithelial portion and inverts through a narrow neck into the roughly egg-shaped papilla, which has an elongated tip. The dermal papilla is connected to the epithelial matrix by a basement membrane. The lowest ranges of matrix cells give rise to three concentric layers of inner root sheath that are arranged on the outside of the thick hair cortex. The slanting nuclei between inner root sheath and fibrous root sheath constitute the outer root sheath (trichilemma) that starts at the lowest pole of the epithelial portion, surrounds the bulb as a thin single layer of cells, and begins to thicken at the upper border of the picture. The trichilemma has a thick basement membrane (the glassy or vitreous membrane of the follicle) tying it to the fibrous root sheath. The lighter staining cells in the center of the hair cortex are medulla which spring from the uppermost matrix cells covering the tip of the papilla. H&E. X400.

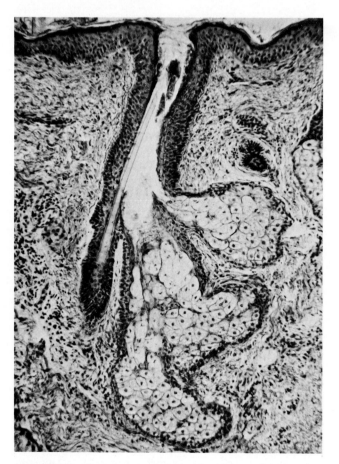

FIGURE 2–25.
Sebaceous follicle of facial skin. Hair root appears as an appendage. The two dark structures in the follicular canal are oblique sections of demodex (see Fig. 18-27). H&E. X135.

quite correct, inasmuch as the follicle is still growing downward and, in so doing, pushes the hair bulb down and away from the hair tip, which remains stationary. Only later are hair and inner sheath pushed upward into the hair canal. The hair becomes free when the inner root sheath and the roof of the hair canal disintegrate.

The first generation of hairs is called *lanugo* and is of similar quality all over the body surface. It usually completes its growth cycle before birth.

The hairs of later generations differ in size and other attributes and are known by a variety of names. Tiny hairs are called *vellus*, stronger ones of the general body surface are known as *terminal hairs*, and thick and long hairs of scalp and other areas have specific Latin names that need not concern us here.

Structure of the Adult Follicle

Strong hairs of scalp, beard, and sexual regions have follicles extending into the hypoderm. The roots of smaller hairs lie in different levels of the dermis, and those of vellus hairs of the face are quite superficial. Sebaceous follicles of the face have tiny appendageal hair roots (Fig. 2-25).

Starting at the business end of the follicle, we see a bulbous thickening (Fig. 2-26) formed by the egg-shaped dermal papilla around which the epithelial hair matrix is arranged like a shell. The matrix and its division products add to the volume of the hair bulb, and the epithelial outer root sheath (trichilemma) forms a thin covering around the whole. The dermal papilla is in contact with the subfollicular dermal pad and the fibrous root sheath by means of a narrow neck through which capillaries enter and exit. The papilla of a growing (anagen) hair is strongly metachromatic and reactive for al-

kaline phosphatase.[36] Epithelial matrix cells around its periphery have little cytoplasm and undergo mitotic division at a high rate, most of the activity being present in the lower half, while the cells of the upper half are mingled with dendritic melanocytes from which the keratinizing hair cells derive their pigment. Albino hair roots have amelanotic melanocytes, while senile white hairs lack melanocytes.

As cells are pushed upward from the matrix, they become slim and elongated, and the cross section of the follicle decreases even though the trichilemma becomes multilayered and thick. Matrix cells mature in six different ways depending on their distance from the base of the papilla (Fig. 2-27). The ring of cells closest to the base forms a single layer of quickly keratinizing elongated cells (Henle's layer) which establishes a firm coat around the soft central parts. The next several ranks of matrix cells produce the much thicker layer of Huxley, which keratinizes at a considerably higher level. Still further up along the periphery of the papilla, two interlocking layers of obliquely oriented cells, the cuticle of the inner root sheath and the cuticle of the hair, are formed. The largest portion of the matrix is used up in producing hair cortex, and the cells above the tip of the papilla give rise to the medulla, which is found only in thick hairs. Oblique sections of a large hair follicle at the level

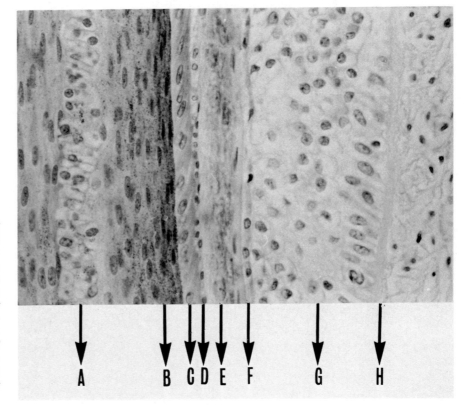

FIGURE 2-27.
Longitudinal section of keratogenous zone of hair and inner root sheath. Hair shaft at left shows medulla (A) within cortex (B). Nuclei of hair cuticle (C) have oblique direction, cell bodies interlock with cuticle of inner sheath (D) with small nuclei. Multiple Huxley's layer (E) and single Henle's layer (F) follow. Trichilemma (G) has large glycogen-filled cells. Its columnar basal cells rest on the vitreous membrane (H), to the right of which are fibers and cells of fibrous root sheath. H&E. X600.

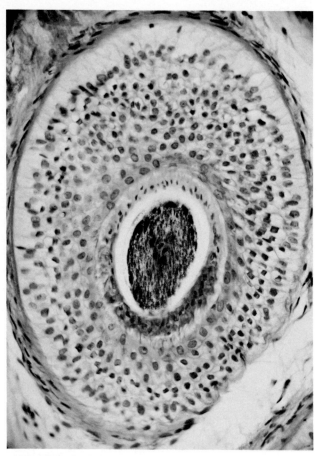

FIGURE 2–28.
Oblique section of scalp hair at level of keratinization of Huxley's layer. Hair with medulla, cortex, and fully keratinized (unstained) cuticle in center. Keratinized Henle's layer (striated) surrounds Huxley's layer, which shows nuclei and dark-staining trichohyalin granules in lower half, pyknotic nuclei only in upper half of picture. Basal cells of outer root sheath are columnar and appear light because they contain much glycogen; central cells are smaller and denser, showing no evidence of keratinization. Small dark nuclei between basal cells belong to amelanotic melanocytes. Direction of nuclei in fibrous root sheath indicates circular and longitudinal layers. H&E. X370.

where Huxley's layer keratinizes (Fig. 2-28) are particularly instructive. The micrograph also shows the vascularized fibrous root sheath and the hyaline (vitreous, glassy) membrane between ectodermal and mesodermal components. The fully keratinized inner root sheath stains very dark blue in O&G sections and has other specific staining reactions (yellow fluorescence with thioflavin T, acid fastness), which permit one to recognize small fragments or single cells under pathologic conditions (Chap. 36).

The fully formed hair and inner root sheath are pushed upward through the relatively stationary tube of stratified epithelium which is the trichilemma (outer root sheath). They enter the isthmus of the follicle above the bulge and the insertion of the arrector muscle. The bulge often is quite inconspicuous in adult hairs, but it may give rise to peculiar branching proliferations[37] resembling miniature trichoepitheliomas, or it may furnish an epithelial tendon (Fig. 2-29) for the muscle, or it may be the source of milia (Chap. 37) through central keratinization. Its site marks the level to which the lower end of the hair ascends in catagen, while the entire portion below disintegrates. The follicular isthmus, thus, is the first portion of the permanent follicle. Its epithelial tube (Fig. 2-24) is surrounded by an intricate net of elastic fibers and by a nerve end organ of cholinesterase-positive sensory fibers which respond to mechanical stimulation transmitted through the hair shaft. The isthmus also is the site where the inner root sheath disintegrates (Straile's zone of sloughing[38]) either at or below the level of the sebaceous duct. Disintegration seems to be due to unknown chemical influences, the fused Henle's and Huxley's layers losing their staining characteristics before they break up. At the same time, the trichilemma which does not keratinize as long as it is in contact with

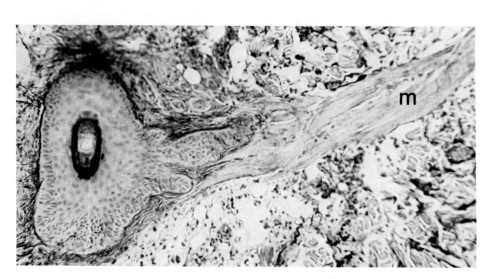

FIGURE 2–29.
Bulge area of a small follicle. Bulge proliferation forms an epithelial tendon for strong arrector muscle (m). Elastic fibers surround follicular isthmus and upper part of bulge and fade out below it. Inner root sheath is dark (blue). O&G.

FIGURE 2–30.
Trichilemmal keratinization. **A.**
Isthmus of anagen follicle, d,
sebaceous duct; i, upper end
of disintegrating inner root
sheath; t, trichilemmal keratin
forming a spur at lower cir-
cumference of sebaceous duct.
Note, keratohyalin (dark) ap-
pears only above sebaceous
duct level in infundibular por-
tion of follicle. H&E. X86. **B.**
Catagen club in transverse
section. Light hair shaft is
surrounded by darker trichi-
lemmal keratin from which it
has retracted in two places
(artifactal cleft). Outer root
sheath epithelium contains
small amounts of glycogen
(dark). Picture resembles a
miniature trichilemmal cyst (Fig.
46-6). PAS-hematoxylin-picric
acid. X352. (From Pinkus. Arch
Dermatol 99:544, 1969.)

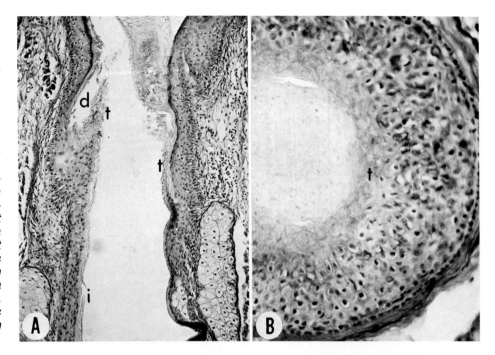

Henle's layer now begins to mature. Trichilemmal keratinization (Fig. 2-30) is a specific seventh form of follicular cell maturation,[39] arising in the stratified epithelium of the outer sheath rather than in the matrix. It produces bulky keratinized cells without the formation of keratohyalin, a property it shares with hard keratins of hair and nail. The keratinizing cells of the inner root sheath and hair medulla, on the other hand, form large eosinophilic droplets of trichohyalin, a substance related to keratohyalin. We shall encounter trichilemmal keratin formation again in the catagen stage of the hair cycle.

The entry of the sebaceous duct marks another change in follicular architecture and function. The duct itself, a short tube of stratified epithelium (Fig. 2-31), keratinizes in epidermoid fashion with formation of keratohyalin and pierces the follicular wall obliquely. Regardless of whether there is only one sebaceous duct or several, the follicular epithelium above this level produces keratohyalin and loose lamellar epidermoid keratin layer, which differs from that of the epidermis on the ultrastructural level.[40] The pilar canal of this infundibular upper portion of the follicle, therefore, might better be termed *pilosebaceous canal*. It exists in sebaceous follicles with rudimentary hair roots as well as in free sebaceous glands of the oral mucosa (Fig. 2-32). The infundibulum extends through the epidermis to the surface and incorporates the remnant of the fetal hair canal. While indistinguishable morphologically from the epidermis with which it is fused, it is a biologic portion of the follicle (acrotrichium[41]) and consists of adnexal rather than

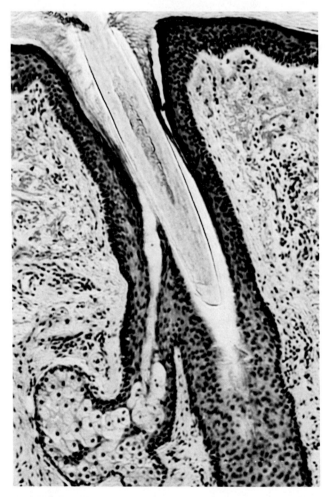

FIGURE 2–31.
Upper hair follicle with sebaceous gland and duct. Oblique
section of medullated hair in piliosebaceous canal. Note
loose epidermoid keratin in infundibulum. H&E. X135.

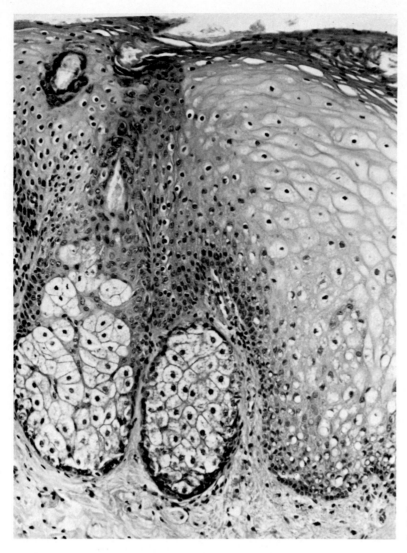

FIGURE 2–32.
Oral mucosa with free sebaceous glands. Note contrast between physiologic parakeratosis of oral surface epithelium and keratinization with keratohyalin of the sebaceous ducts traversing it. H&E. X135.

epidermal keratinocytes, a fact that gains significance in wound healing and in neoplastic processes.

Fibrous Root Sheath. The entire hair follicle, from its beginning, is enveloped in mesodermal stroma. Mesodermal cells accumulate below the early ectodermal germ (Fig. 2-24) and accompany it downward through the dermis into the subcutaneous fat tissue, participating in the formation and growth of the *hair germ* (p. 23). In adult life, the dermal papilla is surrounded by the bell-shaped epithelial matrix, contains nourishing blood vessels, and seems to instruct the matrix cells in which direction to keratinize.[42] It is connected to the fibrous root sheath through the neck of the papilla (Fig. 2-26) which in strong hairs often contains an accumulation of fine elastic fibers, the Arao-Perkins body,[43] which has diagnostic significance in alopecia. The fibrous root sheath consists of circular and longitudinal collagen fibers with their fibro-

blasts and also carries capillary blood vessels. It varies in thickness and becomes very prominent in the catagen phase of the hair cycle and also in some forms of alopecia (Chap. 18). It is joined to the basal cells of the outer epithelial root sheath by a prominent basal membrane (Figs. 2-26 and 2-27) that stains with PAS and often is metachromatic. This is the vitreous (glassy) membrane of the hair follicle. The fibrous root sheath normally does not contain elastic fibers in the lower, transient portion of the follicle but shows a dense elastic component above the insertion of the hair muscle at the bulge (Fig. 2-29). This elastic coat, mixed with nerve fibers, extends upward around the isthmus to the level of the sebaceous duct. Higher up, it is represented by loosely arranged fibers around the pilosebaceous canal. The relation of fibrous root sheath to follicular epithelium is quite different from the dermoepidermal junction (pp. 16–18). It is similar to the relation of stroma and epithelium in benign adnexal tumors and in basal cell epithelioma.

Sebaceous Gland

The normal gland (Figs. 2-31 and 2-32)[44] has one peripheral (basal) layer of flat small cells, all inner layers being lipidized. Early atrophy is manifested by more bulky basal cells and less bulky and less completely lipidized inner cells. Multiple layers of nonlipidized outer cells are definitely pathologic. The contour of the gland is rounded, and continuous collapse of some lobes and formation of new ones give sebaceous glands a variety of shapes and cause vascular stroma to be enclosed deep in some glands. The most central cells disintegrate (holocrine secretion), and the debris is extruded as sebum through the duct which consists of stratified epithelium keratinizing in epidermoid fashion. The size of facial sebaceous glands increases with age,[45] but their proliferative activity decreases. Presence of demodex folliculorum deep in normal sebaceous glands is so common that one can discount its pathologic significance in most cases.

A not uncommon malformation of vellus hair follicles of the face results from the replacement of the sebaceous gland by a two-layered sheet of basal cells, which surrounds the middle portion of the hair root like a skirt or cloak (mantle hair of F. Pinkus) and is seen in histologic sections as epithelial spurs flanking the isthmus (Figs. 18-18B and 18-20A). According to Epstein and Kligman,[46] the epithelium of the mantle may give rise to milia through central keratinization.

Apocrine Gland

Apocrine ducts start as thin tubes high in the follicular wall (Fig. 2-33A) or, occasionally, in the epidermis next to a follicle (displacement). The duct is short and inconspicuous and soon ends at the upper limit of the secretory tubule, which coils up in the deep dermis and subcutaneous fat tissue. The duct has two concentric layers of cuboidal cells and resembles the eccrine duct in routine sections. It also has a similar set of enzymes in histochemical preparations[47,48] (Table 2-3). The secretory portion (Fig. 2-23B, C) consists of an inner layer of eosinophilic cells, which vary from flat to columnar according to the phase of the secretion cycle, and an outer layer of elongated myoepithelial cells. The apocrine tube has a much larger lumen than the eccrine gland and has a different set of enzymes (Table 2-3). It is encased in a network of reticulum and elastic fibers outside the PAS-positive basement membrane. Secretory cells have a round, vesicular nucleus near the base and copious cytoplasm containing a variety of granules. Projection of the api-

TABLE 2–3.
Histochemically Demonstrated Enzyme Activities in the Apocrine and Eccrine Apparatuses

Enzyme	Intraepithelial Duct		Intradermal Duct		Secretory Portion	
	Apocrine*	Eccrine	Apocrine	Eccrine	Apocrine	Eccrine
Amylophosphorylase and branching enzyme	+ + +	+ + +	+ + +	+ + +	− to (±)	+ + +
Succinic and malic dehydrogenases	?†	?	−	+ + +	+	+ + +
Leucine aminopeptidase	?	?	+	+ + +	+ +	+ + +
Acid phosphatase	?	?	+ +	+ + +	+ +	+ + +
Alkaline phosphatase	?	?	−	−	+ + + (in myoepithelial cells)	+ + +
Beta-glucuronidase	?	?	+	+	+ + +	+
Indoxyl esterase	?	?	−	+	+ +	+
Acetyl cholinesterase	?	?	−	−	− to + + (in peripheral nerve fibers)	+ + +

Modified from Hashimoto and Lever[47] with additional data from Švob.[48]
*Refers to the portion embedded in the wall of the hair follicle.
†Indicates that no data are available.

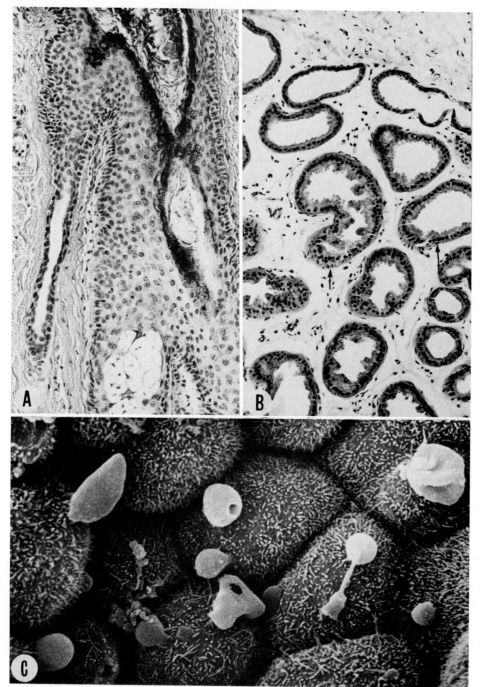

FIGURE 2–33.
Apocrine gland. **A.** *Pilar complex of normal facial skin showing apocrine duct entering a hair follicle above sebaceous gland. Van Gieson. X135.* **B.** *Multiple sections of axillary apocrine coil showing that secretory cells may vary from flat to columnar in same unit. Nuclei of myoepithelial cells are visible wherever tubule is cut tangentially (arrows).* **C.** *Scanning electron micrograph of surface of apocrine secretory epithelium shows the bulging surface cap of the cells beset with microvilli. Some drops of secretion adhere to the cell surface. X4420. (Courtesy of Dr. W. H. Wilborn.)*

cal cytoplasm into the lumen gave rise to the concept of apocrine secretion by decapitation. Although this view has been corrected by electron microscopic studies, the fact remains that apocrine sweat contains corpuscular elements which give it a milky or colored quality. Inspection of Figure 2-1A, representing axillary skin, shows the differences in size and morphology of apocrine and eccrine glands.

Apocrine glands are concentrated in the axillae and anogenital regions but are distributed more widely than is commonly admitted (Fig. 38-1). Glands are encountered too commonly on the face (Fig. 2-33A), scalp, and anterior trunk to be considered abnormal (ectopic). The ceruminous glands of the ear canal[49] and the glands of Moll of the eyelids are modified apocrine glands.

Arrector Muscle

M. arrector pili (Fig. 2-29) is a smooth muscle which may vary from one thin strand to several bulky cords. Under pathologic conditions, there seems to be an inverse relation between size of follicle and muscle. Skin with atrophic hair follicles, whether it be on scalp or lower legs, often contains surprisingly large muscles. Hypertrophy of the muscle is found in pityriasis rubra pilaris (Chap. 18). The arrector typically contains elastic fibers which run parallel to the muscle fibers and form elastic tendons at both ends. Because students often have difficulty differentiating smooth muscle from nerves, we like to point out that muscle bundles usually appear straight in longitudinal section, while nerves appear wavy. Schwann cell nuclei are shorter than the long, rod-shaped nuclei of smooth muscle, and the latter may assume zigzag shape if the fiber is contracted during fixation. In cross sections, both types of nuclei look small and round, but the muscle nucleus is in the center of the fiber, while nerve fibers show the axon as a tiny and faintly stained dot in the center of the empty-appearing myelin sheath. O&G stain shows elastic fibers associated with muscle, but not with nerve, and shows muscular cytoplasm blue, while nerves appear pink. Other special stains are available if doubt persists.

Haarscheibe

Described by F. Pinkus[50] as a half millimeter round dermoepidermal disk in close vicinity to hairs and recognized as a nerve end organ, the haarscheibe (hair disk, Fig. 2-24) remained an anatomic curiosity until a few years ago, when neurophysiologists identified it as a slow-adapting touch receptor in mammalian skin. It is not easily recognized in routine sections but may be seen as a stretch of slightly elevated and thickened epidermis, limited by long epithelial ridges at either end. Electron microscopy has confirmed the existence of many tactile Merkel cells in the basal layer. The little organ has a well-vascularized dermal component in which a thick myelinated nerve arborizes and makes contact with the Merkel cells. Its Schwann cells contain melanin granules.[51] Benign neoplasia of this least conspicuous component of the pilar apparatus has recently been described (Chaps. 36 and 41).

Hair Cycle

No hair grows forever. The proliferative phase (anagen) lasts a few weeks in vellus and terminal hairs, several years in long scalp hairs, but invariably it is followed by a resting phase (telogen). The intricate processes (Fig. 2-34) accompanying the period of subsiding growth (catagen) and the beginning of new hair growth at the end of telogen pro-

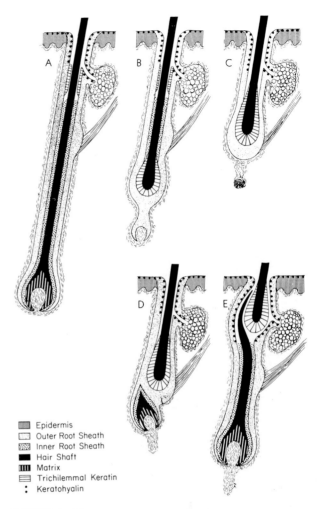

Epidermis
Outer Root Sheath
Inner Root Sheath
Hair Shaft
Matrix
Trichilemmal Keratin
Keratohyalin

FIGURE 2–34.
Diagram of hair cycle. **A.** *Anagen.* **B.** *Catagen.* **C.** *Telogen.* **D.** *Early anagen.* **E.** *Telogen effluvium.*

duce a great variety of histologic pictures, with which one has to become familiar lest one misinterpret the haphazard cuts presented in routine sections. The first sign of subsiding hair growth is loss of metachromasia of the dermal papilla, which can be recognized in O&G sections. Mitotic activity stops, and the hair matrix retracts from the papilla. The now inactive melanocytes remain in the papilla except at the time when a hair changes to senile whiteness. At that crucial time, all melanocytes are caught in the dying, retracting hair and are lost to the next hair germ.

The entire lower follicle collapses, its epithelial part becoming a thin cord, while the mesodermal part is wrinkled in thick folds. The hair itself escapes upward, formation of internal root sheath ceasing before that of cortex, and the lower end of the hair shaft now becomes surrounded by keratinizing trichilemma (Fig. 2-30) which adds its specific dense keratin to form the club.[52] Pictures (Fig. 2-35) that have been described as brushlike spread-

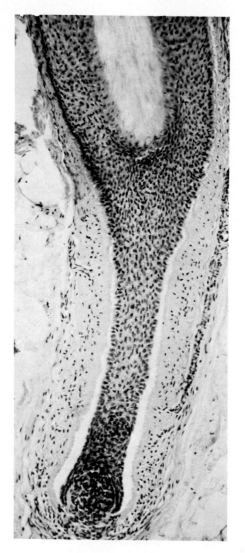

FIGURE 2–35.
Catagen follicle. Atrophing dermal papilla at lower end is connected with trichilemmal sac containing early club hair (at top) by epithelial hair stem, which will shorten and disappear in telogen. Fibrous root sheath (separated by artifactal left from epithelium) is thickened. Note darker-staining nucleated trichilemmal cells beginning to lay down anchoring hair club material around the lower end of the light-staining hair shaft. H&E. X135.

ing of keratinized hair cells actually mean convergence of keratinizing trichilemmal cells into the catagen club, a picture bearing strong similarity to that seen in young trichilemmal cysts (Chap. 37). The hair thus becomes anchored at the level of the bulge, where it is surrounded in full telogen by a smooth contoured trichilemmal sac from which the folds of the fibrous sheath extend downward.

Papilla and matrix are inconspicuous during telogen, which may last from two to six months. When regrowth of hair begins, the new germ closely resembles the fetal hair germ except that it

now forms at the base of the trichilemmal sac. Its axis is at an angle with the axis of the old hair, a useful sign in telling a follicle in early anagen from a catagen follicle. The hair matrix and papilla push downward through the channel marked by the collapsed fibrous sheath, and only later, the tip of the new hair protected by its inner root sheath pushes upward past the old club hair and loosens it from its moorings. The old hair usually falls out before the new one reaches the surface, but occasionally both hairs may be present in the follicle at the same time. This phenomenon is exaggerated in trichostasis spinulosa (Chap. 46), where a dozen or more dead hairs may remain in the follicle. This general scheme of the hair cycle has recently been challenged by Inaba and his co-workers,[53] who found that axillary hair of Japanese is newly formed in the region of the sebaceous duct when dermal papilla and the entire lower part of the hair follicle have been surgically removed. This phenomenon, known so far only in the vibrissae (tactile hairs) of lower mammals, needs further investigation.

THE ECCRINE GLAND

Contrary to the apocrine type, eccrine glands, the true sweat apparatus of man, originate directly from the epidermis independent of hair follicles. The fetal eccrine germ first appears as a crowding of basal cells, similar to the hair germ, but it grows down straight into the dermis as a slender cord with a knobby end. It begins to coil when it reaches the subcutaneous tissue. The eccrine epithelium also grows upward through the epidermis. The epithelial cord acquires a lumen in the seventh or eighth fetal month, and the entire eccrine apparatus then consists of four main portions: the spiraling intraepidermal eccrine sweat duct unit (acrosyringium), the straight intradermal duct, which actually continues the spiral but has an unpredictable course, the coiled duct, and the secretory portion. The latter two form about equal parts of the sweat coil, so that the two old terms, *syrinx* for the duct and *spirema* for the coil, overlap in their meaning (Chap. 38). In skin containing relatively numerous eccrine glands, the coils are found at two levels: superficial ones in the deep dermis and deep ones in the subcutaneous tissue.

The acrosyringium has two or more layers of cells which are distinctly different from the surrounding epidermal keratinocytes of the sweat duct ridge (p. 14). The unit forms a spiral, which seems to have a constant length, being almost straight in acanthotic epidermis and tightly coiled in atrophic

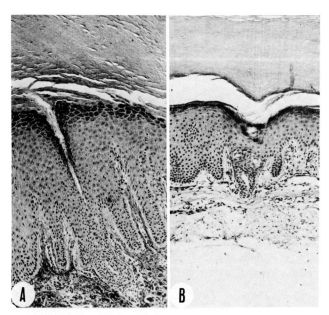

FIGURE 2–36.
*Intraepidermal eccrine sweat duct unit (acrosyringium) in acanthotic (**A**) and atrophic (**B**) palmar epidermis. Respective straightening and coiling of unit suggest that it has a definite length. (From Pinkus. J Invest Dermatol 2:175, 1939.)*

skin (Figs. 2-36 and 14-11). Its nonpigmented keratinized cells are exfoliated on the surface and are replenished by new cells forming in a subepidermal matrix zone,[54] in which mitoses appear in greater number (Fig. 2-37) during periods of rapid turnover, e.g., after tape stripping. The lumen of the intra-epidermal duct is slitlike or star shaped and coated with a PAS-positive, diastase-resistant cuticle. As the cells move up with the epidermis, they begin to form keratohyalin and acidophilic keratin (Fig. 2-12) at a level below the keratogenous zone of the epidermis itself. The intradermal duct consists of a thin fibrous sheath, which is much less conspicuous than the fibrous hair root sheath, and of two concentric layers of cuboidal epithelial cells, of which the outer ones may undergo mitosis. The lumen is covered with a PAS-positive cuticle. The epithelial cells contain much glycogen, which is apt to disappear with profuse sweating. Histochemically demonstrable enzyme activities are listed in Table 2-3.

The lumina of both duct and secretory part usually are smaller than one half of the total diameter of the tube, but the junction of the two portions often shows a fusiform widening, the ampulla.[55] The secreting portion has a much less regular lining than the duct. Its outer layer of myoepithelial cells is inconspicuous, while the inner layer has two components, the light and the dark cells, which may have a staggered arrangement. While no granules are visible in H&E sections, O&G stains will often reveal dark blue, coarse granules which are also acid-fast and show in Ziehl-Neelsen preparations. PAS-positive granules have been described in myxedematous patients.[56] The lumen often contains PAS-positive masses. The stroma of the coil consists of loose connective tissue, which may contain fat cells even when the coil is located in the

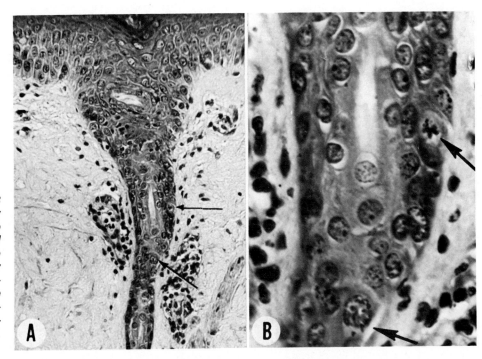

FIGURE 2–37.
*Subepidermal eccrine duct 48 hours after removal of horny layer by tape stripping. Two mitoses (arrows) and several nuclei in early prophase are seen. Mitoses being extremely rare in normal ducts, this micrograph indicates that there is a matrix zone for acrosyringium which has been activated by the stripping. **A**. H&E. X180. **B**. X400.*

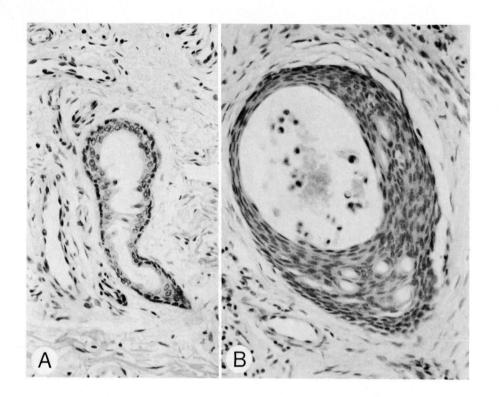

FIGURE 2–38.
Eccrine ducts obstructed by scar formation in dermis form small cysts with evidence of spiraling tendency. H&E. **A.** *X125.* **B.** *X400.*

dermis rather than in subcutaneous fat tissue. The stroma may be metachromatic and alcian blue positive and is quite vascular. There is a definite basement zone around the secretory epithelium in which fine reticular and elastic fibers form a basket impregnated with PAS-positive material.

Although the kinetics of the acrosyringeal cells and their replacement by mitotic division of dermal duct cells have been clarified by the work of Christophers and Braun-Falco,[57] much remains to be learned about the regeneration of the eccrine apparatus. When the duct is severed experimentally in the mid-dermis,[58] the deep stump proliferates and forms small cysts with spiraling lumen, a phenomenon also observed when ducts are obstructed by squamous cell carcinoma or other pathologic processes[59] (Fig. 2-38). Ductal epithelium participates in wound healing and forms new epidermis. On the other hand, when ducts are interrupted by subepidermal bullae, they often form small keratinizing cysts (sweat duct milia), which are exfoliated spontaneously. It seems possible that all sweat duct cells gradually move upward along the basement membrane and eventually are converted into acrosyringeal cells and exfoliated. Nothing is known about regeneration of the secretory cells. Occasional mitoses may be found in sections, and epithelium of eccrine coils shows vigorous proliferative activity in tissue culture.[60]

One morphologic abnormality is occasionally encountered in the secretory portion. The cyto-

plasm of the cells appears foamy and light staining. Acid phosphatase activity is increased,[61] but although a single patient reported to us that his sweating was diminished, no clear association with sweat dysfunction could be established.* Similar vacuolated cells were observed in a child affected with adrenoleukodystrophy.[62]

INTRAEPIDERMAL DENDRITIC CELLS

Melanocytes

Normal epidermis contains dendritic cells at the dermoepidermal junction and between the prickle cells. The former are known as clear cells of Masson in nonpigmented skin, usually are dopa-positive, and contain melanin granules in pigmented skin. They are the melanocytes (Fig. 2-39), neuroectodermal symbionts (see Fig. 2-2, and p. 15) in the epidermis. See Chapter 32 for additional cytologic details.

Melanocytes contribute melanin granules to the epidermal keratinocytes just as they do to keratinizing hair cells. Their number varies from approxi-

*In very recent work it was reported that the sweat of two persons having this anomaly is deficient in a substance allowing thin spreading of secreted sweat and produced by the dark cells of normal glands (Grosshans E, Juillard J, Libert JP, et al. J Invest Dermatol 74:455, 1980).

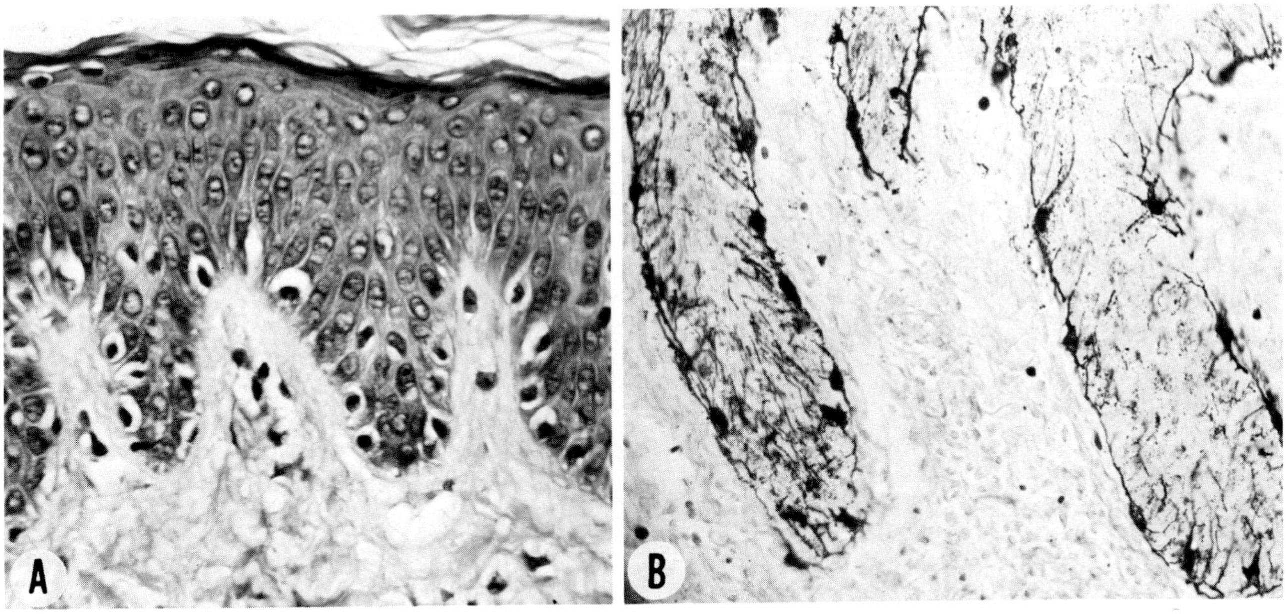

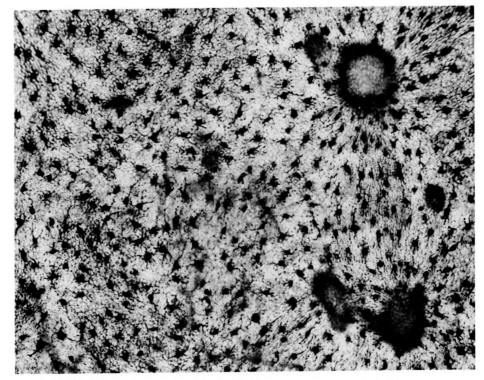

FIGURE 2–39.
Epidermal melanocytes. **A.** *Masson's clear cells in almost nonpigmented normal epidermis. H&E. X370.* **B.** *Pigment block in acanthotic epidermis of eczematous dermatitis. Melanocytes are full of pigment which outlines their dendrites. Masson-Fontana silver reaction. X370.*

mately 500 to 2000 per sq mm of surface in different areas of the skin (Fig. 2-40). It is, however, almost equal in the skin of all human races, the difference in epidermal pigmentation being mainly one of function. More melanin is being produced more continuously by every melanocyte in dark-skinned individuals. In addition, highly active melanocytes produce larger melanosomes, regardless of whether activity is stimulated by genetic factors or by irradiation.[63] Small melanosomes are pack-

FIGURE 2–40.
Lower surface of an epidermal sheet separated from dermis by immersion in sodium bromide solution and stained with dopa.[65] The black rings are outlets of hair follicle and sweat ducts. The fairly even distribution of dendritic melanocytes and the faint polygonal outlines of basal keratinocytes are shown. X200 (approx).

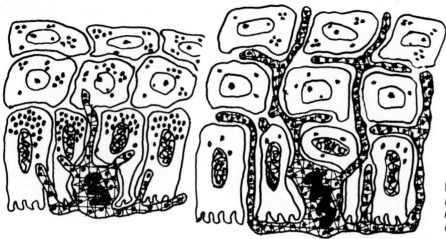

FIGURE 2–41.
Diagram illustrating the epidermal melanin unit (left) and its disruption in disease due to pigment block (right).

aged into lysosomes in prickle cells and are degraded before they reach the horny layer. Melanosomes larger than approximately 0.35 μ, on the other hand, remain single and unaltered.[64] Melanocytes are capable of phagocytosis and accumulate lipid droplets in epidermis overlying xanthomas.[65]

In normal black skin, melanocytes are not very conspicuous between the heavily pigmented basal cells unless they protrude toward the dermis. Each melanocyte seems to be associated with about 10 basal cells, with which it forms the epidermal melanin unit.[66] In dermatitis, this symbiotic relationship is easily disturbed (Fig. 2-41). Transfer of melanin into keratinocytes is blocked,[67] and the melanocytes become engorged and highly dendritic (Fig. 2-39B). The dispersion of melanin granules in the dendrites contributes to the clinical darkening of inflamed skin in blacks, while in histologic sections, the epidermis appears paler because the edematous keratinocytes contain less melanin.

Langerhans Cells

High-level dendritic cells (Table 2-2) are known as Langerhans cells (Fig. 2-42), are dopa negative, do

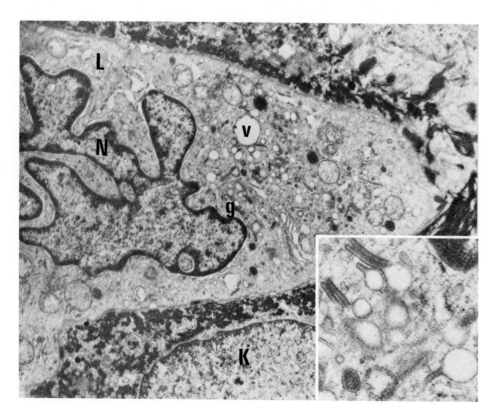

FIGURE 2–42.
Langerhans cell (L) between keratinocytes (K). Electron micrograph X11,200 shows the deeply indented nucleus (N). Vacuoles (V) and Birbeck granules (g), with their tennis-racquet shape, are visible. Inset shows details of granules. (Courtesy of Dr. A. P. Lupulescu.)

not contain melanin, and are usually demonstrated by gold chloride and ATPase techniques, although one can recognize them in routine sections with a fair degree of confidence (Fig. 2-4). They are a separate race of nonkeratinocytes not derived from neural crest, but from the bone marrow, and are able to undergo mitotic division.

Research activity has greatly increased since their role in immunologic disease has been recognized.[68,69] New techniques for their demonstration have been developed,[70,71] but their outstanding characteristic, besides a deeply indented nucleus, is the Langerhans cell granule (Birbeck granule), demonstrated and investigated by electron microscopists. This body has been found also in cells in the dermis, in lymph nodes, and especially in the specific cells of histiocytosis X (Chap. 24).

Merkel Cells

Merkel cells appear to be modified keratinocytes. They were described in the early anatomic literature as tactile cells in connection with intraepidermal nerve endings and have recently been shown by electron microscopy to contain characteristic dense granules.[72] They are concentrated in the haarscheibe and possess sparse desmosomes, which connect them to neighboring basal cells. They are difficult to identify in routine sections. There is very recent evidence that they are the tumor cells of trabeculated carcinoma of the skin (Chap. 40), and they also have been found in pagetoid reticulosis of Woringer and Kolopp (Chap. 44).

REFERENCES

1. Montagna W, Parakkal PF: The Structure and Function of Skin, 3rd ed. New York, Academic Press, 1974
2. Pinkus H: Anatomy and Embryology of the Skin. In Andrade R, Gumport SL, Popkin GL, Rees TD (eds): Cancer of the Skin. Philadelphia, Saunders, 1976
3. Montagna W, Freedberg IM (eds): Cutaneous Biology 1950–1975. J Invest Dermatol 67:1–230, 1976
4. Pinkus H, Tanay A: Embryologie der Haut. In Jadassohn J: Handbuch der Haut-und-Geschlechtskrankheiten, Ergänzungswerk, 1, 1. Berlin, Springer-Verlag, 1968
5. Holbrook KA: Human epidermal embryogenesis. Int J Dermatol 18: 329, 1979
6. Flaxman BA: Cell identification in primary cell cultures from skin. In Vitro 10:112, 1974
7. Breathnach AS: Development and differentiation of dermal cells in man. J Invest Dermatol 71:2, 1978
8. Brough AJ, Jones D, Page RH, Mizukami I: Dermal erythropoiesis in neonatal infants: a manifestation of intrauterine viral disease. Pediatrics 40:627, 1967
9. Deutsch TA, Esterly NB: Elastic fibers in fetal dermis. J Invest Dermatol 65:320, 1976
10. Mishima Y, Pinkus H: Electron microscopy of keratin layer stripped human epidermis. J Invest Dermatol 50:89, 1968
11. Findlay GH: Blue skin. Br J Dermatol 83:127, 1970
12. Plewig G, Marples RR: Regional differences of cell sizes in the human stratum corneum. J Invest Dermatol 54:13, 1970
13. Goldschmidt, H, Thew MA: Exfoliative cytology of psoriasis and other common dermatoses. Quantitative analysis of parakeratotic horny cells in 266 patients. Arch Dermatol 106:476, 1972
14. Madsen A: Diagnostic scale analysis of desquamating dermatoses. Acta Derm Venereol 52:415, 1972
15. Wright N: Cell population kinetics in human epidermis. Int J Dermatol 16:449, 1977
16. Schell H: Zur Zellkinetik der Epidermis aus biorhythmischer Sicht. Zentralblatt Haut Geschl Kr 141:149, 1979 [lengthy bibliography]
17. Grove GL: Epidermal cell kinetics in psoriasis. Int J Dermatol 18:111, 1979
18. Swann MM: The control of cell division: a review, II. Cancer Res 18:1118, 1958
19. Pinkus H: The direction of growth of human epidermis. Br J Dermatol 83:556, 1970
20. Pinkus H: Die Makroskopische Anatomie der Haut. In Jadassohn J: Handbuch der Haut-und Geschlechtskrankheiten, Ergänzungswerk 1, 2. Berlin, Springer-Verlag, 1965, p 1
21. Tring FC, Murgatroyd LB: Surface microtopography of normal human skin. Arch Dermatol 109:223, 1974
22. Hodge SJ, Freeman RG: The basal lamina in skin disease. Int J Dermatol 17:261, 1978
23. Sweet RD: Orientations. Trans St Johns Hosp Dermatol Soc 57:135, 1971
24. Reed RJ, Ackerman AB: Pathology of the adventitial dermis: anatomic observations and biologic speculations. Hum Pathol 4:207, 1973
25. Cooper JH: Histochemical observations on elastic sheath-elastic fibril system of dermis. J Invest Dermatol 52:169, 1969
26. Pinkus H, Mehregan AH, Staricco RG: Elastic globes in human skin. J Invest Dermatol 45:81, 1965
27. Hashimoto K: Normal and abnormal connective tissue of the human skin. I. Fibroblast and collagen. Int J Dermatol 17:457, 1978
28. Braverman IM, Yen A: Ultrastructure of the human dermal microcirculation. II. J Invest Dermatol 68:44, 1977
29. Pierce RH, Grimmer BJ: Age and the chemical constitution of normal human dermis. J Invest Dermatol 58:347, 1972
30. Šmahel J, Charvát A: Fatty tissue in plastic surgery. Acta Chir Plast 6:223, 1964
31. Smith U, Sjostrom L, Bjorntorp P: Comparison of two methods for determining human adipose cell size. J Lipid Res 13:822, 1972
32. Whimster JW: Morbid anatomy and the skin. Trans St Johns Hosp Dermatol Soc 54:11, 1968
33. Pinkus H: Cutis punctata linearis colli. Arch Dermatol 114:625, 1978
34. Pinkus H: Embryology of hair. In Montagna W, Ellis RA (eds): The Biology of Hair Growth. New York, Academic Press, 1958, p 1
35. Holbrook KA, Odland GF: Structure of the human fe-

tal hair canal and initial hair eruption. J Invest Dermatol 71:385, 1978

36. Kopf AW: The distribution of alkaline phosphatase in normal and pathologic human skin. Arch Dermatol 75:1, 1957

37. Madsen A: Studies on the "bulge" (Wulst) in superficial basal cell epitheliomas. Arch Dermatol 89:698, 1964

38. Straile WE: Root sheath-dermal papilla relationships and the control of hair growth. In Lyne AG, Short BF (eds): Biology of the Skin and Hair Growth. Sydney, Angus & Robertson, 1965

39. Pinkus H: "Sebaceous cysts" are trichilemmal cysts. Arch Dermatol 99:544, 1969

40. Knutson DD: Ultrastructural observations in acne vulgaris: the normal sebaceous follicle and acne lesions. J Invest Dermatol 62:288, 1974

41. Duperrat B, Mascaro JM: Une tumeur bénigne développée aux dépens de l'acrotrichium ou partie intraépidermique de follicle pilaire: porome folliculaire (acanthome folliculaire intraépidermique; acrotrichoma). Dermatologica 126:291, 1963

42. Pinkus H: Static and dynamic histology and histochemistry of hair growth. In Baccaredda-Boy A, Moretti G, Frey JR (eds): Biopathology of Pattern Alopecia. Basel, S. Karger, 1968

43. Arao T, Perkins EM Jr: The interrelation of elastic tissue and human hair follicles. In Montagna W, Dobson RL (eds): Hair Growth. Oxford, New York, Pergamon Press, 1969, pp 433–440

44. Montagna W, Bell M, Strauss JJ (eds): Sebaceous glands and acne vulgaris. J Invest Dermatol 62:117, 1974

45. Plewig G, Kligman AM: Proliferative activity of the sebaceous gland of the aged. J Invest Dermatol 70:314, 1978

46. Epstein W, Gligman AM: The pathogenesis of milia and benign tumors of the skin. J Invest Dermatol 26:1, 1956

47. Hashimoto K, Lever WF: Appendage Tumors of the Skin. Springfield, Ill, Thomas, 1968

48. Švob M: Histochemistry of sweat glands. Radovi Akad Nauka BiH 16:71, 1972

49. Perry ET: The Human Ear Canal. Springfield, Ill, Thomas, 1957

50. Pinkus F: Über Hautsinnesorgane neben dem menschlichen Haar (Haarscheiben) und ihre vergleichend-anatomische Bedeutung. Arch Mikr Anat Entwickl Gesch 65:121, 1904

51. Kawamura T, Ishibashi Y, Mori S: Haarscheibe, with special reference to its Merkel cells and perineurale Pigmenthülle. Jpn J Dermatol (Ser B) 81:363, 1971

52. Pinkus H: Factors in the formation of club hair. In Brown AC, Crounse RG (eds): Hair, Trace Elements, and Human Illness. New York, Praeger, 1980.

53. Inaba M, Anthony J, McKinstry C: Histologic study of the regeneration of axillary hair after removal with subcutaneous tissue shaver. J Invest Dermatol 72:224, 1979

54. Christophers E, Plewig G: Formation of the acrosyringium. Arch Dermatol 107:378, 1973

55. Loewenthal LJA: The eccrine ampulla: morphology and function. J Invest Dermatol 36:171, 1961

56. Dobson RL, Abele DC: Cytologic changes in the eccrine sweat gland in hypothyroidism. J Invest Dematol 37:457, 1961

57. Christophers E, Braun-Falco O: Zur Zellreduplikation in ekkrinen Schweissdrüsen vor and nach Stripping. Arch Klin Exp Dermatol 228:220, 1967

58. Lobitz WC Jr, Holyoke JB, Brophy D: Response of the human eccrine sweat duct to dermal injury. J Invest Dermatol 26:247, 1956

59. Santa Cruz DJ, Clausen K: Atypical sweat duct hyperplasia accompanying keratoacanthoma. Dermatologica 154:156, 1977

60. Pinkus H: Notes on structure and biological properties of human epidermis and sweat gland cells in tissue culture and in the organism. Arch Exp Zellforsch 22:47, 1938

61. Rupec M: Zur Ultrastruktur and sauren Phosphatase-Aktivität in den Schweissdrüsen mit "clear reticulated cytoplasm." Arch Dermatol Res 258:193, 1977

62. Martin JJ, Ceuterick C, Martin L, Libert J: Skin and conjunctival biopsies in adrenoleukodystrophy. Acta Neuropathol (Berlin) 38:247, 1977

63. Toda K, Pathak MA, Parrish JA, et al.: Alteration of racial differences in melanosome distribution in human epidermis after exposure to ultraviolet light. Nature [New Biol] 236:143, 1972

64. Olson RL, Gaylor J, Everett MA: Skin color, melanin, and erythema. Arch Dermatol 108:541, 1973

65. Silvers DD, Becker LE, Helwig EB: Epidermal melanocytes in eruptive xanthomas. An ultrastructural study. Arch Dermatol 107:847, 1973

66. Duchon J, Fitzpatrick TB, Seiji M: Melanin 1968: some definitions and problems. In Kopf AW, Andrade R (eds): Year Book of Dermatology, 1967–1968. Chicago, Year Book, 1968

67. Pinkus H, Staricco RG, Kropp PJ, Fan J: The symbiosis of melanocytes and human epidermis under normal and abnormal conditions. In Gordon M: Pigment Cell Biology. New York, Academic Press, 1959

68. Silberberg-Sinakin I, Baer RL, Thorbekke GJ: Langerhans cells. A review of their nature with emphasis on their immunologic functions. Prog Allergy 24:268, 1978

69. Juhlin L (ed): The Langerhans cell and contact dermatitis. Acta Derm Venereol [Suppl] (Stockh) 79:1, 1978

70. Juhlin L, Shelley WB: New staining techniques for the Langerhans cell. Acta Derm Venereol 57:289, 1977

71. Sjöberg, S, Axelsson S, Falck B, Jacobson S, Ringberg A: A new method for the visualization of the epidermal Langerhans cell and its application on normal and allergic skin. Acta Derm Venereol [Suppl] (Stockh) 79:23, 1978

72. Winkelmann RK, Breathnach AB: The Merkel cell. J Invest Dermatol 60:2, 1973

CHAPTER

3

Technical Data, Including Pitfalls and Artifacts

Clinical examination of skin lesions provides to the dermatologist the gross pathologic description upon which a differential diagnosis can be made. However, histopathologic examination is sometimes needed for definitive diagnosis. Dermal pathology has developed into a subspecialty to which many pathologically oriented dermatologists and general pathologists with special interest in dermatology have contributed a vast amount of information. In order to use this knowledge most efficiently, clinician and pathologist must correlate their data and efforts. The clinician should provide detailed information when he submits a specimen. This must include age and sex of the patient, shade of skin color essential for judging pigmentary change, exact site of the biopsied lesion (Chap. 2), and a concise history and description of the dermatosis. Clinical diagnosis or a list of differential diagnoses should be given without fear of influencing the judgment of the pathologist, who is just as ready to disprove as to support the clinical diagnosis.[1]

It is essential also for every dermatologist to be, to some degree, laboratory oriented. Clinicians should be aware of the practical importance of proper selection of skin lesions for histologic examination, the correct methods for performing biopsy, and the steps involved in tissue preparation. They should be acquainted with factors producing various artifacts and the ways to prevent these changes. They should know about special stains and their indication for diagnosis of skin disorders. These are the subjects of discussion in this chapter.

SELECTION OF SITE AND LESION FOR BIOPSY

Selection of a lesion representative of a generalized eruption depends mainly on the type of efflorescence.[2]

In a *vesiculobullous dermatitis*, an early lesion not older than 24 to 48 hours is desirable. After this period, a significant amount of reparative epithelial change will take place at the floor of the blister, which may dislocate the bulla from its primary site. Presence of intact epidermis in the roof of an early bulla is an important point for differential diagnosis. This sign may be completely invalidated in older lesions. When only large bullous lesions are present, a punch or, preferably, an excisional biopsy specimen should be taken from the edge of a new lesion extending into the normal skin, so that sections will include the area of attachment of the roof of the bulla.

When the eruption is characterized by lesions in various stages of development, it is essential to select a well-developed lesion, neither too early nor too late in the state of regression. If the eruption shows gradual evolution of lesions, multiple biopsies of various stages are most informative.

Eruptions with actively progressing borders usually assume a circular, circinate, or serpiginous shape. From such lesions, a fusiform* excisional bi-

---

*While the term "elliptical" is used routinely, excisional biopsy specimens usually have a fusiform outline. In many cases, it is technically simpler and cosmetically more satisfactory to make a diamond-shaped or hexagonal incision.

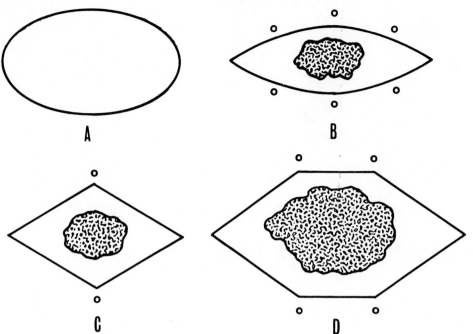

FIGURE 3–1.
Diagram of skin incisions. **A.** *An ellipse is never the shape of a biopsy specimen.* **B.** *A fusiform excision is often used. It requires several interrupted sutures for adequate closure.* **C.** *Four straight incisions produce a diamond that can be closed with one suture. This procedure encourages the beginner to cut straight down through the entire thickness of the skin.* **D.** *If the lesion is large, it is outlined by two parallel incisions, which are then connected to produce a hexagon. Two interrupted sutures are usually sufficient for closure.* (From Pinkus. Cutis 20:609, 1977.)

opsy is most desirable (Fig. 3-1). The specimen should start in normal skin, cross the active border, and include part of the central portion. This procedure eliminates the problem of misorientating the specimen during paraffin embedding and of missing the active tissue changes in the histologic sections. For example, if a round punch biopsy is obtained from the border of a ring of porokeratosis of Mibelli, the specimen may be embedded in a way that the sections are taken parallel to the rim of the lesion and the characteristic cornoid lamella is either completely missed or may be represented in a few sections in the form of a bandlike area of parakeratosis.

In the group of skin lesions characterized by areas of *atrophy* or *sclerosis*, an elliptical excision biopsy is most desirable. The biopsy should be taken from the border of the lesion and include equal parts of normal and diseased skin, and it should be deep enough to include the entire thickness of the skin and part of the subcutaneous fat tissue. As a second choice, one may obtain two punch biopsies, one from the inside of the lesion and one from normal skin at the periphery of the lesion. Such punch biopsies should be embedded side by side to provide normal and diseased area for comparative studies.

If several lesions of similar character are available, one should select a site above the knee for biopsy. Histologic signs of stasis vascular changes may be present below the knee even in young persons and may interfere with proper diagnosis. Pso-

riatic plaques or other inflammatory dermatoses over the extensor surface of elbows or knees are often complicated by lichenification. Biopsy specimens taken from other areas may be more diagnostic.

Severely excoriated lesions are not desirable for histologic examination. Excoriation (Fig. 3-2) produces areas of loss of the epidermis and upper portion of the corium, and in skin lesions involving mainly these two areas, an excoriated lesion is completely nondiagnostic. This is a great problem in dermatitis herpetiformis, lichen urticatus, and other very pruritic diseases.

BIOPSY PROCEDURE

When a lesion has been selected for biopsy, one may clean the skin surface by very gentle application of an alcohol sponge, taking care not to separate any scale or crust. Local anesthesia is best obtained by infiltration under the lesion of 2 percent lidocaine solution or other suitable anesthetic. Addition of Suprarenin in 1:100,000 strength greatly reduces bleeding and is rarely contraindicated. A 2-ml or 5-ml syringe and a No. 26 needle are suitable. The injection should be made deep into the corium and subcutaneous tissue. Dermojet has been used for injecting anesthetic solution into the skin. Unfortunately, this method of local anesthesia has produced artifactual changes within the

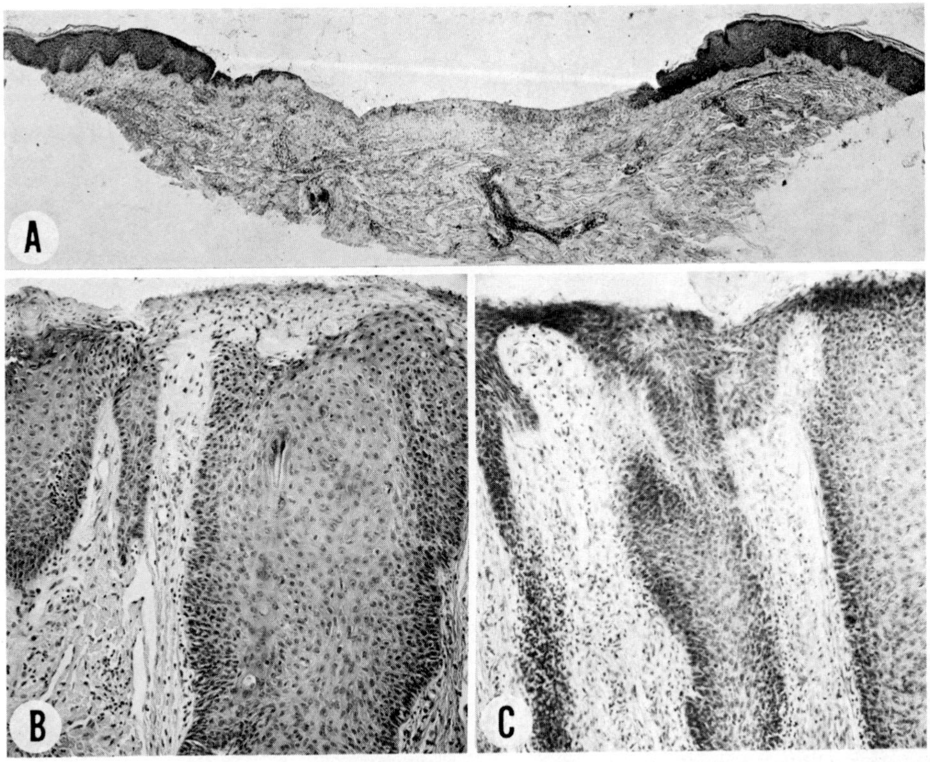

FIGURE 3–2.
Excoriations. **A.** *Deep excoriation has removed entire epidermis. Absence of significant inflammatory infiltrate in dermis suggests that ulceration is not due to a preexistent pathologic process. H&E. X41.* **B** *and* **C.** *Hypertrophic lichen simplex chronicus with evidence of excoriation which has removed suprapapillary plate and exposed papillary heads. H&E. X82.*

epidermis and corium in the form of multiple empty vacuoles (Fig. 3-3) in the fixed tissue sections.

Punch Biopsy and Excisional Biopsy

A 3- to 4-mm punch biopsy provides an adequate amount of tissue for diagnosis of most skin lesions. The biopsy should include the entire thickness of the corium and part of the subcutaneous fat tissue. Excisional biopsy is most desirable when the tissue should be sectioned in a specific direction and is most informative in skin lesions with active borders or in atrophodermas. An excisional specimen should be immediately placed corium down on a piece of paper or cardboard to which it will adhere. This step will prevent the tissue from curling. When the specimen is narrow, contraction of the

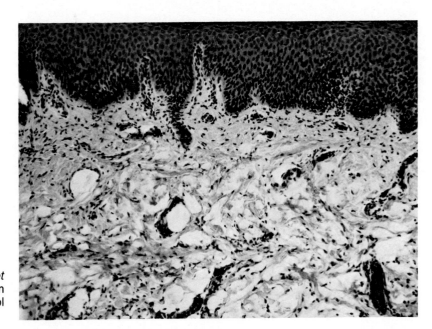

FIGURE 3–3.
Vacuoles in dermis resulting from Dermojet injection of anesthetic. H&E. X135. (From Mehregan and Pinkus. Arch Dermatol 94:218, 1966.)

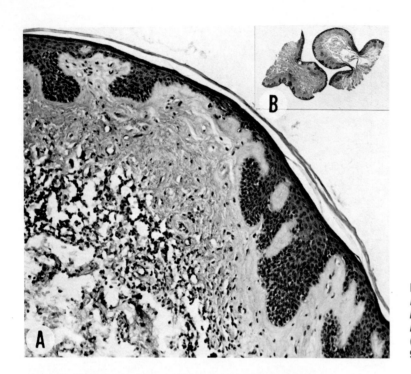

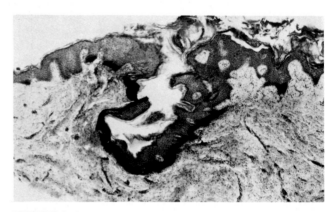

FIGURE 3–4.
*Lesion of lichen sclerosus et atrophicus which has been deformed into a pedunculated mass by forceps pressure. **A.** H&E. X100. **B.** H&E. X5. (From Mehregan and Pinkus. Arch Dermatol 94:218, 1966.)*

dermis may produce so much overhang and curvature of the epidermis that sections show the epidermis cut at a variety of angles (see Fig. 3-15).

Various types of artifacts may be produced during the biopsy of skin lesions. Forceps pressure may deform a flat piece of skin into a seemingly pedunculated mass (Fig. 3-4). If the deep portion of a punch biopsy specimen is squeezed by forceps, the collagen bundles in the corium will show pseudosclerotic changes (Fig. 3-5) resembling scleroderma. If a toothed forceps is clamped firmly on the skin within the biopsy area, a sinuslike intrusion of epidermis into the corium may result (Fig. 3-6). This artifact usually can be recognized by its rectangular

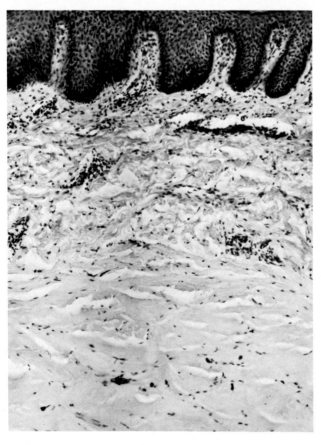

FIGURE 3–5.
Pseudosclerodermatous changes in deep dermis due to forceps injury. H&E. X135. (From Mehregan and Pinkus Arch Dermatol 94:218, 1966.)

FIGURE 3–6.
Pseudosinus produced by toothed forceps. H&E. X75 (From Mehregan and Pinkus. Arch Dermatol 94:218, 1966.)

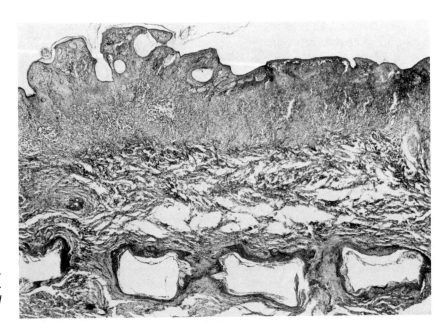

FIGURE 3–7.
Pseudocysts produced by toothed forceps. Note square outline and compression of epidermis and dermis around holes. H&E. X30.

shape and because it is surrounded by compressed collagenous tissue (Fig. 3-7). Traumatic separation of the epidermis from the dermis (Fig. 3-8; see Fig. 3-19) may occur during biopsy, especially in skin lesions where the connection of epidermis to corium is defective, as in cases of lichen planus, porphyria, and epidermolysis bullosa.

Superficial and Deep Biopsy

Superficial shave biopsy, including the epidermis and papillary layer of the corium, is acceptable in some instances of superficial dermatoses, such as psoriasis, or certain neoplasms, such as flat warts, benign cellular nevi, or seborrheic verrucae. In most inflammatory disorders, metabolic disturbances, and tumors, however, a deep biopsy including the entire thickness of the skin is necessary. An even deeper biopsy (Fig. 3-9) is essential for diagnosis of those skin diseases in which the pathologic changes reside in the lower portion of the corium and subcutaneous fat tissue. These include all types of nodular lesions of the leg and the group of panniculitides. Thickness of the skin in various areas should be taken into consideration. In taking

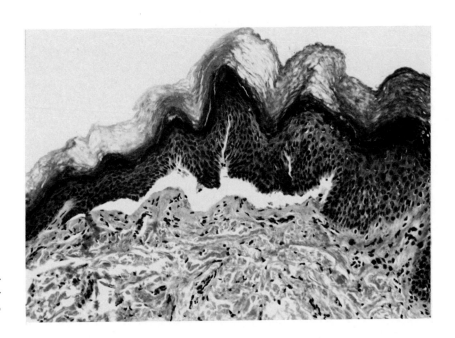

FIGURE 3–8.
Dermalepidermal separation due to biopsy trauma. H&E. X135. (From Mehregan and Pinkus. Arch Dermatol 94:218, 1966.)

a biopsy from a lesion of palm or sole, one may obtain a piece of tissue which appears relatively thick and adequate and yet includes nothing more than the thick keratin of these areas.

The cutaneous punch should be pressed into the skin with a rotary motion until one feels it sink into the softer fat tissue. On withdrawal of the instrument, the plug of skin then usually pops out of the wound. It can be lifted up gently with forceps without exerting pressure, and its base can be snipped through easily with scissors. On the other hand, if the incision is made only part way through the dermis, it takes much more effort to dissect the base with scissors. Wound healing is improved by full-thickness punching. The defect can be sutured more easily if no tough dermal tissue remains in its base. If the site is left open, it will heal more quickly because granulation springs mainly from the better vascularized subcutaneous tissue.

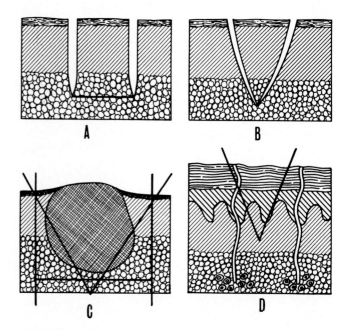

FIGURE 3–10.
*Diagram showing correct and incorrect incisions. **A.** Correct vertical knife incisions extending into subcutaneous fat tissue. Completion of excision by scissors is easy. **B.** Incorrect wedging of incisions produces an insufficient amount of deep tissues. **C.** The same types of incision produce complete and incomplete removal of a globular tumor. **D.** Wedge incisions in the thick skin of palms and soles often do not penetrate the dermis. (From Pinkus H. Cutis 20:609, 1977.)*

If a knife is used, the blade should cut vertically through the skin into fat tissue for the same reasons (Fig. 3-10). Vertical incision also avoids the common mistake of obtaining a tissue wedge with a narrow base rather than a rectangular block. We remind the beginner that, in well-anesthetized skin, a deep incision does not hurt the patient more than a shallow one and may save him the trauma of a second procedure, which could be made necessary by an inadequate first specimen. The cosmetic result of a deep biopsy will be better because the wound edges can be brought together more easily by suture without undue tension. The danger of arterial bleeding is minimal, and oozing of blood can almost always be stopped by firm compression for about 7 minutes.

Curette Biopsy

Material obtained from curettage of a lesion may be submitted for histologic examination. One should attempt to obtain some larger pieces of tissue early during the procedure in order to prevent loss of minute pieces and to facilitate embedding of the specimen in correct position. The material for tis-

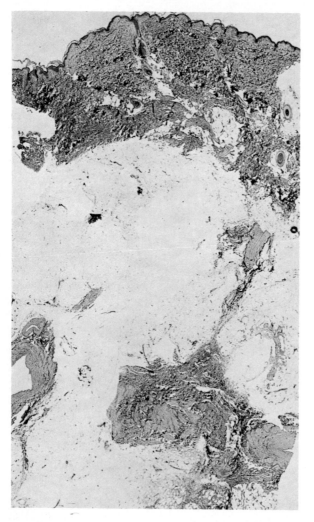

FIGURE 3–9.
Ideal biopsy specimen for diagnosis of cutaneous-subcutaneous lesion. Diagnosis: erythema nodosum. H&E. X9.

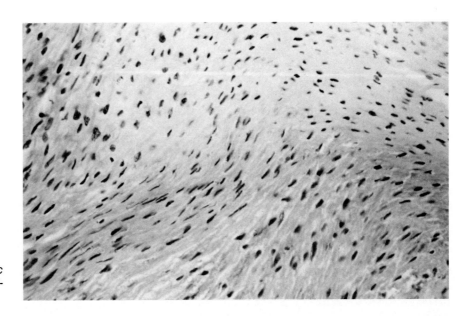

FIGURE 3–11.
Polarization of cell nuclei by electric current produced in a verruca vulgaris. H&E. X400.

sue examination by curettage should be taken before the lesion is electrodesiccated. The electric current produces severe artifactual changes characterized by marked dehydration of the tissue and by elongation of cell nuclei in the direction of the current (polarization of cells) (Fig. 3-11). Tissue samples can be obtained from a nodular lesion by utilizing a dendritic dental broach for identification of the cell infiltrate or such organisms as Leishman bodies.[3] Another artifact observed in curetted basal cell epitheliomas is characterized by squeezing out the solid epithelial tumor masses, leaving behind empty spaces within the fibrous mesodermal stroma which then may resemble a lymphangioma (Fig. 3-12). Similarly, whole lobes of sebaceous glands may be squeezed out of a hair follicle (Fig. 3-13). This can also occur as a natural phenomenon.[4]

Microscopically Controlled Excision

A modified Mohs chemosurgery technique eliminates the necessity of zinc chloride paste fixation.[5] Freshly excised tissue is divided into several segments, mapped, and processed by frozen sectioning in a cryostat.[6]

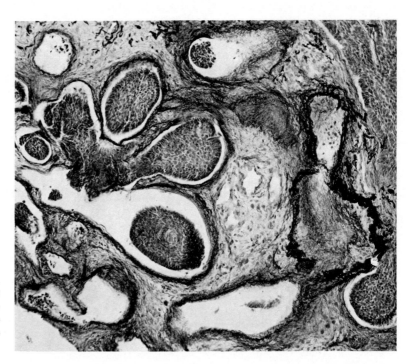

FIGURE 3–12.
Squeezing effect on basal cell epithelioma. Epithelial nests have been separated from their stroma and some have been lost, causing impression of angioma. In this case, tumor stroma contains newly formed elastic fibers. O&G. X135.

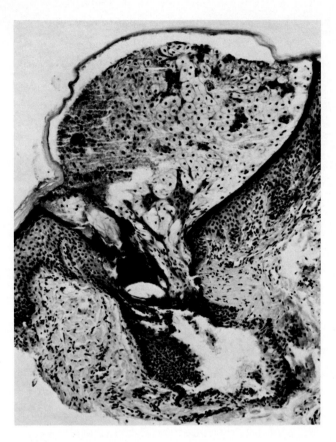

FIGURE 3–13.
Subcorneal displacement of sebaceous gland. H&E. X135.
(From Mehregan and Pinkus. Arch Dermatol 94:218, 1966.)

FIXATION

The biopsy specimen should be placed immediately into a fixative solution. Various fixatives are available for routine purposes, 10 percent formalin or, preferably, neutral buffered formaldehyde solutions being convenient and effective. These fixatives are prepared as follows:

10 Percent Formalin Solution

Concentrated formaldehyde solution (40 percent)	100	ml
Tap water	900	ml

Neutral Buffered Formaldehyde Solution (pH 7.0)

Concentrated formaldehyde solution (40 percent)	100	ml
Tap water	900	ml
Acid sodium phosphate, monohydrate	4	gm
Anhydrous disodium phosphate	6.5	gm

During the winter season, in the northern United States, for example, if a specimen placed in formalin fixative is soon deposited in an outdoor mailbox, the tissue may freeze while undergoing fixation. Numerous ice crystals form, which later become manifest (Fig. 3-14) in the tissue sections as intracellular empty vacuoles. If the process of

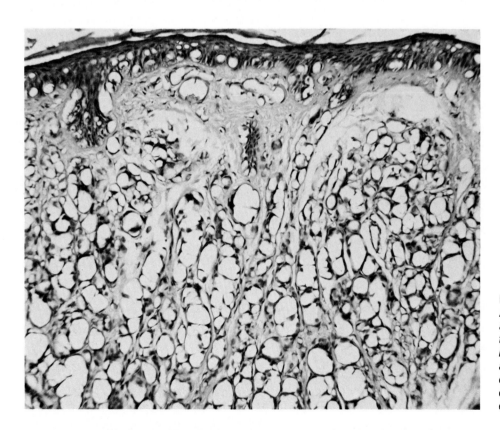

FIGURE 3–14.
Artifact caused by formalin fixation proceeding at freezing temperature. This section of an intradermal nevus cell nevus is almost unrecognizable because of vacuole formation in epidermal cells and nevocytes. H&E. X180.

freezing takes place slowly, larger ice crystals and intracellular vacuoles are formed, which may render the specimen completely unsuitable for interpretation. To prevent this artifact, one should keep specimens in formalin solution at room temperature for at least six hours before exposing them to freezing temperatures. This period allows adequate tissue fixation, and later freezing will not produce disturbing changes. Alcoholic fixatives may be substituted during the cold winter months, since they do not freeze except under arctic conditions. Alcoholic formalin (formol-alcohol) fixative is prepared as follows:

Concentrated formaldehyde solution (40 percent)	100 ml
95 percent ethyl alcohol	900 ml

Seventy percent ethyl or isopropyl alcohol may be used as a fixative. The alcoholic fixatives produce some shrinkage of the tissue and should not be used if frozen sections for fat stain are desired.

A disturbing phenomenon occurring with the use of nonbuffered formalin is formation of formalin pigment (acid formaldehyde hematin) by the action of acid aqueous solution of formaldehyde on blood-rich tissue. It can be prevented by buffering the fixative to a pH above 6. Formalin pigment appears as dark brown microcrystalline particles, refractile under polarized light. It occurs largely within the vascular spaces among apparently intact or laked erythrocytes and also extravascularly within phagocytes.[7] The pigment may be removed from the tissue sections by either Verocay's method[8] or Kardasewitsch's method.[9] In the Verocay method, sections are deparaffinized by two changes each in xylene and absolute ethyl alcohol and then immersed for 10 minutes in 0.01 percent potassium hydroxide in 80 percent ethyl alcohol. The sections are then washed for 5 minutes in two changes of water. In the Kardasewitsch method, sections are immersed in 1 to 5 percent solution of ammonium hydroxide in 70 percent ethyl alcohol for a period of 5 minutes to 4 hours. Iron pigment deposition in tissue may occur when formalin solution is contaminated by a rusted container.

Adequate fixation time depends on the thickness of the specimen. Fixation progresses from the periphery of the tissue, and the central portion is fixed last. Fixatives do not penetrate intact epidermis easily but reach it from the dermal side. Punch biopsies up to 4 mm in thickness do not need trimming, but larger punches may be divided into two pieces to produce a flat surface for embedding and to reduce the thickness of the specimen. From large excisional specimens, one may cut 3-mm-thick strips. Ordinarily, the amount of fixative solution should be about 20 times the volume of the specimen.

TISSUE PROCESSING AND PREPARATION OF THE HISTOLOGIC SECTIONS

Every specimen received in a histopathology laboratory should be given an accession number and also be identified by a short gross description. Small punch biopsies up to 4 mm usually do not require trimming. Larger punch specimens may be trimmed at one edge or divided into two pieces through the center of the specimen to provide a flat surface for embedding. Elliptical excisional specimens not wider than 4 mm also do not require trimming. Larger pieces, however, may be trimmed from one side. It is often requested of the pathologist to check an excised suspected neoplasm for completeness of the removal of the tumor. We divide such an elliptical specimen through the smaller diameter into several thin slices and embed these side by side. In the sections from these pieces, one will look for evidence of tumor extension to the lateral and lower border of the specimen. If the clinical diagnosis suggests a disease in which fat stain may be necessary, one portion of the specimen may be stored in formalin solution in a cool place for frozen sections.

Dehydration

Each laboratory uses a timetable and method for dehydration, clearing, and paraffin embedding of the specimens to suit conditions. Basically, the formalin-fixed specimens pass through graded alcohol to become dehydrated, then through two or three changes of xylol or chloroform to become defatted and cleared, and finally through two or three changes of paraffin at a temperature of 60C, the entire process requiring about 24 hours. One can shorten the time by placing the fixed specimens into tetrahydrofuran and changing the fluid twice at 1.5-hour intervals.[10] The tissue specimens are then placed into three changes of paraffin in a 60C oven. A modified paraffin substance (Paraplast) is much superior to paraffin for embedding.

Embedding

Embedding of skin specimens requires special attention. The epidermal surface of each specimen must be identified, and then the specimen is placed

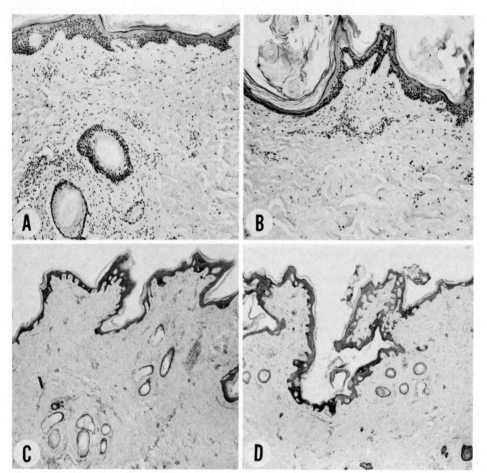

FIGURE 3–15.
Four pieces cut from normal skin, embedded at angles varying from vertical in **A** *to 45° in* **D**. *H&E. X60.* (From Mehregan and Pinkus. Arch Dermatol 94:218, 1966.)

into a mold or a container holding the melted Paraplast in such a manner that the surface of the skin is in a completely upright position. Figure 3-15 shows sections of pieces of normal abdominal skin embedded in the correct upright and also in incorrect tangential positions. Note the increasing degree of papillomatous appearance of the epidermis and papillary connective tissue in wrongly embedded specimens. If the specimen is embedded with the epidermal surface lying down flat, early sections will show a sheet of epidermis containing small islands representing cross sections of the connective tissue papillae. Deeper sections will contain only the corium and show the cutaneous adnexa in cross section.

Cutting

After cooling and hardening, the Paraplast blocks are trimmed to desirable size and may be mounted on wood blocks. The specimens should be placed into the microtome in such a manner that the edge of the knife will hit the epidermis first. The epidermis, especially if thick and hyperkeratotic, represents the area of greatest resistance. If the relatively soft corium is cut first and then the knife edge meets the resistant area, artifactual separation may occur between these two parts. In addition, particles of connective tissue fibers or other intradermal material may be carried into the epidermis by the edge of the knife. We set the microtome at 10 μ for routine purposes because the skin is a notoriously difficult tissue to cut, and thinner sections do not give better definition of detail. The thicker sections actually provide a slightly better three-dimensional impression, which is important in the interpretation of skin structure.

In preparation of the skin sections, the result is greatly dependent upon the condition of the microtome and knife. Microtomes should be cleaned at the end of the working day and lubricated regularly. The microtome knife should be carefully cleaned and sharpened by honing. Commercial knife sharpeners may be used if the knife is dull or deep nicks are present. A dull knife will cut alternating thick and thin sections. Irregularities over the cutting edge of the knife may produce linear scratch marks in tissue sections (Fig. 3-16).

Attempts should be made to cut ribbons of con-

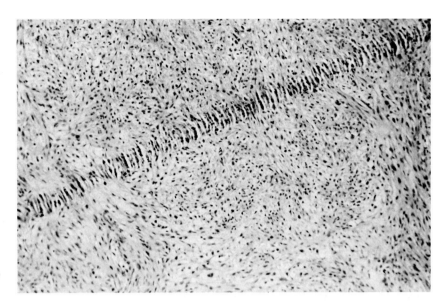

FIGURE 3–16.
Scratch mark produced by a nick in the knife blade. H&E. X400.

secutive sections from the paraffin blocks and to mount all of them on slides (serial sections). It is desirable to prepare several slides of each specimen so that at least 30 to 100 consecutive sections are

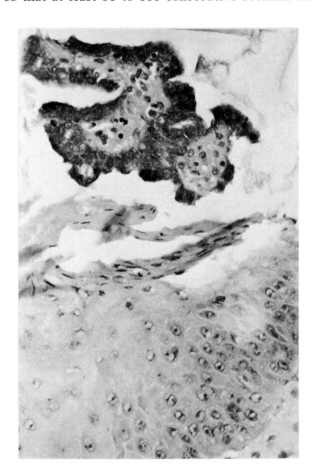

FIGURE 3–17.
Piece of endometrium above epidermis, showing contamination from waterbath.

available for routine and special stains. Ribbons cut from paraffin sections are floated on a waterbath, cut into pieces of desirable length, and mounted on microscopic slides. The surface of the water should be cleaned after each specimen to prevent contamination (Fig. 3-17). The temperature of the bath should be regulated to prevent overheating and, thus, overstretching of the sections. Excess water is wiped off the slides, and the slides are placed in a warm oven to dry for several hours. If they are not properly dried, sections may become detached from the slides during staining.

STAINS

Hematoxylin and eosin (H&E) is the most widely used stain in histopathology laboratories. This stain is sufficient for diagnosis of many skin diseases. It is, however, not a complete stain, since it does not demonstrate some important tissue components, such as elastic fibers or mast cells, does not differentiate between melanin and hemosiderin pigments, and shows fungal mycelia, cocci, and amyloid poorly. To provide this additional information, we use as our second routine stain the acid orcein-Giemsa (O&G) method. We find that its routine use improves our diagnostic ability in many cases and makes recutting of blocks for special stains unnecessary in many instances. A look at the index of this book will show how often information gained from this stain is referred to in the text. The most commonly used special stains in our laboratory are periodic acid-Schiff (PAS) stain using amylase digestion for microorganisms, a modified Mowry stain using PAS, alcian blue, and

TABLE 3–1.
Staining Reactions of Some Tissue Constituents

Tissue Constituents	Stains	Results
Collagen	Van Gieson	Collagen, red; muscle and nerves, yellow
	Masson's trichrome	Collagen, blue; muscle, red
	Hematoxylin-eosin	Collagen, pink; nuclei, blue
Elastic fibers	Acid orcein-Giemsa	Elastic fibers, dark brown; collagen, pink; melanin, black; hemosiderin, greenish yellow; mast cell granules, deep purple
	Aldehyde fuchsin	Elastic fibers, deep purple; also sulfated AMPS (mast cell granules) and certain epithelial mucins, deep purple
Reticulum	Gomori's or Wilder's	Reticulum fibers, black; also melanin and nerves, black
Glycogen	Periodic acid-Schiff (PAS) reaction	Glycogen, magenta red; also fungous wall and certain mucopolysaccharides, red
Acid mucopolysaccharides (AMPS)	Alcian blue	AMPS, light blue
	Colloidal iron	AMPS, light blue
	Toluidine blue	AMPS, metachromatic purple
Fungi	Digested PAS	Fungous walls, red
	Grocott's methenamine silver	Fungous walls, black
Bacteria	Gram	Gram-positive bacteria, blue; gram-negative bacteria, red
	Fite	Acid-fast bacilli, red
Melanin	Masson's ammoniacal silver nitrate	Melanin, black
	Acid orcein-Giemsa	Melanin, greenish black
Iron (hemosiderin pigment)	Prussian blue and Turnbull's reactions	Tissue ferric and ferrous iron, deep blue
Calcium	Von Kossa	Calcium salts, dark brown to black
	Alizarin red	Calcium-Alizarin compound, red
Amyloid	Crystal violet	Amyloid, red
	Congo red	Amyloid, red with green birefringence
	Acid orcein-Giemsa	Amyloid, light blue

picric acid for glycogen and neutral and acid mucopolysaccharides,[11] and the Fite method for acid-fast bacilli. In the remainder of this chapter, hematoxylin-eosin, acid orcein-Giemsa, and periodic acid-Schiff stains are described in detail. Other stains useful in dermal pathology (Table 3-1) are briefly summarized. For more information we refer you to the books of Pearse,[12] Barka and Anderson,[13] Lillie,[14] and the *Manual of Histologic Staining Methods of the Armed Forces Institute of Pathology.*[15]

Hematoxylin and Eosin Stain

Fixation

May be used after any fixation

Technique

Paraffin, celloidin, or frozen sections

Solutions

HARRIS' HEMATOXYLIN:

Hematoxylin crystals	5.0	gm
Alcohol, 95 percent	50.0	ml
Ammonium or potassium alum	100.0	gm
Distilled water	1000.0	ml
Mercuric oxide	2.5	gm

Dissolve the hematoxylin in the alcohol, the alum in the water by the aid of heat. Mix the two solutions. Bring the mixture to a boil as rapidly as possible and then remove from the heat and add the mercuric oxide. Reheat the solution until it becomes dark purple, about 1 minute, and promptly remove the container from the flame and plunge it into a basin of cold water. The solution is ready to use when cool.

ACID ALCOHOL

70 percent alcohol	1000.0	ml
Hydrochloric acid, concentrated	10.0	ml

ALCOHOLIC EOSIN SOLUTION

Eosin Y, water soluble	2.0	gm
Distilled water	160.0	ml
Alcohol, 95 percent	640.0	ml

Dissolve eosin Y in the distilled water, then add the 95 percent alcohol. If a deeper shade is desired, add a drop of acetic acid to each 100 ml of solution.

Staining Procedure

1. Xylene, absolute alcohol, 95 percent alcohol, 70 percent alcohol, to distilled water.
2. Harris' hematoxylin for 10 minutes.
3. Rinse in tap water.
4. Differentiate in acid alcohol—3 to 10 dips. Check the differentiation with the microscope—nuclei should be distinct and the background very light or colorless.*
5. Wash in running tap water for 10 to 20 minutes.
6. Stain with eosin from 15 seconds to 2 minutes depending on the age of the eosin and the depth of counterstain desired.
7. 95 percent alcohol.
8. Absolute alcohol—at least two changes.
9. Xylene—two changes.
10. Mount in Permount or other suitable medium.

Results

Nuclei—purple to blue
Cytoplasm—pink
Keratohyalin—dark purple
Collagen—pink
Elastic fibers—unstained
Calcium—dark purple or blue
Muscle fibers—pink.

Acid Orcein and Giemsa Stain (Pinkus and Hunter)[16]

Fixation

Formalin or alcohol. Fixatives containing chromate or mercury are not suitable.

Solutions

A. Dissolve 0.2 gm of Orcein Synthetic Harleco (Harleco, Inc., Philadelphia) in 100 ml 70 percent ethyl alcohol; add 0.6 ml concentrated hydrochloric acid. Solution is ready for use immediately and improves on standing. It has a long shelf life but becomes exhausted by frequent use.
B. Dilute Giemsa solution: one drop of any good Giemsa stock solution for each 20 ml of distilled water. A phosphate buffer solution adjusted to pH 7.0 may be used if distilled water is too acid.
C. A few drops of 1 percent alcoholic solution of eosin yellow are added to 95 percent alcohol for decolorization of excessively blue sections.

Staining Procedure

1. Deparaffinize sections in xylene and bring through absolute and 95 percent alcohol into 70 percent alcohol.
2. Immerse in solution A for 30 to 60 minutes. This new synthetic orcein stains elastic fibers specifically and produces very little background staining. The background may be completely decolorized by short immersion of the stained sections in absolute alcohol or 0.1 percent acid alcohol. This is rarely necessary.
3. Wash in running tap water for 10 minutes.
4. Stain for 12 to 15 hours (preferably overnight) in solution B. Do not hurry this step. The various tissue components pick the various shades out of a very dilute solution if given enough time. One may speed up this step by having the sections stained for 1 hour in 1 percent Giemsa solution in an oven at 60C.[17]
5. Wipe excess fluid off slides. Generally the sections are now stained blue. The excess blue is removed by dehydrating the sections in 95 percent alcohol to which a few drops of solution C have been added. How much eosin should be used depends on the degree of overstaining and is learned by experience. If the sections have almost the desired rose-pink color of the collagen when they come out of the Giemsa solution, omit eosin altogether in this step.
6. Remove sections when the collagen of the skin begins to turn pink from blue. Finish dehydration and decolorization in two changes of absolute alcohol.
7. Two changes of xylene.
8. Mount in Permount or other suitable medium.

Results

The nuclei should be deep blue; cytoplasm of epidermis, smooth muscle, and other cells, light blue;

---

*We have replaced this step by immersing the slides in 1 percent aqueous solution of hydrochloric acid for 1 to 2 minutes. By avoiding surface tension changes between water and alcohol, the danger of sections becoming detached is minimized.

collagen, rose-pink; elastic fibers, dark brown to black. Mast cell granules and some acid mucinous substances stain metachromatically purple,* but glandular mucin stains grayish blue, and myxedema does not stain at all. Melanin is dark green, almost black; hemosiderin, yellow-brown or light grass green. Red blood cells and eosinophilic granules are bright red; cytoplasm of plasma cells, dark blue or grayish blue. Amyloid stains a clear sky blue under ideal conditions but may be light grayish blue, while other hyaline substances stain pink. Fibrin and fibrinoid material are greenish blue. Unna's elacin and collastin assume various shades from black to gray to blue. Trichohyalin is red; the fully keratinized inner root sheath, deep dark blue; the glassy membrane of the hair follicle, often metachromatic lavender. Keratohyalin of the epidermis usually does not stain very well, but nuclei of parakeratotic stratum corneum often stain much more distinctly than with hematoxylin. Bacteria, fungal hyphae and spores, and other microorganisms are dark blue.

Other Elastic Fiber Stains

Other elastic fiber stains are described briefly. In Verhoeff's iodine-iron hematoxylin, elastic fibers stain in black color, as do nuclei and some other substances. Young and very thin elastic fibers (elaunin fibers) stain poorly or not at all. Weigert's resorcin fuchsin stain demonstrates the elastic fibers in black color. Fullmer's orcinol new fuchsin stains elastic fibers in deep violet color. Gomori's aldehyde fuchsin is listed with the acid mucopolysaccharide stains later in this chapter.

Periodic Acid-Schiff (PAS) Reaction of Hotchkiss and McManus

The PAS reaction is a fundamental stain in carbohydrate histochemistry. In this reaction, aldehyde radicals are created by mild periodic acid oxidation in the tissue sections. The free aldehyde radicals then react with Schiff reagent, forming a red to magenta color compound.

---

*Substances staining purple with Giemsa solution have an affinity for the reddish azure components of the dye mixture and do not represent true metachromatic staining. The visible effect, however, is similar. It is restricted to sulfated mucin substances.

Solutions

SCHIFF'S LEUCOFUCHSIN SOLUTION

Dissolve 1.0 gm basic fuchsin in 200.0 ml hot distilled water. Bring to boiling point. Cool to 50C. Filter and add 20.0 ml normal hydrochloric acid. Cool further, and add 1.0 gm anhydrous sodium bisulfite or sodium metabisulfite. Keep in the dark for 48 hours until solution becomes straw-colored. To completely decolorize, add 0.5 gm activated charcoal, shake vigorously for 2 minutes, and filter. Solution should be colorless. Store in refrigerator.

To test Schiff's leucofuchsin solution, pour a few drops of Schiff's solution into 10 ml of 37 to 40 percent formaldehyde in a watch glass. If the solution turns reddish purple rapidly, it is good. If the reaction is delayed and the resultant color deep blue purple, the solution is breaking down.

0.5 PERCENT PERIODIC ACID SOLUTION

Periodic acid crystals	0.5	gm
Distilled water	100.0	ml

NORMAL HYDROCHLORIC ACID SOLUTION

Hydrochloric acid, conc., sp gr 1.19	83.5	ml
Distilled water	916.5	ml

0.5 PERCENT AQUEOUS LIGHT GREEN COUNTERSTAIN

Light green	0.5	gm
Distilled water	100.0	ml
(Harris's hematoxylin can also be used as counterstain)		

DIASTASE SOLUTION

Diastase of malt	1.0	gm
Buffer solution	100.0	ml

BUFFER SOLUTION

NaCl	8.0	gm
Disodium phosphate	1.3	gm
Sodium phosphate monobasic	0.8	gm
Distilled water	1.0	liter

Staining Procedure

1. Xylene.
2. Absolute alcohol.
3. Alcohol, 95 percent.
4. Alcohol, 70 percent.
5. Rinse in distilled water.
6. Periodic acid solution for 5 minutes (oxidizer).
7. Rinse in distilled water.
8. Place in Schiff's leucofuchsin for 10 minutes.
9. Place in running tap water for 10 minutes for pink color to develop.

10. Stain in Harris' hematoxylin for 2 minutes, or light green counterstain for a few seconds. Light green is recommended for counterstaining sections for the demonstration of fungi.
11. Rinse in tap water.
12. Alcohol, 70 percent.
13. Alcohol, 95 percent.
14. Absolute alcohol, two changes.
15. Xylene, two changes.
16. Mount in Permount.

Results

Glycogen, some mucins, reticulin, fibrin of thrombi, colloid droplets, most basement membranes, amyloid, and other elements show a positive reaction—rose to purplish red. Bacterial and fungal cell walls are deep magenta red; nuclei, blue (with hematoxylin); background, pale green (with light green).

PAS stain demonstrates glycogen and other carbohydrates in tissue sections. Glycogen may be removed by the enzyme diastase in 1 percent aqueous solution. The sections are placed in the enzyme solution for a period of 30 minutes at 37C and are then washed in distilled water. Treated sections and sections on a control slide are stained by PAS method. If the PAS-positive material present in the control sections is completely absent in the sections subjected to diastase digestion, the material is glycogen. Otherwise, it is considered a PAS-positive, diastase-resistant material. Most mucopolysaccharides except acid mucopolysaccharides (such as hyaluronic acid and chondroitin sulfate) will give positive reactions. Sialomucin and some mast cell granules are PAS-positive. Starch granules, a common contaminant of tissue sections, also are stained. PAS reaction with diastase digestion may be used for demonstration of deep or superficial fungous infections, especially in cases of sporotrichosis or where the number of organisms is small.

Alcian Blue Stain (Mowry)

In this stain,[11] a 0.1 to 1 percent solution of alcian blue 8GS in 3 percent acetic acid is used. By changing the pH values of the solution, distinction can be made[18] between sulfated and nonsulfated groups of acid mucopolysaccharides (AMPS). At pH 2.5 to 3.0, most acid mucopolysaccharides stain a blue color. But at a very low pH value (0.4), only strongly acidic groups, such as sulfated AMPS (chondroitin sulfate and heparin), will give a positive reaction. The nonsulfated AMPS and sialomucin fail to react at this low pH.

A combination of alcian blue and periodic acid-Schiff (AB-PAS) counterstained with picric acid is a very colorful and informative stain for demonstration of acid and neutral mucopolysaccharides in dermal mucinosis and alopecia mucinosa.

Colloidal Iron Stain

In Mowry's modification[11] of Hale's method, tissue sections are exposed to colloidal iron solution. The reaction is probably based on binding of colloidal iron to acidic groups. Demonstration of bound iron is made by the ferrocyanide-hydrochloric acid method. AMPS produce a blue to light green color.

Toluidine Blue Stain

This stain is used for demonstration of metachromasia. Metachromasia may be defined as a staining reaction in which a dye selectively stains certain tissue substances in a color that differs from the color of the dye itself. The production of metachromasia depends on the presence of free electronegative charges of certain minimal density. AMPS, nucleic acids, and other acidic groups if present in sufficient quantity will produce metachromasia.[12] A 0.1 percent toluidine blue solution at pH 1.0 to 6.0 is used for demonstration of metachromasia. At pH values 3 to 6, tissue rich in hyaluronic acid will show metachromasia. At pH values 1.5 and below, only strongly acidic compounds, such as sulfated AMPS, will give metachromasia.[18]

Aldehyde Fuchsin (Gomori) [19]

This stain may be used for demonstration of elastic fibers and certain groups of AMPS. The elastic fibers stain in a deep violet to purple color. The same color reaction is produced by mast cell granules, sialomucin of epithelial origin, and, to a lesser degree, by chondroitin sulfate. The stain is most useful for demonstrating mucin production in cases of extramammary Paget's disease.

Enzyme Digestion

Amylase (see above) may be used for digestion of glycogen in association with PAS stain. Two other enzymes are available for investigation of AMPS. Bacterial or, more commonly, bovine testicular *hyaluronidase* is used for removal of hyaluronic acid from the tissue sections. Digestion is then followed by either the alcian blue or colloidal iron stain. *Sialidase* (neuraminidase) is used for decomposition of sialomucin in the tissue sections. *Ribonuclease* removes ribonucleic acid (RNA) from tissue sections.

Reticulum

Either Gomori's[20] or Wilder's[21] modification of the Bielschowsky-Maresch's silver method may be used. The reticulum fibers stain in the form of delicate dark brown to black fibrils.

Amyloid

Amyloid deposits may be demonstrated by one of the following methods: Highman's crystal violet[22] will stain amyloid metachromatic in a reddish purple color. Bennhold's congo red stain,[15] examined under polarized light, shows green birefringence.[23] O&G stains amyloid light blue. Amyloid is also weakly PAS-positive.

Lipids

Formalin calcium fixation of the specimen for a period not longer than two or three days is recommended,[13] but routine formalin is adequate for ordinary diagnostic purposes. Frozen sections are stained by either the oil red 0 or Sudan black method. The lipids stain deep red or greenish black, respectively. The clinician must alert the laboratory to prevent processing the specimen through lipid solvents if a fat stain is desired.

Iron

Prussian blue and Turnbull's reaction are commonly used. Prussian blue reaction is based on the reaction of tissue ferric iron (Fe^{+++}) with potassium ferrocyanide in acid solution and formation of ferric-ferrocyanide with a deep blue color in the tissue sections. Turnbull's reaction is similar. In this method, ferrous iron (Fe^{++}) is demonstrated by reacting with potassium ferricyanide, resulting in the formation of a deep blue color. The tissue sections are best counterstained with nuclear fast red.

Melanin

This pigment has a light to dark brown color in H&E stain. Exposure to a 1 to 2 percent silver nitrate solution specifically darkens melanin.[14] Fontana-Masson's ammoniacal silver nitrate technique can be used for combined demonstration of melanin and premelanin.[24] This reaction is based on the reducing capacity of the melanosome skeleton and precipitation of black silver protein compound. A similar reaction is produced by Gomori's methenamine silver stain.[25] Azure in the O&G stain causes melanin granules to appear greenish black and makes special stains unnecessary if it is used as a routine stain. Melanin pigment can be bleached out of the tissue sections by long exposure to 10 percent hydrogen peroxide or 0.5 percent potassium permanganate solution.

Tyrosinase (dopa-oxidase) reaction: for demonstration of this enzyme, slices of rapidly frozen tissue or specimens fixed for a short time in cold formalin may be used. Special arrangements, therefore, must be made with the laboratory if the clinician desires this type of examination. The reaction takes place in two phases. In the first phase, L-tyrosin is slowly converted to L-dopa, and in the second phase, L-dopa is rapidly transformed into intermediate compounds and finally into melanin pigment.

Calcium

Two methods are commonly used for demonstration of calcium in tissue sections.

1. The *Von Kossa method* is based on the combination of silver with anions of insoluble salts which may be phosphate, oxalate, sulfate, chloride, or sulfocyanide and reduction to metallic silver by exposure to light.[26] In practice, it demonstrates insoluble salts of calcium.
2. *Alizarin red S:* In this method a 2 percent solution of alizarin red S adjusted to pH 4.1 to 4.3 with diluted ammonia is used. An orange-red calcium-alizarin compound is formed in 1 to 5 minutes.[26]

Silver and Other Metals

In the hematoxylin-eosin stain, silver appears as dark brown to black colored granules representing a silver-protein complex. Silver may be removed by placing the sections in 1 percent potassium ferricyanide in 20 percent sodium thiosulfate solution.[12] Silver can also be demonstrated by dark-field examination of the tissue sections. Mercury[27] and gold[28] have similar properties.

Silica

Silica can be demonstrated by polarization microscopy. Polarization may be produced in any microscope by the use of two pieces of Polaroid, which is available in large sheets in photo or laboratory supply stores. One piece is introduced into the pathway of the light within or below the condenser system. Another piece may be simply placed on top of the slide. With rotation of one of these two pieces, the light field becomes darker, and double refractile crystals of silica become apparent.

Stains for Fungi

PAS stain after digestion with diastase can be used for demonstration of superficial and deep fungi. Grocott stain[29] also has been widely used. In this method, the organisms stain dark brown to black. Mucicarmin has been recommended for the demonstration of *Cryptococcus neoformans*.[30]

Bacterial Stains

Most bacilli and cocci show up well in O&G-stained sections. Ziehl-Neelsen's carbolfuchsin and methylene blue stain is used for demonstration of acid-fast bacteria in smears or tissue sections. Acid-fast bacilli and ceroid stain red. Cell nuclei are blue, and mast cell granules take a blue-violet color. Certain granules in sweat glands (Chap. 2) and keratinized hair and inner root sheath (Chap. 2) also are apt to retain the red color. Hansen's bacilli need special precautions and are best demonstrated by the Fite method.[31]

Gram stain can be used on smears or tissue sections; gram-positive bacteria stain blue-black, and gram-negative organisms stain red.

PREPARATION OF TZANCK SMEAR AND TISSUE IMPRINTS

Preparation of Tzanck smears is simple and can be done as a routine office procedure. Smears should be taken from an early vesiculobullous lesion which shows no sign of secondary infection. The top of the bulla is separated by the tip of a surgical blade. The contents of the bulla and material obtained by gentle scraping of the floor of the bulla are collected by the edge of the blade and spread evenly over a glass slide. The preparation may be air dried or fixed by dipping four or five times into 95 percent ethyl alcohol. The slide is stained by a few drops of stock Giemsa solution for 2 or 3 minutes or by Paragon multiple stain for frozen sections.[32] Tissue imprints may be prepared by touching the punch biopsy specimen to a clean, dry glass slide in multiple spots. The slides are air dried and stained by either the Giemsa or Wright stain.[33] They are then rinsed in distilled water, air dried, and coverslipped for examination under the high, dry power of the microscope or, if necessary, under oil immersion.

FOREIGN BODIES

Various foreign materials may be observed in the examination of tissue sections. Some of these have been introduced into the skin at variable times before biopsy and may have produced a variety of tissue reactions.[34] Others arrive during tissue processing. Silica and other substances producing granulomatous reactions will be discussed in Chapter 20. Wood and other plant material are highly birefringent and can be thus identified. Pencil lead, other forms of carbon, and other substances, such as cinnabar, are encountered in accidental or purposeful tattoos (Chap. 27). Silver and other metals were mentioned earlier. Suture material may have been left in the tissue from previous surgery or may have been placed by the surgeon with the purpose of tissue orientation. Formalin pigment, previously mentioned in this chapter, may form as the result of formalin fixation of blood-rich tissues. Starch granules, plant hairs,[35] alternaria spores, fungous hyphae, and pollen are ordinary tissue contaminants (Figs. 3-18 and 3-19).

ARTIFACTS

In addition to being aware of the artifacts that may result from the biopsy procedure and tissue processing, the dermatopathologist must be cognizant of tissue alterations which arise in vivo but are not classifiable as dermatoses in the usual sense of the word. One of these, excoriation, was illustrated at the beginning of this chapter. There are other physical and medicamentous influences that may produce characteristic changes. Suction[36] may induce

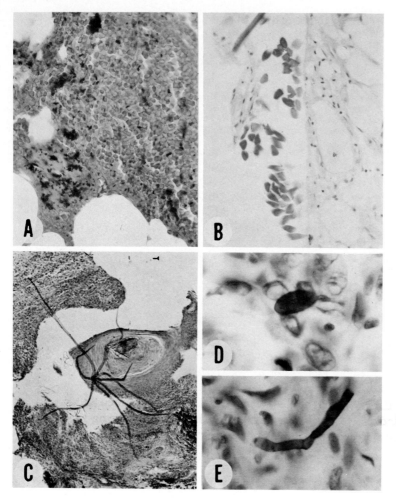

FIGURE 3–18.
Foreign bodies encountered in tissue sections.
A. *Formalin pigment in hemorrhagic tissue. H&E.
X280.* **B.** *Suture material, probably nylon thread.
H&E. X180.* **C.** *Plant hair contaminant. O&G.
X60. (From Pinkus. Arch Dermatol 100:96, 1969.)*
D. *Alternaria spore. H&E. X400.* **E.** *Fungous my-
celium. H&E. X400.*

paranuclear vacuoles and, later, dermoepidermal
separation. Friction[37] leads to rupture of cell membranes following intercellular edema. Electric current produces severe deformity of cells (Fig. 3-11).

Sunburn leads to the formation of characertistic
pyknotic cells in the epidermis.[38] Freezing was
shown many years ago to induce multinucleated
epidermal giant cells. The chemical action of po-

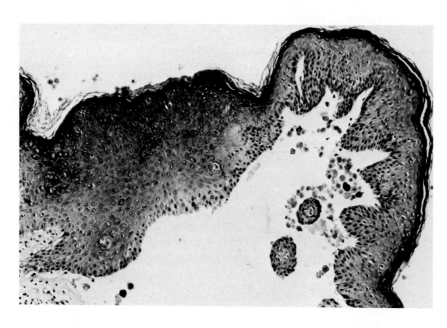

FIGURE 3–19.
*Starch granules in artificial cleft be-
tween epidermis and dermis. Artifact is
indicated by emptiness of space except for dislodged hair follicles and foreign bodies. The latter are identified as
starch by size, roundish or polygonal
shape, and dark center which represents air bubble. They could be further
identified by positive reaction to PAS.
H&E. X135.*

dophyllin in the treatment of warts causes characteristic clumped mitoses (Fig. 31-9), and systemic administration of methotrexate and hydroxyurea has been shown to produce peculiar pyknotic prickle cells with eosinophilic cytoplasm in psoriatic epidermis.[39] The application of cantharidin leads to acantholysis, and the list could be greatly prolonged. The pathologist should suspect that any unusual and bizarre changes in epidermis and dermis may be due to accidental or intentional artifact. Being able to identify some specific alterations will make him very useful to the clinician in obscure cases (Chap. 16).

REFERENCES

1. Pinkus H; Skin biopsy: a field of interaction between clinician and pathologist. Cutis 20:609, 1977
2. Mehregan AH, Pinkus H: Artifacts in dermal histopathology. Arch Dermatol 94:218, 1966
3. Griffiths WAD, Dutz W: Repeated tissue sampling with a dental broach. Br J Dermatol 93:43, 1975
4. Weigand DA: Transfollicular extrusion of sebaceous glands: natural phenomenon or artifact? A case report. J. Cutan Pathol 3:239, 1976
5. Tromovitch TA, Stegman SJ: Microscopic-controlled excision of cutaneous tumors. Chemosurgery fresh tissue technique. Cancer 41:653, 1978
6. Fritsch WC, and Ceilley RL: The use of the cryostat for histographic surgery. J Cutan Pathol 4:154, 1977
7. Ackerman AB, Penneys NS: Formalin pigment in skin. Arch Dermatol 102:318, 1970
8. Verocay J: Beseitigung der "Formolniederschläge" aus mikroskopischen Schnitten. Zentralbl Allg Pathol 19:769, 1908
9. Kardasewitsch B: Eine Methode zur Beseitigung der Formalin-Sedimente aus mikroskopischen Präparaten. Z Wiss Mikr 42:322, 1925
10. Malkinson FD, Potter B: Use of tetrahydrofuran for routine and rapid dehydration and clearing. Arch Dermatol 82:798, 1960
11. Mowry RW: The special value of methods that color both acidic and vicinal hydroxyl groups in the histochemical study of mucins, with revised directions for the colloidal iron stain, the use of alcian blue G8X and their combinations with the periodic acid-Schiff reaction. Ann NY Acad Sci 106:402, 1963
12. Pearse AGE: Histochemistry, Theoretical and Applied, 2nd ed. Boston, Little, Brown, 1960
13. Barka T, Anderson PJ: Histochemistry: Theory, Practice and Bibliography. New York, Harper & Row, 1963
14. Lillie RD: Histologic Technic and Practical Histochemistry. New York, McGraw-Hill, 1965
15. Luna LG: Manual of Histologic Staining Methods of the Armed Forces Institute of Pathology, 3rd ed. New York, McGraw-Hill, 1968
16. Pinkus H, Hunter R: Simplified acid orcein and Giemsa technique for routine staining of skin sections. Arch Dermatol 82:699, 1960
17. Krobock E, Rahbari H, Mehregan AH: Acid orcein and Giemsa stain. Modification of a valuable stain for dermatologic specimens. J Cutan Pathol 5:37, 1978
18. Johnson WC, Johnson FB, Helwig EB: Effect of varying the pH on reactions for acid mucopolysaccharides. J Histochem Cytochem 10:684, 1962
19. Gomori G: Aldehyde fuchsin: a new stain for elastic tissue. Am J Clin Pathol 20:665, 1950
20. Gomori G: Silver impregnation of reticulum in paraffin sections. Am J Pathol 13:993, 1937
21. Wilder HC: An improved technique for silver impregnation of reticulum fibers. Am J Pathol 11:817, 1935
22. Highman B: Improved methods for demonstrating amyloid in paraffin sections. Arch Pathol 41:559, 1946
23. Hashimoto K, Gross BG, Lever WF: Lichen anyloidosus. Histochemical and electron microscopic studies. J Invest Dermatol 45:204, 1965
24. Mishima Y: New technique for comprehensive demonstration of melanin, premelanin, and tyrosinase sites: combined dopa-premelanin reaction. J Invest Dermatol 34:355, 1960
25. Gomori G: Chemical character of the enterochromaffin cells. Arch Pathol 45:48, 1948
26. McGee-Russell SM: Histochemical methods for calcium. J Histochem Cytochem 6:22, 1958
27. Burge KM, Winkelmann RL: Mercury pigmentation: an electron microscopic study. Arch Dermatol 102:51, 1970
28. Cox AJ: Gold in the dermis following gold therapy for rheumatoid arthritis. Arch Dermatol 108:655, 1973
29. Grocott RG: A stain for fungi in tissue sections and smears. Using Gomori's methenamine-silver nitrate technic. Am J Clin Pathol 25:975, 1955
30. Lopez JF, Lebron RF: *Cryptococcus neoformans:* their identification in body fluids and cultures by mucicarmin stain (Mayer). Bol Asoc Med PR 64:203, 1972
31. Fite GL, Cambre PJ, Turner MH: Procedure for demonstrating lepra bacilli in paraffin sections. Arch Pathol 43:624, 1947
32. Barr RJ: Cutaneous cytology. Int J Dermatol 17:552, 1978
33. King DT, Sun NCJ: Touch preparation in diagnosis of skin disorders. Arch Dermatol 115:1034, 1979
34. Mehregan AH, Faghri B: Implantation dermatoses. Acta Derm Venereol (Stockh) 54:61, 1974
35. Pinkus H; Stellate plant hair contaminant in the laboratory. Arch Dermatol 100:96, 1969
36. Hunter JAA, McVittie E, Comaish JS: Light and electron microscopic studies of physical injuries to the skin. I. Suction. Br J Dermatol 90:481, 1974
37. Hunter JAA, McVittie E, Comaish JS: Light and electron microscopic studies of physical injuries to the skin. II. Friction. Br J Dermatol 90:491, 1974
38. Daniels F Jr, Brophy D, Lobitz WC Jr: Histochemical responses of human skin following ultraviolet irradiation. J Invest Dermatol 37:351, 1961
39. Smith C, Gelfant S: Effects of methotrexate and hydroxyurea on psoriatic epidermis. Arch Dermatol 110:70, 1974

Immunofluorescence of the Skin

During the past decade, immunofluorescent study of the skin has evolved from a laboratory research tool into a reliable aid in diagnosis and classification of a variety of diseases, including pemphigus, bullous pemphigoid, dermatitis herpetiformis, lupus erythematosus, and vasculitis. Distinctive immune responses and staining patterns have been recognized corresponding to the primary histopathology of each disease. A brief summary of direct and indirect immunofluorescent techniques and their interpretations are presented in this chapter.

INDIRECT AND DIRECT TECHNIQUES

The indirect immunofluorescent test (Table 4-1) is a serologic procedure similar to the antinuclear antibody and FTA-abs tests. This procedure is used for the detection of intercellular substance and basement membrane zone antibodies, or pemphigus and pemphigoid antibodies. For the indirect immunofluorescent test, 10 to 20 ml of the patient's serum kept at room temperature should be sent to the laboratory. Unfixed frozen sections of human skin are used as substrate. After incubation of the sections with the diluted serum to be tested, the sections are stained with antiserums to human IgG, IgM, and IgA, and with complement conjugated with fluorescein isothiocyanate. Following buffered rinses, the sections are examined with a microscope equipped with an ultraviolet light (UVL) source.

The direct immunofluorescent test is used for the detection of bound immunoglobulins IgG, IgA, IgM, and complement in skin sections of lesions from patients with bullous diseases, lupus erythematosus, or vasculitis. This test is not a true serologic procedure but is a histologic technique for the localization of immunoglobulins and complement in tissues. Unfixed skin biopsy specimens are cut in a cryostat at $-20C$ and are stained with fluorescein isothiocyanate antiserum to either IgG, IgA, IgM, or complement. After incubation and buffered rinses, the slides are examined with the UVL-equipped microscope.

Biopsy technique for immunofluorescent study is very important. In vesiculobullous diseases, perilesional skin should be submitted instead of an intact blister. Serum should also be provided for the indirect test to detect pemphigus or pemphigoid antibodies. A normal skin specimen from the buttock area may be included, especially if dermatitis herpetiformis is suspected. In evaluation of a patient for systemic lupus erythematosus (SLE), the most complete immunopathologic correlation can be made if three biopsy specimens are submitted for direct immunofluorescent tests: one of a skin lesion, another of a sun-exposed normal skin area for differentiation of discoid lupus erythematosus (DLE), and a third specimen from an unexposed

TABLE 4–1.
Indirect and Direct Immunofluorescent Tests in Bullous Dermatoses

	Indirect (serum)	Direct (skin)		ANA
		Involved	Uninvolved	
Intercellular pattern: mainly IgG				
Pemphigus vulgaris	+	+	+	−
Pemphigus vegetans	+	+	+	−
Pemphigus erythematosus	+	+	+	±
Pemphigus foliaceus	+	+	+	−
Basement membrane zone pattern: mainly IgG and C3				
Bullous pemphigoid	+	+	+	−
Cicatricial pemphigoid	±	+	+	−
Herpes gestationis	±	+	−	−
Bullous SLE	−	+	+	+
Granular papillary or linear dermoepidermal deposits of IgA				
Dermatitis herpetiformis	±	+	+	−
Bullous disease of childhood	−	+	±	−

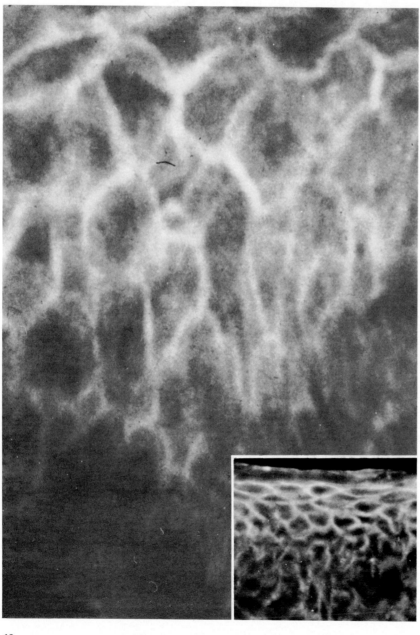

FIGURE 4–1.
Pemphigus vulgaris. DIF test on involved skin shows intercellular pattern of IgG deposition. (Courtesy of Dr. T. F. Downham, II.)

normal skin, such as from the buttock, for prognosis. To establish the presence of immunofluorescent vasculitis, a biopsy specimen of a lesion not older than 24 to 48 hours is necessary.[1-3] Skin specimens are now placed in Michel's transport solution and no longer require transportation in liquid nitrogen or dry ice.[4]

Immunofluorescent tests are a major contribution in the diagnosis and management of the pemphigus group of diseases and lupus erythematosus.

PEMPHIGUS GROUP

Phemphigus vulgaris, vegetans, foliaceus, and erythematosus are characterized by the presence of pemphigus antibodies in serum which reacts with the intercellular substance using the indirect immunofluorescent technique (Fig. 4–1). The direct test also shows a positive intercellular substance pattern. These antibodies are disease specific. However, occasional, low-titer, false-positive tests have been detected in postburn patients, individuals with allergic reactions to penicillin, and in dermatophytosis. Pemphigus antibodies are not present in Hailey and Hailey's disease.[5] Pemphigus antibody titers are largely dependent upon the type of substrate used and may not necessarily correlate with the disease activity.[6,7] However, following of antibody titers during the treatment and management of the disease is recommended, keeping in mind that clinical correlation is essential for good therapeutic results.

Pemphigus foliaceus may show subcorneal intercellular antibodies in the anatomic site of the blister.[8] Patients with pemphigus erythematosus have fixed (direct immunofluorescence) IgG and complement at the dermoepidermal junction only in the involved facial skin areas. All skin areas, however, show typical intercellular IgG deposits characteristic of pemphigus.[9]

Bullous pemphigoid shows a linear or tubular band at the basement membrane in 70 to 80 percent of patients utilizing the indirect immunofluorescent technique. Fixed immunoglobulin binding by the direct method, however, can be demonstrated in 90 to 95 percent of patients with active lesions (Fig. 4-2). The serum titer of pemphigoid antibodies does not parallel the course of the disease.

Cicatricial pemphigoid shows basement membrane zone antibodies circulating or fixed, similar to bullous pemphigoid within the involved areas of conjunctiva, oral mucosa, or skin.[5]

Dermatitis herpetiformis shows granular deposits of IgA and, occasionally, IgG in the papillary dermis and, less frequently, at the basement zone adjacent to the blister. Complement may also be present. Linear IgA deposits may be present in the uninvolved skin, and some patients may have circulating basement membrane zone antibodies of the IgA type.[10]

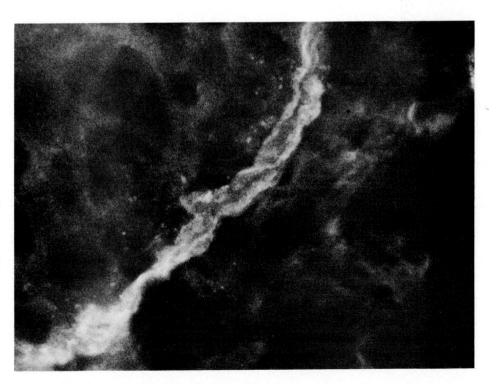

FIGURE 4–2.
Bullous pemphigoid tubular band. Skin adjacent to the bulla incubated with fluorescein-conjugated goat antihuman pooled immunoglobulins shows a sharply marginated twisted band with a dark center, giving a hollow tubular appearance at the dermoepidermal junction. (From Burnham et al. Arch Dermatol 102:42, 1970. Copyright © 1970 American Medical Association.)

TABLE 4–2.
Direct Immunofluorescence of Skin in Lupus Erythematosus

	Involved	Unexposed Normal Skin	Sun-Exposed Normal Skin
Discoid LE	+ Homogeneous pattern	−	−
SLE	+ Homogeneous or thready pattern	+ Stippled pattern	+
Vasculitis	+ Blood vessels	−	−

In herpes gestationis, sera of patients contain an IgG antibody which localizes to the basement membrane, similar to the situation in bullous pemphigoid.[11]

Direct immunofluorescent preparations utilizing skin lesions are also useful for the diagnosis of chronic bullous dermatosis of childhood.[12,13]

LUPUS ERYTHEMATOSUS

In lupus erythematosus, immunofluorescent tests aid in diagnosis and prognosis (Table 4–2). The fluorescent lupus band is a granular band along the basement membrane which may show three patterns: homogeneous, thready, or stippled. There ap-

pears to be a correlation between the type of clinical lesion and the pattern of the band. The homogeneous band is seen in clinical hyperkeratotic and atrophic lesions of DLE and SLE but not in the clinically normal skin areas of SLE patients (Fig. 4-3). The thready pattern is present in diffuse erythematous and edematous plaques and in new lesions of chronic discoid lupus erythematosus (Fig. 4-4). The stippled pattern appears in clinically normal skin of SLE patients (Fig. 4-5). The uninvolved skin of patients with SLE shows a positive band in 50 to 60 percent of the biopsy specimens. No lupus band is present in the normal skin of patients with DLE. Involved skin of SLE patients shows a positive lupus band in 90 to 95 percent of cases and in 85 to 90 percent of patients with DLE lesions. Sun-exposed normal skin of patients with SLE shows a lupus band in 80 percent of the biopsy specimens.[14-19] The lupus band test is useful when development of systemic lupus erythematosus in a patient with chronic discoid lesions is suspected. The presence of a lupus band in the uninvolved skin of patients with SLE may be of prognostic significance, indicating renal involvement.[20] Occasionally, a false-positive lupus band may occur in patients with polymorphous light eruption, rosacea, or facial telangiectasia.[21]

Immune vasculitis, sometimes associated with collagen vascular diseases, such as SLE, shows deposition of immunoglobulins and complement in the wall of blood vessels, utilizing the direct immunofluorescent technique.[22]

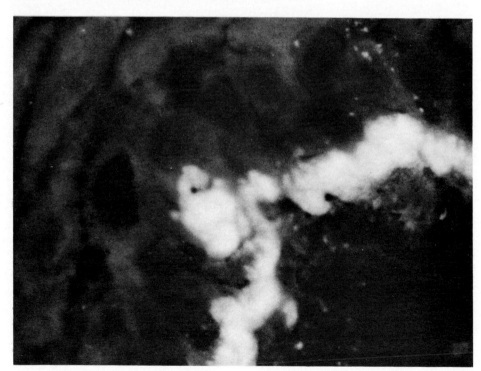

FIGURE 4–3.
Lupus erythematosus homogeneous band. Atrophic skin lesion of a patient with SLE incubated with fluorescein-conjugated goat antihuman IgG shows a brightly fluorescent, well-demarcated, and solid homogeneous band at the dermoepidermal junction. (From Burnham and Fine. Arch Dermatol 99:413, 1969. Copyright © 1969 American Medical Association.)

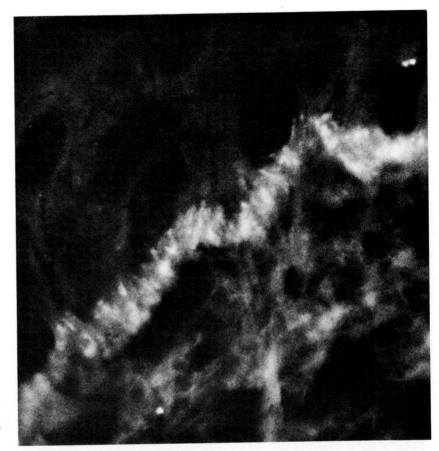

FIGURE 4–4.
Lupus erythematosus thready band. Diffuse erythematous lesion of arm of a patient with SLE incubated with fluorescein-conjugated goat antihuman IgG demonstrates the thready band and an underlying weaker homogeneous fluorescence at the dermoepidermal junction. (From Burnham et al. Arch Dermatol 102:42, 1970. Copyright © 1970 American Medical Association.)

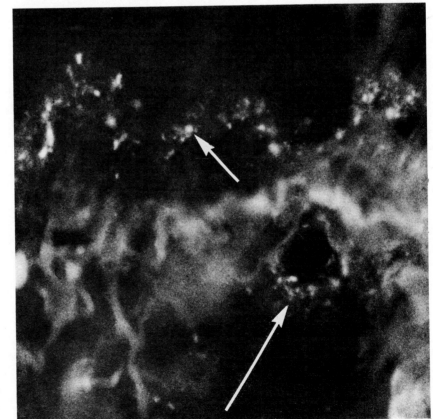

FIGURE 4–5.
Lupus erythematosus stippled band. Clinically normal skin of patient with SLE incubated with fluorescein-conjugated goat antihuman pooled immunoglobulins shows discontinuous stippled band and elongated threadlike stipples at the dermoepidermal junction. Stipples are also present in the wall of a capillary blood vessel (arrows). (From Burnham and Fine. Arch Dermatol 103:24, 1971. Copyright © 1971 American Medical Association.)

REFERENCES

1. Beutner EH, Chorzelski TD, Bean SF, et al.: Immunopathology of the Skin. Labeled Antibody Studies. Stroudsburg, Pa. Dowden, Hutchinson & Ross, 1973
2. Fry L, Seah PP: Immunological Aspects of Skin Diseases. New York, Wiley, 1974
3. Beutner EH, Chorzelski TD, Jordon RE: Autosensitization in Pemphigus and Bullous Pemphigoid. Springfield, Ill., Thomas, 1970
4. Michel B, Milner Y, David K: Preservation of tissue fixed immunoglobulins in skin: Biopsies of patients with lupus erythematosus and bullous diseases. J Invest Dermatol 59:449, 1973
5. Lever WF: Pemphigus and pemphigoid. J Am Acad Dermatol 1:2, 1979
6. Judd KP, Lever WF: Correlation of antibodies in skin and serum with disease activity in pemphigus. Arch Dermatol 115:428, 1979
7. Judd KP, Mescon H: Comparison of differential substrates useful for indirect immunofluorescence testing of sera of patients with active pemphigus. J Invest Dermatol 72:314, 1979
8. Bystryn JC, Abel E, DeFeo C: Pemphigus foliaceus. Arch Dermatol 110:857, 1974
9. Chorzelski TP, Jablonska S, Blasczyk M: Immunopathological investigations in the Senear-Usher syndrome (co-existence of pemphigus and lupus erythematosus). Br J Dermatol 80:211, 1968
10. Katz SI, Strober W: The pathogenesis of dermatitis herpetiformis. J Invest Dermatol 70:63, 1978
11. Katz SI, Hertz KC, Yaoita H: Herpes gestationis: Immunopathology and characterization of the herpes gestationis factor. J Clin Invest 57:1434, 1976
12. Prystkowsky S, Gilliam JN: Benign chronic bullous dermatosis of childhood. Arch Dermatol 112:837, 1976
13. Esterly NB, Furey NL, Kirschner BS, et al.: Chronic bullous dermatosis of childhood. Arch Dermatol 113:42, 1977
14. Burnham TK, Neblett TR, Fine R: The application of the fluorescent antibody technique to the investigation of lupus erythematosus and various dermatoses. J Invest Dermatol 41:451, 1963
15. Tan EM, Kunkel HG: An immunofluorescent study of the skin lesions in systemic lupus erythematosus. Arthritis Rheum 1:37, 1966
16. Burnham TK, Fine R: The immunofluorescent "band" test for lupus erythematosus. III. Employing clinically normal skin. Arch Dermatol 103:24, 1971
17. Tuffanelli DL: Lupus erythematosus. Arch Dermatol 106:553, 1972
18. Monroe EW: Lupus band test. Arch Dermatol 113:830, 1977
19. Provost TT: Subsets in systemic lupus erythematosus. J Invest Dermatol 72:110, 1979
20. Gilliam JN, Cheatum DE, Huron ER, et al.: Immunoglobulin in clinically uninvolved skin in systemic lupus erythematosus (associated with renal disease). J Clin Invest 53:1434, 1974
21. Fisher DA: Polymorphic light eruption and lupus erythematosus. Differential diagnosis by fluorescent microscopy. Arch Dermatol 101:458, 1970
22. Schroeter AL, Copeman PWM, Jordon RE, et al.: Immunofluorescence of cutaneous vasculitis associated with systemic disease. Arch Dermatol 104:254, 1971

CHAPTER

5

General Pathology: Terminology

Many phenomena encountered in dermatohistopathology are unique to the skin and are best described in specific terms not often used in general pathology. Exact definition and application of these terms aid greatly in precise description and communication.

Similarly, it is advisable to follow a systematic pattern in the description of skin sections. Every normal constituent of the skin should be mentioned in order to show that it has not been overlooked. It is convenient to start at the surface and work down toward the subcutaneous layer, but a few modifications are recommended. If a section represents a tumor, either of the epidermis or of the dermis, this is best stated at the outset. A good description of a skin section should make it possible for the reader to visualize the pathologic change, and the statement that we are dealing with a tumor and where it is located is very helpful in this respect. Also, if the principal abnormal feature is located deep in the dermis or subcutis, it is wise to mention this right away, before proceeding with the routine detailed description.

Another modification that we recommend is to begin with the living major portion of the epidermis. Start with the rete malpighi or prickle cell layer, then trace these cells in their natural course through the granular into the horny layer. This is followed, if necessary, by details concerning the condition of the basal layer and junction. Papillary and subpapillary portions of the dermis are de-

scribed next, then the reticular portion (mid-dermis and deep dermis), and finally the subcutaneous fat tissue, if the submitting dermatologist or surgeon was circumspect enough to include it in his biopsy. Absence of the deeper layers should be recorded, as they often contain invaluable clues to the diagnosis which in their absence may remain unclear. The outlined scheme will be followed in this chapter, and photomicrographs of various skin diseases (some found in succeeding chapters) will be used to illustrate and name the phenomena of cutaneous general pathology.

There are several reasons for our recommendations. Unless we can be content with the short statement, "The epidermis shows no significant changes," we have to keep in mind that all pathobiologic alterations of the epidermis start in its living portion. All changes in the horny layer (with the exception of external trauma) are initiated in the prickle cell layers. The basal layer, on the other hand, less frequently shows tangible pathology, and if it does, this is best discussed in terms of its two principal functions: as a regenerative layer and as a part of the epidermodermal junction.

Another reason is the fact that the true baseline in the structural organization of the skin is the superficial dermis at the base of the papillae, as shown so vividly in Figure 2-10 and mentioned in Chapter 2. The normal epidermis resembles a moldable cover over the dermis and fills all the spaces between the papillae. In pathologic biology, if the papillae become edematous or hypertrophic, they elevate the epidermis above them, the rete ridges becoming exaggerated. When the epidermis becomes hyperplastic, it also thickens toward the outside of the body. If its ridges grow high and large, the spaces between them are filled by the accommodating papillae, and the suprapapillary plate is pushed up. With very few exceptions (see lichen simplex chronicus in Chap. 7 and pseudoepitheliomatous proliferation in Chap. 34), there is no downgrowth of rete ridges, and this often misused descriptive term should be applied with the utmost caution.

EPIDERMIS

General Configuration

The epidermis may be thicker or thinner than normal. Figure 5-1A is taken from a case of chronic eczematous dermatitis. The epidermis is thicker than normal and contains a larger number of prickle cells. It exhibits *acanthosis* (akanthos, Greek for spine or prickle), which is defined as epidermal *hyperplasia* through overabundance of prickle cells. Figure 5-1B, in contrast, shows a thick epidermis consisting of relatively few and very large prickle cells. This state is best called epidermal *hypertrophy* (sometimes called *pseudoacanthosis*). A rough estimate of the number of prickle

cells can be obtained by counting the number of nuclei along a vertical line between basal layer and granular (or parakeratotic) layers. Normally, four to seven nuclei are present, depending on whether one chooses the area above a papilla or that in a rete ridge. In Figure 5-1A, 10 to 12 nuclei are found in a vertical row in a ridge, 4 to 5 above the papilla. In Figure 5-1B, the range is 4 to 7, indicating that there is no overproduction (hyperplasia) of cells. Epidermal *atrophy* and *hypoplasia* are shown in Figure 5-2. The number and vertical diameter of cells are diminished, and, at the same time, rete ridges are short or absent. Note that hyperplasia, hypertrophy, hypoplasia, and atrophy are judged by the number and size of the prickle cells. The basal layer by definition is always single, as pointed out in Chapter 2. The condition of its cells must be described separately and will be discussed later.

The condition of the *rete ridges* and the *suprapapillary plate* (that part of the epidermis above a line connecting the tips of the papillae) should be noted separately. The latter can be thick or thin. The ridges may be absent, short, long, thin, thick, clubbed, or pointed. They may be even or uneven in length and width. A word of caution is necessary. Because we ordinarily examine thin vertical sections, rete ridges may be cut at any angle. Cross sections look like pegs, but tangential and oblique sections may look like very broad blocks. It is only from comparing size and shape of ridges in a long section, or better in serial sections, that one

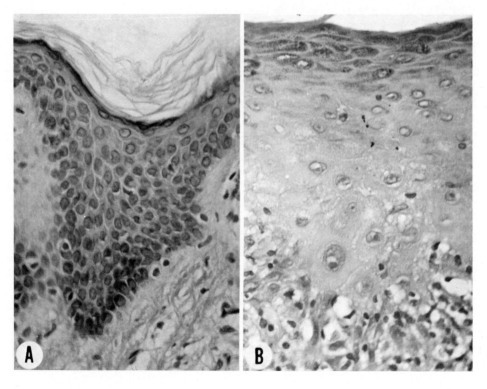

FIGURE 5–1.
Hyperplasia and hypertrophy of epidermis. **A.** *Mildly acanthotic epidermis of chronic lichenification.* **B.** *Hypertrophic epidermis of lichen planus. Compare number and size of keratinocytes in these photos taken at identical magnification. H&E. X352.*

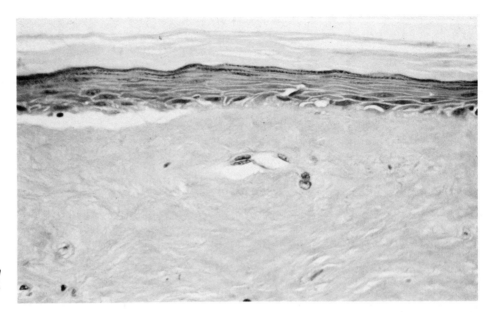

FIGURE 5–2.
Epidermal atrophy in lichen sclerosus et atrophicus. H&E. X370.

can get an approximate estimate of their true configuration in any biopsy specimen. For this purpose the split skin preparations of Oberste-Lehn[1] (Semper preparations, Horstmann) are highly instructive (Fig. 5-3). The tendency to describe any acanthotic epidermis as "psoriasiform" is regrettable (Chap. 8).

Special Features in the Prickle Cell Layer. Prickle cells may be smaller than normal (atrophic) but more commonly are larger, either through *hypertrophy* or *intracellular edema.* The size of the nucleus in nonneoplastic disease varies within narrow limits. It has been well shown that every prickle cell nucleus contains approximately the same amount of chromatin (diploid). Therefore, a smaller nucleus will stain darker than a larger one. The size of the cell body varies considerably, and whether this is due to hypertrophy or edema is difficult to judge in routine sections. The depth of staining is a poor indicator. Prickle cells of acanthotic epidermis may contain much glycogen (Fig. 5-4) and, therefore, may appear pale in H&E and other stains without being edematous. A high degree of intracellular edema usually is indicated by

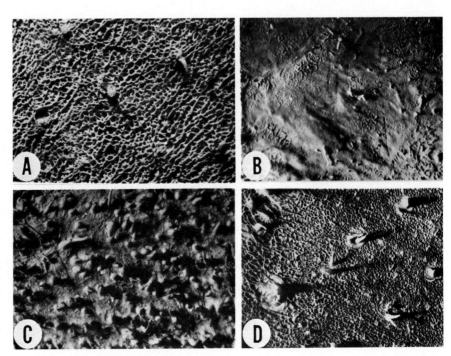

FIGURE 5–3.
Lower surface of epidermis in various skin diseases. Specimens prepared by Dr. H. Oberste-Lehn according to Horstmann's method and photographed in oblique incident light. The projecting peglike structures are the stumps of hair roots and sweat ducts. **A.** *Psoriasis. Note even pattern of accentuated rete ridges.* **B.** *Lichen planus. Note atrophy of ridges.* **C.** *Chronic discoid lupus erythematosus. Large number of small facial hair follicles, distended by keratinous plugs.* **D.** *Lichen simplex chronicus at left, normal skin at right. Gradually increasing hyperplasia of rete ridges becoming excessive in left upper corner. (From Pinkus.* Arch Dermatol 82:681, 1960.)

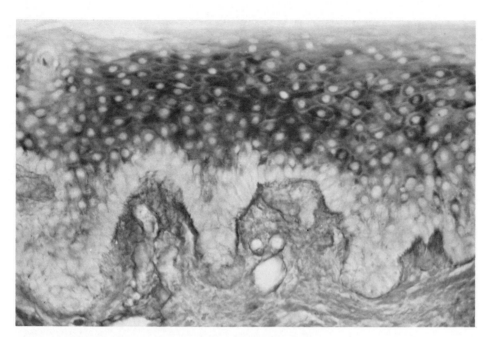

FIGURE 5–4.
Glycogen (dark because PAS-positive) in acanthotic epidermis. Note absence of glycogen in basal cells and in keratinizing layers. PAS-light green. X285.

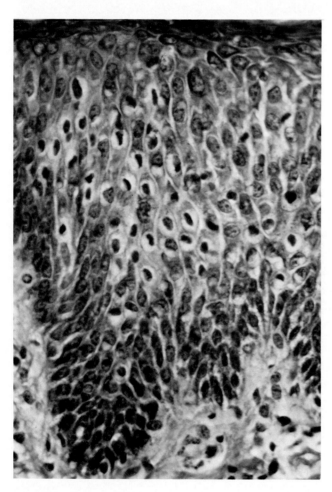

FIGURE 5–5.
Intracellular edema producing perinuclear halos. H&E. X465.

a perinuclear or paranuclear empty space due to retraction of the nucleus from the tonofibril-containing peripheral cytoplasm during routine fixation (Fig. 5-5).

More important for diagnostic purposes are the presence, quantity, and distribution of *intercellular edema*. This widens the intercellular spaces and accentuates the intercellular bridges (Figs. 2-5 and 7-4). The relationship of intercellular bridges, desmosomes, and tonofibrils was discussed in Chapter 2. It should be noted in description whether edema is diffuse or focal. A pronounced degree of intercellular edema is called *spongiosis* because it makes an epidermal section resemble a sponge (Fig. 5-6). Once the overstretched intercellular bridges rupture, *vesiculation* is initiated. *Intraepidermal vesicles* of this type are referred to as *spongiotic vesicles*.

Vesiculation plays an important part in clinical diagnosis, and the pathologist is often called upon to decide the type and location of the vesicle. A classification and differentiation of vesiculating processes will be given in Chapter 11. Here we point out that vesicles and bullae can arise at any level within and just below the epidermis. They may be *subcorneal* (above the granular layer, Fig. 11-14), *intragranular* (Fig. 11-16), *intraepidermal* (Fig. 7-5), and *subepidermal*. Subepidermal vesicles can result from separation at the dermoepidermal junction (Fig. 11-7), sometimes in association with basal cell degeneration (Fig. 9-4), or they may be *intradermal bullae* resulting from *bullous edema* of the papillae (Fig. 10-4).

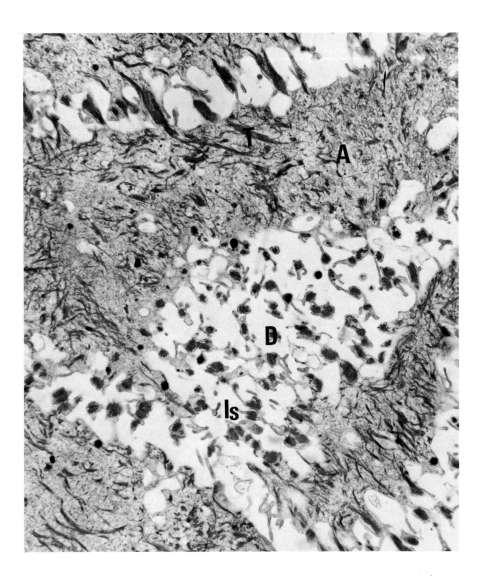

FIGURE 5–6.
Spongiosis. Intercellular edema more severe than in Figure 2-6. Intercellular space (Is) filled with partly broken intercellular bridges (D) and microvilli. Tonofilaments (T) in cytoplasm (A) extend to intercellular bridges. Electron micrograph. X8000. (Courtesy of Dr. A.P. Lupulescu.)

Intraepidermal vesicles and bullae may result from spongiosis through rupture of stretched intercellular bridges or from acantholysis (dissolution and disappearance of intercellular connections, Fig. 11-1) or from necrosis and disappearance of entire cells. The latter is the mechanism of *reticulating degeneration*, which is particularly common in viral diseases (Fig. 12-1). Empty spaces within or below the epidermis that do not contain recognizable fluid and may be due to retraction of separated elements during fixation are referred to as *clefts* (e.g., Fig. 28-1 in Darier's disease, also lichen planus). Flat, flaccid vesicles resulting from acantholysis are called *lacunae* (e.g., in Hailey-Hailey's disease, Fig. 28-5). Unique processes are the edema and rupture of hypertrophic granular cells (Figs. 29-4, and 29-6), leading to the bullae of epidermolytic hyperkeratosis (bullous form of ichthyosiform erythroderma), and the basal cell disintegration of epidermolysis bullosa.

Not only tissue fluid but formed elements of various types may be present within the epidermis. Inflammatory cells, including neutrophilic and eosinophilic polymorphonuclears as well as lymphocytes, easily enter through temporary breaks (Fig. 8-7) in the basement membrane (*exocytosis*). They may migrate singly in the intercellular spaces or may accumulate in vesicles. Accumulations of polymorphonuclear cells between the damaged cells of the suprapapillary plate of psoriasiform tissue reactions (Fig. 8-12) are known as *spongiform pustules* (Kogoj). Groups of pyknotic leukocytes found in the keratinizing layers are known as *Munro microabscesses* (Fig. 8-3). Other cells, such as mast cells, but particularly reticuloendothelial and lymphomatous cells, invade the epidermis. This is an important diagnostic feature in histiocytosis X (monocytes and Langerhans cells, Fig. 24-1) and in mycosis fungoides (atypical mononuclear cells, Pautrier abscesses, Fig. 44-5). Red blood cells also get into the epidermis, as do fragments of elastic and collagenous fibers and clumps of amyloid. These and other nonmotile elements are gradually pushed outward with the stream of keratinocytes and are eliminated on the surface (*transepidermal elimination*).[2,3] Transepidermal elimination should, however, be kept separate from transepidermal perforation, which is a much more massive process (pp. 74–75).

Stratum Granulosum and Stratum Corneum. Vertical sections of normal epidermis usually show one or two rows of granular (keratohyalin) cells except on the acral parts of the extremities, where this layer is thicker. Multiple layers of granular cells are described as *hypergranulosis*. Reduction (*hypogranulosis*) or absence of granular layer is abnormal and should always be mentioned in description.

Hypergranulosis and absence of granular layer may be found together in one section, in alternating or focal distribution. Because it may be of diagnostic significance, the state of the granular layer in topical relation to rete ridges or papillae should be mentioned: e.g., in Figure 5-7, the granular layer is absent from the *suprapapillary* portions, while it is thickened in the *interpapillary* stretches.

The horny layer (stratum corneum) varies considerably in width and compactness in different parts of the normal skin (Fig. 2-1).[4] It is, therefore, very important to know exactly from which locality a biopsy specimen has been obtained. *Hyperkeratosis* means increased thickness of the horny layer. It may be *orthokeratotic* (consisting of mor-

phologically normal cells without nuclei) or *parakeratotic* (containing pyknotic nuclei). Hyperkeratosis may be *relative* in comparison to the atrophic or hypoplastic prickle cell layer, or it may be *absolute*, and often it is both. The normal horny layer often is described as having a basketweave appearance because our routine sections stain mainly the cell walls, while the body of the cell appears empty. This state is exaggerated in some diseases, e.g., verruca plana. In other sections (Fig. 9-1), the horny layer looks compact or compressed, similar to that of palms and soles. A compressed horny layer may be relatively thin and yet represent hyperkeratosis. In other conditions (e.g., psoriasis), we encounter a lamellated stratum corneum, composed of alternating layers of orthokeratosis and parakeratosis (Fig. 8-8).

Scale and Crust. Hyperkeratosis usually corresponds to the clinical aspect of scaliness, especially if it is parakeratotic or lamellated. One can often judge the clinical characteristics in the sections. The large lamellar scales of psoriasis tend to separate in histologic sections; the fine branny scale of seborrheic dermatitis appears as *moundlike* foci (Fig. 8-2). The thin, disklike scale of pityriasis lichenoides chronica can be recognized and is a help in diagnosis (Fig. 13-3).

If tissue fluid (serum) is mixed with horny material, usually of parakeratotic type, a *scale-crust* results (Fig. 5-8). The inspissated and dried-up serum appears in the sections as amorphous material that is eosinophilic and usually PAS-positive. The term *colloid keratosis*[5] has been applied to

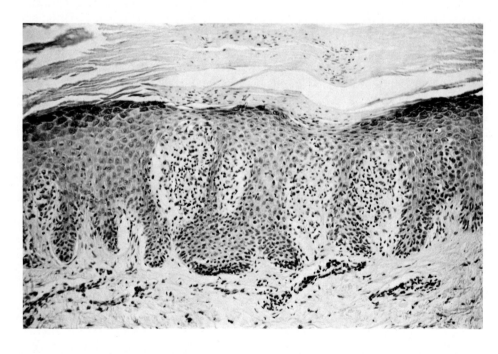

FIGURE 5–7.
Psoriasiform lesion showing association of parakeratosis and loss of granular layer with heads of papillae. H&E. X135.

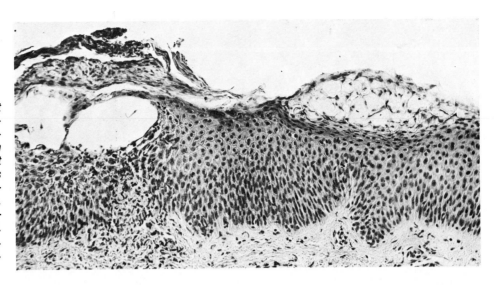

FIGURE 5–8.
Two types of parakeratotic crust in cases of seborrheic dermatitis. At left, dense parakeratotic lamellae are mixed with pyknotic leukocytic nuclei. At right, coagulated serum is caught between cells and produces a spongy appearance. H&E. X126. (From Sutton. Diseases of the Skin, 11th ed. 1956. Courtesy of Dr. R. L. Sutton, Jr. Contributed by H. Pinkus.)

conditions in which large blobs of dense PAS-positive material are found in the hyperplastic horny layer (Fig. 46-16).

An essential part of the examination of the horny layer is a search for microorganisms, such as fungi and bacteria, which may solve an otherwise puzzling histopathologic picture. Hyphae and spores are sometimes visible in H&E sections and are easily recognized in O&G sections (Fig. 13-1A), although it must be admitted that the PAS procedure furnishes a much more dramatic demonstration (Figs. 13-1B and 13-2). Bacteria also are stained by the Giemsa solution. Scabies mites (Fig. 13-11) and various foreign particles that may or may not have significance may be found in the stratum corneum. It is worthwhile to examine red and white blood cells that adhere to the skin surface. They may give a clue to sickling or other erythrocyte abnormalities and to leukemia, even if the small vessels in the skin do not contain blood.

Disturbances in the Basal Layer. It must be said at the outset that nothing has caused more confusion in dermatopathology than the indiscriminate application of the designation "basal cell" to any epithelial cell that has a relatively small dark nucleus and scant cytoplasm (Chap. 2). The concept of basal cell carcinoma as a tumor of basal cells and opposed to spinous or squamous cell carcinoma as a tumor composed of prickle cells has had repercussions extending into other fields of pathology and has injected dualistic concepts into biologic and embryologic investigations. Fortunately, the electron microscopists have reconfirmed classic concepts and have securely established the unity of all keratinocytes. Basal cells, prickle cells, and keratinized cells are the same strain of cell at different ages, just as the slim adolescent changes into the paunchy middle-ager and the shriveled old màn (Fig. 5-9). This simile, of course, cannot be pursued too far. The germinal basal cell is eternally young. It does not produce progeny but splits into two cells equal to itself. That one of these daughters usually goes on to maturation and death may be explained by its becoming separated from immaturity-preserving contact with the dermis.

The numerous applications of the term *basal cell* and suggested substitutes are listed in Table 2-2. In most instances, substitution of *basaloid cell* is acceptable and self-explanatory. It has become

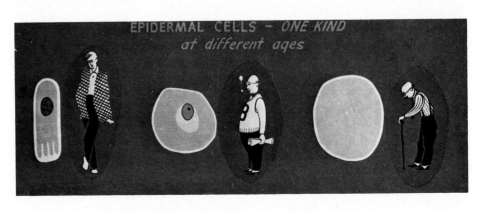

FIGURE 5–9.
Three ages of man and keratinocyte. (From Pinkus and Steele. AMA Scientific Exhibits, 1955. Courtesy of Grune & Stratton.)

abundantly clear that similarity in H&E-stained paraffin sections does not mean morphologic or functional or biologic identity of small, dark-staining epithelial cells.

The term *basal cell* is then reserved for cells in the *basal layer* of the epidermis or at the periphery of adnexal structures. Cells that are in contact with subserving mesoderm, in most circumstances, are also the only type of cell undergoing mitotic division. However, if mitotic activity is greatly increased, e.g., in psoriasis, two or three strata of the epidermis may contain mitoses[6] and form the *germinal layer* (stratum germinativum) of the hyperplastic epidermis. The cells of these layers may be relatively small and immature; they are basaloid cells (seborrheic verruca, Chap. 33).

Basal cells of normal or abnormal epidermis may be *flat* (Fig. 5-2), *cuboidal*, or *columnar* (Figs. 5-4 and 5-8). In most instances, it suffices to state that the layer is intact. In some diseases, basal cells are said to undergo *liquefaction degeneration* (Fig. 9-6) or *hyalinization* (Fig. 9-4). An organized basal layer may be absent for short or longer stretches of the epidermis, and cells having the morphologic appearance of prickle cells border on the dense inflammatory infiltrate present in all these cases. Usually, this phenomenon is associated with *subepidermal cleft* formation (see lichen planus, lupus erythematosus). The peripheral cells of squamous cell carcinoma usually have little morphologic resemblance to basal cells.

Melanocytes. The basal layer normally contains a complement of melanocytes. Their number being fairly constant for any given area, an unusual scarcity or abundance may have pathologic significance. However, individual sections may show great variations, and judgment must be based on examination of a series of sections. One also has to remember that nonpigmented basal melanocytes are indistinguishable by light microscopy from similarly situated Langerhans cells (Chap. 30).

Melanin in granular form is normally present in basal cells, except in very light skin. It is also found (Fig. 2-12) in prickle cells and horny cells of more darkly pigmented skins. The decision whether absence or presence of melanin has pathologic significance depends on clinical information, which is essential. Many skins under a variety of chronic inflammatory conditions present *pigment block* (Fig. 2-41). The keratinocytes seem unable to accept melanin from the melanocytes, which become engorged with pigment (Figs. 2-39 and 2-41) and highly dendritic. The epidermal melanin unit becomes dissociated (Chap. 30). Failure of pigment transfer on a congenital basis was found to be the cause of universal dyschromatosis in two Bantu.[7] Other disturbances of melanization will be discussed in the corresponding chapters, especially Chapter 30.

Dyskeratosis, Dysplasia, Anaplasia

These terms need special discussion because their significance has changed over the years, and they are often loosely applied. Without going into historical details, it may be said that *dyskeratosis* has a very specific meaning and is practically synonymous with *individual cell keratinization*. In certain diseases, e.g., Darier's (Fig. 28-1) and Bowen's (Fig. 34-11), individual cells become separated from their neighbors through acantholysis. They may proceed to keratinize as round isolated bodies (*corps ronds, grains*) (Fig. 5-10). Some authors distinguish between *benign* and *malignant dyskeratosis*. Thus, Darier's disease is said to be characterized by benign dyskeratosis and Bowen's disease by the malignant counterpart. However, any cell on its way toward keratinization has no malignant potentialities, and diagnosis of benign or malignant in these diseases is based on other criteria.

Cytologic characteristics, which stigmatize Bowen's dermatosis (Fig. 34-11) as carcinoma-insitu usually are called *anaplasia*. This term was introduced to convey the concept that cancer results from a reversion of normal adult cells to embryonic cells. It is obvious that the significance of the word has been changed completely in present usage. There is no similarity between the highly atypical, uneven, and often hyperchromatic cells of Bowen's disease and the well-organized, though immature, cells of the embryo. In the skin at least, it is preferable to substitute *dysplasia* for anaplasia as a descriptive term. More details will be given in Chapter 34 on precanceroses. A certain degree of uneven size and irregular arrangement of basal and prickle cells may exist without diagnostic significance, especially in atrophic epidermis or in instances of heavy exocytosis. Considerable experience is needed to differentiate such changes from true neoplastic dysplasia, and multiple sections should be examined in doubtful cases. Inasmuch as carcinoma-insitu of the skin is not a highly dangerous condition, it is better to err on the conservative side and to ask for rebiopsy at a later date, should the clinical lesion persist. *Multinucleated epidermal giant cells* (Fig. 5-11) are encountered occasionally without diagnostic implications and may be present in dysplastic conditions, especially Bowen's disease, in viral infections (see Fig. 5-16D), and as a result of freezing.

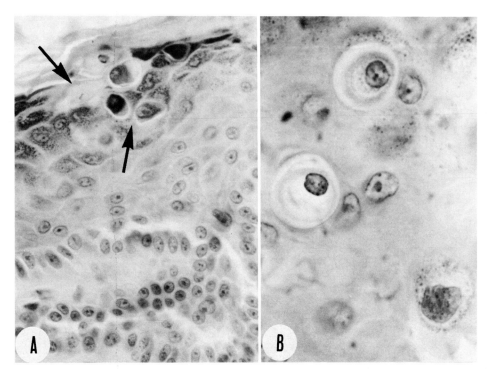

FIGURE 5–10.
Darier's disease. **A.** *Supra-basal cleft as sign of acanthol-ysis. Dyskeratotic cells near granular layer. Corps ronds have a nucleus within a cyto-plasm which is separated from surrounding cells by a cleft (lower arrow). Grain is a kera-tinized body with remnant of a nucleus (upper arrow). H&E. X600.* **B.** *Several corps ronds, one (lower right) with kerato-hyaline granules. H&E. X800.*

Cell Death

Epidermal cells normally die through the intricate maturation process of keratinization. The most common deviation from this process is *parakera-tosis*, usually encountered in inflammation, in which no keratohyalin is formed and the nuclei persist as flat stainable disks. Several other forms of cell death were mentioned in the preceding paragraphs or will be discussed under specific diseases (reticulating and ballooning degeneration in viral diseases, acantholytic degeneration in pemphigus,

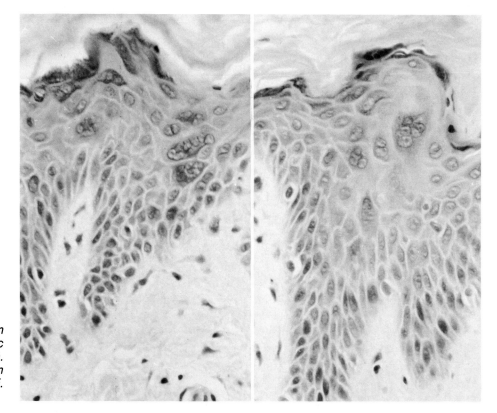

FIGURE 5–11.
Multinucleated giant cells in epidermis have no diagnostic significance in many cases. These examples were found in lichenified dermatitis. H&E. X600.

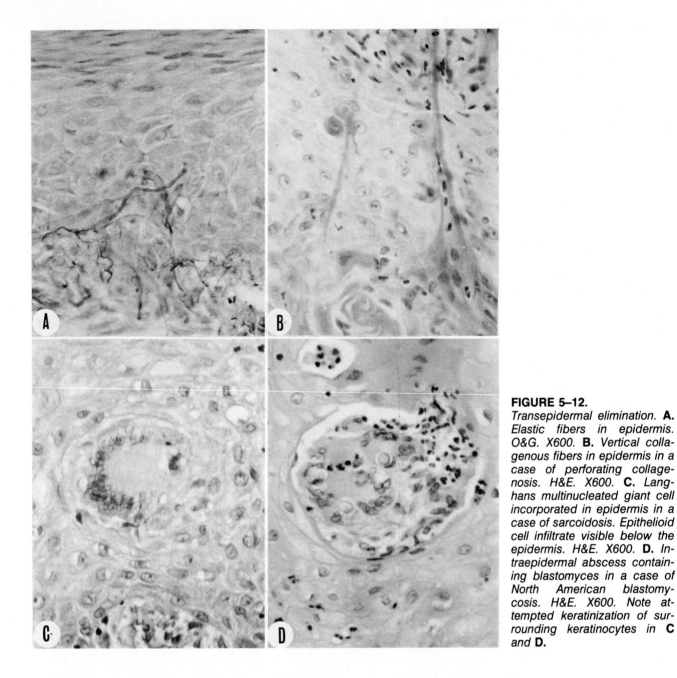

FIGURE 5–12.
Transepidermal elimination. **A.** *Elastic fibers in epidermis. O&G. X600.* **B.** *Vertical collagenous fibers in epidermis in a case of perforating collagenosis. H&E. X600.* **C.** *Langhans multinucleated giant cell incorporated in epidermis in a case of sarcoidosis. Epithelioid cell infiltrate visible below the epidermis. H&E. X600.* **D.** *Intraepidermal abscess containing blastomyces in a case of North American blastomycosis. H&E. X600. Note attempted keratinization of surrounding keratinocytes in* **C** *and* **D.**

epidermolytic hyperkeratosis, basal cell disappearance in epidermolysis bullosa, and lichenoid tissue reactions). Cell-sized hyaline bodies in lichen planus and other diseases are known as *Civatte bodies* (Fig. 9-6), and peculiar pyknotic prickle cells have been described after ultraviolet irradiation and following podophyllin treatment of condyloma acuminatum (Fig. 31-9B). Other types of tissue cells, especially in neoplasms but also in embryologic development (e.g., hair germ), undergo a peculiar type of pyknosis and fragmentation to which the botanical term *apoptosis* has been applied,[8] intimating the concept of programmed cell destruction as a countermeasure to mitotic cell multiplication.

Transepithelial Elimination

Under a variety of circumstances, nonepidermal elements enter the epidermis from the dermis and are eliminated to the outside (Fig. 5-12). This process of *transepithelial elimination* was discussed in detail by Mehregan.[2] Four subdivisions may be made. The entry of motile cells, such as neutrophils or treponemas, may be called transmigration (exocytosis, p. 69). The entry of nonmotile cells, such as erythrocytes, or of nonirritating particles, such as amyloid or carbon, through a break in the basement membrane leads to their being surrounded by epithelial cells and gradually being moved outward with the stream of keratinocytes until they are incorporated in the horny layer and exfoliated. If the particles are small, no definite disturbance of epidermal architecture will occur. A third type of transepithelial elimination involves larger blocks of material, which may be a foreign body, such as calcium, or may be a devitalized portion of the dermis, such as collagen or elastic fibers or a mass of necrotic tissue, more or less infiltrated with inflammatory cells. These materials press against the epidermis from below and cause damage. Damage may vary from precocious keratinization forming a shell around the foreign body to definite epidermal necrosis and superficial ulceration. Ulceration secondarily induces epidermal repair and hyperplasia and leads to eventual elimination and healing.

Smaller defects of this type appear as intraepidermal channels, as in perforating elastosis or collagenosis, but larger defects, as found in perforating granuloma annulare, merge with the processes of ulceration (Chap. 17), in which considerable portions of epidermis are sloughed off. Where the borderline should be drawn is a matter of definition. A fourth type of transepithelial elimination involves hair follicles, as in perforating folliculitis. Here the follicular epithelium surrounds a mass of necrotized and inflamed dermis and incorporates it into the follicular lumen. This bolus formation is followed by slow elimination to the surface. A similar process was recently described for the necrobiotic material of granuloma annulare.[9]

DERMIS

Basement Membrane

The junction or interface between epithelial and mesodermal structures was discussed in Chapter 2. In routine sections stained either with H&E or O&G, the only plainly visible basement membrane is the *vitreous membrane* of the hair follicle (Figs. 2-26, 2-27, and 2-28). The PAS procedure, on the other hand, shows red lines at the lower border of the epidermis (Fig. 2-14), around the periphery of hair follicles and sweat glands, and also around capillary blood vessels. It should be kept in mind that other substances also take the stain (Chap. 3).

The PAS-positive subepidermal basement membrane may be *thickened* or *reduplicated* in lupus erythematosus and other dermatoses and then becomes visible in H&E sections as a hyaline eosinophilic band. The region of the basement membrane has assumed great significance in immunofluorescent studies because autoantibodies, immune complexes, and other substances may be bound here (Chap. 4). In many inflammatory dermatoses, such as psoriasis, close observation will show small breaks in the basement membrane (Fig. 8-7). Every time a leukocyte crosses from dermis into epidermis, the basement membrane is pierced. Breaks in the basement membrane do not enable epidermal basal cells to invade the dermis; examination of the membrane, however, does have significance in tumor pathology. Benign epithelial tumors and basal cell epitheliomas usually have PAS-positive membranes. Squamous cell carcinomas usually have none, and basement membrane disappears when a precancerous keratosis becomes invasive (Chap. 34).

Pars Papillaris

In descriptive histopathology, *papillae* and *subpapillary layer* should be mentioned separately. Papillae can be absent, short, long, narrow, wide, club-shaped, edematous, or even branching. If they are sufficiently long to elevate the covering (suprapapillary) portion of the epidermis above the general level of the skin surface (Figs. 33-1 and 33-5), the term *papillomatosis* is appropriate. A tumor consisting of such elongated and possibly branching papillae and their epidermal cover is called a *cutaneous papilloma*. A cellular nevus (Fig. 32-21) or other specific tumor may have *papillomatous configuration*.

The condition of the *intrapapillary capillaries* should be mentioned separately, when indicated. They may be tortuous, engorged, or hyalinized or may form tufts. Foreign substances, such as hyalin, amyloid, or melanin, may be present in the papillae.

The subpapillary layer, including the subpapillary precapillary and postcapillary vessels, should then be described. It may be diffusely edematous or show perivascular edema. The latter may be obvious as an empty space around vessels, or if cellular infiltrate is present, it is evident in the spacing or separation of the cells in an empty-appearing area. This feature differentiates the lymphocytic infiltrate of lupus erythematosus (Fig. 14-1) from the closely packed lymphocytic mass of leukemia (Fig. 44-2). Blood vessels may show thin or swollen endothelia, may be wide open, engorged, or ectatic. Their walls may be *hyalinized* or thickened through apposition of outer cell layers. For additional details see Chapter 15.

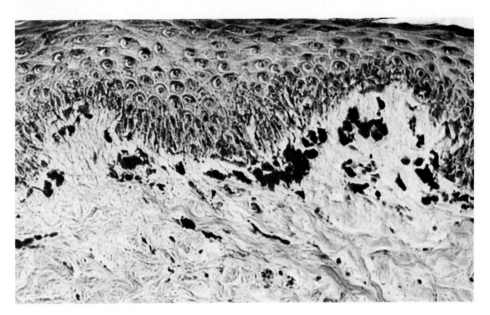

FIGURE 5–13.
Melanophages (macrophages containing clumped melanin) in a case of postinflammatory pigmentation. H&E. X180. (From Sutton. Diseases of the Skin, 11th ed, 1956. Courtesy of Dr. R. L. Sutton, Jr. Contributed by H. Pinkus.)

The usually thin collagen fibrils of the subpapillary layer may be sclerosed, homogeneous, or, on the contrary, separated by edema. Macrophages containing either melanin (*melanophages*, Fig. 5-13) or hemosiderin are found not infrequently. If the presence of melanophages is associated with absence of epidermal pigment, the term *incontinentia pigmenti* may be used.

Red blood cells are fairly commonly seen outside vessels in biopsies of a variety of inflammatory dermatoses, especially in punch biopsy specimens. *Extravasation* may be the result of surgical trauma, especially when vascular walls are weakened by inflammation. Only if erythrocytes are found in various stages of disintegration and possibly associated with hemosiderin is one justified in considering a preexisting *purpuric* condition. Presence of red cells within the epidermis also justifies that assumption. A few small round cells (lymphocytes) and an occasional neutrophilic or eosinophilic leukocyte are of no pathologic significance. Any appreciable number should be evaluated. Neutrophils have a short life span, and their nuclei begin to become *pyknotic* or disintegrate into nuclear dust (Fig. 15-2) after a few days in the tissue (*leukocytoclasia*). In other cases, nuclear dust may be the result of breakdown of lymphocytes or other cells. Mast cells occur normally but are difficult to identify in H&E sections, although O&G sections show them clearly. To judge pathologic increase requires considerable experience. Presence of mast cells in the stroma of benign or malignant epithelial tumors or nevus cell nevi has no diagnostic significance.

Pars Reticularis

The major portion of the dermis, constituted by relatively coarse collagen bundles, thick elastic fibers, and a small number of fibrocytes, is much less frequently involved in cutaneous disease than is the pars papillaris. As a rule, none of the common inflammatory dermatoses, such as eczematous dermatitis, psoriasis, or lichen planus, affects the pars reticularis with more than an extension of lymphocytic infiltrate around smaller vessels. If significant inflammatory infiltrate is present, it may be associated with hair follicles and sweat glands, or it may be diffuse. Its distribution and composition must be noted because the pars reticularis is the common seat of *granulomatous inflammation*. In addition to polymorphonuclear leukocytes, eosinophils, and lymphocytes, we commonly encounter plasma cells and histiocytes in all their various disguises.

Lymphocytes. The term *lymphocyte* has been used rather indiscriminately for many years to identify a small cell with a roundish dark nucleus. One has to realize, however, that any cell, whether fibroblast, histiocyte, or smooth muscle cell, when cut exactly across, will resemble a lymphocyte. Second, pathologists can identify lymphocytes with fair ease if they see a small cell in a lymph node. Identification of such cells in the skin is much more difficult, as new techniques have proved. It is fortunate that enzyme cytochemical and immunologic methods are now available to tell apart not only lymphocytes from monocytes, but T lympho-

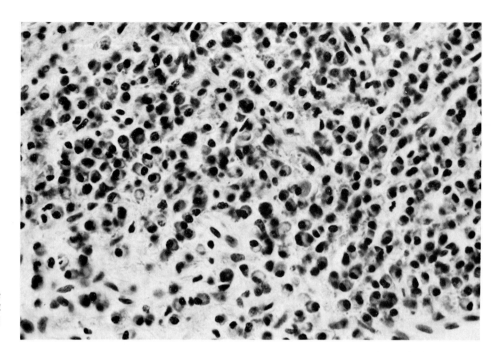

FIGURE 5–14.
Plasma cells in cutaneous plasmacytoma (see Chap. 44 and Figs. 20-11 and 44-1.) H&E. X800.

cytes from B lymphocytes in properly prepared sections of a variety of skin diseases.[10,11] These methods are not yet available for routine use, but their results warn us to use the words *lymphocyte, lymphohistiocytic,* and *lymphoreticular infiltrate* with greater caution. *Small round cell* seems to be a safe circumvention if one is not sure.

Plasma Cells. Plasma cells (Figs. 5-14, 20-11, and 44-1), are derived from B lymphocytes and secrete immunoglobulins. They are easily identified by their larger nucleus, possessing coarse chromatin particles and sitting eccentrically in a round or ovid cell body. The latter is basophilic and is apt to retain hematoxylin unless the sections are thoroughly decolorized. The cytoplasm stains prominently dark blue or grayish blue in O&G sections but does not exhibit granularity or metachromasia, in distinction from mast cells. Usually, there is a lighter staining *paranuclear zone.* Plasma cells undergoing a peculiar type of hyalinization are known as *Russell bodies* (Fig. 5-15).

Histiocytes and Multinucleated Giant Cells. Histiocytes were considered members of Aschoff's reticuloendothelial system, generally benign cells, and the precursors of macrophages (Sec. IV). Modern hematologists have chosen to replace the name "reticulum cell" with *histiocyte* and to point out that many malignant lymphomas are *malignant histiocytomas* rather than "reticulum cell sarco-

mas" (Chap. 44). Early precursor cells are monoblasts in the bone marrow, which develop into *monocytes* in the blood and into mature *tissue macrophages* (another synonym for histiocytes) and into Langerhans cells. In the quiescent state, skin histiocytes are difficult to differentiate from fibroblasts, although their nuclei may be slightly larger, and they have more cytoplasm. It is appropriate to

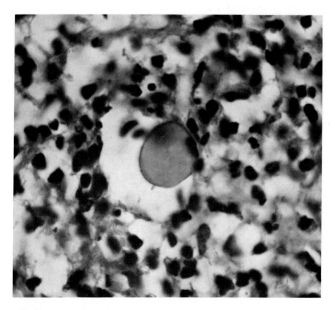

FIGURE 5–15.
Russell body in rhinoscleroma, a granulomatous disease characterized by mixed infiltrate containing many plasma cells. H&E. X800.

say *fixed tissue type cell*, if one cannot identify a cell as either a fibroblast or a histiocyte. When histiocytes contain phagocytized substances, we call them by specific names, such as *melanophages* or *lipophages*. The latter are usually called *foam* cells (Fig. 23-2). Cells containing no visible inclusions in H&E sections may be shown to harbor acid-fast bacilli by special stain. These and other microorganisms are discussed in the chapters on granulomatous inflammation. If histiocytes with large homogeneous cell bodies aggregate closely without intervening connective tissue fibers, they are described as *epithelioid cells*, a term that can be used only in the plural form. Nodular aggregates of epithelioid cells often are called *tubercles* (Figs. 20-1 and 20-13) regardless of etiology.

Multinucleated large histiocytes, which probably originate through fusion of several cells more often than from repeated nuclear division,[12] are known as *multinucleated giant cells*, a term that should be used in its entirety because there also are *mononuclear giant cells* of different significance (Chap. 44). Multinucleated giant cells may be of *Langhans type* (Fig. 5-16A, nuclei form a horseshoe), of *foreign body type* (Fig. 5-16C, nuclei in irregular clusters), or of *Touton type* (Fig. 5-16B, nuclei form a circle between central and peripheral portions of the cytoplasm which usually is foamy). While these variants are most commonly associated with specific disorders (Sec. IV), the association is by no means absolute. Some multinucleated giant cells contain peculiar *asteroid bodies* (Fig. 5-17) which are not pathognomonic for any specific disease. Fragments of elastic fibers and a variety of crystalline and amorphous foreign substances may be enclosed in multinucleated histiocytes.

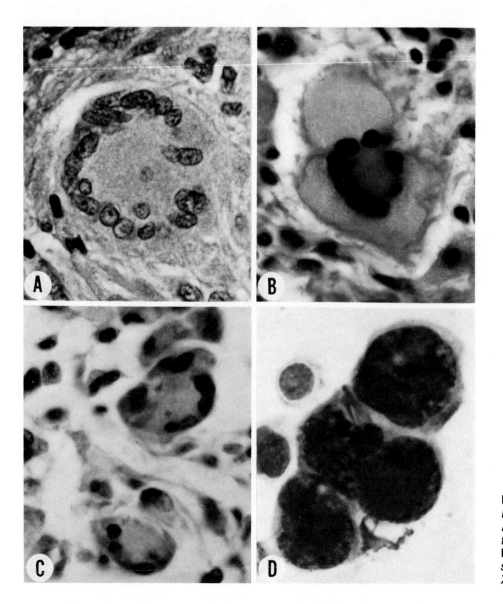

FIGURE 5–16.
Multinucleated giant cells. **A.** *Langhans type.* **B.** *Touton type.* **C.** *Foreign body type.* **D.** *Epidermal cells in Tzanck smear of zoster.* **A, B, C.** *H&E. X800.* **D.** *Giemsa. X800.*

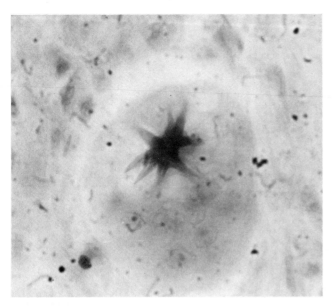

FIGURE 5–17.
Crystalline asteroid body in multinucleated giant cell (nuclei are out of focus). O&G. X1000.

Tumor Cells. Various types of *tumor cells* may occur in the dermis singly or in groups, cords, nests, or masses. They should be described according to their characteristics. The term "sheets of tumor cells" should be avoided because it describes only the two-dimensional appearance of a mass of cells in a thin section.

Noncellular Components. In order to recognize and evaluate structural abnormalities of the noncellular components of the dermis, the student should carefully examine their normal appearance in the many biopsy specimens which exhibit no significant alterations. It is not easy to determine *edema* or *sclerosis* unless one is thoroughly familiar with normal variation and is aware also of the technical fallacies mentioned in Chapter 3. Any marked degree of edema, especially *myxedema* (Fig. 25-9) and *lymphedema* (Fig. 25-8), will not only widen interfascicular spaces but split the collagen bundles into thinner ones or into fibers. The tissue will stain diffusely blue in O&G sections if myxedema is present. Alcian blue will reveal blue-staining fine fibrils.

In the evaluation of elastic fibers, their three-dimensional distribution in the skin must be kept in mind. Short pieces with sharp edges mean that a fiber has been cut transversely (Fig. 5-18) by the microtome knife. *Fragmentation of elastic fibers* (Chap. 26) is very difficult to prove because they weave in and out of the thin section, and the rounded end of a truly fragmented fiber is a rare

sight. Roughness, unevenness along their length, and curling are encountered occasionally and may be significant. The characteristic change of pseudoxanthoma elasticum (Fig. 26-2) is best compared to a heap of *raveled wool thread*, as Zola Cooper used to say. Dissolution into short pieces and granules is found in rare cases of *elastolysis* (Fig. 26-3). The most frequent pathologic change of elastic fibers is their complete absence in localized areas. Inasmuch as elastic fibers are not easily formed anew, their absence often indicates past inflammatory, and especially granulomatous, processes. If new fibers are formed, they usually remain much thinner and are apt to form parallel strands (e.g., striae, Fig. 26-11) or an irregular meshwork (old lesions of lupus erythematosus). Elastic fibers give valuable diagnostic clues in many cases and should be examined routinely (see O&G stain in Chap. 3).

Pathologic changes of blood vessels and nerves are similar to those of other organs. Alterations of hair follicles, sweat glands, and subcutaneous fat tissue will be discussed in their respective chapters.

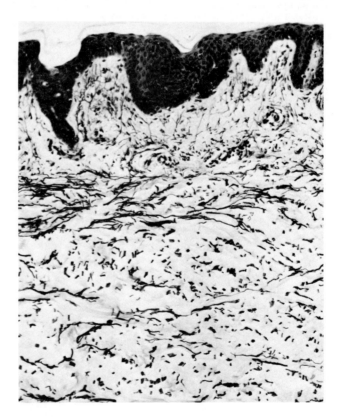

FIGURE 5–18.
Pseudofragmentation of elastic fibers. These are normal elastic fibers cut by microtome knife into fragments of different length owing to their three-dimensional orientation in tissue. Note the difference in thickness and arrangement between the fibers of pars reticularis and pars papillaris (see Fig. 2-17). O&G. X135.

REFERENCES

1. Oberste-Lehn H: Dermoepidermal interface. Arch Dermatol 86:770, 1962
2. Mehregan AH: Transepithelial elimination. In Mali JWH (ed): Current Problems in Dermatology. Basel, S. Karger, 1970, Vol 3, pp 124-147
3. Malak JA, Kurban AK: Catharsis: an excretory function of the epidermis. Br J Dermatol 84:516, 1971
4. Anderson RL, Cassidy JM: Variations in physical dimensions and chemical composition of human stratum corneum. J Invest Dermatol 61:30, 1973
5. Alkiewicz J, Lebioda J, Rokita Z: Über Kolloidkeratose. Dermatol Monatsschr 158:329, 1972
6. Van Scott EJ, Ekel TM: Kinetics of hyperplasia in psoriasis. Arch Dermatol 88:373, 1963
7. Findlay GH, Whiting DA: Universal dyschromatosis. Br J Dermatol 85 [Suppl 7] 66, 1971
8. Kerr JFR, Wullie AH, Currie AR: Apoptosis: a biological phenomenon with wide-ranging implications in tissue kinetics. Br J Cancer 26:239, 1972
9. Bardach HG: Granuloma annulare with transfollicular perforation. J Cutan Pathol 4:99, 1977
10. Burg G, Braun-Falco O: Cutaneous non-Hodgkin lymphoma: re-evaluation of histology using enzyme cytochemical and immunologic studies. Int J Dermatol 17:496, 1978
11. Souteyraud P, Thivolet J, Alaria A, Schmitt D, Parrott H: Étude immunocytologique des lymphomas cutanés malins. Essai de classification. Dermatologica 157:269, 1978
12. Black MM, Epstein WL: Formation of multinucleate giant cells in organized epithelioid cell granulomas. Am J Pathol 74:263, 1974

CHAPTER

6

Systematics of Histopathologic Interpretation

In the preceding chapter, a systematic course of description of a skin section was outlined. In order to make a diagnosis from this morphologic analysis, one should also follow a systematic course of mental analysis. Some diagnoses are so obvious that a short glance through the low-power lens is sufficient. However, one should never be satisfied with a snap diagnosis because closer examination may show features that modify or reverse the first impression. It is human nature that a first opinion gives a bias to the mind, and the beginner is apt to search out features favorable to his opinion and to overlook unfavorable ones. Therefore, it is highly recommended in any case, after arriving at a diagnosis, to ask two searching questions: What else could it be? What speaks against my diagnosis? One should act as the devil's advocate to one's own interpretation. Moreover, the dermatopathologist has no right to make a diagnosis of *nonspecific* dermatitis or inflammation. Every biopsy specimen is a sample of some specific process, but the visible changes may be *noncharacteristic* and may not permit a diagnosis. Similarly, if one is dealing with granulomatous inflammation, the expression *of undetermined etiology* should be used instead of "nonspecific."

TECHNIQUE

For an ideal interpretation, there are two prerequisites. The section should include all of the skin and some of the subcutaneous tissue, and it should be large enough to show all spaced skin structures, such as hair complexes and sweat glands. Even then, one should examine multiple, and preferably serial, sections in order to be sure that the features of the first section are characteristic of the entire biopsy specimen. With the commonly encountered 4-mm punch, examination of at least 30 serial sections is highly desirable. Only a few of these may include a follicle or a sweat gland or may show the most characteristic alterations, especially the center of the clinical lesion. A 2-mm punch (never an ideal specimen) should be sectioned practically from end to end, and of a 6-mm punch or larger excisional biopsy, enough sections should be prepared to insure a representative sample. This can be made easier by dividing the specimen as outlined in Chapter 3.

One should always look at the slide first with the naked eye to see how large the sections are and whether there are perhaps sections of several tissue fragments. If the sections are large, one may want to examine them by using the inverted eyepiece of the microscope as a magnifying glass. The next step must be scanning of the sections under low power. Beginners should be instructed that they may go to high power if their attention is attracted by a detail that they cannot identify with the scanning lens, but that they should quickly revert to the low magnification until they have scanned all the sections on the slide, preferably all the slides available, and certainly all the stains—in our laboratory, routinely H&E and O&G.

CATEGORIZING

Once we have satisfied ourselves that we have seen everything the clinician was good enough to provide, it is best to decide first into which of the major categories of disease the lesion belongs, then to subcategorize until a specific diagnosis is decided upon.

Thus, we try to decide first whether the section represents a tumor or an inflammatory process or neither and whether the epidermis or the dermis is involved mainly. Sometimes, this decision cannot be made immediately, or it may have to be reversed later, but in most cases it is fairly easy and permits one to concentrate on only one major portion of the pathologic field. Tumors and certain metabolic or degenerative diseases then are categorized according to rules given in later chapters.

Inflammatory lesions often can be assigned without too much difficulty to one of two subgroups. Involvement of only the papillary part of the dermis speaks for nongranulomatous processes, while granulomatous inflammation practically always involves also the pars reticularis. Exceptions, such as lupus erythematosus, a nongranulomatous disease involving most of the dermis, and lichen nitidus, a granuloma involving papillae only, are recognized just because of their exceptional features. It is always much easier to ascertain the seat of an inflammatory or neoplastic process by looking for the differential characteristics of superficial and deep elastic fibers in O&G sections. This is one of the most valuable features of the routine use of this stain. Specific instances will be found in several chapters.

A special point for consideration is the involvement of hair follicles in inflammatory disease. Not infrequently, examination of the first section and even of several sections presents a puzzling picture until a subsequent section reveals a follicle in the center of the lesion. The same is true, though much less frequently, for sweat glands. Involvement of larger blood vessels, on the other hand, is

sometimes overlooked because their structure may be so altered as to be almost unrecognizable (Fig. 15-4A) in H&E sections. Here, O&G stain (Fig. 15-4B) not only is apt to show remnants of the elastic coat but usually permits identification of vein or artery by the specific arrangement of the fibers.

Lesions that are neither inflammatory nor neoplastic but consist of specific alteration of connective tissue fibers or deposits of unusual substances, such as mucin and amyloid, require a high level of suspicion in many cases. Here again, except in the case of calcification, the O&G stain usually is more revealing than the H&E, but special procedures may be called for.

Anybody who teaches students and residents will have the experience that the diagnosis of epithelial tumors is easiest, that of mesodermal tumors and specific granulomatous lesions next in line. The greatest difficulty is encountered in the field of simple inflammation, and this, unfortunately, includes the greatest number of all skin lesions encountered in clinical practice and roughly half of the specimens submitted for histologic diagnosis. Even the expert often is stumped and frequently can do no better than to favor one diagnosis over one or several others. If it seems impossible to arrive at a positive diagnosis, it is often helpful to use the negative approach and to rule out all the dermatoses one feels could not be represented by the specimen. By doing so, one can often narrow the diagnosis down to a reasonable choice or even to a single possibility. In this connection, it must be stressed that in the interpretation of tissue reactions, and even of tumors, we are laying down rules, not laws. In the chapters that follow, the words "usually," "often," and "rarely" will be found only too frequently, and we assure the reader that we eliminated them in many places in order not to appear too indecisive. The beginner may be led astray by putting too much stress on a conspicuous but insignificant feature; the pundit may know so many exceptions that his willingness to make a definite diagnosis sags. It is the task of the successful diagnostician to thread his way between the two extremes.[1]

CLINICOPATHOLOGIC COORDINATION

Because a simple report of subacute or chronic dermatitis is of no value to the practicing skin specialist, the dermatopathologist must be familiar with clinical dermatology as well, and he must insist on the clinician's cooperation in submitting sufficient information and a clinical or differential diagnosis. Practitioners who believe that the pathologist should arrive at a diagnosis objectively and not be influenced by clinical data or opinions should realize that the pathologist cannot give the best service to either physician or patient unless he knows the entire story. We gently remind the clinician that we are just as happy to disprove his diagnosis as to support it. The attitude of not a few practitioners, who neglect to supply even such basic facts as the patient's age, sex, or shade of skin, is deplorable.

Clinical information should include the physician's and the patient's name for identification. Sex and age are essential in judging the general characteristics of the skin specimen and sometimes are helpful in diagnostic deliberations. The question for color or shade of skin is not discriminatory when a cutaneous biopsy must be examined. Details, such as blond, brunet, olive, Oriental, light or dark Negro, and American Indian, are much more helpful than white, Caucasian, colored, or black in judging whether the amount of pigment in the section is normal or abnormal for the individual. The exact anatomic site of biopsy is highly important in view of the great topical differences encountered in the skin (Chap. 2). A simple sketch is helpful.

A concise clinical history is of inestimable value for the pathologist in throwing out completely inapplicable diagnoses or explaining unusual features. The same is even more true of a clinical description of the eruption. Finally, there should be a clinical diagnosis or a list of differential diagnoses. By comparing the clinician's list with his own, the pathologist may be able to rule out certain diagnoses, to favor others, and perhaps to come up with a single one that fits clinical and pathologic data alike. Cooperation between clinician and pathologist is more important in the field of skin disease than in almost any other field if the patient is to derive the greatest benefit from the biopsy.

Some time ago, an attempt was made to give a broad presentation of dermatohistopathology under the aspect of cooperation between clinician and pathologist. A number of dermatopathologists were asked to discuss a particular field under the heading: How useful is a biopsy in this particular field of disease? The outcome was presented in two special issues of the journal *Cutis* on dermatopathology.[2,3]

Figure 6-1 should help students in their differ-

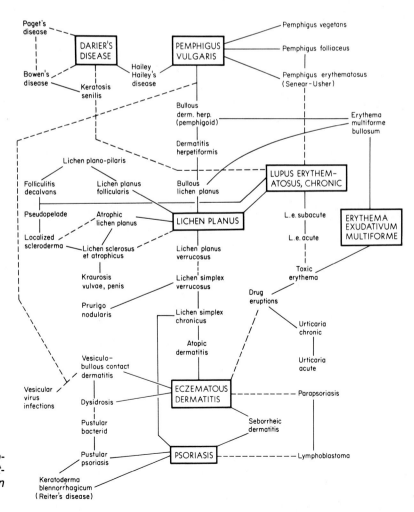

FIGURE 6–1.
Diagrammatic representation of histomorphologic similarities of tissue reaction and resulting differential diagnostic considerations in inflammatory skin diseases.

ential diagnostic deliberations. It lists the most common types of tissue reaction as centers of gravity or foci of crystallization, e.g., eczematous dermatitis and psoriasis. Other diagnoses are arranged in between according to the degree of morphologic similarity in tissue sections. Nosologic relations are not necessarily implied. Solid lines indicate common differential problems, dashed lines uncommon ones. While the diagram may seem confusing at first, we hope its study will help the student to be aware of diagnostic possibilities. One example is the morphologic row from eczematous dermatitis to lichen planus. Chronic dermatitis with lichenification resembles lichen simplex chronicus, and this, in turn, resembles verrucous lichen planus.

REFERENCES

1. Pinkus H: Four-dimensional histopathology. Arch Dermatol 82:681, 1960
2. Pinkus H (ed): Special issue: Dermatopathology, Part I. Cutis 20 (5), 1977
3. Pinkus H (ed): Special issue: Dermatopathology, Part II. Cutis 21 (2), 1978

SECTION

II

SUPERFICIAL INFLAMMATORY PROCESSES

Superficial as well as *inflammatory* are used here in a very wide sense. We include lesions which histologically have their seat predominantly in the pars papillaris of the dermis, with or without involvement of the epidermis, and which are not neoplastic or obviously granulomatous. Inasmuch as the word *dermatitis* means inflammation of skin, we do not use it as a specific diagnostic term but always add a modifying adjective, such as *eczematous* or *seborrheic*. We exclude from this section lesions in which the pathognomonic disturbance is alteration of the noncellular components of the dermis or deposition of metabolic products, such as amyloid or calcium.

We deal, therefore, with the most common dermatoses, such as eczematous dermatitis, psoriasis, lichen planus, drug eruptions, and the so-called papulosquamous lesions. Many of these are caused by known external or internal agents to which the skin reacts. In others, the cause is unknown, but we can conceive of them as reactions to injury, as will be pointed out in the individual discussions. Reaction to injury is the most basic definition of inflammation[1] and gives us the courage to include all these dermatoses under one heading. Reaction to injury also is the common denominator under

which we can try to analyze the colorful variety of lesions that we encounter in this group. The concept of reaction to injury explains why the skin may respond to a great variety of agents with identical or similar alterations. Great as its repertoire is, the skin has a limited number of expressions. Erythema exudativum multiforme may be the response to a dozen or more different agents and contact-type eczematous dermatitis to thousands of sensitizing externa.

The histopathologist, therefore, deals with the expression of tissue reaction, and in each individual biopsy section we deal with one fixed moment of the reaction, one that the clinician chooses more or less judiciously from several or many lesions in various stages of development. Our ability to diagnose a disease from the tissue reaction depends on interpretation and is influenced by our knowledge of clinical dermatology, our concept of the disease in question, and our individual experience with the limits of variability of the disease. The pathologist and the submitting clinician must be aware that the report rendered includes interpretation. In our laboratory we sum up our findings, not under the heading of "microscopic diagnosis" but as "conclusions," and we are not ashamed if occasionally we have to revise our conclusions on the basis of fol-low-up information.

The following chapters, then, will bear such headings as "eczematous reactions," and "psoriasi-form reactions," rather than the names of individual diseases.

REFERENCE

1. Forbus WD: Reaction to Injury. Pathology for Students of Disease Based on the Functional and Morphological Responses of Tissues to Injurious Agents. 2 vols. Baltimore, Williams & Wilkins, 1943, 1952.

CHAPTER
7

Eczematous Tissue Reactions

Under this heading are included lesions encountered in all types of contact dermatitis, in atopic dermatitis, lichen simplex chronicus, and dyshidrosiform dermatitis. Exfoliative dermatitis and prurigo will be considered. Seborrheic dermatitis, asteatotic dermatitis, and the related nummular eczema will be discussed in the differential diagnosis of psoriasiform tissue reactions (Chap. 8). Stasis dermatitis will be considered under the heading of vasculitides (Chap. 15) and photosensitivity reactions in the differential diagnosis of lupus erythematosus (Chap. 14). Eczematous tissue reactions are also encountered in some of the papulosquamous diseases discussed in Chapter 13.

"Eczema" is an old word which has been used in the clinic with so many meanings that it has become practically meaningless. *Eczematous tissue reaction*, however, has a well-defined connotation: It is the epidermal reaction to injurious agents encountered typically in contact dermatitis due to sensitization. The dermal reaction is secondary and rather noncharacteristic, except that it involves the blood vessels of the superficial plexus, as do many other dermatoses. The typical epidermal change involves four principal features: intercellular edema, acanthosis, parakeratosis, and exocytosis, all present in a focal, spotty distribution. From these changes are derived others, such as vesiculation and lichenification, but an occasional throwback to the four cardinal features identifies a lesion as *eczematous tissue reaction*. To eliminate this term from our nomenclature deprives us of a useful unifying concept.

CONTACT DERMATITIS

Primary Irritant Type

Contact dermatitis is commonly divided into *primary irritant* and *sensitization dermatitis*. When a primary irritant is not strong enough to cause necrosis, it is apt to produce more damage to superficial living cells than to deeper structures. The reaction to the injury will consist of exudation of fluid and polymorphonuclear cells from the blood capillaries into the epidermis, which becomes edematous and may show cell degeneration. Figure 7-1 illustrates the site of a patch test 48 hours after application of a primary irritant. Horny and granular layers show no or minor morphologic alterations because cell bodies and intercellular connections are quite rigid in these strata. Electron microscopic examination is needed to reveal changes.[1] The upper strata of prickle cells are separated by spongiotic edema and inflammatory cells, with the production of an intraepidermal vesicle. There is a degree of acanthosis, suggesting that mitotic proliferation has started to replace the damaged upper layers. There is some edema of the papillae, and leukocytes are emerging from the dilated capillaries. Mild lymphocytic infiltrate is present in the papillar layer.

Epidermal Regeneration. In primary irritant dermatitis, the outpouring of fluid and scavenger cells is due to the presence of chemically damaged epithelium, but the basic repair mechanism of the

87

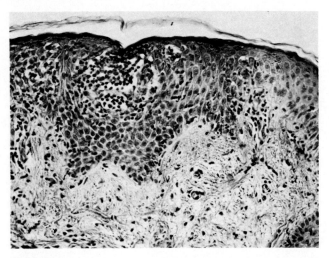

FIGURE 7–1.
Primary irritant type of contact dermatitis. Patch test with sodium lauryl sulfate after 48 hours. H&E. X135.

epidermis is similar when we remove the horny layer by tape stripping,[2] thus exposing the prickle cells to dehydration. In this case, edema and exudate remain minimal, and the regenerative sequence is more clearly seen (Fig. 7-2A to F). One-half hour after stripping, the uppermost cells look parakeratotic as they begin to dry out. Most of the prickle cells eventually are involved in this process, while the basal cells become very large. Their

edematous appearance is due to accumulation of glycogen. After 36 to 48 hours, a great burst of mitotic activity develops in the basal layer and replaces, within a few days, the cells lost through stripping and dehydration. A new and usually hyperplastic granular layer is formed, followed by maturation of a new horny layer. Most of the original epidermis is exfoliated as a parakeratotic scale.

Pictures of this type are occasionally encountered in biopsy sections and can be interpreted as accelerated epidermal regeneration if one is familiar with them. In contact dermatitis and other inflammations, the picture is variously modified, but the basic process persists. Old and damaged material is eliminated toward the surface and is replaced, often in excess, by mitotic division of germinal cells at the base of the epidermis. Awareness of this process makes it possible to interpret fixed sections in terms of temporal sequence.

Sensitization Dermatitis

If contact dermatitis is due to a substance to which the skin was sensitized previously, the picture (Fig. 7-3 A to D) differs from the primary irritant type. Experimentation and electron microscopy[3–5] have shown that epidermal Langerhans cells recognize and bind contact allergens and probably carry them

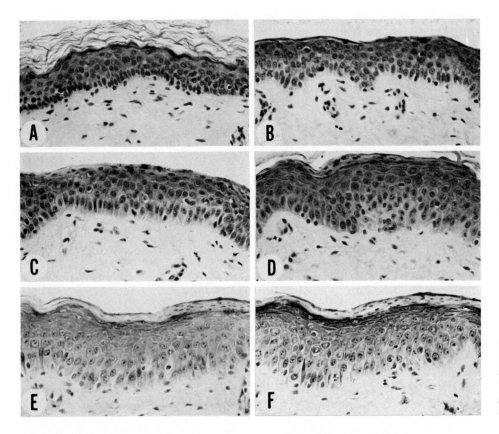

FIGURE 7–2.
Epidermal response to tape stripping. **A.** *Control.* **B.** *After 12 hours.* **C.** *After 24 hours.* **D.** *After 36 hours.* **E** *and* **F.** *After 48 hours. H&E. X205.*

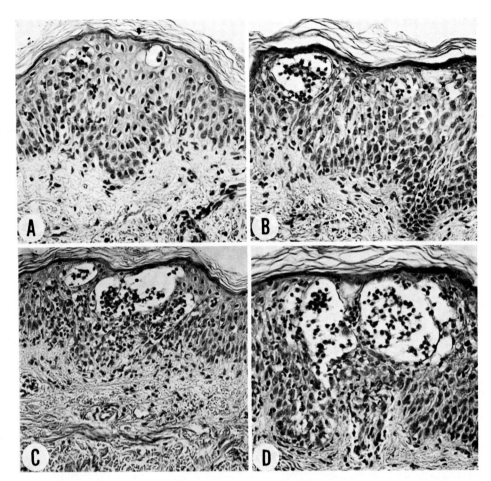

FIGURE 7–3.
Sensitization-type contact dermatitis. Figures represent several fields from a 48-hour patch test reaction to 5 percent nickel sulfate solution. Compare with Figure 7-7, showing dermal sensitivity reaction to nickel sulfate in another patient. Some vesicles contain mainly degenerating epithelial cells. Such pictures should not be confused with Pautrier abscesses of mycosis fungoides (Fig. 44-5B). H&E. X128.

to lymph nodes. On subsequent exposure to the allergen, sensitized lymphocytes enter the epidermis from below and cause the eczematous reaction. Therefore, edema and cell damage are found early in the lower prickle cell layers. The upper layers are involved by extension and because the damaged cells are carried quickly toward the outside. Simultaneously, the epidermis will react with excessive regeneration, and acanthosis and accentuation of rete ridges result. Unless the damaging contact is a fleeting one, new cells will sustain damage, and the process of edema, spongiosis, and vesiculation will be found in different stages of development and varying degrees of severity throughout the epidermis.

The cardinal epidermal features of sensitization-type contact dermatitis are (1) edema, which is mainly intercellular and may lead to spongiosis and vesiculation, (2) acanthosis, (3) parakeratosis, and (4) exocytosis, including lymphocytes and polymorphonuclear cells. A highly important fifth feature is the focal, spotty character of all these changes, in horizontal and vertical direction. As one scans a section from end to end, one encounters relatively normal portions interspersed with areas of spongiosis and intraepidermal vesiculation. Different

ages of such changes can be inferred from their vertical distribution. Dermal changes are edema and cellular infiltrate in papillae and subpapillary layer. Lymphocytes predominate; eosinophils may be few or fairly numerous; neutrophils are absent except inside dilated blood vessels. Closer examination reveals degranulation of mast cells and basophils as an essential early change.[6]

Acute Contact Dermatitis

Figure 7-4 illustrates a case of acute contact dermatitis due to a drawing ointment applied to the skin near the knee four days previously. The onset of dermatitis within 24 hours and the character of the response are evidence of previous sensitization. The focal distribution of the cardinal features is well shown. It is interesting to note that the original thick horny layer of the knee is present intact above the inflamed epidermis. This fact provides objective evidence that the dermatitis can be only a few days old. The malpighian layer is about 10 times thicker than normal, not only through edema and vesiculation but through an actual increase in

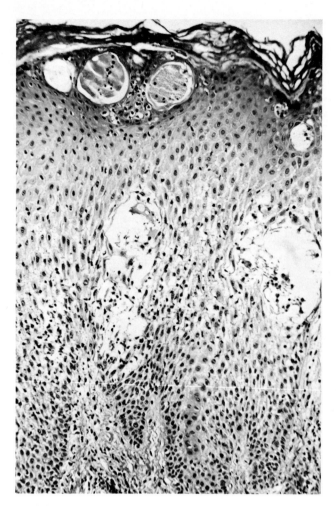

FIGURE 7–4.
Acute sensitization-type contact dermatitis, 4 days after application of a drawing ointment to skin near knee. H&E. X135.

stratum corneum is lost, and the surface is covered by parakeratotic scale or scale-crust. The granular layer disappears quickly but may return just as quickly in subsiding areas. This feature adds to the impression of spottiness. Because focal conditions may change repeatedly, parakeratosis may be underlaid by a new granular layer, and orthokeratotic lamellae may alternate with parakeratotic material.

Interesting modifications are introduced when the dermatitis is due to spicules that have mechanically irritating as well as sensitizing properties. Mineral wool,[7] fiberglass, possibly coated with epoxy resins,[8] and the hairs of caterpillars containing a sensitizing substance[9] are examples. Both the epidermal damage and the dermal response may be modified.

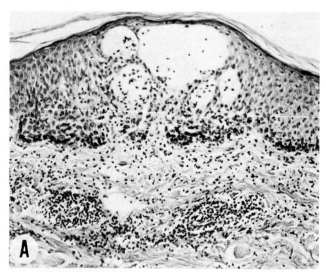

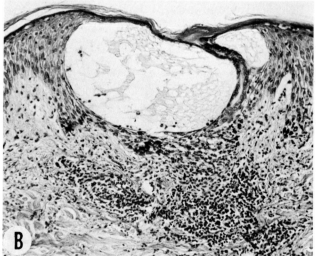

FIGURE 7–5.
*Acute vesicular contact dermatitis without much acanthosis. **B.** Note sweat duct winding its way between vesicles. H&E. X185.*

the number of cells. It is truly acanthotic, and mitotic division of basal cells could be demonstrated in the sections but is not illustrated in the photomicrograph. The vesicles in the higher layers are smaller and contain dense basophilic material. This indicates that they are beginning to dry up and are older and have moved up from deeper layers. In contrast to the impressive epidermal changes, those of the dermis are mild and noncharacteristic.

The combination of the four cardinal features varies with duration and severity of the dermatitis. The fifth feature, spottiness, is always evident. In a mild case of acute dermatitis, there may be vesiculation and relatively little acanthosis, as illustrated in Figure 7-5. In more prolonged cases, acanthosis becomes more prominent, but the epidermis may not be as thick because there is less edema. After the first few days, any trace of the normal

Chronic Contact Dermatitis

In chronic contact dermatitis (Fig. 7-6), vesiculation often is completely absent, and evidence of intercellular edema may be scant. Even parakeratosis and loss of granular layer may be minor. Acanthosis is the outstanding feature. The picture then is that of lichenification and merges with that of lichenification originating from other causes. Minor differences will be discussed under atopic dermatitis, lichen simplex circumscriptus, and psoriasis.

Histologic examination makes it evident that the clinical thickening and stiffness of the skin in lichenification are due mainly to acanthosis and hyperkeratosis. The characteristic coarse folds are due to the uneven size and shape of rete ridges and a degree of papillomatosis. Inflammatory infiltrate may be minor and restricted to the periphery of small subpapillary vessels. The latter usually show no appreciable thickening of their walls, a feature often found in lichenified atopic dermatitis and circumscribed lichen simplex.

The histologic features of contact dermatitis are best studied in biopsy specimens obtained from clear-cut cases. In everyday diagnostic work, they may not be so convincing because the picture may have been modified by topical applications, by scratching, or by systemic steroid treatment. Combination of atopic dermatitis with acute medica-mentous contact dermatitis, or chronic contact dermatitis lichenified by scratching may puzzle the most astute observer. An outstanding example is diaper dermatitis.[10]

One should remember that histologic pictures closely resembling the eczematous tissue reaction can be caused by infectious organisms, ranging from diphtheria bacilli[11] to dermatophytes (Chap. 13), if they remain in the surface layers of the skin. Unrelated papulosquamous eruptions, especially pityriasis rosea (Chap. 13), and seborrheic dermatitis (Chap. 8) also may mimic eczematous dermatitis.

Dermal Contact Sensitivity Reaction

The situation becomes even more complicated by the introduction of the concept of the dermal type of contact sensitivity reaction. These cases[12,13] are often caused by nickel or neomycin but possibly by many other substances. The clinical picture may imitate atopic dermatitis. Histologically (Fig. 7-7), epidermal changes may be minor[14] and, if present, are restricted to acanthosis with some parakeratosis. Infiltrate in the dermis is prominent, usually perivascular, often nodular, and frequently not restricted to the pars papillaris. There usually is a mixture of lymphocytes, plasma cells, and eosinophils. Fixed-tissue-type cells or larger mononuclear

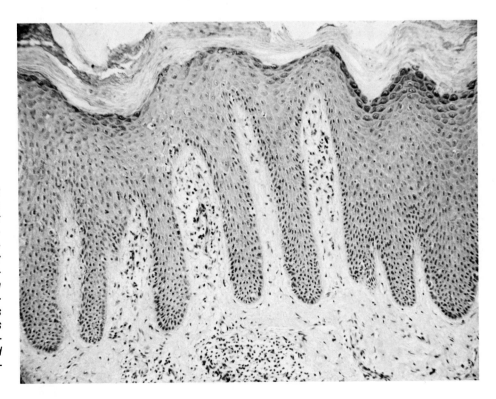

FIGURE 7–6.
Lichenified chronic contact dermatitis. Rete ridges even and long as in psoriasis, but suprapapillary thick and without Munro abscesses. Granular layer almost intact, partly thickened. Only minor indication of intercellular edema in left half of picture. Some parakeratosis indicates earlier loss of granular layer. No excess mitotic activity. Mild inflammatory infiltrate in papilla and subpapillary layer. No exocytosis. H&E. X135.

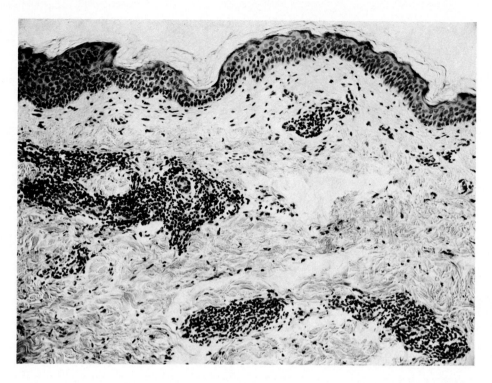

FIGURE 7–7.
Dermal contact sensitivity reaction. Patch test with nickel sulfate after 48 hours in a nickel-sensitive patient. Compare with Figure 7-3, which represents epidermal response to nickel sulfate in another patient. H&E. X135.

round cells may contribute aspects of a granulomatous, or even lymphomatous, infiltrate. This impression is enhanced by immigration of mononuclear cells into the epidermis. The dermal type of contact sensitivity reaction can be a stumbling block to clinician and pathologist alike. It should always be considered in the differential diagnosis of chronic itching dermatoses, in which the suspicion of mycosis fungoides arises.[15] Photosensitivity dermatitis also may produce the picture of dermal sensitivity reaction (Chap. 14).

DYSHIDROSIFORM DERMATITIS

The term *dyshidrosiform* is chosen because there is no histologic involvement of sweat ducts in the lesions usually diagnosed as dyshidrosis or pompholyx by clinicians. Pathologic changes of sweat ducts are readily demonstrable in miliaria (Chap. 19), but the sweat ducts thread their way between the vesicles of dyshidrosiform dermatitis. This type of tissue reaction (Fig. 7-8) is simple vesicular eczematous dermatitis modified by the terrain of thick

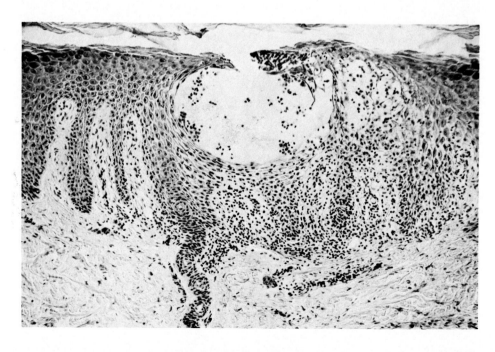

FIGURE 7–8.
Dyshidrosiform type of eczematous dermatitis. This specimen was obtained from acral skin with relatively thin horny layer. Note sweat duct not involved in vesiculation. H&E. X135.

epidermis covered by a thick, horny layer. Spongiotic vesicles forming in the normally bulky rete of palms and soles (Fig. 2-1C) have room to grow and are prevented from rupturing by the physiologic hyperkeratosis of these regions. Differential diagnosis of other vesiculopustular lesions of palms and soles is discussed in Chapter 8 (Fig. 8-13).

ATOPIC DERMATITIS

Pure atopic dermatitis (Fig. 7-9), if this exists (the effects of scratching are practically always evident), either in infants or older children, rarely presents vesicles or even much intercellular edema but has acanthosis, parakeratosis, and some exocytosis. Acanthosis usually is quite even, the epidermal cells are relatively small, and mitoses are significantly increased[16] and are present in suprabasal layers. In older cases, the pictures resemble that of chronic lichenification. One outstanding feature of atopic skin is a peculiar prominence of the walls of small subpapillary vessels.[17] It is due to endothelial thickening and apposition of a few peripheral cells, nothing very definite but recognizable if one pays attention to it. It is an expression of the factor of vascular reaction (Chap. 10). The quantity of inflammatory infiltrate varies according to the activity of the process at the time of biopsy. The cells are lymphocytes and histiocytes: eosinophils may or may not be present, and mast cells are increased in number.

Atopic dermatitis, because of its chronicity, often leads to a loss of superficial elastic fibers and later to some increase of collagen and to fibrosis. An elastic fiber stain, therefore, is helpful. The rather characteristic histologic features of excoriation (Chap. 3, Fig. 3-2) are frequently present in all types of eczematous tissue reaction, but especially in atopic dermatitis and lichenification; one must learn to recognize them.

EXFOLIATIVE DERMATITIS

Exfoliative dermatitis is a clinical term applied to generalized involvement of the skin with erythema, swelling, and diffuse copious scaling. The presence of exfoliating scales differentiates this dermatosis from certain forms of universal erythroderma (Chap. 44), although the two terms are sometimes used interchangeably. The histopathologist must try to determine whether the clinical picture has developed as the most severe manifestation of eczematous dermatitis, psoriasis, or drug sensitivity reaction or whether it represents cutaneous lymphoma. Rarer disorders, such as pityriasis rubra pilaris (Chap. 18) and ichthyosiform erythroderma (Chap. 29), also may come into differential diagnosis. It is usually not too difficult to come to a conclusion on the basis of careful histologic examination if the differential features mentioned in this and the other pertinent chapters are taken into consideration.

PRURIGO

Prurigo is one of the old dermatologic terms that were attached to various diseases by different authors. Thus *prurigo Besnier* is considered a synonym for atopic dermatitis. *Prurigo ferox* and *prurigo hiemalis* are obsolete; the latter probably is synonymous with asteatotic dermatitis. *Prurigo nodularis* will be discussed on pages 95 to 96. That leaves *prurigo simplex*, a clinical diagnosis made rarely by some and more frequently by others in patients who have ill-defined and very pruritic papular lesions with a great deal of excoriation.[18] The histopathologist usually is requested to rule out dermatitis herpetiformis, chronic eczematous dermatitis, and papular urticaria. Histologic conclusions often are vitiated by evidence of severe excoriation (Chap. 3). Typical features of dermatitis

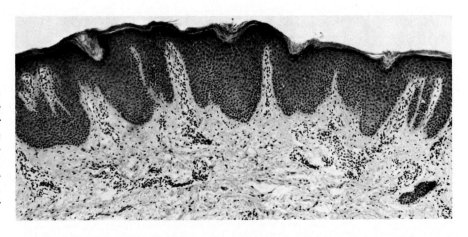

FIGURE 7–9.
Atopic dermatitis (flexural eczema) in a child, which did not present clinical evidence of excoriation or irritation. Note relatively small size of prickle cells in the absence of intracellular and intercellular edema. Uneven ridges and thick suprapapillary plate differ from psoriasis. H&E. X90. (From Pinkus. Ann Allergy 12:671, 1954.)

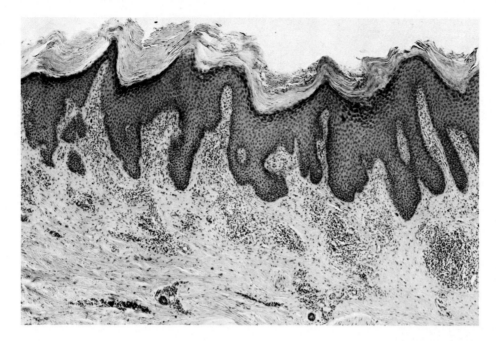

FIGURE 7–10.
Lichen simplex chronicus circumscriptus. Note mild papillomatosis, uneven rete ridges, and papillae, hypergranulosis, and hyperkeratosis with only small foci of parakeratosis. Dermal infiltrate concentrated around small blood vessels, the lumina and walls of which are recognizable at this relatively low magnification. H&E. X75.

herpetiformis (Chap. 11) settle the diagnosis, but their absence does not rule out that protean disease. In order to support a diagnosis of prurigo simplex, one looks for eczematous changes in the epidermis but does not expect vesiculation. Differentiation from an excoriated lesion of papular urticaria (Chap. 10) is virtually impossible. Thus, the histologic analysis of prurigo simplex is highly unsatisfactory and cannot furnish more than a rather lame statement that histologic features are compatible with the clinical diagnosis but do not rule out the other diseases mentioned.

LICHEN SIMPLEX CHRONICUS

Contact dermatitis as well as atopic dermatitis may lead to lichenification. Being concerned with tissue reactions, we need not discuss the controversial subject of neurodermatitis beyond stating that chronic itching leads to chronic scratching and rubbing and that the histologic picture reflects the effects. The purest example of this type of tissue reaction is represented by solid plaques of circumscribed lichen simplex chronicus (Fig. 7-10) as they are found in the ulnar and tibial regions and the nape of the neck. Its chief components are epidermal hyperplasia, fibrosis of superficial dermis, and thickening of the walls of small blood vessels. Inflammatory infiltrate usually is minor and may be absent.

Epidermal hyperplasia of the type to be described now should not be called psoriasiform. It is, to the

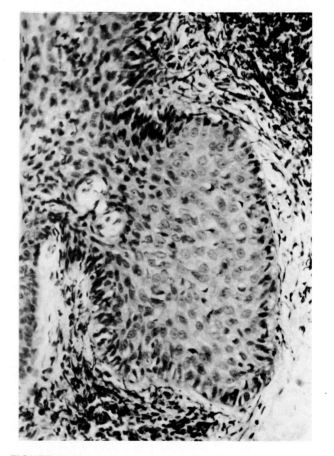

FIGURE 7–11.
Chronic alarm reaction of sebaceous gland, which is transformed into a solid epithelial mass with only a few lipidized cells near the junction with the hair follicle. Heavy inflammatory infiltrate. H&E. X220. (From Mehregan. J Am Acad Dermatol 1:56, 1979.)

contrary, to be distinguished from psoriasiform reactions as described in the next chapter. It is characterized by acanthosis, hypergranulosis, and orthokeratotic hyperkeratosis and may be considered the attainment of a new level of homeostasis in the chronically stimulated epidermis. In experiments with tritium-labeled thymidine, Marks and Wells[19] found that the labeling index measuring cells in the DNA-synthesizing phase is at least as high as in psoriasis (Chap. 8) but that the life span of cells, measured by their transit time through the stratum spinosum, is much longer. They explain this, in part, by the greater mass of the epidermis and, in part, by the fact that some of the labeled cells in the higher strata probably are Langerhans cells and not keratinocytes. The suprapapillary plate in lichen simplex is indeed thick in contrast to psoriasis, and the rete ridges are long and massive but uneven in size (Figs. 5-3 and 7-10). The epidermal surface often shows minor degrees of papillomatosis due to elongation of dermal papillae. Ordinarily, edema, hypogranulosis, and parakeratosis are absent. Their focal presence signifies activity of the underlying eczematous process or response to acute injury by excoriation or infection. In all these respects the lichenified epidermis is quite distinct from psoriatic epidermis, with its evenly long rete ridges, thin suprapapillary plate, and elongated papillae with dilated capillaries. Papillae and subpapillary layers contain vessels that appear rigid and thick walled through apposition of cells and fibers. The pars papillaris may show generalized fibrosis and loss of elastic fibers as the result of many bouts of inflammatory and mechanical injury and repair. Sebaceous glands may be transformed into solid epidermoid plugs (chronic alarm reaction, Chap. 2) (Figs. 7-11 and 7-12), and this feature often adds to the faulty impression of pseudoepitheliomatous downgrowth of epidermis.

PICKER'S NODULE AND PRURIGO NODULARIS

All these features are exaggerated in lesions diagnosed as *giant lichenification* and *Picker's nodule*[20] (Fig. 7-13). Also in this group is *prurigo nodularis*. Authors vary in drawing the limits of this diagnosis. Multiple circumscribed nodular lesions of the lichen simplex chronicus type are relatively frequent in black patients. We prefer to diagnose these cases as *hypertrophic* or *verrucous lichen simplex* and reserve the diagnosis of prurigo nodularis to rare cases in which a definite hyperplasia of cutaneous nerves can be demonstrated. Ordinarily, one cannot recognize nerves in H&E sections above the

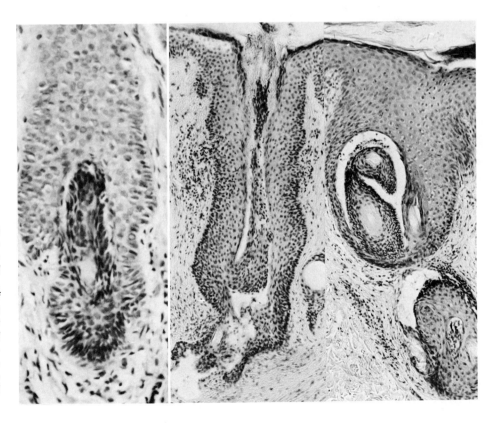

FIGURE 7–12.
Alarm reaction of hair follicles and sebaceous glands in lichen simplex chronicus. Reduction in size, premature and displaced keratinization of hair, absence of lipidization of glands, and extrusion of parts of follicular contents. Relatively mild inflammatory infiltrate and partial devitalization of epidermis point to effects of excoriation. H&E. X125. (From Mehregan. J Am Acad Dermatol 1:56, 1979.)

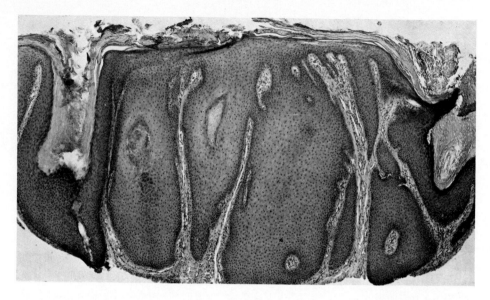

FIGURE 7–13.
Hypertrophic lichen simplex chronicus (Picker's nodule). Some of the massive epithelial structures are rete ridges, others are hyperplastic walls of hair follicles and possibly sweat ducts. Note fibrosis and vascularity of stroma. H&E. X41. (From Mehregan. Dermatol Digest 4:55, 1965.)

mid-dermis. In true prurigo nodularis, however, sizable nerve trunks reach the pars papillaris, as pointed out by Pautrier[21] and Cowan.[22]

REFERENCES

1. Lupulescu AP, Birmingham DJ, Pinkus H: An electron microscopic study of human epidermis after acetone and kerosene administration. J Invest Dermatol 60:33, 1973
2. Pinkus H: Examination of the epidermis by the strip method. II. Biometric data on regeneration of the human epidermis. J Invest Dermatol 19:431, 1952
3. Cormane RM, Husz S, Hammerlinck FF: Immunoglobulin and complement-bearing lymphocytes in eczema. Br J Dermatol 88:307, 1973
4. Silberberg-Sinakin, I, Thorbecke SJ, Baer RL, Rosenthal SA, Berezowsky V: Antigen-bearing Langerhans cells in skin, dermal lymphatics, and in lymph nodes. Cell Immunol 25:137, 1976
5. Shelley WB, Juhlin L: Selective uptake of contact allergens by the Langerhans cell. Arch Dermatol 113:187, 1977
6. Dvorak HF, Mihm MC, Dvorak AM: Morphology of delayed-type hypersensitivity reactions in man. J Invest Dermatol 67:391, 1976
7. Björnberg A, Löwhagen G-B: Patch testing with mineral wool (Rockwool). Acta Derm Venerol (Stockh) 57:257, 1977
8. Cuypers JMC, Hoedemaeker PJ, Nater JP, DeJong MGM: The histopathology of fiberglass dermatitis in relation to von Hebra's concept of eczema. Contact Dermatol 1:88, 1975
9. DeJong MCMJ, Hoedemaeker PJ, Jongebloood WJ, Nater JP: Investigative studies of the dermatitis caused by the larva of the brown-tail moth (*Euproctis chrysorrhaea* Linn). II. Histopathology of skin lesions and scanning electron microscopy of their causative setae. Arch Dermatol Res 255:177, 1976
10. Montes LF: The histopathology of diaper dermatitis. J Cutan Pathol 5:1, 1978
11. Robert P: Les lésions histologiques de la dipthérie cutanée superficielle de type eczématoide. Dermatologica 94:334, 1947
12. Epstein S: Epidermal and dermal reactions in a case of sensitivity to nickel. J Invest Dermatol 38:37, 1962
13. Epstein S: Contact dermatitis due to nickel and chromate. Observations on dermal delayed (tuberculin-type) sensitivity. Arch Dermatol 73:236, 1956
14. Rudner EJ, Hudson P, Mehregan AH: Sensibilidad por contacto dermico: evaluación clinica y dermatopatologica. Arch Argent Dermatol 22:69, 1972
15. Gomez Orbaneja J, Iglesias Diaz L, Sanchez Lozano JL, Conde Salozar L: Lymphomatoid contact dermatitis. A syndrome produced by epicutaneous hypersensitivity with clinical features and a histopathologic picture similar to that of mycosis fungoides. Contact Dermatol 2:139, 1976
16. Van Neste D, Lachapelle J-M, Desmons F: Dermatite atopique. Étude histologique des lésions cutanées et historadioautographie après incorporation de thymidine tritrée. Ann Dermatol Venereol 106:327, 1979
17. Mihm MC Jr, Soter NA, Dvorak HF, Austen KF: The structure of normal skin and the morphology of atopic eczema. J Invest Dermatol 67:305, 1976
18. Kocsard E: The problem of prurigo. Australas J Dermatol 6:156, 1962
19. Marks R, Wells GC: Lichen simplex. Morphodynamic correlates. Br J Dermatol 88:249, 1973
20. Mehregan AH: Picker's nodule. Dermatol Digest 4:55, 1965
21. Pautrier LM: Le névrome de la lichenification circonscrite nodulaire chronique. Ann Dermatol Syphiligr 5:897, 1934
22. Cowan MA: Neurohistological changes in prurigo nodularis. Arch Dermatol 89:754, 1964

area of hairy-chested men. Sections of this lesion (Fig. 8-2) shows the epidermis mildly to moderately acanthotic, with somewhat uneven development of ridges and papillae. There is perivascular infiltrate in the subpapillary layer and, on the surface focal parakeratosis, which often takes the shape of tapering *mounds* and may contain a few pyknotic leukocytes. It is only when one examines serial sections that one becomes aware of the constant association of the parakeratotic areas with the suprapapillary thin portions of the epidermis. Papilla and overlying rete may not look particularly abnormal below a well-developed mound because in these areas one sees the last, exfoliating stage of a tiny inflammatory focus. One has to look closely to find the earlier stages, which are reconstructed in the series shown in Figure 8-3. The very earliest stage of the cyle is a highly edematous papilla with engorged capillary; the epidermis appears unaltered. In the next stage, fluid and a few polymorphonuclear cells enter the suprapapillary plate and cause some intercellular edema. This is followed by loss of granular layer and formation of parakeratotic cells between which the fluid and granulocytes are trapped. Meanwhile, the papillary edema has subsided, and the papilla may become quite inconspicuous. Edema of the suprapapillary plate at first produces a flat mound, which then increases in height by the accumulation of parakeratotic cells and the products of the squirting papilla. Still later, normal horny cells are produced, and the granular layer is reconstituted. The parakeratotic mound now becomes a lenticular focus in the stratum corneum and is eliminated onto the surface.

Individual papillae squirt and subside at different times in seborrheic dermatitis and thus produce focal mounds. Their number, size, and degree of admixture of inflammatory products vary greatly with the intensity of the dermatitis. The described petaloid form is intermediate, being chronic but relatively mild. In acute seborrheic dermatitis, larger parakeratotic crusts may form, the epidermis may become quite acanthotic and spongiotic, and there may be formation of small spongiotic vesicles in the edematous suprapapillary plate (Fig. 5-8). In the follicular form, spongiosis and abscess formation also involve the upper hair follicle and give rise to the characteristic, tiny, pointed pustules of the clinical picture (Fig. 8-4). In other cases of seborrheic dermatitis, the rete ridges may become long and the suprapapillary plate so thin that the tips of the papillae are covered only by parakeratotic material. This picture, which is usually associated with much epidermal and dermal edema and inflammatory infiltrate, merges by degrees into that of *nummular eczema* (pg. 107).[3]

On the other hand, a fresh lesion of seborrheic dermatitis, impressive clinically by its swollen appearance, may be very disappointing under the microscope, where vascular engorgement and dermal edema have been lost in the paraffin-embedded sections. Sometimes one has to look for a few early parakeratotic mounds and a few emigrating leukocytes in order to make a diagnosis. It is a good rule to think of seborrheic dermatitis whenever the clinician describes a florid lesion and the microscopist sees practically normal skin.

Perioral Dermatitis. A recalcitrant, erythematous, scaly, and papular eruption, originally described as light-sensitive seborrheid,[4] has become an increasingly vexing problem to dermatologists. Biopsies are done in order to rule out rosacea, lupus erythematosus, and seborrheic dermatitis. The histologic changes[5] are not pathognomonic (Fig. 8-4) and resemble eczematous dermatitis with parakeratotic scaling and spongiotic edema in epidermis and follicular epithelium, the latter causing a re-

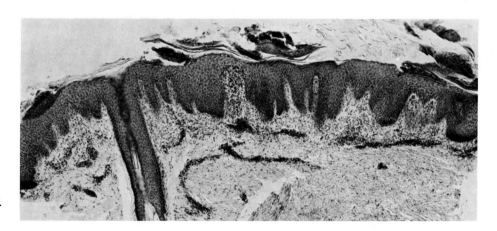

FIGURE 8–2.
Seborrheic dermatitis. H&E. X60.

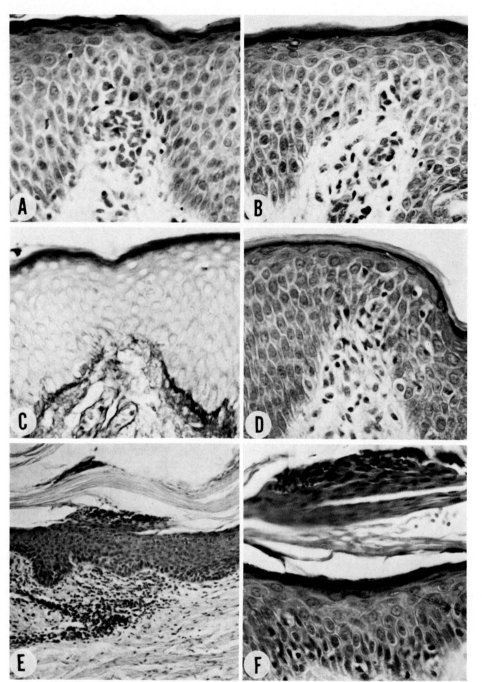

FIGURE 8–3.
Cycle of suprapapillary exudate in seborrheic dermatitis. **A, B,** *and* **D.** *Early stages before parakeratosis develops. H&E. X400.* **C.** *Temporary break in basement membrane. Alcian blue-PAS. X400.* **E.** *Later stage in which a parakeratotic mound includes polymorphonuclear leukocytes, while papilla has become inconspicuous. Lenticular parakeratotic inclusion in horny layer is end product of a previous squirt. H&E. X135.* **F.** *Details of microabscess in a parakeratotic mound which has been lifted up by normal horny material underlaid by a granular layer. H&E. X400.*

semblance to follicular seborrheic dermatitis. Scattered dermal infiltrate consists of lymphocytes, some histiocytes, and occasional plasma cells. The disorder is related to long-continued application of corticosteroid ointments.

ASTEATOTIC DERMATITIS

The differential diagnosis of seborrheic dermatitis may have to include pemphigus erythematosus in rare instances, but a common source of error is the close resemblance of the microscopic picture of asteatotic dermatitis (*winter eczema*). The latter usually has less acanthosis, but all other features are quite similar, and asteatotic (xerotic) dermatitis also may merge histologically and clinically into the picture of nummular eczema in aggravated cases (Fig. 8-5). The presence or absence of well-formed sebaceous glands is helpful in differential diagnosis but requires examination of multiple sections in order to judge the size of glands fairly.

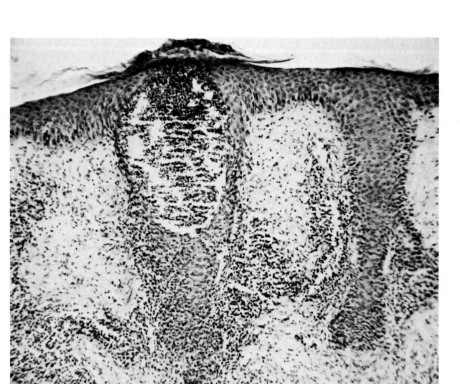

FIGURE 8–4.
Perioral dermatitis. Heavy involvement of upper portion of hair follicle and admixture of polymorphonuclear leukocytes to the generally lymphocytic infiltrate make the picture similar to the follicular type of seborrheic dermatitis. H&E. X135.

PSORIASIS

Classic

Typical lesions of psoriasis (Fig. 8-6) are characterized by a high degree of acanthosis of the rete ridges, which are evenly long and alternate in the section with long edematous and often club-shaped papillae. The suprapapillary plate is thin, and the surface is covered by a lamellated scale in which orthokeratotic and parakeratotic areas alternate. Papillary capillaries appear rigid and tortuous, and there is a rather small amount of perivascular lymphocytic infiltrate in the subpapillary layer. The

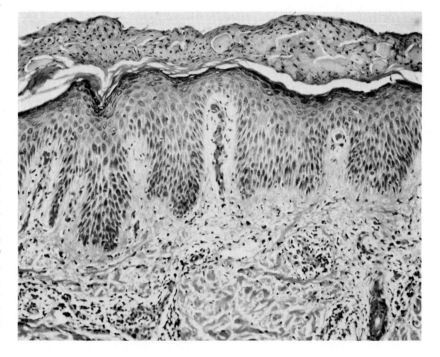

FIGURE 8–5.
Asteatotic dermatitis. Note the generally eczematous character of the changes in this specimen, which obviously was obtained at a moment when a much more exudative phase had been replaced by normalizing processes expressed in acanthosis and hypergranulosis. Highly edematous papilla with prominent vessel below relatively thin suprapapillary plate and eddies in the parakeratotic scale-crust are reminders of the cyclic character of the acute process. Minimal perivascular infiltrate also speaks against a true eczematous dermatitis. H&E. X135.

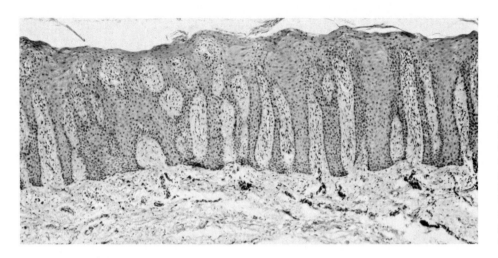

FIGURE 8–6.
Psoriasis, plaque. Only fragments of the scale are present because the lamellated psoriatic stratum corneum easily disintegrates during histologic processing. While some papillae are shown full length, others are cut obliquely and only the upper or the lower portions appear in the section. H&E. X70.

presence of small accumulations of pyknotic neutrophilic leukocytes in the horny layer (*Munro abscesses*[6]) completes the picture. This generalized description is quite adequate for the diagnosis of typical cases but says nothing about the pathobiology of the psoriatic process, nor is it helpful in atypical cases or in the numerous variants of psoriasis.

Examination of sections for evidence of squirting papillae is revealing in both respects. It is easy to find a cycle of events very similar to that in seborrheic dermatitis, except that the amount of serum discharged from the tip of a papilla usually is smaller and the number of leukocytes larger. Lymphocytes and neutrophils often migrate individually through breaks in the basement membrane (Fig. 8-7A) into the suprapapillary plate, then aggregate in the parakeratotic mound, where we call them a *microabscess* (Fig. 8-8). The rhythmic discharges from one papilla seem to last a little longer,

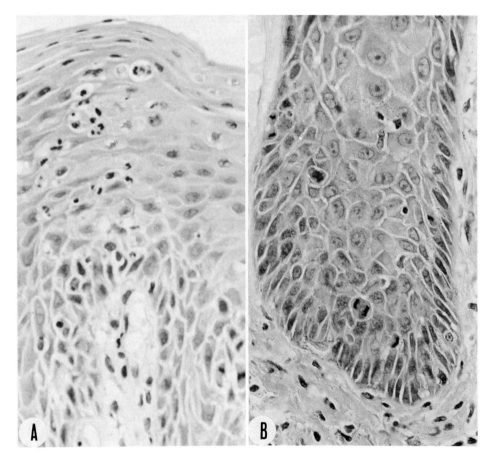

FIGURE 8–7.
*Details of upper (suprapapillary) and lower (ridge) portion of psoriatic epidermis. **A.** Migration of individual leukocytes from tip of papilla into and through suprapapillary plate associated with loss of granular layer and parakeratosis (compare with Fig. 8–3). **B.** Lower part of long rete ridge stains darker (no edema) and shows several mitoses, indicating division of epidermis into a vigorously proliferating lower portion and a damaged and rapidly exfoliating upper portion. H&E. X400.*

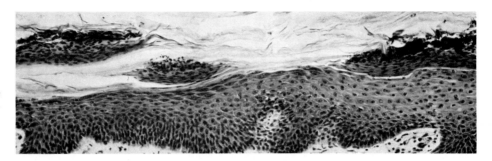

FIGURE 8–8.
Layered scale consisting of thin orthokeratotic lamellae and lenticular parakeratotic formations harboring microabscesses. H&E. X135.

and they repeat themselves at shorter intervals so that one may find two or several cycles, one above the other in different stages of development. Moreover, numerous papillae squirt in close vicinity.

These phenomena seem to explain most of the features of psoriasis. The papillae, and especially their tips, remain in a state of edema and engorgement of capillaries. Polymorphonuclear leukocytes are often visible in the vascular lumen, but rarely in the dermis and practically never in the rete ridges, which are solid without much evidence of edema. (Fig. 8-7B). Instead, leukocytes are found between the living cells of the suprapapillary plate above papillary tips (Fig. 8-9) and between the parakeratotic cells of mounds and lenticular inclusions within the horny layer, which thus becomes lamellar. If one follows one lamella sideways through the length of the section, one sees it swell up (Fig. 8-8) into a lentil-shaped mass of parakeratotic cells, farther on subside and continue as an orthokeratotic thin lamella for a stretch, then become parakeratotic again. The trapping of air between the lamel-

lae contributes to the silvery aspect of the clinical lesion. The inflammatory process varies in intensity from spot to spot and from time to time. Most important, it is always associated with heads of papillae. These events are obscured in the center of very active chronic plaques of psoriasis because of the rapid succession of squirts from many papillae. Intelligent and careful examination is needed to recognize them. Manifest clinical psoriasis is a rhythmic, repeated pathologic event, not a continuous one.

Recent research in psoriasis has concentrated on the epidermis and has led to the postulates that faulty control of epidermal proliferation is the primary disturbance and that a shortened life span of the keratinocytes may lead to incomplete (parakeratotic) maturation. The presence of inflammatory factors has been largely disregarded. One may, however, equally well postulate that the constantly repeated inflammatory insult to the suprapapillary epithelial cells, which leads to their premature death, forces the rete ridges, which remain undam-

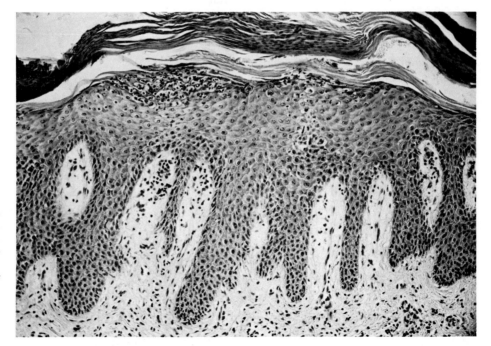

FIGURE 8–9.
Psoriasis with spongiform pustule. Suprapapillary plate appears thick in section because head of squirting papilla is not encountered in section. Stream of leukocytes in right half of picture indicates that a papillary head would be encountered in one of subsequent serial sections. H&E. X135.

aged, to become hyperplastic and to speed up mitotic division (Fig. 8-7B) in an effort to replace the prematurely lost suprapapillary portion. Either hypothesis will explain the data that mitoses are about 10 times as common in psoriasis as in normal epidermis and occur not only in the basal layer but in two to three rows of basaloid germinal cells,[7] and that turnover of the epidermal population is correspondingly speeded up. Similar conditions have been found in control studies of atopic dermatitis and lichen simplex chronicus (see Chap. 7). It is not possible at this time to prove which phenomenon is primary, but as a mental aid in diagnosis, the thought is helpful that mitotic speedup is secondary to epithelial damage, which is secondary to papillary squirting (Fig. 8-10). Very recent investigations of early and later manifestations of psoriasis have led several authors[8,9] to the tentative conclusion that psoriatic epidermal hyperplasia may develop in association with antecedent and persisting events in the dermis. Blood and lymph capillaries show characteristic abnormalities in psoriasis[10,11] and do not become normal even after treatment.

The presence of macrophages, lymphocytes, and mast cells in early and developed lesions of psoriasis and the role of specific antigenic substances in psoriatic horny layer need further investigation but do not influence histologic diagnosis.[12]

Variants

Most of the variants of psoriasis can be understood as variations of the interlocking sequence of events illustrated in Figure 8-10. If papillary exudate and subsequent acanthosis are reduced in quantity, we encounter the picture of *seborrheic psoriasis* or may have difficulty in making a decision between psoriasis and seborrheic dermatitis. The latter is

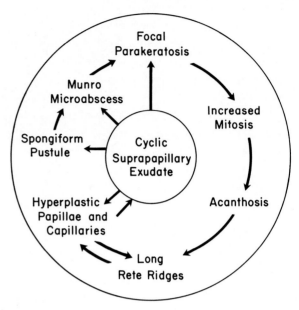

FIGURE 8–10.
Diagram illustrating the hypothesis that cyclic suprapapillary exudate is the main driving force of the established psoriatic process (regardless of possibility that some abnormality in the epidermis may initiate the exudate). According to this view, damage to superficial epidermal layers secondarily induces regenerative mitotic activity in the rete ridges and other histologic changes. (Adapted from Pinkus. Arch Dermatol 107:840, 1973.)

more likely if rete ridges are uneven and if spongiotic edema is evident. Psoriasis is practically ruled out if spongiosis affects the ridges.

We come closer to the features of *pustular psoriasis* when the amount of exocytosis increases. This is often seen in cases of acute psoriatic flare-up, when each new lesion clinically appears as a tiny pustule, then spreads into a scaly erythematous papule. Histologically (Fig. 8-11), we see an aggregate of discharging papillae capped by a huge parakeratotic mound. At this stage, the suprapapillary plate is paradoxically thickened, due mainly to

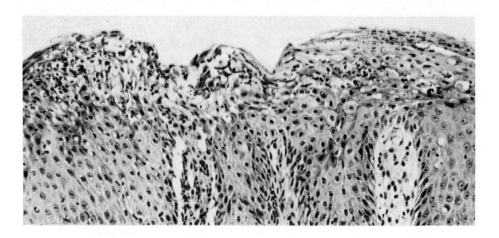

FIGURE 8–11.
Very early, clinically pustular lesion in an acute burst of psoriasis. While suprapapillary plate is relatively thick, most of keratinocytes are damaged and are in process of being converted into parakeratotic elements. H&E. X280. (From Sutton. Diseases of the Skin, 11th ed, 1956. Courtesy of Dr. R. L. Sutton, Jr. Contributed by H. Pinkus.)

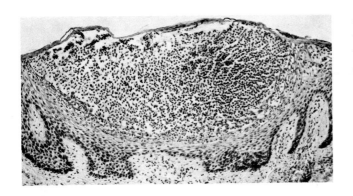

FIGURE 8–12.
Pustular psoriasis of von Zumbusch type. Note spongiform pustulation in the shoulder of this early lesion characterized by massive leukocytic exudate and minimal acanthosis (mitotic activity). H&E. X90.

edema. Such cases simply represent an exaggeration of the exudative process of typical psoriasis. However, the picture is not too different in cases of *generalized pustular psoriasis* of the von Zumbusch type, except that the acanthotic response of the epidermis is much reduced. Microabscesses become macroabscesses (Fig. 8-12), and their precursor state among the still living epidermal cells represents Kogoj's *spongiform pustule* (Fig. 8-9).[13]

The spongiform pustule is the hallmark of Hallopeau's *acrodermatitis continua*. Personal experience convinces us as clinicians that this dermatosis is a variant of psoriasis.

Impetigo Herpetiformis. Almost indistinguishable from generalized pustular psoriasis, either clinically or histologically, is a rare disease called *impetigo herpetiformis*. Originally described as a severe affection of pregnant women, it has also been found in nonpregnant women and in men. It is related to hypoparathyroidism,[14,15] and cases exhibiting no disturbance of calcium–phosphorus metabolism probably should be labeled pustular psoriasis.[16] Histologically, there is a tendency to dissociation in the upper epidermal layers affected with spongiform pustulation, and some rounded acantholytic cells are found in the macropustule (Chap. 11). In this respect, impetigo herpetiformis resembles the *subcorneal pustular dermatosis* of Sneddon and Wilkinson (Chap. 11).

Psoriasis of Palms and Soles: Pustulosis Palmaris et Plantaris. Another special case is *pustular psoriasis of palms and soles*. Here, the concept of suprapapillary exudation helps in the differential diagnosis from *pustulosis palmaris et plantaris* and *dyshidrosiform eczematous dermatitis*. The vesicle

of the latter (Fig. 7-8) is derived from spongiotic intraepidermal edema, and the roof of the blister contains living epidermal cells unless the entire rete is destroyed. The former two (Fig. 8-13) begin in the superficial epidermal layers and soon become subcorneal. The entire rete malpighi is compressed in the bottom of the blister. True pustular psoriasis has at least some evidence of the spongiform pustule in the shoulders of the lesion (Fig. 8-14) or in the septa between adjoining cavities. This sign is absent in pustulosis palmaris et plantaris, which is a rare condition synonymous with *Andrews' pustular bacterid* and not related to psoriasis.[17,18] It is unfortunate that in the literature no clear distinction is made between cases of psoriasis with pustules on hands and feet and the isolated occurrence of a pustular eruption in these localities.

One should not forget that there is another type of volar psoriasis. The clinical picture resembles a dry eczematous eruption, and it is often biopsied for differentiation from occupational dermatitis. In this type, suprapapillary exudate and all accompanying changes are reduced to a minimum. The naturally thick epidermis shows little acanthosis, and the thick horny layer contains only a few scattered lenticular foci of parakeratotic cells and pyknotic leukocytes. Capillaries may be wide, but subepidermal inflammation is almost absent.

Psoriatic Erythroderma. The psoriatic eruption may progress to universal erythroderma or exfoliative dermatitis. The clinical picture is indistinguishable from other forms of erythroderma, especially in malignant lymphoma (Chap. 44). Histologically, however, the picture is that of classic psoriasis with acanthosis, parakeratosis, and Munro abscesses, while there is relatively little cellular infiltrate in the upper dermis.

Psoriasis of Oral Mucosa. The question of psoriasis of the oral mucosa and its possible relationship to geographic tongue will be discussed in Chapter 45.

REITER'S DISEASE

The last member of the family of psoriasiform reactions (Fig. 8-1) is the keratotic or crusted lesion of Reiter's disease. (*Keratoderma blennorrhagicum* on the basis of chronic gonorrhea is histologically indistinguishable.) Figure 8-15 shows a typical but relatively small lesion from the palm. The old thick horny layer has been lifted up by a truncated cone of parakeratotic crust, which actually repre-

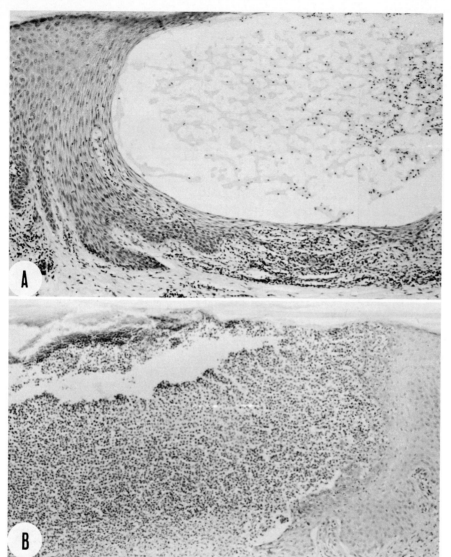

FIGURE 8–13.
Comparison of pustulosis palmaris et plantaris and true pustular psoriasis at low power. **A.** *The vesicopustule probably began intraepidermally and compressed keratinocytes all around it without evidence of spongiosis (Fig. 7–8) or spongiform pustulation visible in* **B.** **B.** *Pustular psoriasis shows a picture identical with Figure 8–12 taken from a lesion of generalized pustular psoriasis. H&E. X125.*

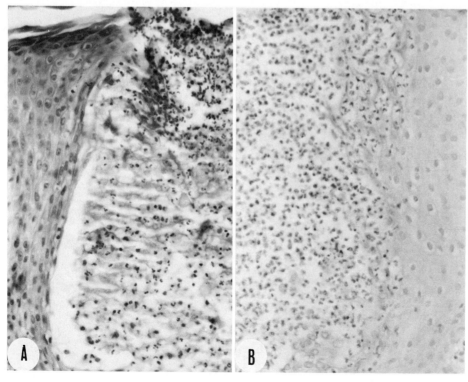

FIGURE 8–14.
Higher magnification of the shoulders of pustules in previous illustration shows the absence **(A)** *and presence* **(B)** *of spongiform pustulation in pustulosis palmaris et plantaris* **(A)** *and pustular psoriasis* **(B)** *of palm. H&E. X250.*

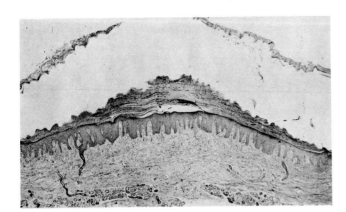

FIGURE 8–15.
Small and relatively dry lesion of Reiter's disease. H&E. X30.

sents a huge mound including dozens of microabscesses and parakeratotic lenticles. The suprapapillary layer is thick because it is highly edematous. If we look for details, we find typical squirting papillae, similar to those of any of the other entities (Fig. 8-16). The difference is quantitative. There is also much edema and inflammatory infiltrate in papillae and the subpapillary layer. In very acute cases, the exudate may almost destroy the suprapapillary plate and may lead to vesiculation under the crust. Lesions of the Reiter syndrome on the glans penis are known as *balanitis circinata*. They closely resemble psoriatic plaques of this area both clinically and histologically. Differential diagnosis must be based on the evaluation of the entire case history.[19]

NUMMULAR ECZEMA

Just as the clinical picture of nummular eczema often develops in an asteatotic or seborrheic soil, so do the histopathologic features suggest an exacerbation of asteatotic and seborrheic dermatitis (Fig. 8-17), with the addition of eczematous features. Edema and leukocytic exudate dominate the picture. Evenly or unevenly sized rete ridges are riddled by spongiosis and exocytosis. The suprapapillary plate may be completely disrupted so that edematous papillary heads are exposed, and the surface is covered by parakeratotic crust containing pyknotic granulocytes and dried serum. Bacterial colonies occasionally are seen in the crust and support the clinical impression of an infectious factor in this disease.[20] Cellular infiltrate consisting of small round cells and granulocytes in the edematous pars papillaris complete the picture, which combines features of the eczematous and psoriasiform tissue reactions.

SULZBERGER–GARBE'S DISEASE

Nine cases of a *distinctive, exudative, discoid and lichenoid chronic dermatosis* were described by Sulzberger and Garbe in 1937. The disease is peculiarly localized in its distribution, being predominantly encountered among middle-aged Jewish males in the New York area. In a recent review,[21] Sulzberger differentiates it from a great variety of other dermatoses, the most important ones being my-

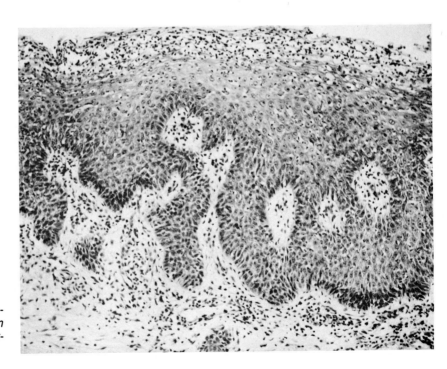

FIGURE 8–16.
More exudative form of Reiter's disease. Transmigration of leukocytes from papillae to disintegrating stratum corneum. H&E. X135.

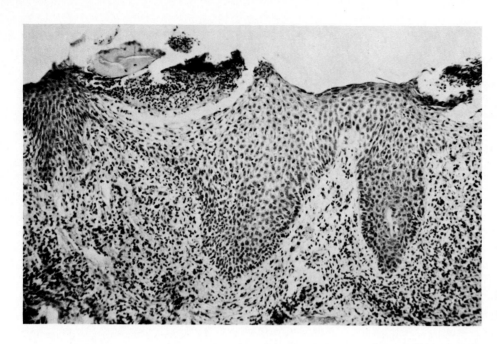

FIGURE 8–17.
Nummular eczema combines eczematous and psoriasiform features. H&E. X135.

cosis fungoides and nummular eczema. We, therefore, discuss it at this point. The epidermal changes resemble those of nummular eczema but are rarely seen unaltered due to the severe pruritus. The arterioles and capillaries of the upper dermis are dilated and have thickened walls. The infiltrate consists of small round cells, fixed tissue type cells, polymorphs, and numerous plasma cells. The latter are found close to vascular walls and are the most characteristic feature except in early lesions. The true pathogenetic relations of this disease are unknown. Fortunately, it responds well to corticosteroids.

REFERENCES

1. Pinkus H: Psoriasiform tissue reactions. Australas J Dermatol 8:31, 1965
2. Pinkus H, Mehregan AH: The primary histologic lesion of seborrheic dermatitis and psoriasis. J Invest Dermatol 46:109, 1966
3. Metz J, Metz G: Ultrastruktur der Epidermis bei seborrhoischem Ekzem. Arch Dermatol Forsch 252:285, 1975
4. Frumess GM, Lewis HM: Light sensitive seborrheic dermatitis. Arch Dermatol 75:245, 1957
5. Marks R, Black MM: Perioral dermatitis. A histopathologic study of 26 cases. Br J Dermatol 84:242, 1971
6. Munro WJ: Note sur l'histopathologie du psoriasis. Ann Dermatol Syphiligr 9:961, 1898
7. Weinstein GD, Frost P: Abnormal cell proliferation in psoriasis. J Invest Dermatol 50:254, 1968
8. Van Scott EJ, Flaxman BA: Lesion kinetics in psoriasis; tissue, cellular, and subcellular compartments. Acta Derm Venereol [Suppl] 73:75, 1973
9. Braun-Falco O: The initial psoriatic lesion. In Farber EM, Cox AJ (eds): Psoriasis, Proceedings of the Second International Symposium of Stanford Univ 1976. New York, Yorke Medical Books, 1976
10. Braverman IM, Yen A: Ultrastructure of the capillary loops in the dermal papillae of psoriasis. J Invest Dermatol 68:53, 1977
11. Staricco RG: Altered capillary response to tape stripping in psoriasis and some other dermatoses: petechial threshold test. Dermatologica 160:315, 1980
12. Farber EM, Cox AJ (eds): Psoriasis, Proceedings of the Second International Symposium of Stanford Univ. 1976. New York, Yorke Medical Books, 1976
13. Colomb B, LaBatie J-P: La pustule spongiforme de Kogoj. Apports de le microscope électronique. Ann Dermatol Venereol 104:707, 1977
14. Leonhardi G, Michel L: Impetigo herpetiformis—ein Symptom des Calciummangels. Arch Klin Exp Dermatol 207:251, 1958
15. Bajaj AK, Swarup V, Gupta OP, Gupta SC: Impetigo herpetiformis. Dermatologica 155:292, 1977
16. Osterling RJ, Nobrega RE, DuBoeuff JA, Van der Mear JB: Impetigo herpetiformis or generalized pustular psoriasis. Arch Dermatol 114:1527, 1978
17. Uehara M, Ofuji S: The morphogenesis of pustulosis palmaris et plantaris. Arch Dermatol 109:518, 1974
18. Pierard J, Kint A: La pustulose palmo-plantaire chronique et recidivante. Etude histologique. Ann Dermatol Venereol 105:681, 1978
19. Perry HO, Mayne JG: Psoriasis and Reiter's syndrome. Arch Dermatol 92:129, 1965
20. Röckl H: Untersuchungen zur Klinik und Pathogenese des Mikrobiellen Ekzems. Hautarzt 7:70, 1956
21. Sulzberger MB: Distinctive exudative discoid and lichenoid chronic dermatosis (Sulzberger and Garbe) re-examined—1978. Br J Dermatol 100:13, 1979

CHAPTER

9

Lichenoid and Poikilodermatous Tissue Reactions

The botanic term *lichen*, signifying dry scurfy forms of lower plant life, has been applied to dry scaly skin disease in such expressions as pityriasis lichenoides or lichenification. The prototype, however, of a lichen of the skin is *lichen planus* (lichen ruber planus). When we call a clinical eruption lichenoid, we usually mean it resembles lichen planus. Similarly, there is a histologic reaction that is typically expressed in the papule and plaque of lichen planus. Clinically atrophic, hypertrophic, and bullous forms of the disease have histologic features easily recognized as variants of this reaction. The lichenoid tissue reaction, however, is also found in nosologically unrelated dermatoses, such as lichen nitidus, certain types of lupus erythematosus, and some solar keratoses. Some of its features are encountered in lichenoid drug eruptions and in erythema dyschromicum perstans. Furthermore, it blends with the tissue reactions characterizing the various types of poikiloderma, a term applied to any clinical picture that combines the four features of telangiectasia, hyperpigmentation, depigmentation, and atrophy in a mottled distribution. Recently, lichen-planus-like tissue reactions have been described in the graft-vs-host reaction.[1] We are thus dealing in this chapter with a heterogeneous assembly of clinical dermatoses, all of which may enter differential diagnosis in the examination of a biopsy specimen. Clinicopathologic correlation is even more essential in this field than in the areas covered in previous chapters, and determination of the correct diagnosis can be a difficult, stimulating, and, in the end, gratifying process.[2,3]

LICHEN PLANUS

The basic histobiologic feature of lichen planus is basal layer damage. Just as we used the suprapapillary exudate to explain most of the other features of psoriasis, so can we derive most of the histologic details of lichen planus by considering that damage to the germinal layer must be reflected in the epidermis and must lead to inflammatory reaction in the subepidermal zone.

Histology

The classic histologic features of lichen planus (Fig. 9-1) include hyperkeratosis, hypergranulosis, and hypertrophy of the rete, liquefaction or colloid degeneration of basal cells, and a bandlike subepider-

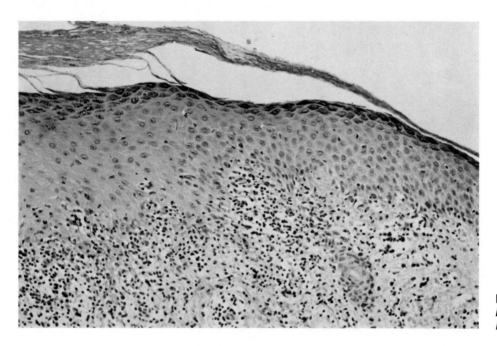

FIGURE 9–1.
Lichen planus, edge of plaque. H&E. X135.

mal lymphocytic infiltrate which invades the lower layers of the epidermis. Focal separation of epidermis and dermis (*Max Joseph spaces*) may occur (Fig. 9-2). Sawtooth-shaped rete ridges and deposition of melanin in dermal macrophages complete the picture (Fig. 9-3).

Damage to the basal layer in lichen planus is manifested in several ways. Normal, regularly aligned, cuboid or columnar basal cells are rarely seen. The lowest cells of the epidermis often look more like prickle cells. Their arrangement is disturbed by the presence of lymphocytes between them. Peculiar round or oval acidophilic bodies

about the size of a basal cell may be present in scant or large numbers within or just below the epidermis (*Civatte bodies*, Fig. 9-4).[4] Occasionally, the impression is gained that most of a rete ridge has been transformed into these colloid bodies, leaving only a pointed sawtooth. Melanocytes are more or less absent or seem degenerating. Melanin granules evidently have been discharged from the damaged basal layer and have been engulfed by macrophages in the subepidermal zone. The darker the skin is normally, the more conspicuous is the feature.

Mitotic figures are rarely seen under the light

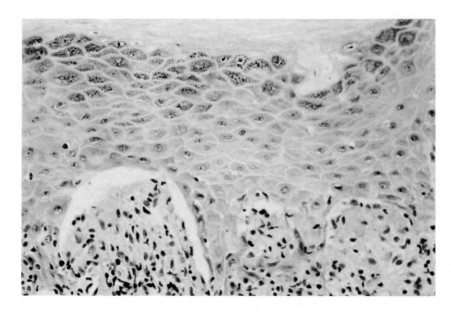

FIGURE 9–2.
Lichen planus. Focal separation between epidermis and dermis due to loss of basal cells (Max Joseph space). Keratohyalin develops halfway through epidermis. Some hyalinized (Civatte) bodies in place of basal cells in right half of picture between inflammatory cells. H&E. X600.

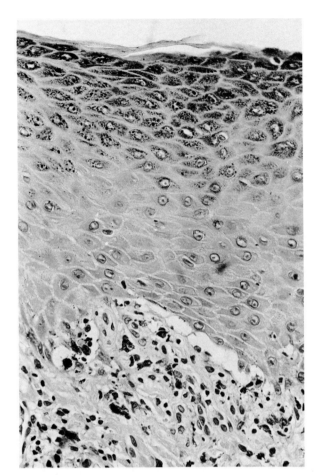

FIGURE 9–3.
Lichen planus. Max Joseph space, thick stratum granulosum, and loss of pigment granules into the dermis, where some are taken up by macrophages. H&E. X600.

microscope in lichen planus, but treatment with tritiated thymidine has shown a greatly increased labeling index,[5] and electron microscopic observations have revealed excessive mitotic activity.[6] The reason for this discrepancy is not clear. It seems likely that many of the labeled cells do not achieve mitosis. The epidermis responds as it always does when mitosis is suppressed: the cells get larger, and the proportion of maturing cells increases.[7] This phenomenon can be observed in human epidermis after the application of small doses of thorium X (Fig. 9-5).[8] There is a reciprocal relationship between mitotic activity and length of epidermal cell life. In psoriasis, high mitotic rate and short life span are associated; in lichen planus, low mitotic rate leads to long retention of cells in a cohesive granular and horny layer. The epidermis may be thick, but actual count reveals that the number of nucleated cells is not much increased (Fig. 5-1B). We are dealing with hypertrophy (pseudoacanthosis) rather than with hyperplasia (acanthosis).

Close inspection and the use of special stains reveal features that set the dermal infiltrate of lichen planus (Fig. 9-6) apart from the plain inflammatory infiltrate of most other superficial dermatoses. While T lymphocytes[9] predominate, plasma cells may be present. Fixed-tissue type cells are always increased in number, most of them being histiocytes, and some containing phagocytized melanin. Others are endothelial cells, the number of capillaries being definitely increased. Elastic fiber stain shows two important facts: the infiltrate is always restricted to the papillary layer, and the superficial

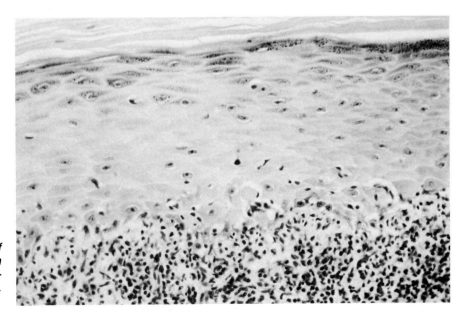

FIGURE 9–4.
Lichen planus. Typical invasion of lower epidermis by lymphocytes, with dissociation of basal layer and formation of Civatte bodies (see Fig. 5-1B). H&E. X600.

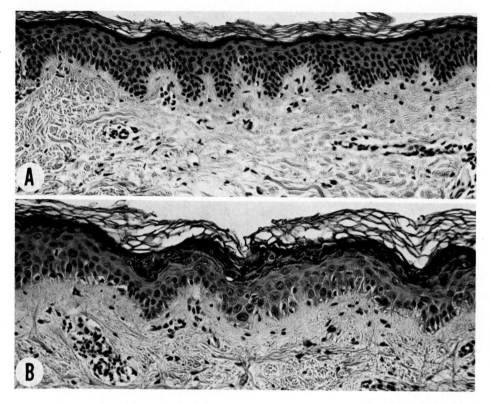

FIGURE 9–5.
Effect of two weekly applications of the alpha ray emitter, thorium X (75 μCi/ml), on normal skin of lateral surface of arm. These small doses did not produce clinical erythema or significant histologic evidence of inflammation. A. Control. B. Mitotic suppression resulting in reduction of living cells and increased proportion of granular and horny cells. H&E. X185. (From Hendren and Pinkus. J Invest Dermatol 22:463, 1954.)

fine elastic fibers usually are destroyed. There are, thus, certain aspects of a granulomatous infiltrate (Sec. IV), and it is not too rare to find an occasional multinucleated giant cell. These features also may be explained as a reaction to the damaged basal layer. The cascade of histobiologic events resulting from basal cell damage is illustrated diagrammatically in Figure 9-7.

An intriguing aspect has been added to the question of lichenoid tissue reactions by the description of lichen-planus-like lesions in the course of chronic graft-vs-host disease.[1] Most authors have described

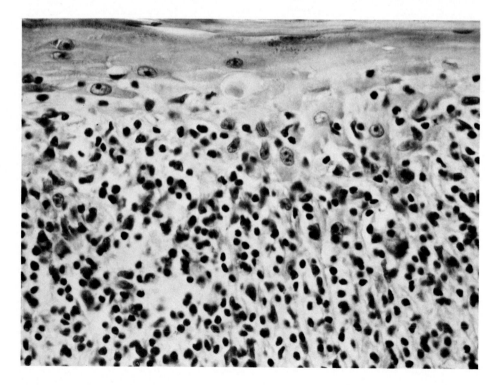

FIGURE 9–6.
Infiltrate of lichen planus. Note obliteration of lower epidermal contour. H&E. X465.

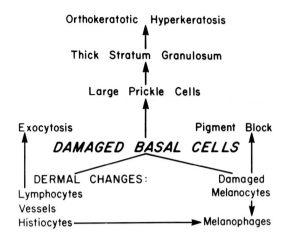

FIGURE 9–7.
Cascade of histobiologic events associated with epidermal basal cell damage. (Adapted from Pinkus. Arch Dermatol 107:840, 1973.)

evidence of aggression of transplanted bone marrow lymphocytes against epidermal basal cells leading to satellite cell necrosis[10] and, in severe cases, to bullous lesions resembling toxic epidermal necrolysis (Chap. 11). It is encouraging to note that, in some cases, basal cell degeneration caused by lymphocytic aggression can reproduce the clinical and histologic picture of lichen planus.

Clinicohistologic Correlation. It is rewarding to correlate the clinical signs of a lichen planus plaque with the histologic ones. Although lichen planus often is counted among the papulosquamous dermatoses, it usually does not have an exfoliating scale but has an adherent horny layer which is removed with difficulty. This phenomenon is explained by facts mentioned on the preceding page. The keratohyaline layer is generally preserved. The whitish Wickham's striae are expressed in the varying thickness of the granular layer. Keratohyline granules reflect and diffuse light (Chap. 2), and their accumulation makes the skin look white. They also influence the transmission of the color of blood, causing a bluish tint. This and the deposition of melanin below the epidermis produce the violaceous hue of the disease. Vascularity of the infiltrate and damage to the basal layer are responsible for a diagnostic procedure well known in France: methodic scraping of a lesion, which will produce the Auspitz phenomenon of capillary bleeding in psoriasis, instead produces subepidermal hemorrhage in lichen planus (Brocq phenomenon[2]). Scraping is also quite painful to the patient, and the paradox that lichen planus patients usually do not have excoriations in spite of intense pruritus is explained by the pain produced by scratching a skin, the free nerve endings of which are in the very layer that is affected by the inflammatory process.

Lichen planus of the mouth and other mucous membranes will be discussed in Chapter 45 and nail involvement in Chapter 46.

Atrophic, Verrucous, and Follicular Lesions

One or the other of the specific histologic features of lichen planus becomes modified in its clinical variants. *Atrophic* (Fig. 9-8) and *annular forms* usu-

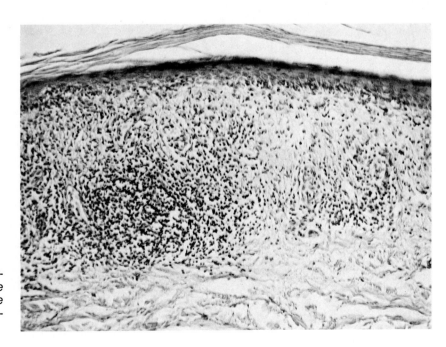

FIGURE 9–8.
Atrophic lichen planus. The active border is at left. Toward the center of the lesion at the right, lymphocytic infiltrate becomes sparse, but basal cell damage persists. H&E. X135.

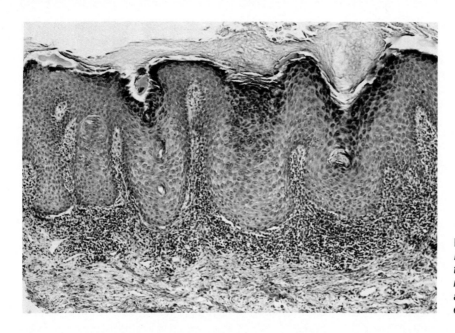

FIGURE 9–9.
Hypertrophic lichen planus. The infiltrate hugs the lower circumference of rete ridges, while the tips of papillae are normal. Note difference in size of epidermal cells.

ally show typical lichen planus features in the periphery, sometimes only for the width of one or two rete ridges. Centrally, the lymphocytic infiltrate is washed out, leaving behind the skeleton of capillary vessels, fixed tissue cells, and macrophages below the now plainly atrophic epidermis. The absence of elastic fibers in this zone is evident in O&G sections and adds to the clinical impression of atrophy. In *hypertrophic* (Fig. 9-9) and *verrucous* cases, on the other hand, the epidermis

seems to overcompensate the damage, and the rete ridges, sweat ducts, and follicular sheaths become truly acanthotic, although preserving their composition of large hypertrophic prickle cells. The infiltrate tends to hug the lower circumference of the ridges, while the suprapapillary portions of the epidermis may appear quite normal, with a good columnar basal layer. This discrepancy is accentuated in *follicular* lichen planus (Fig. 9-10), in which the infiltrate hugs the damaged basal layer of the follic-

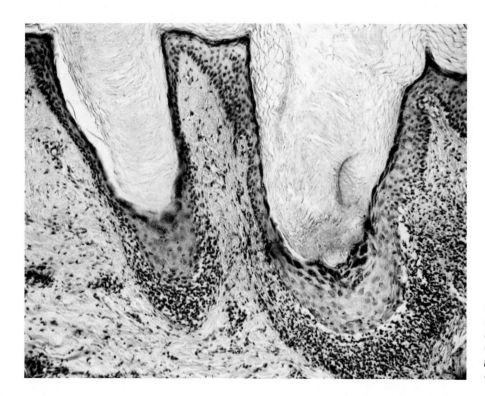

FIGURE 9–10.
Lichen planopilaris. Note almost normal condition of interfollicular epidermis and rounded horny plugs in cup-shaped follicles. H&E. X135.

ular sheaths. The hair root usually atrophies completely, and the entire follicle is converted into a cup-shaped bag filled with a keratin plug. It is characteristic for lichen planus that the keratin plug is ovoid and often wider below the surface (Fig. 14-6), in contrast to the conical or tack-shaped plug of lupus erythematosus. The *Graham–Little syndrome* of scarring alopecia of the scalp seems to be closely related to, if not identical with, lichen planopilaris.

Bullous Lesions

The rare bullous form of lichen planus has found a variety of interpretations. There is little doubt that in older times overtreatment with arsenic could provoke inflammatory edema and that the preformed cleft at the junction led to a bullous exacerbation.[11] There was, however, always a question whether *lichen planus pemphigoides*, in which bullae arise on normal skin and are associated with papular lichen planus, represents an association of the dry skin disease with *dermatitis herpetiformis* or *bullous pemphigoid*. This question has been raised again by immunofluorescent demonstration of immunoglobulins at the basement membrane and of eosinophils in the blister fluid.[12] Further studies will be needed to settle the issue.

Pigmented Lichen Planus, Lichen Pigmentosus and Erythema Dyschromicum Perstans

Healing lichen planus often leaves behind a slightly atrophic, hyperpigmented skin. The pigment is melanin deposited in macrophages and resembles that found in other instances of *postinflammatory pigmentation* (Fig. 5-13 and Chap. 30). The pigmentation may persist for many months, even in cases in which the inflammatory phase was minimal (*lichen invisible pigmenté* of Gougerot).[13,14] The histologic diagnosis may be approached by looking for occasional foci of basal cell damage, for loss of superficial elastic fibers, and for increased vascularity.

Clinical and histologic features of healing lichen planus are simulated by two other dermatoses, *lichen pigmentosus* as described in Japan[15] and recently in India,[16] and *erythema dyschromicum perstans*,[17] originally indentified in South America as *dermatosis cenicienta*.[18] Erythema dyschromicum perstans (Fig. 9-11) was also observed later in the United States,[19] mainly in people of Mexican or Mediterranean extraction, in the form of long-standing macular pigmentation preceded clinically by a mild erythematous and scaly phase and exhibiting histologically occasional foci of basal cell damage, with associated epidermal consequences, mild round cell infiltrate, and pronounced macrophage pigmentation. We suspect,[2] on the basis of our biopsy material, that this dermatosis may be the response to some unidentified environmental noxious agent. It may occur also in light-skinned people,[20,21] where histologic diagnosis may become difficult because there is much less deposition of melanin in macrophages.

LICHEN PLANUS ACTINICUS AND LICHENOID ACTINIC KERATOSIS

Lichenoid tissue reaction in response to sun exposure has been observed in two distinct clinical forms. *Lichen planus actinicus* or *tropicus* has been reported in subtropical countries,[22] and recently in Kenya as *lichenoid melanodermatitis*.[23] It seems to differ from other variants only in its localization on sun-exposed skin. On the other hand, solitary lesions, associated with other manifestations of actinic damage and exhibiting a tissue reaction almost indistinguishable from lichen planus (Fig. 9-12), were described independently by three teams of authors.[24-26] Clinical correlation is extremely important in making the diagnosis of *lichenoid actinic keratosis*, although a mild degree of epithelial dysplasia often arouses suspicion. Inflamed lesions of lentigo senilis (Chap. 32) may be very similar.[27]

POIKILODERMA

We agree with others[28,29] that *poikiloderma atrophicans vasculare* is not a nosologic entity and that we should relate poikilodermatous manifestations to the underlying diseases, which include mycosis fungoides or its precursors, parapsoriasis of the plaque, lichenoid and retiform varieties, and, on the other hand, dermatomyositis and lupus erythematosus. In addition, *poikiloderma of Civatte*, the related *Riehl's melanosis* (melanodermatitis toxica), *congenital poikiloderma of Thomson*,[30] *dyskeratosis congenita*,[31] and two familial forms, *hereditary sclerosing poikiloderma* and *acrokeratotic poikiloderma*, share certain clinical and histologic features.[32] Pinta (Chap. 20) may have to be considered. The clinical differential diagnosis includes *chronic X-ray dermatitis* (Chap. 15) and erythromelanosis follicularis colli (Chap. 30).

The distinctive histologic marker of all forms of

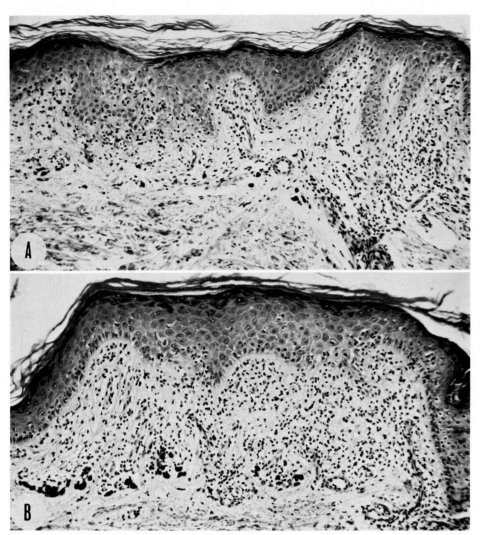

FIGURE 9–11.
Erythema dyschromicum per-stans, as seen in a North American Indian. **A.** *An early lesion showing poikiloderma-tous changes of focal basal cell degeneration in relation to spotty inflammatory infiltrate and ectasia of blood and lymph capillaries.* **B.** *An older stage resembling atrophying lichen planus except for the relatively thick epidermis. Note melano-phages at lower border of fad-ing infiltrate. H&E. X180.*

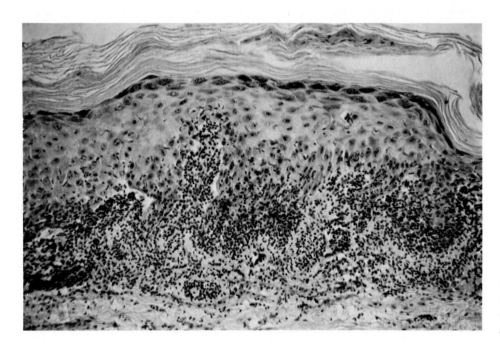

FIGURE 9–12.
Lichen planuslike actinic kera-tosis. Note involvement of tips of papillae and small focus of parakeratosis. H&E. X135.

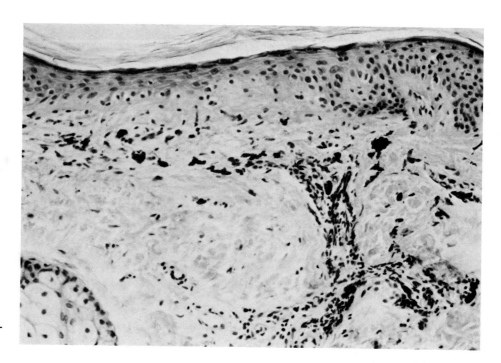

FIGURE 9–13.
Poikiloderma atrophicans vasculare. H&E. X285.

this group is focal basal cell damage, so-called liquefaction degeneration, with the cascade of events that we found in the lichenoid tissue reaction, only in milder form, and spotty distribution corresponding to the clinical mottling. There is variable epidermal thickness from slight hyperplasia to definite atrophy. Epidermal pigmentation is focal, and there is macrophage pigmentation (Fig. 9-13). Spotty telangiectasia and loss of superficial elastic fibers complete the picture of the poikilodermatous tissue reaction, to which the underlying dermatoses add their distinctive features. Thus, the appearances illustrated in Figs. 5-13, 9-11A, 14-2, and 14-3 should evoke the thought that one is dealing with poikiloderma.

The confusion arising from so many dermatoses resembling each other clinically and histologically is perhaps closer to a solution if one considers the recent literature on graft-vs-host reaction.[33] Poikilodermatous features with sclerosis are described in many cases. Basal cell damage may be the underlying feature, leading to a variety of clinical and histologic consequences. Investigations of individual cases with modern immunofluorescent and histochemical methods may bring some clarity in the next five years.

LICHEN RUBER MONILIFORMIS (KAPOSI)

This old dermatosis, always observed as individual rare cases, has been described under a variety of names, *keratosis lichenoides chronica* (Fig. 9-14)

being the most modern one.[34] The clinical picture is striking: bands of moniliform firm papules forming a netlike pattern. The histologic picture of some cases has been similar to lichen planus, and in other cases it has varied widely. In a case[35] involving the lower extremities of a young woman, a most unexpected solution offered itself. After unsuccessful treatment for many years, the introduction of a new tranquilizing drug (chlorpromazine) led to remarkable improvement. The patient's younger brother has epidermolysis bullosa simplex, and the patient admitted scratching at repeatedly forming milia (obstructed sweat ducts) on her legs. In this one case, the moniliform eruption was an artifact.

LICHEN NITIDUS

The supposed nosologic relation of lichen nitidus to lichen planus is based on the fact that a very early lichen planus papule may indeed be almost indistinguishable from a lichen nitidus papule under the microscope. However, the lichen planus papule invariably grows and becomes confluent with others to form a plaque, while the lichen nitidus lesion never exceeds a certain small size, and the papules retain their individuality even if closely grouped.[36] In addition, the typical lichen nitidus papule (Fig. 9-15) has a central parakeratotic cap, often associated with a slight clinical depression of the epidermis. This feature is exaggerated in palmar lesions[37] and has considerable diagnostic significance because it is practically never found in li-

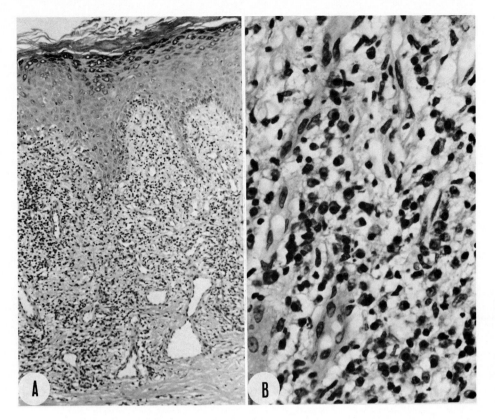

FIGURE 9–14.
*Keratosis lichenoides chronica. **A.** Picture resembles lichen planus, but the infiltrate is not so dense. **B.** Mixed infiltrate includes many plasma cells. (From Nabai and Mehregan. J Am Acad Dermatol 2:217, 1980.)*

chen planus. The common denominator of both dermatoses appears to be damage to basal cells and/or melanocytes. The dermal reaction in lichen nitidus is definitely granulomatous. Often, especially in pigmented skin, it contains a multinucleated giant cell full of melanin. In contrast to lichen planus, there are no deposits of γ-globulin.[38] The almost globular little granuloma resembles a ball pressed against the epidermis from below. The epidermis is thin, completely free of pigment, and

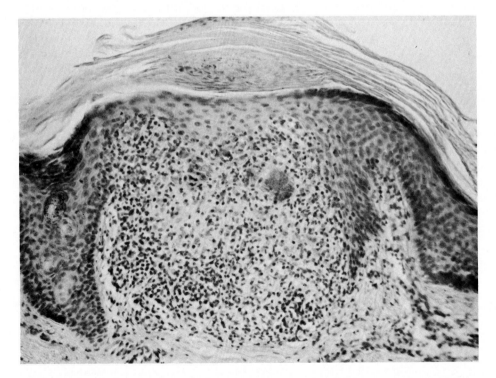

FIGURE 9–15.
Lichen nitidus papule in characteristic (but not universal) location close to a sweat duct. Note absence of granular layer and parakeratosis. The infiltrate appears granulomatous and contains a multinucleated giant cell. Pictures of this type suggested relations to tuberculosis to earlier observers, a concept which is now forgotten. H&E. X180.

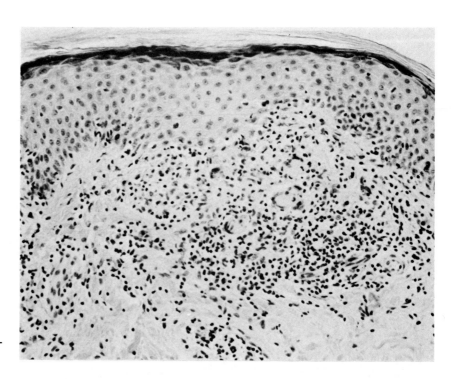

FIGURE 9–16.
Lichenoid eruption due to gold injections. H&E. X150.

lacks a basal layer. In the diagnostic examination for lichen nitidus, it is essential to have serial sections. Otherwise, one may miss the small papule or get only a misleading tangential cut.

LICHENOID DRUG ERUPTIONS AND OTHER LICHENOID LESIONS

The clinical impression of a lichenoid drug eruption is often reflected histologically in hyperkeratosis of the epidermis and spotty damage to basal cells (Fig. 9-16). However, the inflammatory infiltrate usually is perivascular and lymphocytic or mixed and does not have the specific localization and composition of lichen planus. Parakeratosis often is present, while it is a rare feature in lichen planus.[39] A startling dermatosis was seen toward the end of World War II in men who had taken chloroquin hydrochloride (Atabrine) for prolonged periods. The histologic picture of this atypical lichenoid dermatitis[40] was variable, with epidermal acanthosis and atrophy, and, in many cases, led to permanent dermal atrophy and to atrophy of sweat ducts and anhidrosis. Psoriasiform lesions showing the histologic picture of lichen planus have been seen after practolol intake.[41] These cases are mentioned here as a reminder that the field of lichenoid tissue reactions probably is not exhausted by the dermatoses discussed in this chapter.

Other dermatoses carrying the name of lichen have quite different histologic features.[3] Lichen simplex has been discussed under the eczematous reactions (Chap. 7); lichen sclerosus et atrophicus will be dealt with in the chapter on scleroderma (Chap. 25), and lichen striatus under the papulosquamous eruptions, where pityriasis lichenoides also will be found (Chap. 13). Still other lichens are listed in the index. It must be mentioned here that the histologic differential diagnosis between lichen planus and lupus erythematosus in extrafacial localization may be extremely difficult (Chap. 14) and that a lichen-planus-like histologic picture may be encountered in syphilis.

REFERENCES

1. Saurat JH, Gluckman E, Bussel A, et al.: The lichen planus-like eruption after bone marrow transplantation. Br J Dermatol 93:675, 1975
2. Pinkus H: Lichenoid tissue reactions. A speculative review of the clinical spectrum of epidermal basal cell damage with special reference to erythema dyschromicum perstans. Arch Dermatol 107:840, 1973
3. Pinkus H: How useful is biopsy in a lichenoid eruption? Cutis 20:651, 1977
4. Ebner H, Gebhart W: Light and electron microscopic differentiation of amyloid and colloid or hyaline bodies. Br J Dermatol 92:637, 1975
5. Ebner H, Gebhart W: Epidermal changes in lichen planus. J Cutan Pathol 3:167, 1976
6. Ebner H, Gebhart W, Lassman H, Jurecka W: The epidermal cell proliferation in lichen planus. Acta Derm Venereol (Stockh) 57:133, 1977
7. Bullough WS: The control of epidermal thickness. Br J Dermatol 87:187, 1972

8. Hendren OS, Pinkus H: Observations on the reaction of chronic inflammatory dermatoses and of normal skin to varied concentrations of thorium X. J Invest Dermatol 22:463, 1954

9. Bjorke JR, Krogh HK: Identification of mononuclear cells in situ in skin lesions of lichen planus. Br J Dermatol 98:605, 1978

10. Grogan TM, Odom RL, Burgen JH: Graft-vs-host reaction. Arch Dermatol 113:806, 1977

11. Juliusberg F: Lichen ruber and pityriasis rubra pilaris. In Jadassohn J (ed): Handbuch der Haut-und Geschlechtskrankheiten. Berlin, Springer-Verlag, 1931, Vol. 7, Part 2, p 36

12. Sobel S, Miller R, Shatin R: Lichen planus pemphigoides. Immunofluorescence findings. Arch Dermatol 112:1280, 1976

13. Bologa EI, Luncan Malene G, Stroe A: Considerations cliniques, histopathologiques et histochimiques sur le lichen plan pigmentaire d'emblée. Arch Belg Dermatol, 28:85, 1972

14. Grupper C, Buisson J, Durepaire R, et al.: Lichen plan invisible de Gougerot. Bull Soc Fr Derm Syphiligr 78:598, 1972

15. Shima T: Supplementative study on lichen pigmentosus. Jpn J Dermatol 66:353, 1956

16. Bhutani LK, Bedi TR, Pandhi RK, et al.: Lichen planus pigmentosus. Dermatologica 149:43, 1974

17. Convit J, Kerdel-Vegas F, Rodriguez G: Erythema dyschromicum perstans. A hitherto undescribed skin disease. J Invest Dermatol 36:457, 1961

18. Ramirez CO: Dermatosis cenicienta. Dermatología Méx 7:232, 1963

19. Knox JM, Dodge BG, Freeman RG: Erythema dyschromicum perstans. Arch Dermatol 97:262, 1968

20. Byrne DA, Berger RS: Erythema dyschromicum perstans; a report of two cases in fair-skinned patients. Acta Derm Venereol (Stockh) 54:65, 1974

21. Holst R, Mobacken H: Erythema dyschromicum perstans (ashy dermatosis). Acta Derm Venereol (Stockh) 54:69, 1974

22. El-Zawahri M: Lichen planus tropicus. Derm Int 4:92, 1965

23. Verhagen ARHB, Koten JW: Lichenoid melanodermatitis. A clinicopathological study of 51 Kenyan patients with so-called tropical lichen planus. Br J Dermatol 101:651, 1979

24. Lumpkin LR, Helwig EB: Solitary lichen planus. Arch Dermatol 93:54, 1966

25. Shapiro L, Ackerman AB: Solitary lichen planus-like keratosis. Dermatologica 132:386, 1966

26. Hirsch P, Marmelzat WL: Lichenoid actinic keratosis. Derm Int 6:101, 1967

27. Mehregan AH: Lentigo senilis and its evolutions. J Invest Dermatol 65:428, 1975

28. Lever WF, Schaumburg-Lever G: Histopathology of the Skin, 5th ed. Philadelphia, Lippincott, 1975

29. Milne JA: An Introduction to the Diagnostic Histopathology of the Skin. London, Edward Arnold, 1972

30. Wozniak KD, Böhm W: Zum Problem der Poikilodermia congenita Thomson. Z Hautkr 47:625, 1972

31. Nazzaro P, Argentieri R, Bassetti F, et al.: Dyskératose congénitale de Zinsser-Cole-Engman, deux cas. Bull Soc Fr Derm Syphiligr 79:242, 1972

32. Greer KE, Weary PE, Nagy R, Robinow M: Hereditary sclerosing poikiloderma. Int J Dermatol 17:316, 1978

33. Claudy AL, Schmitt D, Freycon F: Graft-vs-host reaction in skin: histological, immunological and ultrastructural studies. Acta Derm Venereol (Stockh) 59:7, 1979

34. Petrozzi JW: Keratosis lichenoides chronica. Possible variant of lichen planus. Arch Dermatol 112:709, 1976

35. Pinkus H: Lichen ruber moniliformis (Kaposi). Arch Dermatol 71:543, 1935

36. Pinkus H, Shair HM: Koebner phenomenon in lichen nitidus. Arch Dermatol 65:82, 1952

37. Weiss RM, Cohen AD: Lichen nitidus of the palms and soles. Arch Dermatol 104:538, 1971

38. Waisman M, Dundon BC, Michel NB: Immunofluorescent studies in lichen nitidus. Arch Dermatol 107:200, 1973

39. Penneys NS, Ackerman AB, Gottlieb NL: Gold dermatitis: a clinical and histopathological study. Arch Dermatol 109:372, 1974

40. Alden HS, Frank LJ: Atypical lichenoid dermatitis. A drug eruption due to quinacrine hydrochloride (Atabrine). Arch Dermatol 56:13, 1947

41. Cochran RET, Thomson J, Fleming K, McQueen A: The psoriasiform eruption induced by practolol. J Cutan Pathol 2:314, 1975

CHAPTER

10

Toxic, Allergic, and Multiform Erythemas

In clinical dermatology, the word *erythema* is attached as a diagnostic term to several manifestations, some of which are characterized only by redness, while others exhibit more or less pronounced swelling and induration and, in some cases, lead to blistering. None of them, however, have scales or other evidence of primary epidermal disease. Correspondingly, in this chapter, emphasis shifts from the epidermis to the dermis, although the epidermis may show highly diagnostic alterations. The diagram of Figure 10-1 illustrates morphologic relations rather than nosologic ones. It is grouped around a vascular reaction which includes endothelial swelling and evidence of vascular permeability in the form of edema and cellular exudate. The latter, as it is common in the skin, consists mainly of small round cells which we call "lymphocytes" for convenience. Usually, there are at least a few eosinophils, while neutrophils may be absent or present. They predominate in Sweet's syndrome. Changes of this type may be found without epidermal changes in acute and chronic urticaria and in eruptions due to drugs. They may be combined with eczematous epidermal reaction in atopic dermatitis and the dermal type of contact sensitivity reaction as discussed in Chapter 7. If there is morphologic evidence of leukocytoclasia, granulomatous infiltration of vessel walls, or vascular necrosis, we deal with a true vasculitis, and these phenomena will be left for Chapter 15. This chapter is devoted mainly to urticaria and to a type of tissue reaction which finds its most complete expression in idiopathic erythema exudativum multiforme. In addition, the role of eosinophils in skin disease will be considered.

URTICARIA

The wheal of *acute urticaria*, in keeping with its fleeting clinical course, is characterized mainly by dermal edema, which is difficult to recognize in paraffin sections, and by some endothelial swelling of small vessels of the superficial plexus and a few eosinophils around them. Somewhat more chronic cases (Fig. 10-2) merge with the picture of toxic erythema, as defined later.

Lichen Urticatus

The tense and quickly excoriated superficial vesicle of so-called *papular urticaria*, also known as *lichen urticatus*, and in Europe by the picturesque and noncommittal name *strophulus*, is a tissue reaction most commonly seen in young children as an allergic reaction to insect bites.[1,2] Inasmuch as the characteristic mid-dermal reaction of ordinary insect bites (see below) is absent, it would seem likely that one or a few bites provoke a crop of ur-

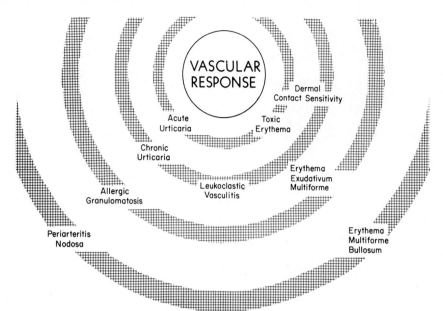

FIGURE 10–1.
Diagram of morphologic relations of various entities involving vascular response and vasculitis, used as a guide in differential diagnosis.

ticated lesions as an allergic reaction in previously affected sites. Histologically, pronounced perivascular infiltrate and edema of the dermis is associated with a spongiotic epidermal vesicle containing eosinophils in lesions that have not been excoriated. The resulting protruding papule is almost conical and strictly limited to the reacting focus (Fig. 10-3). A somewhat similar picture may be encountered in minor viral exanthems (Chap. 12).

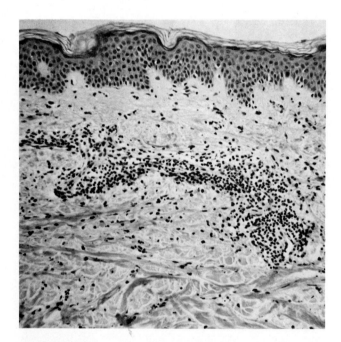

FIGURE 10–2.
Chronic urticaria, representing purest type of reversible inflammatory vascular response of superficial plexus. H&E. X135.

Insect Bites

The histologic hallmark of real insect (mosquito, flea) bites is a mid-dermal center of reaction, which corresponds to the site of deposition of the toxin and may vary from plain edema to tissue necrosis surrounded by heavy perivascular infiltrate including round cells, fragmenting polymorphs, and often eosinophils. Depending on the severity of the damage and the allergic response of the host, features of true vasculitis and of granulomatous inflammation may be present (Chaps. 15 and 21). Long-lasting reactions to arthropod bites are discussed in Chapter 44.

ERYTHEMA EXUDATIVUM MULTIFORME

We are dealing here with the typical Hebra type of erythema multiforme, which has sudden onset and spontaneously involutes within a few weeks. Those cases that formerly were considered chronic forms of erythema multiforme and are now recognized as bullous pemphigoid will be considered in Chapter 11.

Figure 10-4 is a low-power view in which the three zones of the clinical *iris lesion* can be identified: peripheral erythema, intermediate swelling, and central bulla with epidermal necrosis. It is noteworthy that in erythema multiforme, in contrast to the punctiform changes scattered through the lesion of eczematous dermatitis and psoriasis, we are dealing with a zonal arrangement. This has to be kept in mind in the examination of a section,

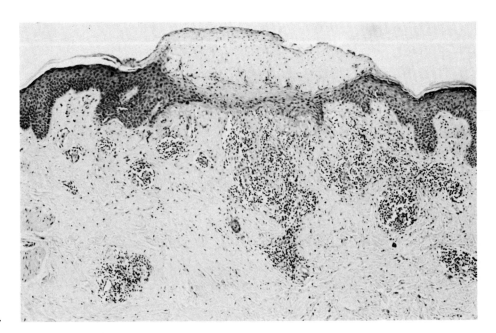

FIGURE 10–3.
Lichen urticatus. H&E. X135.

which preferably should come from a radial biopsy specimen, including all zones.[3]

The earliest changes in the advancing rim of the lesion are inflammatory infiltrate around small subpapillary vessels. The infiltrate often contains neutrophils in addition to lymphocytes; the percentage of eosinophils varies but usually is not high. The inflammatory changes may also affect the pars reticularis. Toward the center, as dermal edema increases, the epidermis also becomes affected by intercellular edema. This stretches all the cells vertical to the skin surface because the stream of exudate is stopped at the granular layer, which, together with the horny layer, remains unaltered. This purely passive edema (Fig. 10-5) of the epidermis is highly characteristic. It does not lead to spongiosis and intraepidermal vesiculation. In other cases, many keratinocytes become pyknotic and

even necrotic (Fig. 10-6), but there is barely any evidence of epidermal proliferation or parakeratosis. Centrally, in the full-blown lesion, bullous edema of the papillae leads to separation between epidermis and dermis. A subepidermal bulla is formed (Table 11-1), the roof of which consists of the entire epidermis in a state of degeneration or necrosis. Shreds of connective tissue fibers often remain attached to the lower epidermal surface. At the same time, the entire thickness of the dermis may become involved with pronounced inflammatory infiltrate, edema, and even hemorrhage. As the lesion extends, the acuteness of the process subsides in the center, the bulla collapses, and the damaged epidermis is eliminated as a necrotic or hemorrhagic crust.

The tissue reaction is similar, whether we are dealing with an idiopathic or postherpetic case of

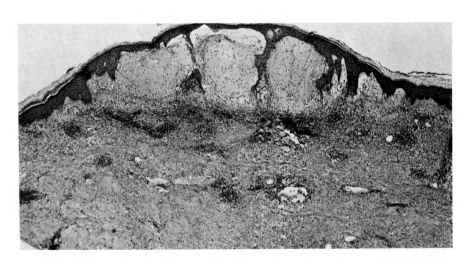

FIGURE 10–4.
Erythema exudativum multiforme exhibiting three concentric regions—vasodilatation (erythema), inflammatory edema, and central subepidermal vesiculation. In later stages, the center of the bulla collapses and dries, producing the clinical target lesion. H&E. X75.

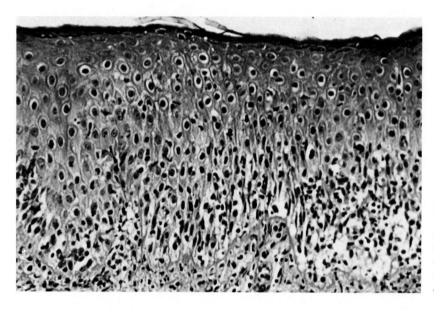

FIGURE 10–5.
Characteristic epidermal edema of erythema multiforme. All cells are elongated vertical to skin surface, nuclei are pyknotic, and there is intracellular and intercellular edema. Granular layer is present, and horny layer, if preserved, would be orthokeratotic. H&E. X180. (From Pinkus. Ann Allergy 12:67, 1954.)

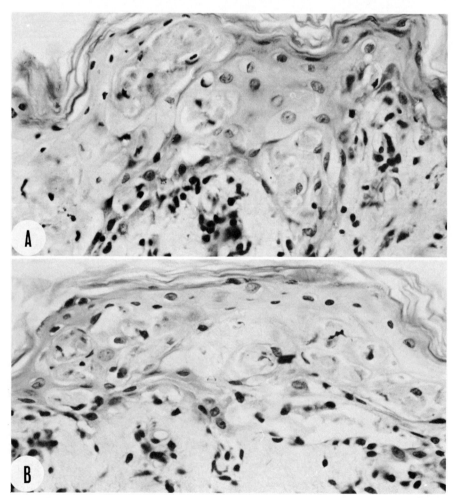

FIGURE 10–6.
Epidermal cell necrosis in erythema multiforme. In these cases, infiltrate in the dermis may be sparse, and the histologic picture may be similar to that of toxic epidermal necrolysis (Chap. 11). This has been called the "epidermal type" of erythema multiforme. H&E. X400.

erythema exudativum multiforme, with a *bullous drug eruption*,[4] or with a lesion secondary to systemic infection. Variations may occur in the number of eosinophils or in the severity of the inflammation. Deposition of immune complexes in the wall of small superficial vessels has been found.[5] Eosinophils may be very numerous, raising the suspicion of bullous disease (Chap. 11). Early and not very severe lesions of *paravaccinia* (Chap. 12) may exhibit features very similar to acute erythema multiforme in the prebullous phase. It must be understood that the bulla is the final and most severe manifestation of erythema exudativum multiforme, that not every lesion proceeds to this stage, and that a biopsy specimen of an early papule may not show a bulla. It is in these cases that epidermal edema of the type illustrated in Figure 10-5 is especially helpful in diagnosis.

Ackerman et al.[6] have emphasized involvement of the dermoepidermal interface with individual necrotized keratinocytes, vacuolar alteration of basal cells (Fig. 10-6), and sparse lymphohistiocytic infiltrate as the earliest manifestations of what they consider the true Hebra type of erythema exudativum multiforme. Orfanos et al.[7] divide erythema multiforme into dermal and epidermal types. There are, no doubt, iris lesions in which inflammatory cellular exudate is practically absent, while the epidermis undergoes acute necrosis and separates from the dermis. The histologic picture, then, is almost indistinguishable from the adult form of *toxic epidermal necrolysis*, which will be discussed in Chapter 11. Iris-type lesions resembling erythema multiforme, but presenting the histologic picture of polyarteritis nodosa, may be found in Kawasaki's disease (Chap. 15).

TOXIC ERYTHEMA

When a biopsy section shows superficial perivascular inflammatory changes without any appreciable epidermal involvement and without evidence of vasculitis, we prefer to label it *toxic erythema* as a generic morphologic diagnosis. In this group are cases of *chronic urticaria* (Fig. 10-2), *erythema marginatum*,[8] *drug eruptions* (Fig. 10-7) of morbilliform, plaque or other papular types, *papular eruptions of pregnancy* (Chap. 11), and the various forms of *erythema perstans*.[9] Histologic differentiation within this group is extremely difficult and must remain tentative, subject to clinical evaluation.

Erythema Annulare Centrifugum

However, many cases of erythema annulare centrifugum (Fig. 10-8) may be identified with some confidence because the infiltrate is unusually heavy and extends into the deeper parts of the dermis. It may resemble Jessner's lymphocytic infiltration (Chap. 14), or it may include larger mononuclear

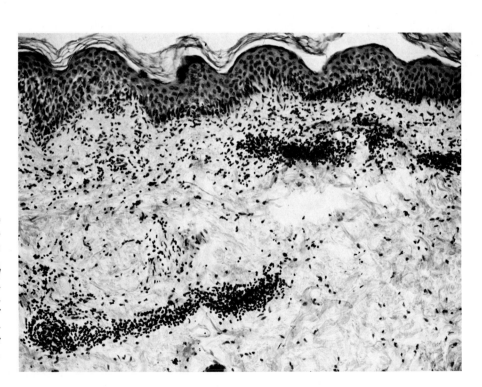

FIGURE 10–7.
Toxic erythema type of drug eruption. While there is some exocytosis and mild intercellular edema in the lower epidermal layers, there is no significant epidermal reaction as in eczematous dermatitis. In differentiation from parapsoriasis en plaques (Figs. 13-7 and 13-8), the infiltrate here is almost purely lymphocytic and may contain some eosinophils. H&E. X135.

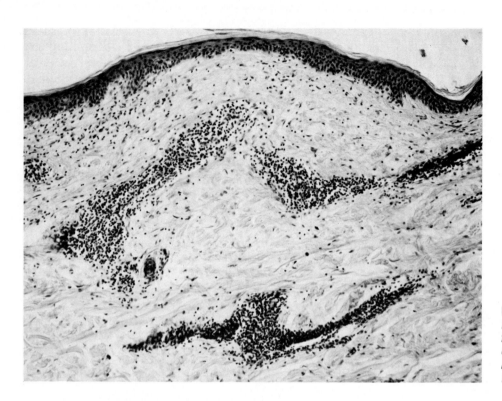

FIGURE 10–8.
Erythema annulare centrifugum. Infiltrate involves the deep vascular plexus. No significant epidermal changes. H&E. X135.

cells and require differentiation from certain types of lymphoma (Chap. 44). Cases have been seen in infants of mothers who had lupus erythematosus.[10]

Erythema Chronicum Migrans

Erythema chronicum migrans has been known in Europe for many years, but recently cases have cropped up in America. It was known to follow tick bite and to be curable with high doses of penicillin. It also can be transferred by inoculation of involved skin. Etiology, however, is undetermined. Recently, it has been found in association with a peculiar type of arthritis.[11] Histologically, there is lymphocytic and histiocytic infiltrate around superficial blood vessels, and a diagnosis can be made only by correlating clinical and histologic features.[12]

Erythema Gyratum Repens

The name *erythema gyratum repens* was given by Gammel[13] to an extraordinary, figurate, scaling erythema that moved from day to day and disappeared after removal of a carcinoma of the breast. In every reported case but one, the eruption was associated with malignancy, in about half of the cases with carcinoma of the bronchus, and improvement usually was noted after successful treatment of the cancer. The one exception is Barber's patient,[14]

who had tuberculosis of the lung. The eruption is remarkable clinically because of its slow movement, configuration, and evidence of a scale on the subsiding border. Histologic examination has not been helpful in explaining this configuration. Mild parakeratosis is reported, in addition to variable superficial dermal infiltrate. Holt and Davies[15] reported an absence of T lymphocytes and coarse granular deposits of IgG and C3 at the basement membrane. The peculiar necrotizing dermatosis associated with carcinoma of the pancreas will be discussed in Chapter 11.

Differential Diagnosis. Differential diagnosis of all forms of toxic erythema includes cases of vasculitis of the small dermal vessels (Chap. 15), papules of secondary syphilis (Chap. 20), the pigmented purpuric eruptions and some other papulosquamous dermatoses (Chap. 13), and dermal contact sensitivity reaction (Chap. 7), which itself may resemble eruptions due to photosensitivity. It is obvious that definite conclusions are extremely difficult in this field and that the histologic diagnosis of toxic erythema should be made by exclusion if no signs of more specific alterations of either epidermis or vessels or other constituents of the dermis can be recognized. When we have settled on the diagnosis "toxic erythema," we often add "compatible with drug eruption" in order to stimulate the clinician to make a thorough search, not only for medicaments but also for the possible role of food additives and other ingested chemicals, which are not classified as drugs.

ACUTE FEBRILE NEUTROPHILIC DERMATOSIS AND ERYSIPELAS

Sweet, who described the dermatosis in 1964,[16] recently reviewed more than 100 published cases of an acute febrile syndrome,[17] in which the patient develops multiple erythematous plaques, not too dissimilar clinically from an acute attack of erythema multiforme. Histologically, there are edema and heavy exudate of polymorphonuclear neutrophilic leukocytes around dermal blood vessels (Fig. 10-9), a picture rarely encountered in the skin except in cases of acute *cellulitis* and *erysipelas.* Demonstration of gram-positive cocci in the latter may assist in differential diagnosis. A similar picture has been reported in the erysipelaslike skin lesions of *familial Mediterranean fever.*[18] Absence of vascular damage and so-called toxic hyalin rules out erythema elevatum diutinum (Chap. 15). The cause of *Sweet's syndrome* is unknown.

HYPEREOSINOPHILIC SYNDROME

The presence of eosinophils in many of the lesions discussed in this chapter makes it advisable to discuss eosinophilia in context, especially since the introduction of the hypereosinophilic syndrome and its various manifestations into the literature.[19] The occurrence of an increased eosinophil count in the peripheral blood triggers a search for allergic reactions, for intestinal parasites, and for dermatitis herpetiformis by the classically trained physician. The finding of eosinophils in tissue sections should stimulate suspicion of entities other than those mentioned in this chapter. It is known that intraepidermal vesicles in the newborn often carry eosinophils (Chap. 18). Urticaria pigmentosa develops eosinophilia after stroking. Eosinophilic spongiosis may be found in pemphigus (Chap. 11). In granulomatous inflammation, eosinophils take on special significance, as discussed in Chapter 21. Kimura's disease or angiolymphoid hyperplasia with eosinophils (Chap. 44) comes to mind. Scabies and tick bites often are rich in eosinophils. Thus, eosinophils in blood or tissues are a warning signal that should be carefully evaluated and put into correlation with other pathologic and clinical signs.

The hypereosinophilic syndrome ranges from cases with frank eosinophilic leukemia to angioedema and urticaria and to almost asymptomatic cases with erythematous skin lesions and abnormal echocardiograms. Each case requires careful evaluation, and one should not forget that a routine H&E stain may show eosinophils very poorly, and O&G stain may be required.

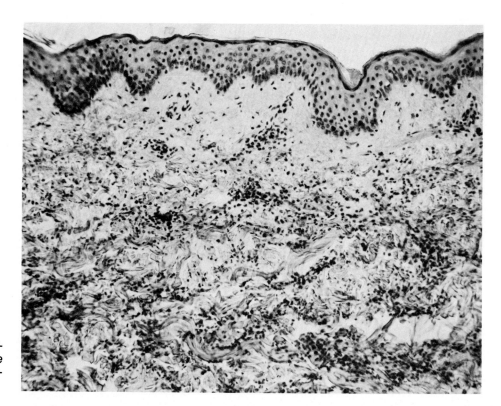

FIGURE 10–9.
Acute febrile neutrophilic dermatosis (Sweet). Most of the cells of the infiltrate have polymorphic nuclei. H&E. X225.

REFERENCES

1. Shaffer F, Jacobson C, Beerman H: Histopathologic correlation of lesions of papular urticaria and positive skin test reactions to insect antigens. Arch Dermatol 70:437, 1954
2. Bazex A, Bazex J, Broussy F, Balas D: Étude anatomopathologique optique et ultra-structurale des papules de prurigo strophulus en phase de début. Bull Soc Fr Derm Syphiligr 82:369, 1975
3. Bedi TR, Pinkus H: Histopathological spectrum of erythema multiforme. BR J Dermatol 95:243, 1976
4. Kauppinen K: Cutaneous reactions to drugs; with special reference to severe bullous mucocutaneous eruptions and sulfonamides. Acta Derm Venereol [Suppl] (Stockh) 68, 1972
5. Kazmierowski JA, Wuepper KD: Erythema multiforme: immune complex vasculitis of the superficial cutaneous microvasculature. J Invest Dermatol 71:366, 1978
6. Ackerman AB, Penneys NS, Clark WH: Erythema multiforme exudativum: distinctive pathological process. Br J Dermatol 84:554, 1971
7. Orfanos CE, Schaumburg-Lever G, Lever WF: Dermal and epidermal types of erythema multiforme. Arch Dermatol 109:682, 1974
8. Brauner GJ, Mihm MC Jr, Des Groseilliers JP: Erythema marginatum in streptococcal endocarditis without rheumatic heart disease. Cutis 12:206, 1973
9. Ellis F, Friedman AA: Erythema annulare centrifugum (Darier's). Arch Dermatol 70:496, 1954
10. Hammar H, Rönnerfält L: Annular erythemas in infants associated with autoimmune disorders in their mothers. Dermatologica 154:115, 1977
11. Dryer RF, Goellner PG, Carney AS: Lyme arthritis in Wisconsin. JAMA 241:498, 1979
12. Goette DK, Odom RB: Erythema chronicum migrans in three soldiers. Int J Dermatol 17:732, 1978
13. Gammel JA: Erythema gyratum repens. Skin manifestations in patient with carcinoma of the breast. Arch Dermatol 66:494, 1952
14. Barber PV, Doyle L, Vickers DM, Hubbard H: Erythema gyratum repens with pulmonary tuberculosis. Br J Dermatol 98:465, 1978
15. Holt PJA, Davies MG: Erythema gyratum repens—an immunologically mediated dermatosis? Br J Dermatol 96:343, 1977
16. Sweet RD: An acute febrile neutrophilic dermatosis. Br J Dermatol 76:349, 1964
17. Sweet RD: Acute febrile neutrophilic dermatosis— 1978. Br J Dermatol 100:93, 1979
18. Azizi E, Fisher BK: Cutaneous manifestations of familial Mediterranean fever. Arch Dermatol 112:364, 1976
19. Kazmierewski JA, Chusid MJ, Parrillo JE, et al.: Dermatologic manifestations of the hypereosinophilic syndrome. Arch Dermatol 114:531, 1978

CHAPTER
11
Vesicular and Bullous Diseases

The skin can produce vesicles and bullae from many different causes, by many different mechanisms, and in all the different layers from the stratum corneum of the epidermis to the stratum papillare of the dermis. The various possibilities are listed in Table 11-1.

Some types of blistering were discussed under eczematous, psoriasiform, lichenoid, and erythematous tissue reactions. Others will be taken up in Chapters 12, 28, 29, and 44. In the present chapter, we deal mainly with *pemphigus vulgaris, dermatitis herpetiformis*, their variants, and other disorders in which the formation of vesicles or bullae is the outstanding characteristic. The entire field has been intensively investigated in recent years, especially by the new techniques of electron microscopy and immunofluorescence,[1] and new data and concepts have been contributed. As could be expected, many of these findings have been helpful in making diagnoses and separating previously confused diseases. Other data have confused lines of separation or have taught us that a patient may suffer from two diseases at the same time.

It has long been known that epidermal cells, when isolated from their neighbors, quickly acquire smooth contours, and desmosomes (prickles, Chap. 2) disappear. We now know that desmosomes split in acantholytic disease, while the joint remains temporarily intact and cells become motile as a result of breaks in the plasma membrane in certain types of injury, such as tape stripping,[2] and perhaps in other dermatoses. Moreover, serum of pemphigus patients contains antibodies against intercellular cement, while these are not present in

other diseases, such as subcorneal pustular dermatosis, in which acantholytic cells may occur. The presence of anti-basement-membrane antibody in patients with bullous pemphigoid correlates well with the light microscopic impression of a clean separation at this level and adds a welcome tool to the differential diagnosis of erythema multiforme and dermatitis herpetiformis in which such antibodies have not been found. Finding and identifying deposits of immunoglobulins and factors of complement at the basement membrane have become helpful procedures. Another new and highly specific feature is the disintegration of basal cells in epidermolysis bullosa simplex, demonstrated by electron microscopy.[3] Many of the details are beyond the scope of histopathologic examination and, therefore, of this book. We must, however, keep in mind that more intricate methods are available and must seek the help of experts in puzzling cases.

ACANTHOLYTIC DISORDERS

While acantholysis is also a basic feature in Hailey-Hailey's and Darier's diseases, these will be discussed in Chapter 28 as inborn errors of epidermal metabolism, and we concentrate here on pemphigus vulgaris and its relatives. Of these, pemphigus vegetans is the closest kin, while pemphigus foliaceus and pemphigus erythematosus, owing to the higher level at which acantholysis occurs, seem to form a separate group histologically as well as clinically. Acrodermatitis enteropathica will be mentioned in differential diagnosis.

TABLE 11–1.
Vesiculobullous Eruptions

Diagnosis	Level of Separation	Characteristics of Epidermis	Histomechanism	Prevalent Inflammatory Cells
Eczematous dermatitis	Prickle layer	Spongiosis	Intercellular edema	Lymphocytes and PMNs
Impetigo	Subcorneal	Mild edema	Exocytosis	PMNs
Subcorneal pustular dermatosis	Subcorneal	Acantholysis, minimal	Exocytosis	PMNs
Pustulosis palmaris et plantaris	Subcorneal	Compressed below bulla	Exocytosis and transmalpighian exudate	PMNs and lymphocytes
Psoriasiform eruptions	Suprapapillary	Spongiform pustule, microabscess	Squirting papilla	PMNs in epidermis, lymphocytes in dermis
Impetigo herpetiformis	Suprapapillary	Spongiform pustule, microabscess	Suprapapillary exudate and acantholysis	PMNs, lymphocytes
Benign familial pemphigus	Suprabasal	Intraepidermal lacunae and budding ridges	Acantholysis	Lymphocytes
Pemphigus vulgaris	Suprabasal	Intraepidermal bulla	Acantholysis	Lymphocytes, some eosinophils
Pemphigus vegetans	Suprabasal, extending into hair follicles	Vegetating hyperplasia, clefts	Acantholysis	Lymphocytes, plasma cells, eosinophils
Pemphigus foliaceus	Subgranular or intragranular	Intraepidermal clefts	Acantholysis	Lymphocytes, some eosinophils
Acrodermatitis enteropathica	Suprabasal or higher	Acanthosis, partial necrosis, parakeratosis	Derangement of lipid metabolism, zinc deficiency	Mixed
Pemphigoid, bullous	Subepidermal	Complete and viable	Junctional separation	Lymphocytes, eosinophils, PMNs
Pemphigoid, cicatricial	Subepidermal	Viable	Junctional separation	Granulation tissue
Dermatitis herpetiformis	Subepidermal	Complete and viable or basal cell necrosis	Papillary necrosis, junctional separation	PMNs, lymphocytes, eosinophils
Chronic bullous dermatosis of childhood	Subepidermal	Viable	Junctional separation	Mixed
Herpes gestationis	Intradermal	Necrosis of basal cells	Papillary edema, HG factor	Mixed, eosinophils
Erythema multiforme	Intradermal	Primary or secondary necrosis	Bullous papillary edema, focal malpighian necrosis	PMNs, lymphocytes
Toxic epidermal necrolysis (TEN), infantile	Intraepidermal	Necrosis of upper half	Staphylococcal toxin	Minimal
TEN, adult type	Subepidermal	Complete necrosis	Drug sensitivity or unknown	Minimal

TABLE 11–1. (continued)

Diagnosis	Level of Separation	Characteristics of Epidermis	Histomechanism	Prevalent Inflammatory Cells
Porphyria cutanea tarda	Subepidermal	Complete and viable	Junctional separation with persistent papillae	Minimal
Epidermolysis bullosa simplex	Subepidermal	Viable above basal layer	Basal cell edema and necrosis	Mild
Epidermolysis dystrophica	Intradermal	Viable	Absence of anchoring fibrils	Variable
Glucagonoma syndrome	Upper epidermal layers	Acanthotic, parakeratotic	Degeneration of upper prickle cells	Polymorphs, mixed
Intranuclear viruses	Prickle layer	Necrotizing, multinucleated giant cells	Reticulating and ballooning degeneration	Mild to severe, lymphocytes, PMNs
Cytoplasmic viruses	Prickle layer	Degenerating	Cellular edema and death	Lymphocytes, PMNs
Bullous incontinentia pigmenti	Prickle layer	Often acanthotic	Toxic?	Eosinophils
Epidermolytic hyperkeratosis	Granular layer	Hyperplastic	Granular cell rupture	Absent
Burn blisters	Subepidermal	Necrotic	Death of epidermis and dermis	Inconspicuous

Pemphigus Vulgaris

Vesiculation in pemphigus is intraepidermal and usually suprabasal. In contrast to the spongiotic edema of eczematous dermatitis which eventually leads to the rupture of intercellular bridges, and also in contrast to the reticulating degeneration of infected epidermal cells in viral diseases (Chap. 12), the bulla of pemphigus results from primary acantholytic separation between keratinocytes above the basal layer. The early stage can be seen under the light microscope as a cleft between basal layer and lower prickle cells and between the latter (Fig. 11-1). Electron microscopic and immunofluorescent observations suggest that the intercellular cement is affected and that desmosomes split before they disappear. Fluid accumulates in the clefts thus created, and the acantholytic cells lie in the bulla like grains of sand. They show peculiar degenerative processes (Fig. 11-2), expressed in a washed-out appearance of the nucleus and a basophilic outer rim of the cytoplasm. Inflammatory infiltrate of moderate amount is usually present in the upper dermis. It is made up of lymphocytes with variable, but usually small, numbers of eosinophils.

The roof of the bulla consists of the fairly intact upper layers of the epidermis, the base of the isolated basal layer, often presenting the appearance of a row of tombstones (Figs. 11-3 and 45-3), still adherent to the dermis. It is important to biopsy early blisters, preferably not older than 24 hours, because later lesions may show too much degeneration of the roof and disintegration of the base or, on the other hand, beginning reepithelization. It is the acantholytic prickle cells and the residual basal cells that are obtained by the Tzanck procedure (Chap. 3) and are seen in the stained smear (Fig. 11-2B).

Pemphigus Vegetans

Acantholysis in pemphigus vegetans usually is suprabasal as in pemphigus vulgaris but becomes very extensive and often descends deep into hair follicles. Simultaneously, the epidermis becomes thickened and papillomatous, and a heavy inflammatory infiltrate develops, characterized by a high percentage of plasma cells in addition to lymphocytes, and often by eosinophils which may form intraepithe-

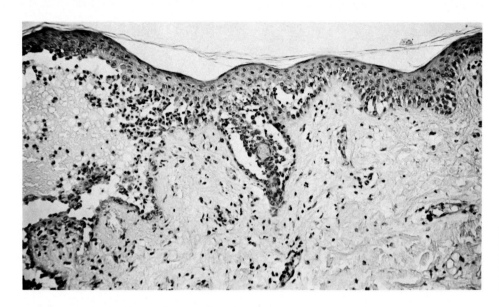

FIGURE 11–1.
Pemphigus vulgaris, edge of bulla. Note acantholysis extending along a sweat duct. H&E. X135.

lial microabscesses. Bullae often are not formed, and the histologic picture (Fig. 11-3) reflects the mushy vegetations seen clinically.

Pemphigus Foliaceus, Pemphigus Erythematosus

The acantholytic cleft usually forms in higher strata, often in the granular layer (Fig. 11-4), in pemphigus foliaceus and the closely related pemphigus erythematosus. Thus, there is no coherent roof to form a bulla, the amount of exudate is usu-

ally less, and a greater thickness of viable epidermis is preserved to protect the dermis. If the acantholytic process repeats itself at short intervals, the multiple foliations of this type of pemphigus result. Antibodies reacting with the higher epidermal layers were demonstrated in the sera of patients.[4]

Fogo Selvagem

The endemic Brazilian pemphigus (fogo selvagem) has been called identical with pemphigus foliaceus[5] or has been attributed to a virus. Histologic studies

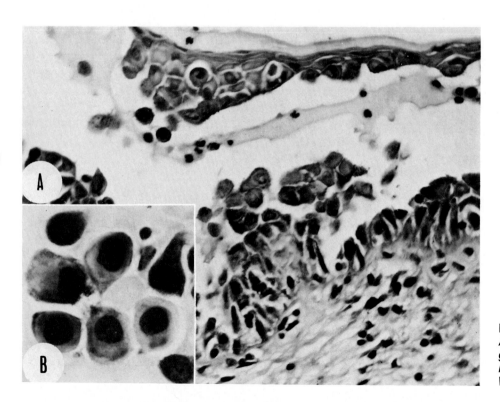

FIGURE 11–2.
*Acantholytic cells in pemphigus vulgaris. **A.** In section. H&E. X465. **B.** Tzanck smear. Wright stain. X800.*

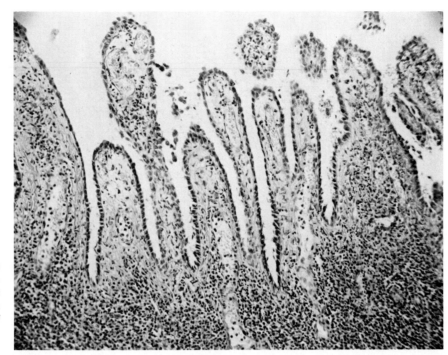

FIGURE 11–3.
Pemphigus vegetans. Upper layers of papillomatous epidermis are completely lost; some acantholytic cells are preserved. Basal layer shows tombstone pattern. Dense infiltrate of round and plasma cells in dermis. H&E. X135.

show no significant differences, but electron microscopic examination of one case showed evidence of dyskeratosis and the presence of viruslike particles.[6]

Eosinophilic Spongiosis. Emmerson and Wilson-Jones[7] reported in 1968 that the skin of patients who later developed pemphigus could present a picture of spongiosis with eosinophils in early stages. This has been confirmed by others,[8,9] and it explains the existence of mixed cases of dermatitis herpetiformis and pemphigus. The existence of this—to the dermatopathologist—very disturbing feature (Fig. 11-5) must be kept in mind. Cases have been reported[10] in which eosinophilic spongiosis was not associated with pemphigus.

Differential Diagnosis. Differentiating features of pemphigus and other dermatoses that may form vesicles, bullae, or pustules are listed in Table 11-1. The most difficult problem in the group of acantholytic lesions is posed by the benign familial pemphigus (Hailey-Hailey's disease). One of the best distinctions is the good preservation of acantholytic cells in that eruption (Fig. 28-3) against the features of cell degeneration in pemphigus vulgaris and vegetans. Individual cell keratinization distinguishes Darier's disease (Table 28-1). In mild forms of pemphigus erythematosus, the epidermal change may resemble the parakeratotic mounds and scale-crusts of seborrheic dermatitis just as the clinical picture does. The presence of acantholytic granular cells should make the diagnosis.

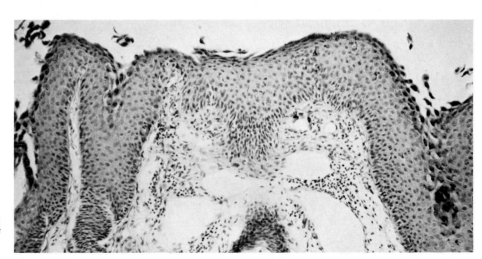

FIGURE 11–4.
Pemphigus foliaceus with acantholytic dissociation of granular layer. H&E. X135.

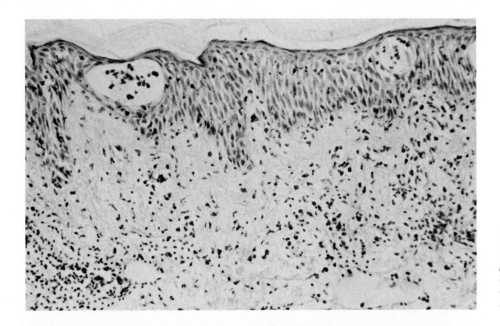

FIGURE 11–5.
Eosinophilic spongiotic pemphigus. Note absence of acantholysis and presence of eosinophils (large dark-appearing cells) in infiltrate. H&E. X225.

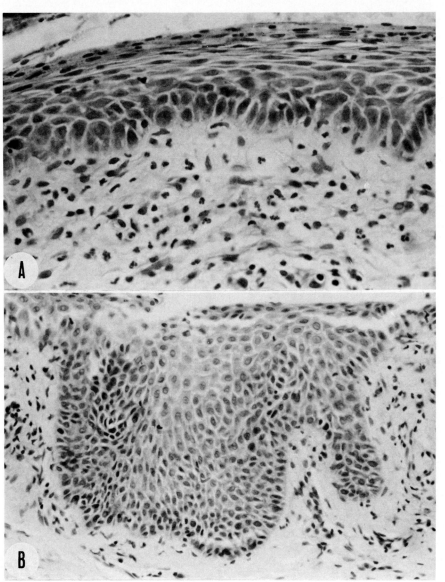

FIGURE 11–6.
*Acrodermatitis enteropathica. **A.** Epidermis rather thin with large uneven basal cells, lack of stratum granulosum, and some exocytosis. This picture may represent epidermal regeneration (see Chap. 5). Moderate inflammatory infiltrate in dermis. **B.** Epidermal hyperplasia with acantholytic cleft formation above basal cells and upper prickle cell layer. H&E. X400.*

The use of D-penicillamine has been followed by eruptions indistinguishable from pemphigus vulgaris or other forms.[11]

Acrodermatitis Enteropathica

A disease in which acantholysis and intraepidermal vesicle formation are found on the basis of deranged lipid metabolism in zinc deficiency is acrodermatitis enteropathica. Acantholysis and the presence of dyskeratotic cells were described quite a few years ago,[12] but electron microscopy has recently revealed[13] severe cytoplasmic disorganization with formation of multiple lipid vacuoles in basal cells and prickle cells. Large portions of the upper epidermis can become necrotic.[14] In addition to acantholysis,[15] there is acanthosis and parakeratosis of variable degree associated with considerable mixed dermal infiltrate (Fig. 11-6). *Candida* has been found in many cases as a secondary invader.

BULLOUS PEMPHIGOID

In contrast to pemphigus vulgaris and its variants, pemphigoid has a subepidermal bulla which seems to be due to a clean split between epidermis and dermis (Fig. 11-7A) similar to the separation one can obtain by the action of enzymes or acids or salts that act on the basement membrane region. The entire epidermis forms the roof of the bulla and shows no degenerative changes (Fig. 11-7B) in early lesions. If the epidermis is pigmented, the lowest layer can be seen to consist of the pigmented and somewhat flattened intact basal cells. The denuded papillary layer forms the base of the bulla. While papillae may still be recognized in very early lesions, they flatten out under the pressure of the fluid contents of the bulla. Inflammatory infiltrate varies greatly from case to case, as does the number of eosinophils which are mixed with lymphocytes and neutrophilic leukocytes. It is obvious that scraping of the blister base in the

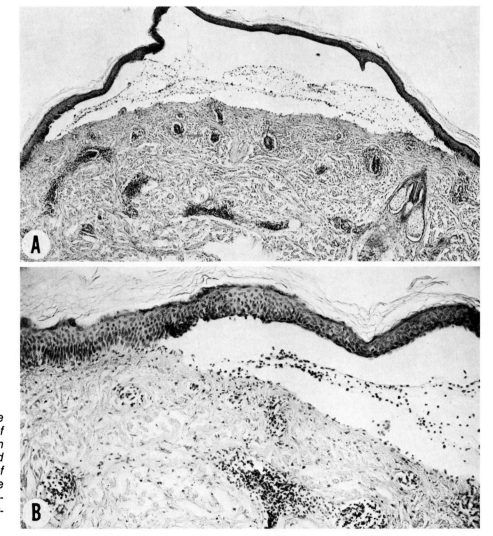

FIGURE 11–7.
Bullous pemphigoid. **A.** *Entire bulla. H&E. X75.* **B.** *Edge of bulla to show clean separation between viable epidermis and intact dermis with flattening of papillae and rete ridges. The bulla contains a mixture of inflammatory cells but no epidermal cells. H&E. X135.*

Tzanck procedure will not procure any epithelial cells. Only inflammatory and red cells will be seen. However, after only 24 hours, reepithelization of the base may begin from the edges and from hair follicles and sweat ducts. Smears from older bullae then may show modulated epithelial cells (Chap. 2), hard to differentiate from acantholytic cells. The patient's serum usually contains antibodies directed to the basement membrane, and immunoglobulins bound to basement membrane can be demonstrated. While these features are helpful in diagnosis, they may also be encountered in atypical cases of various types.[16] The association of bullous pemphigoid with systemic lupus erythematosus,[17] psoriasis,[18] and other diseases has been reported.

CICATRICIAL PEMPHIGOID

Although the pemphigoid lesions of mucous membranes are discussed later in Chapter 45, it must be

mentioned that some patients have extensive skin lesions that lead to scarring (Brunsting-Perry type).[19] The histologic origin of the scarring fibrosis is not clear but is expressed in the formation of some superficial vascularity and granulation tissue in contrast to the reactionless apposition of the new epidermis to the underlying dermis in bullous pemphigoid. There are immunoglobulin deposits at the junction.

DERMATITIS HERPETIFORMIS

Duhring's disease (Fig. 11-8)[20] probably has the most variable picture of all the bullous dermatoses.[21] Vesicles and bullae of greatly varying size are encountered. While separation is subepidermal in principle, the growing vesicle may dissect between epidermal layers (tension bulla). Eosinophilia, while often pronounced, is not as constant as

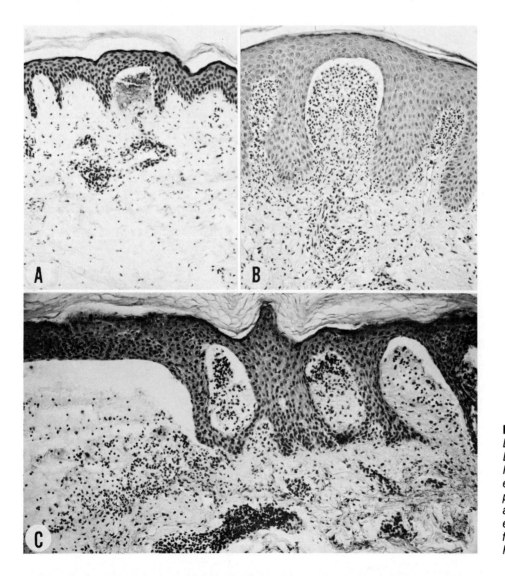

FIGURE 11–8.
Dermatitis herpetiformis. **A.** *Basophilic papillary necrosis. H&E. X90.* **B.** *Neutrophilic and eosinophilic leukocytes in papilla and early epidermal separation. H&E. X135.* **C.** *Confluence of primary vesicles to form the subepidermal bulla. H&E. X135.*

classic descriptions suggest. The most diagnostic feature of dermatitis herpetiformis is present before the vesicle develops, giving a clue to its histogenesis. This feature is a small accumulation of neutrophilic and occasional eosinophilic leukocytes in the tips of individual papillae, which often have a basophilic tinge. The papillary tissue seems to disintegrate, and the epidermis becomes separated. Confluence of several such foci leads to the formation of vesicles.[22] Thus, considerably more damage is done to the dermis than in pemphigoid, bearing out the statement of Oberste-Lehn[23] that inspection of the dermoepidermal interface in split skin preparations shows characteristic differences between the two diseases.

Immunofluorescence shows constant deposition of IgA at the dermoepidermal junction,[24] sometimes accompanied by other immunoglobulins or components of serum. IgA is deposited in granular form in the tips of papillae. More rarely, it is found in linear form along the junction,[25] which suggests a separation of such cases and reapproachment to the chronic bullous dermatosis of children.

CHRONIC BULLOUS DERMATOSIS OF CHILDHOOD

Bullous chronic eruptions are rare in children. While many of them are probably dermatitis herpetiformis, others show atypical clinical and laboratory data, and their therapeutic response varies sufficiently to make the diagnosis doubtful and to bring up the question of a juvenile bullous pemphigoid. Immunofluorescent and electron microscopic studies have been both helpful and confusing. In 1970, Jordon and associates[26] first suggested a separate designation for these cases. More recently, Chorzelski and Jablonska[27] have analyzed 27 cases of blistering eruptions in children and concluded that 12 were dermatitis herpetiformis, 6 were bullous pemphigoid, and 8 were characterized by linear deposits of IgA at the basement membrane. These patients had no gluten-sensitive enteropathy and responded much better to combined treatment with corticosteroids and sulfones than to either alone. They also resembled the adult patients who had linear deposits of IgA. Histologically, there was separation of epidermis from the dermis with a mixed inflammatory infiltrate but no polymorphonuclear abscesses in the papillae. One can hope that these studies have confirmed the existence of a separate chronic bullous disease of children and also of some adults.[25]

DERMATOSES OF PREGNANCY

Two diseases, *impetigo herpetiformis* and *herpes gestationis*, have long been known to be related to pregnancy and to endanger the life of the mother or the fetus. Recently, two nonbullous disorders, *papular dermatitis of pregnancy*[28] and *autoimmune progesterone dermatitis of pregnancy*,[29] have been added. The last named case was exceptional, as the eruption was not pruritic and was characterized by intense eosinophilic infiltrate.

Spangler et al.[28] did not give a histopathologic description of their cases. In our own experience,[30] *pruritic papules of pregnancy* are characterized by lymphohistiocytic infiltrates around the small vessels of the superficial dermis, with some extension around deeper vessels. There is an admixture of polymorphs and eosinophils. The epidermis shows some parakeratosis and crust formation as the result of excoriation, but there is no evidence of subepidermal or supraepidermal bulla. The changes are those of toxic erythema (Chap. 10).[31]

Impetigo herpetiformis resembles generalized pustular psoriasis so closely in its clinical and histologic features that their identity has been postulated (Chap. 8). Presence of acantholytic cells in the zone of spongiform pustulation and disturbances in calcium–phosphorus metabolism in impetigo herpetiformis seem to remain distinguishing features.

Vesicular pruritic eruptions in pregnancy (herpes gestationis) (Fig. 11-9) vary greatly in severity. In the last five years, there have been several publications that clarify the histopathologic picture and pathogenesis. The sera of most patients contain a specific complement-fixing factor—herpes gestationis factor (HGF)—that binds to immunoglobulins and complement deposited in linear fashion along the basement membrane.[32] The histologic picture[33,34] shows a mixed inflammatory cell infiltrate containing eosinophils around the vessels of the superficial and deep plexus and pronounced dermal papillary edema, leading to subepidermal vesiculation with necrosis of basal cells, which may resemble Civatte bodies of lichen planus. Eosinophils may be found in spongiotic foci in the epidermis. This picture is sufficiently different from erythema multiforme, dermatitis herpetiformis, and bullous pemphigoid to establish herpes gestationis as a disease entity, in association with the characteristic immunofluorescent findings.

TOXIC EPIDERMAL NECROLYSIS

Lyell's syndrome,[35] which is clinically characterized by large areas of epidermis becoming detached

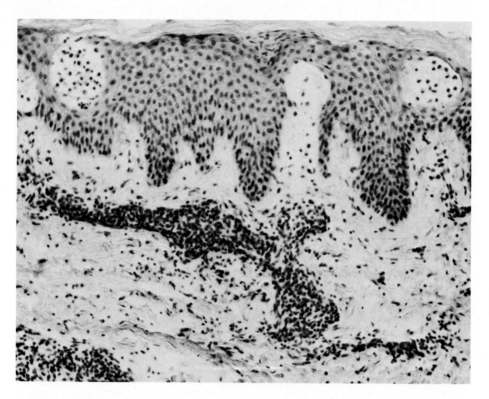

FIGURE 11–9.
Herpes gestationis. In this case, there is subepidermal and intraepidermal vesiculation, moderate acanthosis with focal loss of granular layer and parakeratosis, and considerable perivascular infiltrate consisting mainly of lymphocytes and some eosinophils. H&E. X180.

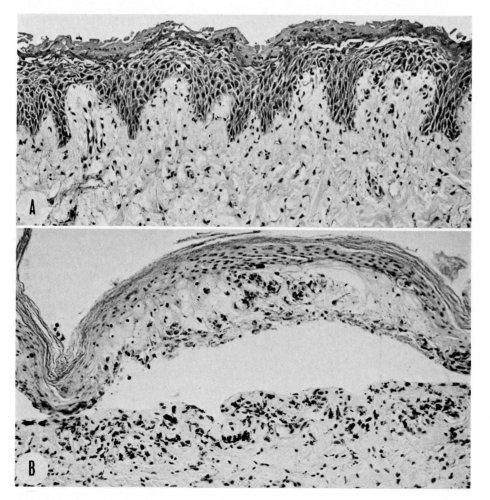

FIGURE 11–10.
*Toxic epidermal necrolysis (Lyell). **A.** Represents a case in which only upper epidermal layers become necrotic, while lower layers exhibit peculiar intercellular edema and cell shrinkage, often seen as an effect of bacterial toxins. **B.** Complete epidermal necrosis (compare to Fig. 10-6). Note relative absence of inflammatory infiltrate in both cases. H&E. X185.*

so that they slide over their base, similar to the appearance of *scalded skin* but without the formation of fluid-filled bullae, seems to become separated into two histologically and pathogenetically distinct groups. In many of the adult cases, a medicamentous cause can be established, the entire thickness of the epidermis becomes necrotic, and the separation is subepidermal (Fig. 11-10B). These features relate this type of case histologically to certain forms of erythema exudativum multiforme (Chap. 10). Most of the cases in infants and a few in adults[36] are caused by staphylococcic toxin and show necrosis of the upper epidermal layers only (Fig. 11-10A). These cases seem identical to *Ritter's disease (dermatitis exfoliativa neonatorum)*. For details see Braun-Falco and Bandmann.[37]

PORPHYRIA CUTANEA TARDA

The bulla of porphyria cutanea tarda is subepidermal (Fig. 11-11)[38] and characterized by two features: almost complete absence of inflammatory infiltrate and persistence of the papillae, which stick up into the blister. It seems possible that the latter feature is due mainly to the tougher weave of the acral skin, where these blisters occur. O&G stain usually shows a heavy elastic fiber support in the papillae. Deposition of PAS-positive, diastase-resistant material and immunoglobulins around superficial blood vessels has been pointed out as characteristic of all porphyric skin lesions.[39] Porphyrialike but reversible changes have been observed after photosensitization due to tetracycline.[40]

Other forms of cutaneous porphyria will be discussed in Chapters 14 and 27.

EPIDERMOLYSIS BULLOSA

The different genetic types of the *mechanobullous diseases*[41] also differ in the site of separation. It must be emphasized that only very early lesions on previously uninvolved skin are suitable for this type of examination. *Epidermolysis bullosa simplex* usually exhibits separation between epidermis and dermis similar to that of porphyria. Electron microscopy, however, has shown that epidermal basal cells disintegrate in this disease.[3] Electron microscopy also has been helpful in more accurate localization of the level of separation in other types. Under the light microscope, the *dystrophic types* may show splits in the basement membrane or intradermal cleft formation (Fig. 11-12) in line with the tendency to fibrosis and scarring. Electron microscopy has shown a primary defect of the anchoring fibrils in the dominant and recessive cases.[42,43] However, the often repeated statement that the bullae of the dystrophic type result from degenerative changes in the dermis should be taken with a grain of salt. Any site previously involved would be expected to show secondary degenerative

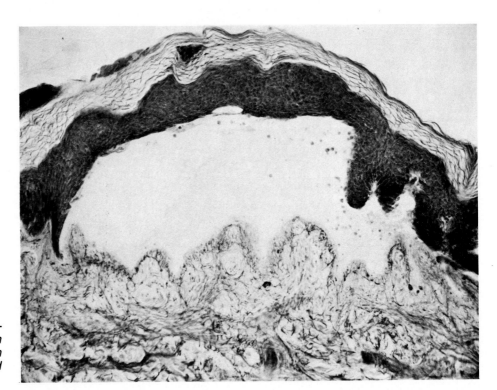

FIGURE 11–11.
Porphyria cutanea tarda. Separation of viable epidermis from almost reactionless dermis with preservation of papillae and elastic fibers. O&G. X135.

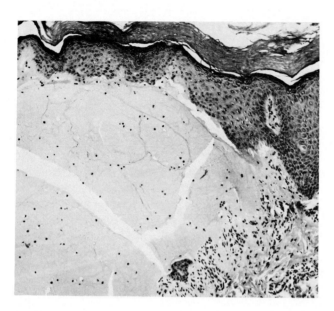

FIGURE 11–12.
Epidermolysis bullosa, dystrophic type, showing adherence of dermal fibers and cells to epidermis. H&E. X135.

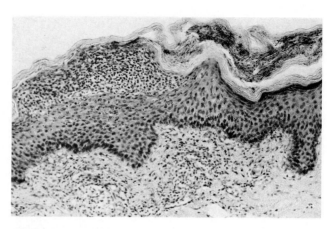

FIGURE 11–13.
Bullous impetigo contagiosa. Transmigration of leukocytes through epidermis and abscess formation below the elevated horny layer at left. At right, pyknotic leukocytes between old and newly formed horny layer. Stratum granulosum absent under fresh lesion, reconstituted under old one. H&E. X250.

dermal changes. Cases of *letalis* (Herlitz) type, renamed *junctional* type because of a clean split between basal cell membrane and basement membrane,[44] also have been found to have similar separations of epithelium and connective tissue in internal organs. A helpful macroscopic clue to the level of separation is the formation of sweat duct milia (Chap. 2) in the dystrophic types. The *localized* type of Weber-Cockayne is said to have suprabasal separation,[45] while more dystrophic forms of *acquired epidermolysis* show intradermal blistering.[46] The peculiar albopapuloid lesions seen in rare

cases will be considered in Chapter 41, and cases combined with congenital localized absence of skin *(Bart's syndrome)* in Chapter 25.

IMPETIGO AND SUBCORNEAL PUSTULAR DERMATOSIS

After proceeding from acantholytic intraepidermal vesiculation to junctional and subepidermal bullae, we must return to the most superficial type, the subcorneal separation, which manifests itself usually as a pustule or purulent bulla. The common-

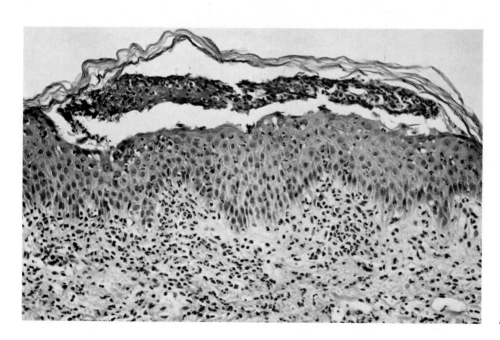

FIGURE 11–14.
Subcorneal pustular dermatosis. H&E. X185.

est, but rarely biopsied, disease in this group is *impetigo contagiosa* (Fig. 11-13), which may form true subcorneal bullae in infants, while in older children and adults, one usually sees only crusts on denuded surfaces. It is important to keep bullous impetigo in mind in the differential diagnosis of *subcorneal pustular dermatosis* (Fig. 11-14) because their histologic pictures are almost indistinguishable.

In both dermatoses, and in a rare variety of chronic impetigolike pyoderma called *dermatitis repens*,[47] we find polymorphonuclear leukocytes migrating through the epidermis and accumulating between granular and horny layers, often without too much disturbance of epidermal architecture.[48] Inflammatory infiltrate in the dermis varies and may be minor. A few acantholytic cells may be found in the blister of Sneddon-Wilkinson's disease, but larger numbers raise a question of pemphigus foliaceus. Immunofluorescent studies will give the answer. It is interesting to note that a patient of ours who was identified in a publication as having subcorneal pustular dermatosis[49] was found to have the von Zumbusch type of psoriasis when she was observed thoroughly at a later date. The differential diagnosis, therefore, must include pustular psoriasis and the closely related impetigo herpetiformis, both of which exhibit spongiform pustulation below the subcorneal accumulation of free granulocytes.

Pustular and crusted clinical lesions are encountered in association with many other dermatoses, especially pruritic ones. We use the term *impetiginization* in cases that are clearly due to superinfection by scratching. Histologically, the picture may be confusing in the absence of clinical information. Presence of colonies of cocci, often already evident in H&E sections and identifiable by O&G or Gram stain, in the superficial pustules and crusts of any inflammatory dermatosis gives a lead to a diagnosis of impetiginization. In other cases, pyodermatous lesions indistinguishable from ordinary impetigo are manifestations of immune deficiency sydromes, such as the *Wiscott-Aldrich syndrome*[50] and *granulomatous disease of childhood*.[51] Table 11-2, slightly modified from one published by Wilkinson,[52] gives a survey of dermatoses associated with polymorphonuclear leukocytes.

TABLE 11–2.
Dermatoses Regularly Associated with Polymorphonuclear Leukocytes

Location of PMNs	Mechanics or Distribution	Disease Entities
Subcorneal	Superficial infection or injury	Impetigo, yeast or fungal infections, chemical injury (nickel, turpentine)
	Unknown cause	Psoriasiform tissue reactions, subcorneal pustular dermatosis
	Secondary	Pustulosis palmaris et plantaris, transepidermal elimination of products of deeper inflammation
Intraepidermal		Psoriasiform tissue reaction, nummular eczema, pustulosis palmaris et plantaris, some viral infections, halogen eruptions, deep fungal infections
Dermal	Adnexal	Staphylococcal infections, acne vulgaris, rosacea, halogen eruptions
	Diffuse	Cellulitis and erysipelas, neutrophilic febrile dermatosis, anthrax, DNA autosensitivity, some bullous diseases
	Vascular	Leukocytoclastic vasculitis, periarteritis nodosa, erythema elevatum diutinum
	Granulomatous	Erythema nodosum (early), all mixed cell granulomas, granuloma faciale, mycosis fungoides

After Wilkinson.[52]

NECROLYTIC MIGRATORY ERYTHEMA

Over the last five years, a characteristic dermatosis has been recognized as a paraneoplastic manifestation of islet cell carcinoma of the pancreas, especially *glucagonoma*. These migrating erythematous lesions had been observed occasionally since 1948, but histologic examination brought out specific changes that were observed in 1973 as *necrolytic migratory erythema*.[53] The disease causes blisters

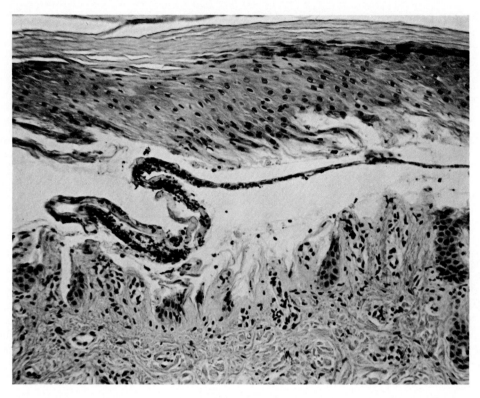

FIGURE 11–15.
Bulla associated with barbiturate coma. Epidermal cells deformed and pyknotic. Papillary connective tissue frayed. Tips of some rete ridges adhere to dermis. Pyknotic polymorphonuclear leukocytes and fibrin in the bulla. The entire aspect suggests separation due to shearing forces. H&E. X180.

that are intraepidermal, situated in the higher prickle cell layer, and associated with transformation of epithelial cells into flat or ballooning elements without keratohyalin.[54] Occasionally, truly acantholytic cells have been observed.[55] Acanthosis varies. Inflammatory infiltrate in the dermis is mild. Polymorphonuclear cells accumulate in the bulla. The differential diagnosis includes acrodermatitis enteropathica and the various bullous dermatoses.

OTHER BULLOUS LESIONS

Bullous eruptions resembling bullous pemphigoid have been reported in association with internal malignant disease. Inasmuch as bullous pemphigoid is a disease of the older age group in which cancer is more common and some bullous eruptions that wax and wane with the ups and downs of the cancer have atypical features, it is advisable to reserve judgment until more of these rare cases have been investigated by modern methods. It may well be that the association of true bullous pemphigoid with malignancy is coincidental[56] and that bullous eruptions of different character[57] are indeed related to cancer. Association of subepidermal bullae with carbon monoxide or barbiturate poisoning (Fig. 11-15), phototoxic bullae from frusemide medication[58] or psoralens, and bullae in diabetes mellitus[59] and a variety of neurologic disorders[60] are being recorded more and more frequently. One should not forget bullae due to burns and friction. All these are subepidermal and may be associated with epidermal damage. These lesions evidently are not related to the disease, bullous pemphigoid. Furthermore, relatively rare bullous eruptions, so-called localized bullous pemphigoid which in some cases may be localized dermatitis herpetiformis,[61] need additional study if they do not show basement membrane fluorescence. It is obvious that some cases of bullous disease can be diagnosed with certainty only after repeated biopsy and thorough clinical observation supported by immunofluorescent procedures.

MUCOUS MEMBRANE LESIONS

The oral manifestations of the bullous diseases and the mucous membrane pemphigoid will be discussed in Chapter 45.

REFERENCES

1. Pearson RW: Advances in the diagnosis and treatment of blistering diseases: a selective review. In Year Book of Dermatology. Chicago, Year Book, 1977

2. Mishima Y, Pinkus H: Electron microscopy of keratin layer stripped human epidermis. J Invest Dermatol 50:89, 1968
3. Pearson RW: Studies on the pathogenesis of epidermolysis bullosa. J Invest Dermatol 39:551, 1962
4. Bystryn J–C: Pemphigus foliaceus. Subcorneal intercellular antibodies of unique specificity. Arch Dermatol 110:857, 1974
5. Guimaraes Proenca N, Rivitti E: Antiepithelial antibodies in Brazilian pemphigus foliaceus. Int J Dermatol 16:799, 1977
6. Lagerholm B, Frithz A: Submicroscopic aspects of the keratinization, dyskeratinization and acantholysis of fogo selvagem. Acta Derm Venereol (Stockh) 58:37, 1978
7. Emmerson RW, Wilson-Jones E: Eosinophilic spongiosis in pemphigus. A report of an unusual histological change in pemphigus. Arch Dermatol 97:252, 1968
8. Knight AG, Black MM, Delaney TJ: Eosinophilic spongiosis. A clinical histological and immunofluorescent correlation. Clin Exp Dermatol 1:141, 1976
9. Degos R, Civatte J, Belaïch S, Bonvalet D: Spongiose à éosinophiles. A propos de deux cas. Bull Soc Fr Dermatol 83:14, 1976
10. Kennedy C, Hodge L, Sanderson KV: Eosinophilic spongiosis: a localized bullous dermatosis unassociated with pemphigus. Clin Exp Dermatol 3:117, 1978
11. Kennedy C, Hodge L, Sanderson KV: Skin changes caused by D-penicillamine treatment of arthritis. Report of three cases with immunological findings. Clin Exp Dermatol 3:107, 1978
12. Piper EL: Acrodermatitis enteropathica in an adult. Arch Dermatol 76:221, 1957
13. Ginsburg R, Robertson A Jr, Michel B: Acrodermatitis enteropathica. Abnormalities of fat metabolism and integumental ultrastructures in infants. Arch Dermatol 112:653, 1976
14. Brazin SA, Johnson WT, Abramson LJ: The acrodermatitis enteropathica-like syndrome. Arch Dermatol 115:597, 1979
15. Juljulian HH, Kurban AK: Acantholysis: a feature of acrodermatitis enteropathica. Arch Dermatol 108:105, 1971
16. Provost TT, Maize JC, Ahmed R, et al.: Unusual subepidermal bullous diseases with immunologic features of bullous pemphigoid. Arch Dermatol 115:156, 1979
17. Kumar V, Binder WL, Schotland E, et al. Coexistence of bullous pemphigoid and systemic lupus erythematosus. Arch Dermatol 114:1187, 1978
18. Koerber WA Jr, Price NF, Watson W: Coexistent psoriasis and bullous pemphigoid. A report of six cases. Arch Dermatol 114:1643, 1978
19. Jacoby WD, Bartholome CW, Ramchaud SC, et al.: Cicatricial pemphigoid (Brunsting-Perry type). Case report and immunofluorescence findings. Arch Dermatol 114:779, 1978
20. Alexander JO'D: Dermatitis herpetiformis. In Rook A (ed): Major Problems in Dermatology, vol 4. London-Philadelphia, Saunders, 1975
21. Eng AM, Moncado B: Bullous pemphigoid and dermatitis herpetiformis. Arch Dermatol 110:51, 1974
22. MacVicar DN, Graham JH, Burgoon CF Jr: Dermatitis herpetiformis, erythema multiforme and bullous pemphigoid: a comparative histopathological and histochemical study. J Invest Dermatol 41:289, 1963
23. Oberste-Lehn H: Dermoepidermal interface: pictorial demonstration of significant changes in skin disease. Arch Dermatol 86:770, 1962
24. Katz SI, Strober W: The pathogenesis of dermatitis herpetiformis. J Invest Dermatol 70:63, 1978
25. Jablonska S, Chorzelski T: Dermatose à IgA linéaire. Ann Derm Venereol 106:651, 1979
26. Jordon RE, Beau SF, Triftshauser CT, Winkelmann RK: Childhood bullous dermatitis herpetiformis. Arch Dermatol 101:629, 1970
27. Chorzelski TP, Jablonska S: IgA linear dermatosis of childhood (chronic bullous disease of childhood). Br J Dermatol 101:535, 1979
28. Spangler AS, Reddy W, Bardanil WA, et al.: Papular dermatitis of pregnancy. A new clinical entity? JAMA 181:577, 1962
29. Bierman SM: Autoimmune progesterone dermatitis of pregnancy. Arch Dermatol 107:896, 1973
30. Rahbari H: Pruritic papules of pregnancy. J Cutan Pathol 5:347, 1978
31. Lawley TJ, Hertz KC, Wade TR, et al.: Pruritic urticarial papules and plaques of pregnancy. JAMA 241:1696, 1979
32. Carruthers JA: Herpes gestationis: a reappraisal. Clin Exp Dermatol 3:199, 1978
33. Hertz KC, Katz SI, Maize J, Ackerman AB: Herpes gestationis. A clinicopathologic study. Arch Dermatol 112:1543, 1976
34. Harrington CI, Bleehen SS: Herpes gestationis: Immunopathological and ultrastructural studies. Br J Dermatol 100:389, 1979
35. Lyell A: Toxic epidermal necrolysis (the scalded skin syndrome). A re-appraisal. Br J Dermatol 100:67, 1979
36. Sturman SW, Malkinson FD: Staphylococcal scalded skin syndrome in an adult and a child. Arch Dermatol 112:1275, 1976
37. Braun-Falco O, Bandmann HJ (eds): Das Lyell-Syndrom. Das Syndrom der "verbrühten" Haut. Bern, Verlag Hans Huber, 1970
38. Cormane RH, Szabò E, Hoo TT: Histopathology of the skin in acquired and hereditary prophyria cutanea tarda. Br J Dermatol 85:531, 1972
39. Epstein JH, Tuffanelli DL, Epstein WL: Cutaneous changes in the porphyrias; a microscopic study. Arch Dermatol 107:689, 1973
40. Epstein JH, Tuffanelli DL, Seibert JS, Epstein WL: Porphyria-like cutaneous changes induced by tetracycline hydrochloride photosensitization. Arch Dermatol 112:661, 1976
41. Bauer EA, Briggaman RA: The mechanobullous diseases (epidermolysis bullosa). In Fitzpatrick TB, et al. (eds): Dermatology in General Medicine, 2nd ed. New York, McGraw-Hill, 1979
42. Anton-Lamprecht I, Schnyder UN: Epidermolysis bullosa dystrophica dominans; ein Defekt der anchoring fibrils? Dermatologica 147:289, 1973
43. Briggaman RA, Wheeler CEJ: Epidermolysis bullosa dystrophica—recessive: a possible role of anchoring fibrils in the pathogenesis. J Invest Dermatol 65:203, 1975
44. Schachner L, Lazarus GS, Dembitzer H: Epidermolysis bullosa hereditaria letalis. Pathology, natural history and therapy. Br J Dermatol 96:51, 1977
45. DesGroseilliers JP, Brisson P: Localized epidermolysis bullosa. Arch Dermatol 109:70, 1974

46. Roenigk HH, Ryan JH, Bergfield WF: Epidermolysis bullosa acquisita. Report of three cases and review of all published cases. Arch Dermatol 103:1, 1971

47. Ashurst PJC: Relapsing pustular eruptions of the hands and feet. Br J Dermatol 76:169, 1964

48. Sneddon IB: Subcorneal pustular dermatosis. Int J Dermatol 16:640, 1977

49. Beck AL, Kipping HL, Crissey JT: Subcorneal pustular dermatosis. Arch Dermatol 83:627, 1961

50. Scher PK: Wiskott–Aldrich syndrome. Cutis 12:566, 1973

51. Bass LJ, Voorhees JJ, Dubin HV, et al.: Chronic granulomatous disease of childhood. Superficial pyoderma as a major dermatologic manifestation. Arch Dermatol 106:68, 1972

52. Wilkinson DS: Pustular dermatoses. Br J Dermatol 81 [Suppl 3]:38, 1969

53. Wilkinson DS: Necrolytic migratory erythema with carcinoma of the pancreas. Trans St Johns Hosp Dermatol Soc 59:244, 1973

54. Kahan RS, Perez-Figaredo RA, Neimanis A: Necrolytic migratory erythema. Distinctive dermatosis of the glucagonoma syndrome. Arch Dermatol 113:792, 1977

55. Swenson KH, Amon RB, Hanifin JM: The glucagonoma syndrome. A distinctive cutaneous marker of systemic disease. Arch Dermatol 114:224, 1978

56. Paslin DA: Bullous pemphigoid and hypernephroma. A critical review of the association of bullous pemphigoid and malignancy. Cutis 12:554, 1973

57. Skog J: Cutaneous manifestations associated with internal malignant tumors with particular reference to vesicular and bullous lesions. Acta Derm Venereol (Stockh) 44:117, 1964

58. Burry JN, Lawrence JR: Phototoxic blisters from high frusemide dosage. Br J Dermatol 94:495, 1976

59. Bernstein JE, Medenica M, Soltani K, Criem SF: Bullous eruption of diabetes mellitus. Arch Dermatol 115:324, 1979

60. Arndt KA, Mihm MC, Parrish JA: Bullae: a cutaneous sign of a variety of neurologic diseases. J Invest Dermatol 60:312, 1973

61. Trepanier Y: Localized bullous dermatitis herpetiformis. Arch Dermatol 101:98, 1970

CHAPTER

12

Inflammatory Virus Diseases

Long-known human diseases characterized by an inflammatory reaction of the skin to viruses are the varicella-herpes group, variola-vaccinia, paravaccinia, ecthyma contagiosum, and rubella, rubeola, and related exanthems. To these have been added "minor" virus rashes caused by Coxsackie and other recently identified agents. The Gianotti–Crosti syndrome also seems to be caused by a virus. For reviews of the entire field see Nasemann[1] and Harman et al.[2] We will deal here only with diagnostic microscopic features. Other viruses that cause mainly epithelial proliferation will be discussed in Chapter 31.

INTRANUCLEAR VIRUSES

Herpes simplex, zoster, and *varicella* have in common not only the intranuclear localization of the virus but also the specific epidermal reaction described as reticulating and ballooning degeneration. Infection and death of individual cells leads to defects in the malpighian layer, which are quickly filled with fluid and produce vesicles of netlike appearance. This process can be best observed in early or mild lesions or in the borders of larger ones, in which the center forms a vesicle characterized by almost complete disintegration of the living parts of the epidermis (Fig. 12-1). In the vesicle are edematous cells and cell groups floating like balloons. Multinucleated epithelial cells are common.

These often huge elements, whether mononucleated or multinucleated, are the characteristic feature in Tzanck smears (Fig. 5-16D). In well-stained preparations, especially with O&G stain, one sees eosinophilic inclusion bodies in some or many nuclei. In H&E sections, the nucleus more commonly has a pale ground-glass appearance with a thin hematoxylin-stained rim (Fig. 12-1).

The vesicle thus is intraepidermal, but the individual features depend very much on the age of the lesion and the acuity of the process. It is remarkable that herpes simplex is apt to produce the most severe destruction accompanied by heavy dermal infiltrate. Varicella (Fig. 12-2) usually has relatively mild and superficial inflammation,[3] while the infiltrate of vesicular zoster is intermediate in amount and extends deep into the subcutaneous tissue, often involving nerve trunks. In hemorrhagic and necrotizing cases of zoster, tissue changes will be, of course, correspondingly severe. In herpes simplex, viral colonization of outer root sheath is not uncommon, and typical cytologic changes may be found more easily there than in the destroyed epidermis. Superinfection of inflamed skin, especially in atopic dermatitis, with herpes simplex virus is known as *Kaposi's varicelliform eruption* or *eczema herpeticum,* which can be differentiated by Tzanck smear from the clinically similar *eczema vaccinatum.*

The demonstration of virus-infected large nuclei in genital ulcers proves herpes simplex even in the

145

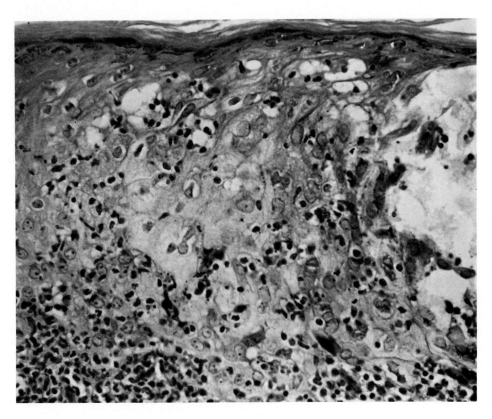

FIGURE 12–1.
Edge of herpes zoster vesicle showing ground-glass appearance of nuclei due to intranuclear inclusions, reticulating degeneration due to complete disappearance of individual cells, and ballooning degeneration with formation of multinucleated giant cells. H&E. X370. (From Sutton. Diseases of the Skin, 11th ed, 1956. Courtesy of Dr. R. L. Sutton, Jr. Contributed by H. Pinkus.)

simultaneous presence of chancroid (Fig. 17-2). On the other hand, one must not forget that large and sometimes multinucleated cells may be found in the epidermis for a variety of nonspecific reasons (Fig. 5-11).

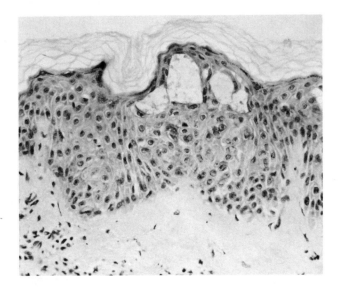

FIGURE 12–2.
Varicella. Relatively mild derangement of epidermis with several small vesicles due to reticulating degeneration of keratinocytes. Horny layer intact, mild inflammatory infiltrate in dermis. H&E. X250.

VARIOLA AND VACCINIA

Smallpox is said to have been eradicated, but *vaccinia* is to be considered in the differential diagnosis of vesicular dermatoses because it may be spread by contamination, as in *eczema vaccinatum*. The mechanism of vesiculation in these two diseases consists of reticulating and ballooning degeneration of prickle cells. The process is slower and starts in the upper layers, with formation of multiloculated vesicles, while edema and inflammatory infiltrate of the dermis may be already well developed. Inclusion bodies, if present, are intracytoplasmic (*Guarneri bodies*).

PARAVACCINIA AND ECTHYMA CONTAGIOSUM

The so-called *milker's nodule* (Fig. 12-3) owes its hard consistency *(stone pox)* to a combination of epidermal acanthosis, high degree of edema, and much cellular infiltrate. Early stages may resemble erythema multiforme with beginning bullous edema of papillae (Chap. 10), but the epidermis does not necrotize but shows vacuolization of the higher prickle cell layers and fingerlike elongation of rete ridges. The vacuolated cells contain eosinophilic

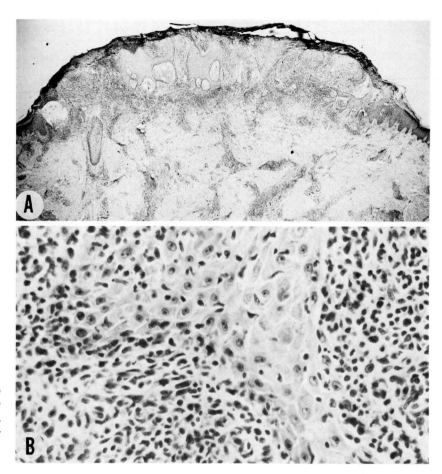

FIGURE 12–3.
A. *Milker's nodule (paravaccinia). Note resemblance to erythema exudativum multiforme at low power. H&E. X14.* **B.** *Acanthosis and mixed, almost granulomatous infiltrate at high power. H&E. X280.*

inclusion bodies in cytoplasm and nucleus. Inflammatory infiltrate (Fig. 12-3) consists of a mixture of polymorphs, lymphocytes, and plasma cells. Most of the infiltrate remains fairly superficial. Virus has been cultured in bovine fetal kidney[4] and resembles that of sheep pox.

Sheep pox or *orf* (Fig. 12-4) exhibits ballooning and reticular degeneration of the epidermis in the early stage and may produce pseudoepitheliomatous proliferation later. The dermis is highly vascular and edematous and contains severe inflammatory infiltrate of mixed character. Eosinophilic inclusion bodies may be demonstrable in the cytoplasm. The virus of *ecthyma contagiosum* is a DNA-containing poxvirus.[5]

MEASLES AND GERMAN MEASLES

The histologic picture of *rubeola* and *rubella* is more or less that of a toxic erythema. Multinucleated epidermal cells may be found in true *measles*,[6] but the pathognomonic mesenchymal cells with numerous nuclei are usually present only in lymphoid tissues. A morbilliform exanthem having

histologic features of polyarteritis nodosa develops in cases of *Kawasaki's disease* (Chap. 15).

COXSACKIE AND ECHO VIRUSES

Exanthems have been described due to various newly identified viruses. Figure 12-5 illustrates a case and shows an intraepidermal vesicle with some degeneration of prickle cells, localized dermal edema and hemorrhage, and some perivascular round cell infiltrate. The histologic picture of all these diseases is of diagnostic value only in coordination with the clinical features and possibly corroborative laboratory evidence of rising antibody titers. The most common clinical differential diagnosis is with drug exanthems, and these rarely produce intraepidermal vesicles or multinucleated giant cells. Lichen urticatus (Chap. 10) and possibly pityriasis rosea (Fig. 13-1) may enter histologic differential diagnosis.

A special case is hand-foot-and-mouth disease, caused by a Coxsackie virus.[7] Histologically, it also shows ballooning and reticulating degeneration of the epidermis with neutrophils and mononuclear

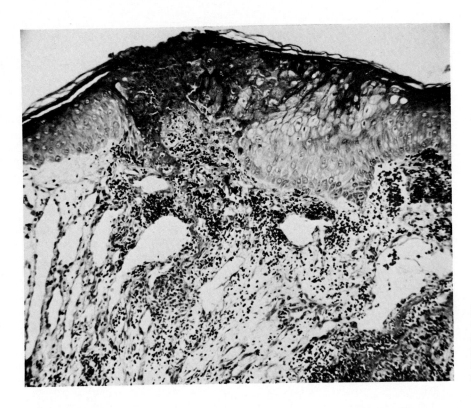

FIGURE 12–4.
Ecthyma contagiosum (orf). Epidermis is in part necrotic and shows beginning proliferative changes. Edema, telangiectasia, and inflammatory infiltrate in dermis. H&E. X135.

cells in the vesicles. The dermis shows a mixed cellular infiltrate.

GIANOTTI-CROSTI SYNDROME

A large body of literature[8] has accumulated concerning *papular acrodermatitis of childhood*, which has been recognized as the skin manifestation of infection with hepatitis B virus. A peculiar feature of the disease is that it has been extensively reported from Europe, and there is one report of an epidemic occurrence in Japan,[9] but there are only a few reports from the United States.[10,11] The reasons for this low incidence in this country of an apparently striking febrile disease in children is unclear. The histologic picture is said to consist of some acanthosis, spongiosis, and parakeratosis of the epidermis and a mixed lymphohistiocytic infiltrate of the upper dermis with Pautrier-like monocytic ac-

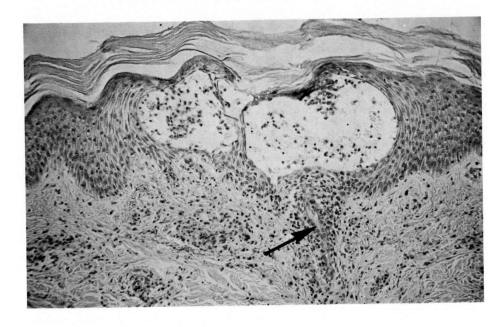

FIGURE 12–5.
Viral exanthem, suspected to be caused by echovirus. H&E. X135. Note sweat duct (arrow) near center of lesion.

cumulations in the epidermis. Therefore, it is, at best, compatible with the clinical diagnosis but not diagnostic.

REFERENCES

1. Nasemann T: Die Virus Krankheiten der Haut. In Marchionini A (ed): Jadassohn's Handbuch der Haut- und Geschlechtskrankheiten, Ergänzungswerk, vol 4, pt 2. Berlin, Springer-Verlag, 1961
2. Harman RRM, Nagington J, Rook A: Virus infections. In Rook A, Wilkinson DS, Ebling FJG (eds): Textbook of Dermatology, 2nd ed. Oxford, Blackwell, 1972
3. McSorley J, Shapiro L, Brownstein MH, et al.: Herpes simplex and varicella-zoster: comparative histopathology of 77 cases. Int J Dermatol 13:69, 1974
4. Leavell UW, Phillips IA: Milker's nodules. Pathogenesis, tissue culture, electron microscopy and calf inoculation. Arch Dermatol 111:1307, 1975
5. Hoxtell E, Gentry WC, Zelickson AS: Human orf with electron microscopic identification of the virus. Cutis 16:899, 1975
6. Ackerman AB, Suringa DWR: Multinucleate epidermal cells in measles. Arch Dermatol 103:180, 1971
7. Kimura A, Abe A, Nakao T: Light and electron microscopic study of skin lesions of patients with hand, foot, and mouth disease. Tohoku J Exp Med 122:237, 1977
8. Gianotti F: Papular acrodermatitis of childhood and other papulo-vesicular acro-located syndromes. Br J Dermatol 100:49, 1979
9. Ishimaru Y, Ishimaru H, Toda G, et al.: An epidemic of infantile papular acrodermatitis (Gianotti's disease) in Japan associated with hepatitis B surface antigen subtype ayw. Lancet 1:707, 1976
10. Rubenstein D, Esterly NB, Fretzin O: The Gianotti-Crosti syndrome. Pediatrics 61:433, 1978
11. Castellano A, Schweitzer R, Tong MJ, Omata M: Papular acrodermatitis of childhood and hepatitis B infection. Arch Dermatol 114:1530, 1978

CHAPTER

13

Miscellaneous Papulosquamous Eruptions

In this chapter are brought together a number of superficial skin diseases that cannot be easily fitted into one of the patterns discussed in previous chapters. Rather than try to call them eczematous, psoriasiform, and so on, we prefer to distinguish them by their particular characteristics.

Because the papulosquamous disorders often have confusing or indistinct clinical features, they constitute a considerable percentage of specimens in a dermatopathologic laboratory. Some answers are easy: Psoriasis and lichen planus may be confused clinically but are at diametric ends of the histologic spectrum. Other differentiations may be difficult because the diseases belong to the same group of tissue reaction, for instance, seborrheic dermatitis and psoriasis. Still others may be unsatisfactory because of the absence of pathognomonic features, as in pityriasis rosea.

The dermatoses to be discussed here are pityriasis rosea, superficial fungous infections, various forms of parapsoriasis, the pigmented purpuric eruptions, lichen striatus, and scabies. We thus include considerably more territory than is covered by the classic clinical group. On the other hand, seborrheic dermatitis, psoriasis, lichen planus, and other possible candidates were discussed in previous chapters. Secondary syphilis will be consid-ered together with other forms of the disease in Section IV.

PITYRIASIS ROSEA

If one biopsies a dozen or more typical cases of pityriasis rosea by taking complete cross sections of small lesions or radial slices extending from normal skin into the center of large ones, one arrives at a fairly consistent concept of the histologic changes. However, most routine biopsies are taken from atypical cases, and often a punch biopsy is submitted without indication of how it should be oriented for favorable sectioning. On such material, conclusions can be stated only as "compatible with, but not diagnostic of" pityriasis rosea.

A well-oriented section of a typical lesion is characterized by definite zonal arrangement. Farthest out, under still normal epidermis, there is mild to moderate edema of the pars papillaris, engorgement of widened subpapillary vessels, and moderate perivascular round cell infiltrate. These changes increase toward the center, and now the epidermis becomes slightly thickened, more through edema than actual acanthosis. At the height of the inflammatory process, there is usually one, sometimes two, small intraepidermal vesicles (Fig. 13-1) of spongiotic type, accompanied by some exocytosis. Adjacent to the vesicle, parakeratosis and loss of granular layer are found for a relatively short distance. As edema and inflammatory infiltrate begin to subside toward the center of the plaque, the parakeratotic scale moves upward and is replaced by normal keratinization in the clearing center. The scale thus has a free end at the central side of the lesion corresponding to the collarette effect of the clinical lesion.

There is nothing really specific about any of these changes. It is only their typical combination and arrangement that make the diagnosis. The changes are of eczematous type, and contact dermatitis, tinea, or drug eruptions, especially gold dermatitis,[1] may produce similar pictures. Perhaps the most impressive feature is the almost regular presence of an intraepidermal vesicle in a clinically dry dermatosis. This feature will help in the differentation from those diseases in which intraepidermal vesicles are practically never found: psoriasis, parapsoriasis, seborrheic dermatitis, and secondary syphilis.

SUPERFICIAL FUNGOUS INFECTIONS

Histologic examination of skin changes caused by dermatophytes in the widest sense illustrates three biologic phenomena. One is that microorganisms do not have to invade living tissue in order to cause inflammation and immune reactions.[2] The second is that the number of demonstrable organisms is inversely related to the degree of inflammatory reaction, and the third is that fungal elements found in tissue sections are not necessarily the cause of the dermatosis but may be secondary parasites or even innocent bystanders. The dermatophytes, with the occasional exception of *Trichophyton rubrum* and *Candida*, live only in the dead horny layers of epidermis, hair, or nail. The inverse relation of number of organisms to inflammatory tissue reaction will be described under the individual diseases, and we shall encounter a related principle in the chapters on granulomatous inflammation (Sec. IV). *Candida* is the outstanding example of an opportunistic organism that may or may not be the principal cause of the dermatosis in which it is encountered. Hyphae and spores of nonpathogenic molds also may be seen in tissue sections and may be mistaken morphologically for dermatophytes. A recent exhaustive review of the dermal pathology of superficial fungous infection is available.[3]

Noninflammatory Lesions

Among the tineas, *tinea versicolor* occupies a singular place, histologically as well as clinically. There is almost complete absence of edema or inflammatory infiltrate. The epidermis also is practi-

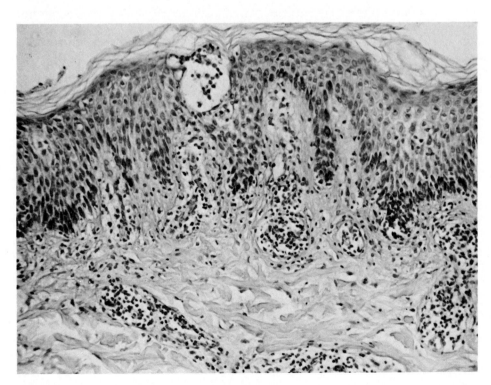

FIGURE 13–1.
Pityriasis rosea showing characteristic solitary intraepidermal vesicle at point of greatest activity. There are two other foci of less severe spongiotic edema, and the epidermis in the left side of the picture shows the earliest stage of parakeratosis, which farther into the lesion (not shown in the photo) will replace the normal horny layer and lead to scale formation. H&E. X180.

cally normal, although it may be slightly thickened. Only the horny layer is definitely thickened. Characteristic filaments and grouped spores usually can be seen in H&E sections, if the observer has learned to examine the stratum corneum with care in any section that does not offer other obvious diagnostic features. The fungi stain beautifully in O&G sections (Fig. 13-2A), and it is hardly ever necessary to call for special stains, such as PAS (Fig. 13-2B). Scanning electron microscopy provides beautiful pictures.[4] The light microscopic impression of lessened epidermal pigmentation has been confirmed by electron microscopic evidence of melanocytic damage.[5] This becomes accentuated in cases of so-called *tinea versicolor alba.*

Two rare conditions which share the features of large numbers of microorganisms and absence of inflammation with tinea versicolor are *tinea nigra palmaris,*[6,7] due to *Cladiosporum* species, and *pitted keratolysis,* from which *Streptomyces* and the organism of erythrasma have been cultured.[8] The more typical clinical forms of *erythrasma* may also

be mentioned here, although the causative microbe has been reclassified as *Corynebacterium minutissimum.* This organism is so small that it can be recognized only by oil immersion examination, and even then identification in thin tissue sections is hazardous. Skin scrapings stained with methylene blue or tape strippings[9] of the horny layer are advisable. The second technique is also the easiest way to demonstrate the tinea versicolor organism.

Tinea Superficialis

Other superficial fungous infections usually are due to *Trichophyton* species and often are of the *tinea circinata* type. They present a more or less eczematous reaction, but the picture frequently is somewhat bizarre, with very spotty spongiosis, acanthosis, and parakeratosis punctuated by occasional intraepidermal vesiculation. Just as in pityriasis rosea, there is a zonal arrangement if the sections are oriented properly, and, again, one cannot

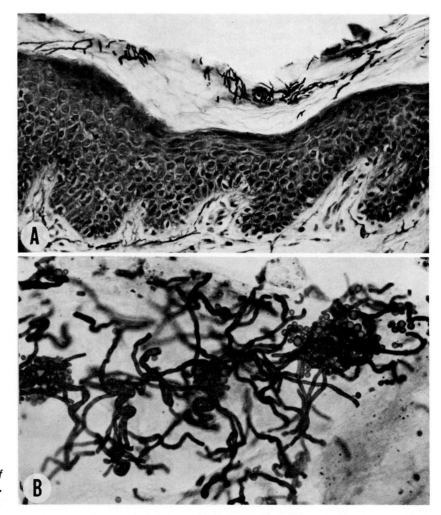

FIGURE 13–2.
Tinea versicolor. **A.** *Demonstration of fungi in honry layer. O&G. X180.* **B.** *Fungi in a scale stained by PAS. X460.*

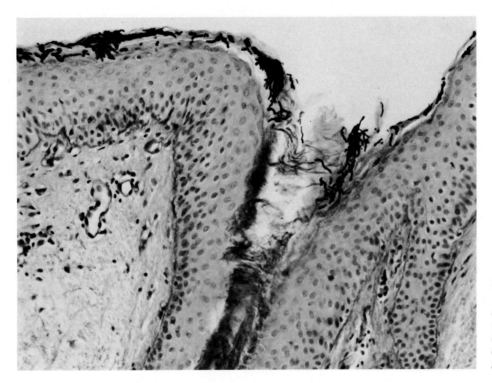

FIGURE 13–3.
Tinea faciei showing mycelia in the horny layer of the epidermis and the follicular infundibulum. Mild reactive changes of epidermis and dermis. PAS-hematoxylin. X225.

rely on this feature in routine material. It is important to keep in mind that mycelia are found only in the horny layer and, often, only in a short stretch peripheral to the inflammatory zone. Mycelia cannot be expected above the area of heaviest inflammation. Although thin paraffin sections are far from ideal objects in the search for dermatophytes, it happens every once in a while that the histopathologist finds dermatophytes (Fig. 13-3) where the clinician either did not think of the diagnosis or was unsuccessful in this search. It is also well to remember that mycelia may be absent from the surface layer but present in the follicular ostium, especially in intertriginous areas. O&G sections usually are satisfactory for finding dermatophytes, but PAS stain should be done in critical cases.

It must not be forgotten that vesiculobullous dermatitides are caused on the feet, especially between the toes, by dermatophytes and by erythrasma,[10] and that mycelia may or may not be present in the surface scale in otherwise eczematous spongiotic epidermal reaction. Other lesions due to dermatophytes and *Candida* will be discussed in Chapters 18 and 45.

PARAPSORIASIS

On both clinical and histologic grounds, we prefer to separate the *guttate* forms of Brocq's parapso-

riasis under the name of *pityriasis lichenoides* from those with larger of ill-defined lesions (*parapsoriasis en plaques, xanthoerythrodermia perstans, parapsoriasis lichenoides*). We feel, however, that pityriasis lichenoides should be subdivided into chronic, subacute, and acute (and possibly varioliform) types and the acute form is not to be set up as a separate species.

Pityriasis Lichenoides

Among the most striking features of the *guttate* lesions under the microscope (Fig. 13-4A) are their sharp definition and their constant size, which hardly ever exceeds the limits of a widefield eyepiece under low power (total magnification X40). This latter feature is one good clue. Another is the character of the scale in the fully developed chronic and subacute lesion, with some modification in the acute form. The scale is flat (Fig. 13-4B), and while it shows parakeratotic inclusions and even occasional microabscesses, it is not split into lamellae as is the psoriatic scale. It either adheres to the underlying epidermis or separates as a whole, a feature typical also in clinical examination. In the acute forms, the scale often is converted into a crust and may contain serum, leukocytes, and red cells. The third outstanding feature is the peculiar, passive behavior of the epidermis. While it may be slightly thickened in the chronic type, it rarely

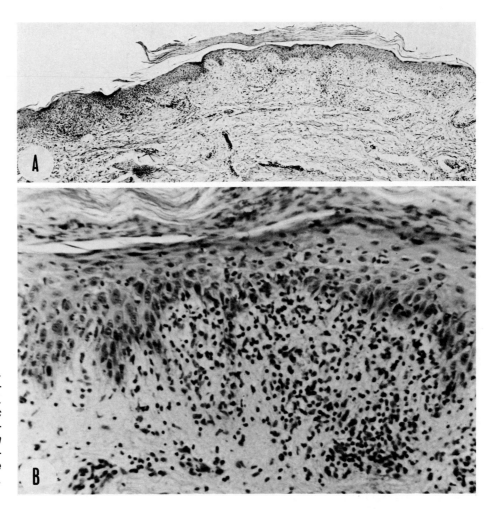

FIGURE 13–4.
Pityriasis lichenoides chronica.
A. *Typical size and appearance at low magnification. H&E. X45.* **B.** *Disklike parakeratotic scale with suggested microabscesses, epidermal invasion by round cells, and perivascular infiltrate. Epidermis is more acanthotic than usual. H&E. X135.*

gives the appearance of active regenerative or reactive inflammatory changes. It just seems to sit there suffering the invasion by inflammatory cells. That these are predominantly round cells is another important difference from psoriasis. The subpapillary dermis exhibits variable degrees of edema and perivascular round cell infiltrate, relatively mild in the *chronic* form and becoming increasingly severe in the *subacute* (Fig. 13-5) and *acute* (Fig. 13-6) types. Black and Marks[11] find many histiocytes and no evidence of vascular disease. Marks et al.[12] also confirm our long-held opinion that the varioliform type is probably a variant of the more chronic form (Juliusberg's disease[13]). It is our impression that the name *Mucha–Habermann disease* has been applied too liberally to cases that show occasional crusted lesions and that it might be more properly reserved for more hyperacute and severely necrotic cases.[14,15] There are many intermediate cases in which the severity of the tissue reaction depends a lot on the individual lesion and the stage in which it was taken for biopsy. In really severe lesions, the entire epidermis and part of the pars papillaris undergo necrosis, and there is hemorrhage associated with much edema and inflammatory infiltrate. A papulonecrotic lesion is produced which has very little in common with the histologic picture of variola.

Thus, the various forms of guttate parapsoriasis are characterized by their typical size, by relatively minor, though characteristic, epidermal participation,[16] and by histiocytic and small round cell infiltrate, which has a peculiar tendency to invade the epidermis. There is no evidence of vasculitis. These latter features tie the histologic picture of pityriasis lichenoides to the other forms of parapsoriasis. For a discussion of recently described lymphomalike lesions (lymphomatoid papulosis) see Chapter 44.

Parapsoriasis en Plaques

It becomes increasingly obvious[17,18] that parapsoriasis en plaques should be divided into two forms with decidedly different prognosis and recognizable clinical and histologic differences. One type, which has been called "digitate dermatosis" and "chronic superficial dermatitis" and which we prefer to call

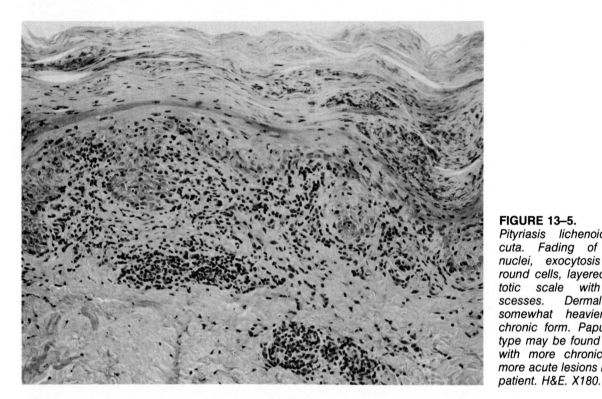

FIGURE 13–5.
Pityriasis lichenoides suba-cuta. Fading of epidermal nuclei, exocytosis of small round cells, layered parakera-totic scale with microab-scesses. Dermal infiltrate somewhat heavier than in chronic form. Papules of this type may be found associated with more chronic and with more acute lesions in the same patient. H&E. X180.

small-plaque parapsoriasis, has no serious signifi-cance, while *large-plaque parapsoriasis* sooner or later progresses toward mycosis fungoides, some-times through the intermediate state of *poikilo-derma* (see below). Histologic differences may not be striking in early lesions but become more pro-nounced as the large-plaque type progresses.

Just as the plaques of parapsoriasis are barely palpable clinically, so may the histologic features be very mild. A practically normal epidermis (Fig. 13-7) has an almost normal horny layer with occa-sional foci of parakeratosis. A few round cells may have migrated into the epidermis, most often sin-gly, only occasionally simulating an eczematous

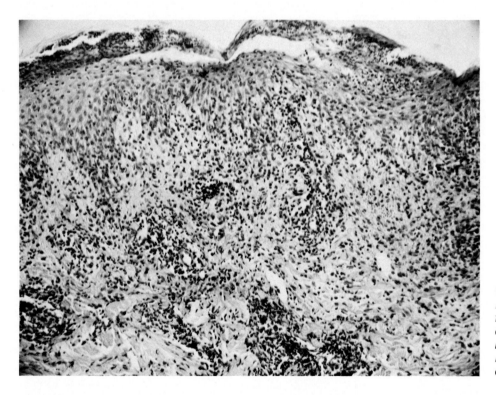

FIGURE 13–6.
Pityriasis lichenoides et varioli-formis acuta. Fairly early lesion of moderate intensity. Begin-ning breakdown of epidermis. Infiltrate consists of mononu-clear cells. H&E. X135.

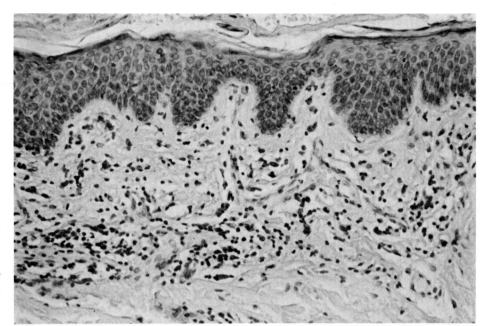

FIGURE 13–7.
Small-plaque form of parapsoriasis. Almost normal epidermis with minimal parakeratosis. Moderate diffuse infiltrate consisting of small round cells and fixed-tissue type cells. No sign of the poikilodermatous tissue reaction. The picture is characterized more by the absence of specific features of other diseases than by any outstanding hallmarks of its own. H&E. X225.

vesicle or a Pautrier abscess (Fig. 13-8A). The subepidermal infiltrate also is mild, somewhat diffuse, and accentuated around subpapillary vessels (Fig. 13-8). It presents one feature characteristic of all types of parapsoriasis: the admixture of a fair proportion of fixed-tissue type cells to small round cells. This phase of parapsoriasis en plaques, therefore, has features that suggest a mild and benign proliferative process of lymphoreticular cells rather than an inflammatory disease. The small-plaque variant remains in this state indefinitely. The large type, if biopsied at intervals, will show a row of progressively heavier alterations. These do not concern the epidermis, although it may be somewhat

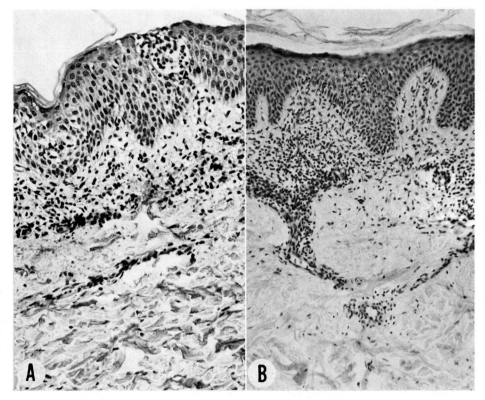

FIGURE 13–8.
*Parapsoriasis en plaques. **A.** Intraepidermal vesicle combining features of eczematous reaction (Fig. 7-3) and Pautrier abscess (Fig. 44-5B) in a lesion exhibiting mild infiltrate and no acanthosis. **B.** Less epidermal invasion in a case with considerable acanthosis and fairly heavy infiltrate. H&E. X135.*

acanthotic and may have more parakeratosis and even an occasional microvesicle. It is the infiltrate that increases in severity and tendency to epidermal invasion (Fig. 13-8B). Its composition of small round cells and fixed-tissue type cells remains unchanged (Fig. 13-9). Careful search may reveal an occasional, very large, and dark-staining nucleus. Eosinophils and plasma cells are rare occurrences. The question that so often prompts biopsy in these cases—Is it still parapsoriasis en plaques or is it changing into mycosis fungoides?—should be answered with great reserve. Actually, the turning point is more sharply defined by the clinical features of pruritus and increased succulence of the plaques than by any histologic feature. More about differential diagnosis will be said in the chapter on lymphoreticular neoplasms (Chap. 44).

Parapsoriasis Lichenoides and Poikiloderma

The histologic features of the rare *lichenoid* and *reticulated* types of parapsoriasis are similar to parapsoriasis en plaques, and may evolve from them, but often tend toward those of *poikiloderma* into which the clinical features also merge.[19] Indeed, parapsoriasis is one of the three diseases which can cause the clinicopathologic symptom complex of *poikiloderma atrophicans vasculare.* Dermatomyositis and lupus erythematosus are the other two (Chap. 9).

PIGMENTED PURPURIC ERUPTIONS

There seems to be little doubt that *Schamberg's* and *Majocchi's diseases* are variants of the same process. *Gougerot-Blum's lichenoid purpuric eruption* and *lichen aureus* have somewhat distinctive features. *Hutchinson's angioma serpiginosum* has been separated[20] as a noninflammatory, purely angiomatous, and very rare entity (Chap. 42).

Schamberg–Majocchi Eruption

The first low-power impression (Fig. 13-10) in a case of Schamberg-Majocchi eruption is that of a peculiarly ragged infiltrate, which is neither diffuse nor strictly perivascular, is widespread in the subpapillary layer but not dense, and is somewhat focal without forming definite papules. The epidermis usually is not much changed, except for focal invasion by inflammatory cells, which may cause some edema and parakeratosis. Closer inspection reveals ectatic small vessels with swollen endothelia, and in favorable sections, one may recognize the hyaline degeneration of vessel walls that is the

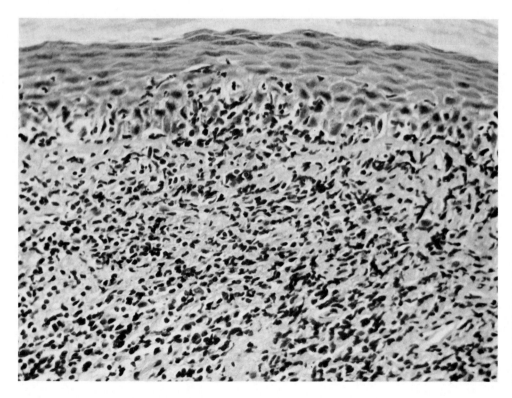

FIGURE 13–9.
Premycotic phase of large-plaque type of parapsoriasis. More diffuse and polymorphous infiltrate with strong tendency to invade the lower layers of the atophic epidermis in a clinically poikilodermatous lesion. H&E. X375.

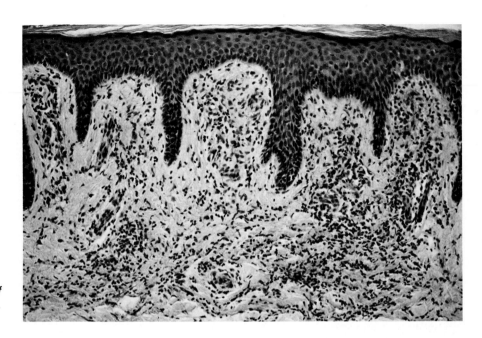

FIGURE 13–10.
Pigmented purpuric eruption of Schamberg-Majocchi type. H&E. X135.

hallmark of these affections. Hemorrhage by diapedesis, decomposed red cells, and hemosiderin deposits complete the picture.

In routine diagnostic work, the two principal clinical features of purpura and pigmentation are of little help. Extravasation of red blood cells is common in skin sections due to surgical trauma, especially in punch biopsy. It is only if disintegrating red cells are recognized that one can diagnose in vivo hemorrhage. Hemosiderin is peculiarly difficult to see in H&E sections, when only small amounts are present. Usually, the clinician will submit a fresh lesion in which the gradual process of conversion of hemoglobin into hemosiderin has barely begun. O&G sections are not helpful either. While they show erythrocytes more clearly, they leave hemosiderin unstained and often obscure in contrast to melanin. Specific stain for iron, therefore, is required if blood pigment has to be demonstrated. However, this is rarely necessary because other histologic features are sufficiently characteristic.

Gougerot-Blum Eruption

Gougerot-Blum eruption usually shows a considerably heavier infiltrate, some epidermal acanthosis, and considerably more invasion by inflammatory cells associated with edema and parakeratosis. Inasmuch as this disease usually forms more persistent plaques, the amount of hemosiderin also is apt to be greater.

Lichen Aureus (Purpuricus)

An often linear (zosteriform) eruption on legs or trunk of young adults has been described under the striking name of *lichen aureus*, although the clinical color is more often the red-brown color of hemosiderosis (lichen purpuricus). The cause is unknown, and the course is protracted as in all the pigmented purpuric eruptions.[21] The histologic features are a mixed round cell–histiocytic infiltrate that is often separated from the epidermis by edematous papillary tissue, and there is no evidence of epidermal invasion. Free red cells and hemosiderin are present in the tissue. The presence of Langerhans cells has been demonstrated[22] in several cases by electron microscopy.

Differential Diagnosis

The differential diagnosis of all pigmented purpuric eruptions, if they are found on the legs below the knees, must include stasis dermatitis (Chap. 15) and drug eruptions. Any medicamentous dermatitis that produces a maculopapular exanthem on other parts of the body is apt to become purpuric on the lower legs and to produce pictures barely distinguishable from Schamberg–Majocchi's disorder. Tufting of capillaries in the papillary layer without evidence of hyalinization of the walls speaks for stasis. Active microvasculitis speaks for an eruption due to medicaments, especially certain sleeping pills.

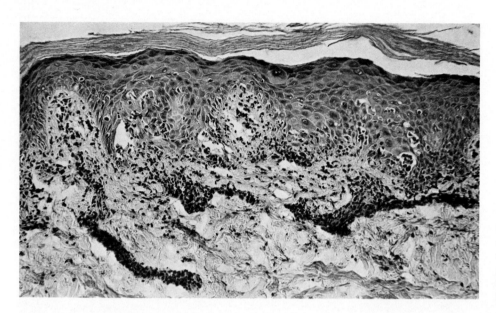

FIGURE 13–11.
Lichen striatus. Note individual cell keratinization and heavy perivascular infiltrate extending below superficial plexus. H&E. X135.

LICHEN STRIATUS

The most typical feature of lichen striatus, its linearity, cannot be appreciated under the microscope. There are, however, certain fairly characteristic histologic features (Fig. 13-11) that can make one suspect the diagnosis even without clinical information. One should keep in mind Felix Pinkus' original analysis[23] that each papule occupies the area of the wheel-spoke-like distribution of the ramifications of one ascending arteriole. There is some similarity to the pigmented purpuric eruptions in the ragged appearance of the infiltrate. However, closer inspection shows that one can delineate fairly well defined papules and that there is an unusually heavy lymphocytic infiltrate around selected subpapillary vessels and their extensions into the middermis. Within the papule, the infiltrate invades the epidermis almost as heavily as in lichen planus but is accentuated in some papillae, while others may be almost free, in contrast to the continuous band of lichen planus infiltrate.[24] The epidermis correspondingly varies in thickness and degree of edema. In later stages,[25] the basal cells de-

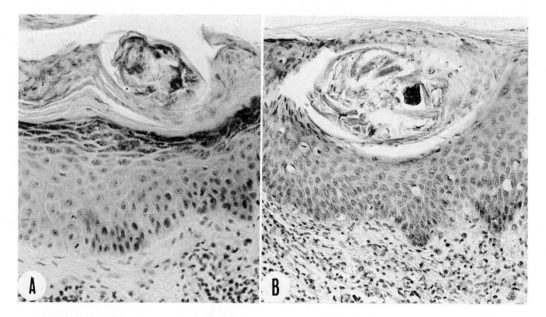

FIGURE 13–12.
*Scabies. **A.**Cross sections of female acari in parakeratotic horny layer of a papule. Mild epidermal and considerable dermal inflammatory reaction. Note spines on abdomen of mite in **B.** H&E. X185.*

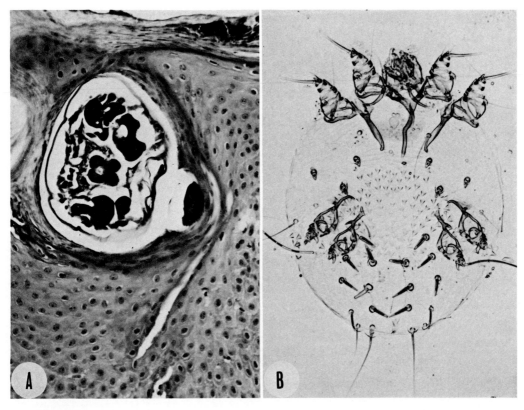

FIGURE 13–13.
Scabies. **A.** *Sectioned mites in the acanthotic epidermis of Norwegian scabies. H&E. X180.* **B.** *Female acarus in native preparation obtained from a burrow. Unstained in water. X400.*

generate and microvesicles result. The desmosomes retract,[26] and individual cells resembling the corps ronds of Darier's disease result in about half of the cases.[27]

SCABIES

The histologic diagnosis of scabies is usually unsatisfactory but sometimes gratifying. Submission of a biopsy specimen means that the clinical diagnosis has been missed. Otherwise, the patient would have been treated with or without demonstration of the acarus (Fig. 13-13B) in a fresh horny layer preparation. Inasmuch as the papulosquamous and often excoriated lesions on the skin of an infested individual usually do not contain the mite—it is mainly found in the characteristic linear burrows— the histologic features are most often quite noncharacteristic eczematous changes. Once in a while, however, an unexpected, peculiar body (Fig. 13-12) is discovered in a circumscribed thickening of the parakeratotic horny layer and can be identified as a sectioned acarus. In even rarer instances, the histopathologist may discover large numbers of mites

in the greatly thickened horny layer of a clinically verrucous lesion from a case of *Norwegian scabies* (Fig. 13-13A). Persistent nodular lesions occur in connection with scabies, as with other arthropods (Chap. 44), and should always be thought of in unclear nodular lesions. No mites are found in these cases.[28]

REFERENCES

1. Penneys NS, Ackerman AB, Gottlieb NL: Gold dermatitis: a clinical and histopathological study. Arch Dermatol 109:372, 1974
2. Jones HE, Reinhardt JH, Rinaldi MG: Acquired immunity to dermatophytes. Arch Dermatol 109:840, 1974
3. Graham JH, Barroso-Tobila C: Derman pathology of superficial fungus infections. In Baker RD (ed): The Pathologic Anatomy of Mycoses. Handbuch der speziellen pathologischen Anatomie und Histologie, vol 3, pt 5. Berlin, New York, Springer-Verlag, 1971
4. Marinaro RE, Gershenbaum MR, Roisen FJ, Papa CM: Tinea versicolor: a scanning electron microscopic view. J Cutan Pathol 5:15, 1978
5. Boiron G, Surlève-Bazeille J-E, Gauthier Y, Maleville J: Étude ultrastructurale de divers stades évolutifs de

pityriasis versicolor. Ann Derm Venereol 105:141, 1978

6. Hitch JM: Tinea nigra palmaris. Report of a case originating in North Carolina. Arch Dermatol 84:318, 1961

7. Itani Z: Tinea nigra palmaris. Mykosen 15:27, 1972

8. Young CN: Pitted keratolysis. Trans St Johns Hosp Dermatol Soc 60:77, 1974

9. Marks R, Ramnarain ND, Bhogal B, et al.: The erythrasma microorganism in situ: studies using the skin surface biopsy technique. J Clin Pathol 25:799, 1972

10. Grigorin D, Delacrétaz J: La forme vesiculo-bulleuse de l'érythrasma interdigito-plantaire. Dermatologica 152:1, 1976

11. Black MM, Marks R: The inflammatory reaction in pityriasis lichenoides. Br J Dermatol 87:533, 1972

12. Marks R, Black MM, Wilson-Jones E: Pityriasis lichenoides: re-appraisal. Br J Dermatol 86:215, 1972

13. Juliusberg F: Die Parapsoriasis Gruppe. Zentralbl Haut Geschlechtskr 45:417, 1933

14. Degos R, Duperrat B, Daniel F: Le parapsoriasis ulcéro-nécrotique hyperthermique. Forme suraiguë du parapsoriasis en gouttes. Ann Dermatol Syphiligr 93:481, 1966

15. Horowitz DC, Rehbein HM: Parapsoriasis (Mucha-Habermann disease). Cutis 12:401, 1973

16. Marks R, Black MM: The epidermal component of pityriasis lichenoides. Br J Dermatol 87:106, 1972

17. Samman PD: The natural history of parapsoriasis en plaques (chronic superficial dermatitis) and prereticulotic poikiloderma. Br J Dermatol 87:405, 1972

18. Hu CH, Winkelmann RK: Digitate dermatosis. A new look at symmetrical, small plaque parapsoriasis. Arch Dermatol 107:65, 1973

19. Bonvalet D, Colan-Gohm K, Belaïch S, et al.: Les différentes formes du parapsoriasis en plaques. A propos de 90 cas. Ann Derm Venereol 104:18, 1977

20. Barker LP, Sachs PM: Angioma serpiginosum. Arch Dermatol 92:613, 1965

21. Waisman M, Waisman M: Lichen aureus. Arch Dermatol 112:696, 1976

22. Schnitzler L, Verret J-L, Schubert B, et al.: Lichen aureus ou lichen purpuricus. A propos de 5 cas. Intérêt de l'étude ultrastructurale. Ann Derm Venereol 104:731, 1977

23. Pinkus F: Über eine besondere Form strichförmiger Hautausschläge. Dermat Z 11:19, 1904

24. Pinkus H: Lichen striatus and lichen planus. Report of a case of simultaneous occurrence, with discussion of nomenclature and mechanics of linear and systematized dermatoses. J Invest Dermatol 11:9, 1948

25. Stewart WM, Lauret P, Pietrini P, Thomine E: "Lichen striatus." Critères histologiques (a propos de 5 cas). Ann Derm Venereol 104:132, 1977

26. Charles R, Johnson BL, Robinson TA: Lichen striatus. A clinical, histologic and electron microscopic study of an unusual case. J Cutan Pathol 1:265, 1974

27. Staricco RG: Lichen striatus. Arch Dermatol 79:311, 1959

28. Fernandez F, Torres A, Ackerman AB: Pathologic findings in human scabies. Arch Dermatol 113:320, 1977

SECTION

III

DEEP INFLAMMATORY PROCESSES

All dermatoses discussed so far involve predominantly the epidermis and the pars papillaris of the dermis. If low-power inspection reveals abnormal aggregates of cells mainly in the pars reticularis or the subcutaneous fat tissue, we can immediately rule out the superficial inflammatory dermatoses. The next step is to ascertain the nature of the abnormally present cells. Epithelial and mesodermal tumor cells, with the exception of some small-cell metastatic carcinomas, are easily recognized. Lymphomatous infiltrates are more difficult to identify, but we shall leave this point for Chapter 44. If the infiltrate consists of a mixture of cells, one should look particularly for any appreciable number of fixed-tissue type cells, which in most cases are histiocytes, and put the lesion into the category of granulomatous inflammation, whether they are present in the form of epithelioid nodules or not (Sec. IV). The next chapters then will deal with deep inflammatory infiltrates composed of small round cells (lymphocytes) mainly. Polymorphonuclear leukocytes and plasma cells may be present.

Classification within the group is made according to the particular structures with which the infiltrate is associated. Thus, we can separate out vasculitides in which sizable blood vessels are affected, inflammation of fat lobes (panniculitis) or interlobar septa, and lesions associated with hair follicles or sweat glands. Finally, there are some dermatoses in which only small vessels seem to serve as the centers of inflammation. The outstanding example of this type is lupus erythematosus.

Lupus Erythematosus and Related Conditions

HISTOLOGY OF LUPUS ERYTHEMATOSUS

Testimony to the close biologic interactions between mesoderm and epithelium, the diagnostic features of all manifestations of cutaneous lupus erythematosus involve changes in the dermis, in the epidermis, and in the pilosebaceous follicles. The changes are qualitatively similar but are combined in varying quantity. Inasmuch as the clinical criteria of discoid and systemic cannot be recognized under the microscope, it seems best to list the histologic forms of the disease as chronic, subacute, and acute (Figs. 14-1, 14-2, and 14-3).

For diagnostic and differential purposes, it is then recommended to look for triads of alteration in epidermis and hair follicles and for five features in the dermis. If all or the majority are present, a diagnosis can be made with considerable assurance, but one has to keep in mind the biologic limitations of some of the criteria. For instance, one cannot expect keratotic plugging of follicles if all the hair roots have been destroyed by the disease. The diagnostic criteria are listed in Table 14-1. Important diagnostic features[1] have been added by immunofluorescent methods[2,3] but they are beyond the scope of this book, as are the intriguing electron microscopic findings of viruslike intracellular inclusions.[4]

Special Features

It may seem strange that epithelial changes play such an important part in the diagnosis of a connective tissue disease. One may resolve this paradox by considering the close interaction between mesoderm and ectoderm. It is also paradoxical that fibrinoid and vascular changes, which play such a prominent part in lupus erythematosus of internal organs, are barely worth looking for in routinely stained sections of skin. One should further realize that many of the diagnostic changes develop slowly. It is generally best to biopsy a well-established lesion of at least several weeks' duration.

The epidermal changes have much similarity to those of lichen planus and, for the same reason, damage to basal cells.[5] This is apt to be more spotty in lupus erythematosus (Fig. 14-2) and restricted to the areas where lymphocytic infiltrate touches the epidermis. Sawtooth appearance of rete ridges is hardly ever seen, and hyaline bodies[6] are extremely rare. Atrophy of the malpighian layer (Fig. 14-3) may be extreme in subacute and acute cases and makes a striking contrast to the thick horny layer, which usually rests on a well-developed or even thickened granular layer. Occasional spots of parakeratosis may be found in the more acute forms due to the vulnerability of the tissues. Some cases of chronic discoid lupus erythematosus, clinically

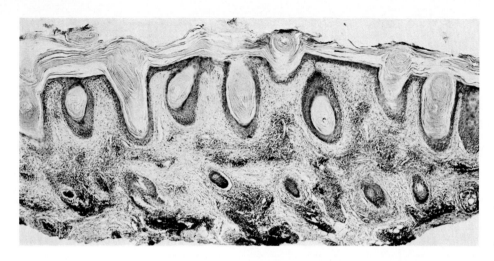

FIGURE 14–1.
Chronic lupus erythematosus of beard. Section shows all typical features except that follicular plugs are less conical than usual. Note orthokeratotic hyperkeratosis and epidermal and sebaceous atrophy. Edema and telangiectasia are more pronounced in the superficial dermis; perivascular lymphocytic infiltrate in the deeper layers.

FIGURE 14–2.
Subacute lupus erythematosus. Note numerous pigmented macrophages below nonpigmented atrophic epidermis (symptomatic incontinentia pigmenti). H&E. X135.

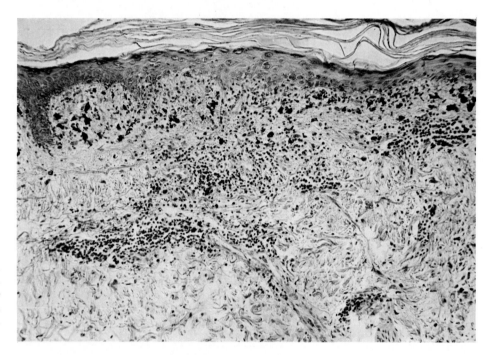

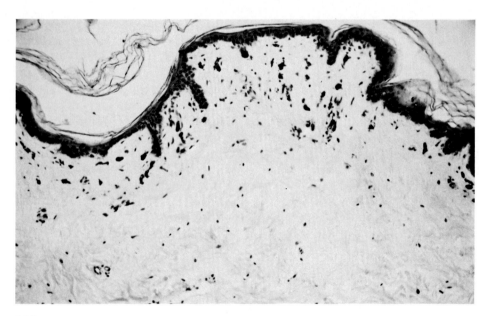

FIGURE 14–3.
Acute lupus erythematosus. Atrophic epidermis with relative hyperkeratosis. Papillary layer highly edematous. Practically no inflammatory infiltrate. Numerous melanophages appear in skin of this black patient. H&E. X180.

TABLE 14–1.
Diagnostic Features of Lupus Erythematosus

Epidermis
Hyperkeratosis and hypergranulosis
Atrophy (rarely hyperplasia) of the malpighian layer
Focal liquefaction necrosis of the basal layer
Pilary Complex
Conical keratotic plugs
Sebaceous atrophy
Pilar atrophy
Dermis
Lymphocytic infiltrate with focal invasion of epidermis
   and follicular sheath
Edema
Telangiectasia
Subepidermal macrophage pigmentation
Focal destruction of elastic fibers

of the verrucous type, show marked acanthosis alternating with atrophic stretches of epidermis. Close inspection of H&E-stained sections may reveal changes of the basement membrane, which are more obvious with the PAS procedure. The membrane is of uneven width but more commonly thickened and even reduplicated. In other areas, it may appear frayed or lost.

The earliest follicular change is sebaceous atrophy. However, even this takes some weeks to develop and usually affects the small superficial glands of the vellus follicles of the face first, while the large, deep-seated glands of the sebaceous folli-

cles may remain of fair size for some time. Therefore, sebaceous atrophy is usually of less diagnostic value in subacute and acute lesions. The keratotic plug also develops gradually but may be quite pronounced in acute cases where general epithelial atrophy is severe. It need not be present in every follicle. Basal layer damage of follicular sheath is seen particularly well on strong scalp hairs associated with a hugging lymphocytic infiltrate similar to that of *lichen planopilaris*. It is an empiric rule that the plug in lupus erythematosus often is conical, while that of follicular lichen planus is rounded and sits in a cup-shaped or even bottle-shaped follicle (Fig. 14-4). Eventually the pilosebaceous structures may disappear completely, leaving behind remnants of fibrous sheath and the hair muscle. In these late stages, one must not expect keratotic plus histologically or carpet-tack scale clinically.

The most prominent dermal sign is the pure lymphocytic infiltrate (Fig. 14-1) that is apt to be present in all layers of the dermis, but most regularly in the middle third. It is arranged around small vessels and, therefore, is mainly found in the vicinity of hair follicles. It is heavy and nodular in chronic cases but differs from the massive infiltrate of a lymphocytic lymphoma by the fact that all cells are neatly spaced rather than packed close. This is a sign of the edema which is present at the same time. A few plasma cells, even an occasional

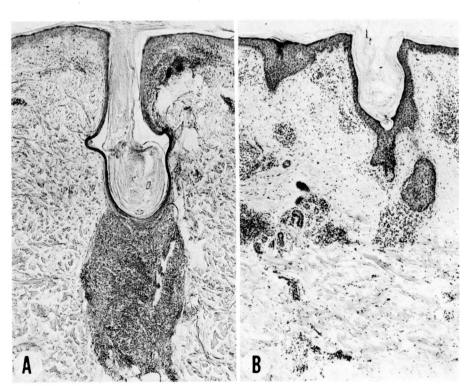

FIGURE 14–4.
*Comparison of follicular plugs. **A.** Lichen planus. H&E. X60. **B.** Chronic lupus erythematosus. H&E. X75. Follicle of lichen planus is cup-shaped or bottle-shaped, plug may extend into middermis, and infiltrate hugs lower pole. Plug of lupus erythematosus usually is conical and restricted to infundibulum. Infiltrate is perivascular and approaches follicular epithelium in various places.*

eosinophil, are permissible, but heavier admixture of these cell types raises doubts. They are more commonly present in the *polymorphous light eruptions*. The infiltrate practically always approaches the epidermis in a few places and is associated with basal cell degeneration. One may have to scan a number of sections to find this feature, but its complete absence favors *Jessner's lymphocytic infiltration*. The infiltrate is in reciprocal relation to the amount of edema as one goes from chronic to subacute and acute lesions. It may be entirely absent in very acute cases which show only a generally red skin clinically. This produces the peculiar picture illustrated in Figure 14-3. A specific stain would reveal considerable amounts of dermal hyaluronic acid[7] in this type of case. Edema is noticeable in various ways: by spacing of the lymphocytes, splitting of collagen bundles, and a peculiarly empty look of the subpapillary zone (Fig. 14-1). Edema usually is associated with telangiectasia, not only of blood vessels but also of lymph vessels. Since the latter are rarely recognized in normal skin or other dermatoses, the presence of open spaces lined only by occasional endothelial cells is a good clue for lupus erythematosus.

As in lichen planus, the damaged basal layer releases melanin granules which are taken up by macrophages. This sign (Figs. 14-2 and 14-3) is apt to be minimal in very fair skin and is striking in brown skin. It has no diagnostic value in itself (symptomatic incontinentia pigmenti, Chap. 5) because it is also present in fixed drug eruptions, Riehl's melanosis, lichen planus, and various other dermatoses, but its presence should make one suspicious.

The fifth dermal feature, spotty absence of elastic fibers, is of considerable diagnostic value in chronic cases. It is due to the fact that elastic fibers are easily destroyed by chronic inflammatory infiltrate and not easily formed anew. Chronic lesions of lupus erythematosus, therefore, will reveal loss of preexisting elastic fibers in areas previously involved by infiltrate. This feature persists long after the lesion has become quiescent and all infiltrate has disappeared. In some cases, especially in young patients, new elastic fibers may be formed, but these are thin and abnormally arranged. Areas of elastic fiber destruction may look quite normal in H&E sections but are conspicuous with O&G stain. The feature may be present in Jessner's lymphocytic infiltration but is rarely seen in polymorphous light eruption.

Variants

In the *hypertrophic* or *verrucous* form of chronic lupus erythematosus, epidermal atrophy may be replaced by considerable acanthosis. However, all other diagnostic features usually are present. *Bullous* lupus erythematosus results very rarely from confluence of basal cell necrosis and excessive superficial edema. On the other hand, the coexistence of bullous pemphigoid and lupus erythematosus has been reported (Chap. 11) and must be investigated by immunofluorescent methods. True *lupus erythematosus profundus* (Figs. 14-5 and 14-6) is rare.[8,9] It does not have any of the epidermal and follicular changes of the usual type, and the deep cutaneous and subcutaneous infiltrate (*lupus panniculitis*) may have a granulomatous character (Chap. 16). Most of the cases formerly diagnosed rather loosely as deep lupus erythematosus are now recognized as Jessner's lymphocytic infiltration. *Lupus erythematosus of the scalp* is to be differentiated from other forms of scarring alopecia (Chap. 18) by the extrafollicular changes in the epidermis and around blood vessels, where lymphocytic infil-

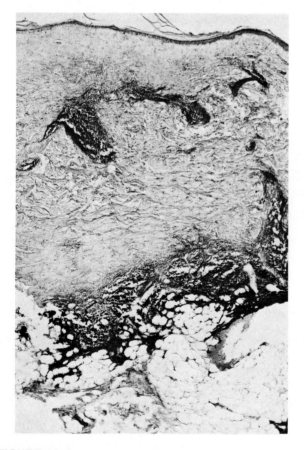

FIGURE 14–5.
Lupus erythematosus profundus. Diagnosis must be based on clinicopathologic correlation. H&E. X30.

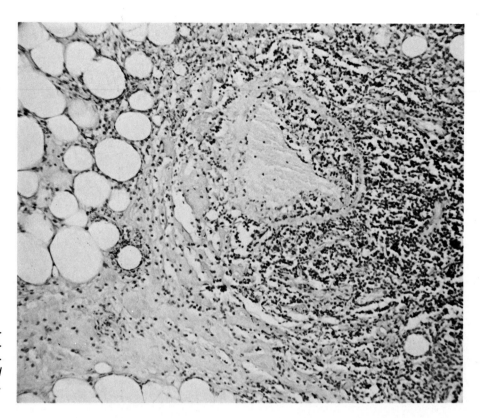

FIGURE 14–6.
Panniculitis of lupus erythematosus profundus. Lymphocytic infiltrate disrupts the structural integrity of a large vein (phlebitis) and extends between fat cells. H&E. X135.

trate and loss of elastic fibers should be looked for. Flat plaques of lupus erythematosus on the body and extremities, where hair follicles are few, may be extremely hard to tell from lichen planus. The distribution of the infiltrate—exclusively superficial in lichen planus, extending deeper around vessels in lupus erythematosus—is the best clue.

The syndrome of *mixed connective tissue disease* may present cutaneous lesions of discoid or systemic lupus erythematosus in a high percentage of cases.[10] There is no histologic differentiation except by immunofluorescence.

Lupus erythematosus of the oral mucosa cannot be differentiated from lichen planus with any degree of assurance (Chap. 45).

JESSNER'S LYMPHOCYTIC INFILTRATION

In spite of the noncharacteristic name and the abortive way[11] in which the disease was announced to the world, Jessner's distinguishing his *lymphocytic infiltration* (Fig. 14-7) from lupus erythematosus was a highly welcome event. We feel with Beare[12] that it is an entity worth differentiating from discoid lupus erythematosus because it has a much better prognosis. The principal histologic deviations are the absence of epidermal involvement and of follicular plugging. Some sebaceous atrophy

and rather extensive loss of elastic fibers may be present. Edema and telangiectasia usually are not pronounced. On the other hand, Jessner's disease can be differentiated from lymphocytoma by the fact that its lymphocytic infiltrate has an inflammatory perivascular character even though it may be nodular and dense in some cases. We, therefore, exclude it from the group of benign lymphoplasias (Chap. 44).

PHOTOSENSITIVITY REACTIONS

One of the more perplexing diagnostic problems is the field of inflammatory tissue reactions related to light sensitivity. Not only are many lesions of lupus erythematosus aggravated or triggered by light, but eruptions caused by actinic exposure have multiplied in recent years owing to the photosensitizing propensities of numerous internal medications and external additives to soaps, bleaches, and cosmetics. Omitting phototoxic lesions in which necrosis of epidermal cells parallels that of other forms of primary irritant dermatitis (Chap. 7), we are confronted with classic *polymorphous light eruptions*, *photocontact dermatitis*, and the recurrent summer eruptions which have to be differentiated from certain forms of *porphyria.* The recurrent summer eruptions of the *hydroa aestivale* and

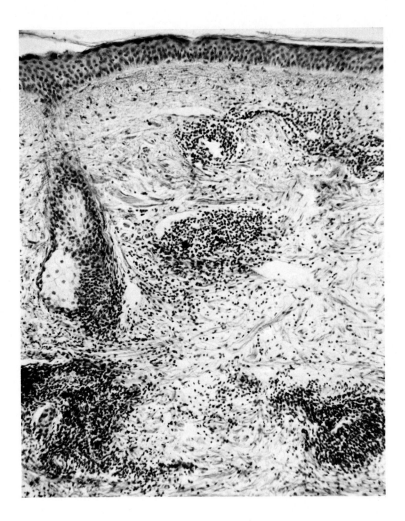

FIGURE 14–7.
Jessner's lymphocytic infiltration. While epidermis is not affected by infiltrate, this does invade follicular sheath, an exceptional feature. There is, however, no sebaceous atrophy or follicular plugging. H&E. X135.

hydroa vacciniforme types suffered reduction in number[13] when it was recognized that many are manifestations of porphyria or protoporphyria. The striking and disturbing clinical symptoms, however, are due to a reticulating degeneration of the epidermis forming vesicles and bullae and often associated with superficial dermal necrosis leading to vacciniform scarring. With the exception of *erythropoietic protoporphyria* in which a specific PAS-positive substance accumulates in the upper dermis (Chap. 27), the common histologic denominator of all these lesions is an inflammatory reaction associated with small vessels in the upper and middle dermis.[14] The deep dermis is involved rarely, but the infiltrate extends definitely into the reticular portion. Therefore, lupus erythematosus and dermal contact sensitivity reactions most commonly enter differential diagnosis.

Polymorphous light eruptions present a cellular infiltrate more polymorphous (mixed) than that of lupus erythematosus. Eosinophils, some plasma cells, and perhaps some neutrophils are encountered. The epidermis is commonly involved in an eczematous manner rather than with atrophy. Hair follicles, sebaceous glands, and elastic fibers are not usually damaged. Histologic differentiation from dermal contact sensitivity reactions (Chap. 7) should not be expected: these lesions are in the same group of tissue reactions, and clinical information or patch testing must give the answer. Reaction to a five-day photo patch test is shown in Figure 14-8. Precancerous changes due to ultraviolet rays will be treated in Chapter 34 and *actinic reticuloid* in Chapter 44.

Pellagra

A different mechanism of light sensitivity causes the cutaneous manifestations of *pellagra* and of *Hartnup's disease*, which have the common denominator of nicotinamide deficiency. In the acute dermatitic stage, there is chronic inflammatory infiltrate, and predominantly subepidermal bullae may form. Later, epidermal hyperkeratosis, parakeratosis, and hyperpigmentation are seen, followed by epidermal atrophy. The dermis often shows the elastic changes of chronic actinic influ-

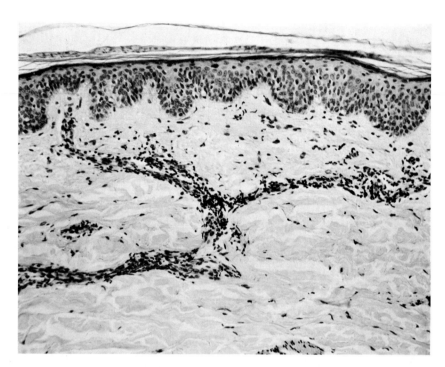

FIGURE 14–8.
Light sensitivity reaction. Photo patch test 5 days after application of 3 MED to sensitized skin. A thin layer of parakeratosis between two orthokeratotic layers remains as evidence that the epidermis has undergone an acute inflammatory phase (in this case, a sunburn reaction) and has recovered, now exhibiting mild acanthosis and a rather thick granular layer. The dermal infiltrate is similar to that of dermal contact sensitivity reaction (Fig. 7-7) and of drug eruption (Fig. 10-7), with which it also shares a tendency to invasion of the epidermis. H&E. X135.

ence (Chap. 26) and may exhibit hyalinization of collagen in the deeper layers.[15] Tissue changes are confirmatory of a clinical diagnosis rather than diagnostic.

DERMATOMYOSITIS

It seems convenient to discuss the skin manifestations of dermatomyositis at this point because they cause diagnostic difficulties with systemic lupus erythematosus. Many of these manifestions are as noncharacteristic histologically as they are clinically. The trained eye, however, looks for evidence of edema, especially around small vessels, and a fairly mild perivascular infiltrate in which plasma cells and an occasional eosinophil join the small round cells (Fig. 14-9). Definite diagnosis is rarely possible in the absence of striated muscle pathology (Fig. 14-10). Occasionally, degenerative changes

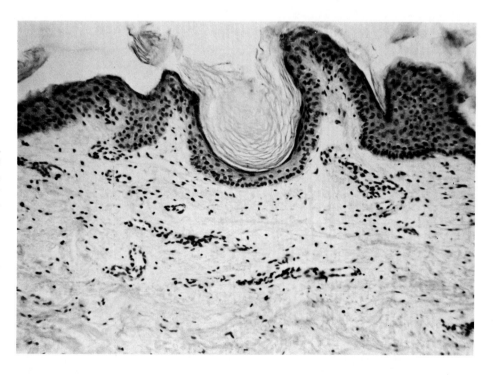

FIGURE 14–9.
Dermatomyositis. The histologic changes are mild and suggestive rather than diagnostic. The epidermis shows no significant (poikilodermatous) changes in this instance. There is dermal edema, which would react with stains for hyaluronic acid. Small blood vessels with prominent endothelial lining are associated with very mild cellular infiltrate, which at high magnification could be shown to contain an occasional plasma cell and rare eosinophil. H&E. X180.

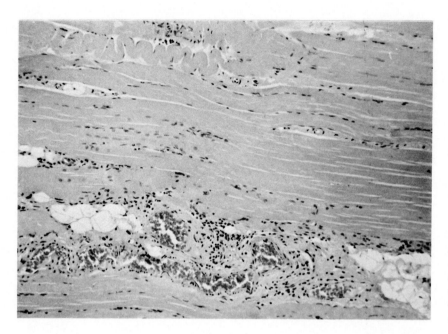

FIGURE 14–10.
Myositis of dermatomyositis. Lymphocytic infiltrate of interstitial connective tissue (containing some fat cells). Severe atrophy of skeletal muscle fibers showing long stretches without nuclei. The diagnosis of dermatomyositis must often be based on muscle biopsy. When obtaining a muscle biopsy specimen, however, the surgeon should not submit the overlying skin as the cutaneous specimen. Instead, a separate specimen should be taken from an area that exhibits clinical changes. H&E. X250.

have been observed in smooth muscle.[16] Hyaluronic acid is surprisingly plentiful in the edematous skin, a feature shared with systemic lupus.[17]

Diagnosis becomes easier when *poikilodermatous* features (Chap. 9) are present. Here again, it is easier to differentiate dermatomyositis from a simple dermatitis than from a poikilodermatous form of lupus erythematosus (Fig. 14-11). The latter is apt to have a heavier and purely lymphocytic infiltrate in the subacute form and much more extensive damage to the basal layer and epidermal atrophy in the acute type. A type of dermatomyositis associated with generalized pityriasis rubra pilaris-like horny plugging of hair follicles has been reported.[18]

REFERENCES

1. Tuffanelli DL: Connective tissue diseases. In Year Book of Dermatology 1978. Chicago, Year Book, 1978
2. Jablonska S (ed): Uses for immunofluorescence tests of skin and sera. Arch Dermatol 111:381, 1975
3. Burnham TK: Antinuclear antibodies. A simplified classification of the nuclear immunofluorescent patterns. Arch Dermatol 114:1343, 1978
4. Wrzolkowa T, Kozakiewicz J: Virus-like structures in the skin in the course of chronic lupus erythematosus. Dermatologica 154:228, 1977
5. Davies MG, Marks R: Evolution of the lesion of discoid lupus erythematosus: a comparison with lichen planus. Br J Dermatol 97:313, 1977
6. Ueki H: Hyaline bodies in subepidermal papillae: immunohistochemical studies in several dermatoses. Arch Dermatol 100:610, 1969

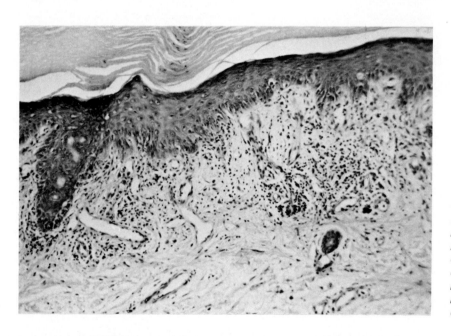

FIGURE 14–11.
Poikilodermatous form of lupus erythematosus. Skin of finger. Telangiectasia, lymphocytic infiltrate, and basal cell damage causing epidermal atrophy (see coiled acrosyringium in atrophic epidermis) are features fitting lupus erythematosus as well as poikilodermatous dermatomyositis. H&E. X250.

7. Panet-Raymond G, Johnson WC: Lupus erythematosus and polymorphous light eruption. Arch Dermatol 108:785, 1973

8. Tuffanelli DL: Lupus erythematosus panniculitis (profundus). Arch Dermatol 103:231, 1971

9. Schnitzler L, Verret J-L, Schubert B, Ginies J-L: Le lupus érythémateux profond. Intérêt de l'étude ultrastructurale. Ann Derm Venereol 105:153, 1978

10. Chubick A, Gilliam JN: A review of mixed connective tissue disease. Int J Dermatol 17:123, 1978

11. Jessner M: Lymphocytic infiltration of the skin. Arch Dermatol 68:447, 1953

12. Beare JM: Lymphocytic infiltration of the skin (Jessner-Kanof). In Rook A, Wilkinson DS, Ebling FJG (eds): Textbook of Dermatology, 2nd ed. Oxford and Edinburgh, Blackwell, 1968, p. 1382

13. Bickers DR, Demar LK, DeLeo V, et al.: Hydroa vacciniforme. Arch Dermatol 114:1193, 1978

14. Stern WK: Anatomic localization of the response to ultraviolet radiation in human skin. Dermatologica 145:361, 1972

15. Moore RA, Spies TD, Cooper ZK: Histopathology of the skin in pellagra. Arch Dermatol 46:100, 1942

16. Dupré A, Bonafé JL, Delsol G, Okiman F: Degenerescence des muscles arrecteurs dans une observation de dermatomyosite. Dermatologica 152:33, 1976

17. Jans JF, Winkelmann RK: Histopathology of the skin in dermatomyositis. Arch Dermatol 97:640, 1968

18. Dupré A, Floutard, Christol B, et al.: Dermatomyosite avec spinulosisme (dermatomyosite type Wong). Ann Dermatol Syphiligr 103:141, 1976

CHAPTER

15

Dermal Vasculitides and Other Vascular Disorders

All inflammatory processes involve blood vessels. True inflammation depends on the presence of blood vessels. Therefore, the terms *vasculitis* or *angiitis* should not be used loosely for those inflammatory changes that we have considered up to now, all of which exhibit reversible endothelial swelling, perivascular edema, and perivascular cell infiltrates. "Vasculitis" means inflammation of the vascular wall. In order to diagnose vasculitis, we need evidence of organic damage to the wall in the form of necrosis, hyalinization, fibrinoid change, or granulomatous involvement. The fact that a vascular wall is occupied by many polymorphonuclear leukocytes is not necessarily evidence of vasculitis: All inflammatory leukocytes go from the bloodstream into the tissue, and they must migrate through the walls of the vessels. Figure 15-1 represents a very early stage of a case of DNA autosensitivity (Chap. 16) in which large numbers of polymorphs were attracted into the site of the reaction and migrated through the walls of small and larger vessels without causing lasting damage to the wall, and without evidence of more than functional alteration of the wall. These pictures therefore simulate, but do not represent, vasculitis.

Identification of endothelial cells is made possible under the electron microscope by the presence of Weibel-Palade bodies,[1] rather large and usually elongated homogeneous structures in the cytoplasm which occur more commonly in young rather than quiescent cells. It is much easier to diagnose vasculitis if there is a vascular wall substantial enough for us to recognize damage in routine sections. Many cutaneous vessels do not fulfill this requirement, and the question of presence or absence of vasculitis remains in doubt. Of the diseases discussed so far, only the pigmented purpuric eruptions are apt to show vasculitic changes in the form of hyalinization of the walls of very small vessels. Vascular damage is difficult to demonstrate in cutaneous lupus erythematosus. In later chapters on granulomatous inflammation (Sec. IV), vasculitis will be encountered more often.

In this chapter, the first tissue reaction to be discussed is leukocytoclastic vasculitis,[2] the more severe expressions of which merge with cutaneous forms of polyarteritis nodosa and other types of necrotizing angiitis[3] (Table 15-1). Embolic and thrombotic phenomena will be discussed next. Other types of vascular disease that do not fit conveniently into other chapters will be given attention. The so-called lymphocytic vasculitis of pityriasis lichenoides acuta (Chap. 13) and of certain drug eruptions comes so close to a heavy perivascular infiltrate that we prefer not to single it out as an entity.

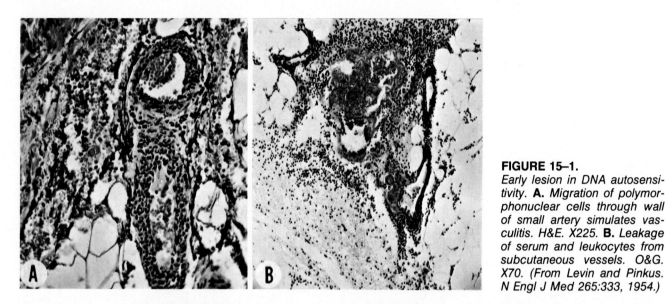

FIGURE 15–1.
*Early lesion in DNA autosensitivity. **A**. Migration of polymorphonuclear cells through wall of small artery simulates vasculitis. H&E. X225. **B**. Leakage of serum and leukocytes from subcutaneous vessels. O&G. X70. (From Levin and Pinkus. N Engl J Med 265:333, 1954.)*

TABLE 15–1.
Clinical Types of Necrotizing Angiitis

Small Vessels: Leukocytoclastic Vasculitis
Ruiter's and Gougerot's allergic vasculitis
Schoenlein-Henoch's purpura
Chronic urticaria
Palpable purpura
Drug-induced reactions
Erythema elevatum diutinum
Kawasaki's disease

Large Vessels: Sensitivity Angiitis
Periarteritis nodosa
Wegener's granulomatosis
Allergic granulomatosis
Chöfflertrain
Temporal arteritis

NECROTIZING ANGIITIS

Leukocytoclastic Vasculitis

Leukocytoclastic vasculitis is recognized by the presence of fragmented leukocytic nuclei (nuclear dust) in and around the vascular wall. The term is applicable to mild forms involving small vessels and often related to drugs and to the more severe forms of sensitivity angiitis which merge into periarteritis nodosa and may involve sizable vessels.[4] Reference is made here to the diagram in Chapter 10 (Fig. 10-1). We repeat that the relations shown in this scheme do not imply nosologic identity but are helpful in making a differential diagnosis by increasing awareness of morphologically similar conditions.

Ruiter's *allergic arteriolitis*[5] is illustrated in Figure 15-2A. It is closely related to, or identical with, *Gougerot's allergides*[6] and affects relatively superficial small vessels. Hyalinization of vascular walls, perivascular edema, nuclear debris, and presence of eosinophils and neutrophils in addition to round cells (Fig. 15-2B) are the outstanding features. Degranulation of mast cells may play a role.[2] The relative predominance of any feature will vary with the age and severity of the individual lesion. The changes are rarely severe enough to cause appreciable tissue necrosis, but hemorrhage may be present. The lesions may appear clinically as chronic urticaria or as palpable purpura.[2] Similar alterations are the histologic substrate of Schoenlein-Henoch's *purpura rheumatica*.[7]

Periarteritis Nodosa

Sensitivity angiitis and polyarteritis nodosa (Fig. 15-3) usually involve somewhat larger and deeper vessels which have sizable walls.[8] Surprisingly, this fact may not help in the diagnosis when H&E sections are examined. The structure of the vessel may be altered so much (Fig. 15-4A) that is is hard to recognize. O&G sections are very helpful (Fig. 15-4B) because the subintimal elastic ring of arteries and the elastic coats of veins are usually well preserved. The histologic hallmark of polyarteritis nodosa is necrosis of all or part of the vascular wall. This occurs early and is accompanied by neutrophilic and eosinophilic infiltrate. It is followed by more chronic inflammation, often by thrombosis, and sometimes by rupture and hemorrhage and eventual replacement by scar tissue. The picture in individual sections, therefore, depends on the stage of the disease, but evidence of destruction of the vessel wall and presence of eosinophils are requirements for diagnosis.

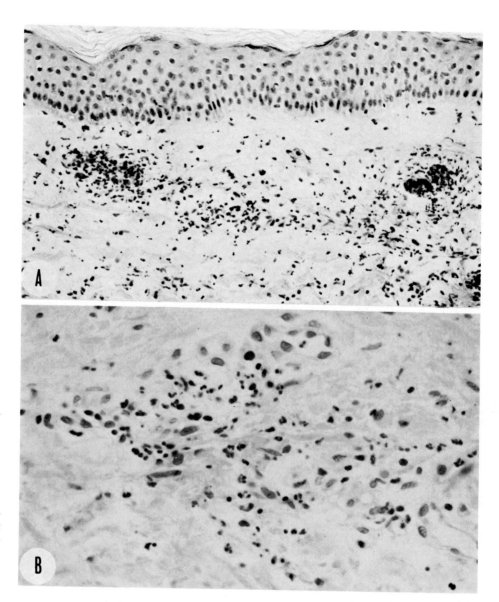

FIGURE 15–2.
*Leukocytoclastic vasculitis. Vessels of the subpapillary plexus are involved. Polymorphonuclear leukocytes break down, leaving nuclear dust. **A.** H&E. X225. **B.** H&E. X465.*

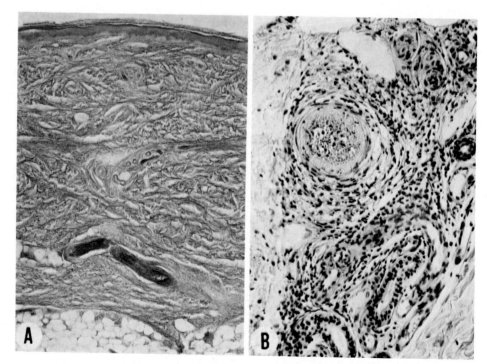

FIGURE 15–3.
*Segmental arteritis in case of clinical livedo racemosa (livedo reticularis). All layers of wall of a deep, medium-sized vessel are involved. **A.** O&G. X70. **B.** H&E. X225.*

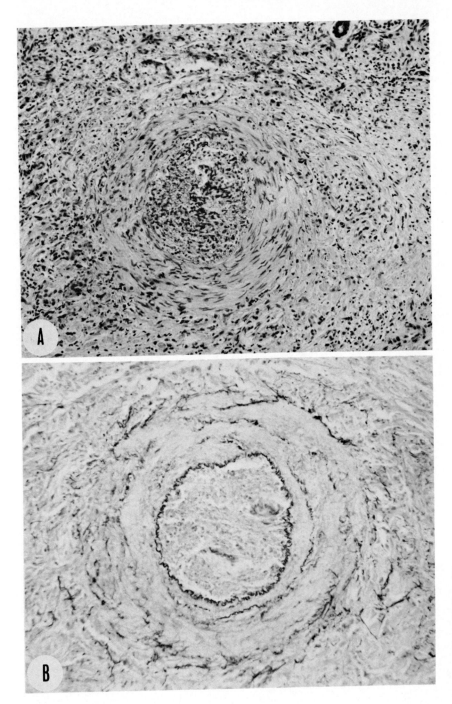

FIGURE 15–4.
Nodular vasculitis. **A.** *The wall of a fairly large vessel of the deep dermal plexus is disrupted by inflammatory infiltrate and its lumen filled by a thrombus. H&E. X120.* **B.** *Elastic fiber stain permits easier identification of the vessel wall and documents partial destruction of fibers. O&G. X120.*

Other Forms

Other forms of necrotizing angiitis with strongly granulomatous tissue reaction have been described as *Wegener's granulomatosis*[9] and *allergic granulomatosis.*[10] Although they may involve the skin with deep-seated nodules, they rarely come to the attention of the dermatopathologist. They cause granulomas with central necrosis that may or may not contain a recognizable vessel and may have aspects of a palisading granuloma (Chap. 22). The various forms of granulomatous and necrotizing vasculitis were discussed by Burton and Burton[11] (the *Chöfflertrain*) and Diaz et al.[12] A special form occasionally seen by dermatologists is temporal arteritis (Fig. 15-5). Mucous membrane manifestations will be mentioned in Chapter 45.

Kawasaki's Disease

An infantile acute febrile *mucocutaneous lymph node syndrome* was described in Japan and later in Hawaii and the continental United States[13] that

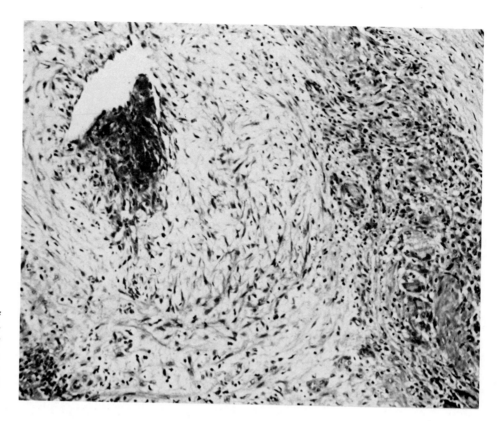

FIGURE 15–5.
Temporal arteritis. A branch of the temporal artery is partly occluded by subendothelial proliferation, and its wall is affected by granulomatous infiltrate, including multinucleated giant cells. H&E. X135.

seems to be related to cutaneous polyarteritis nodosa. Children affected are usually younger than 5 years of age and develop a polymorphous scarlatiniform, morbilliform, or erythema multiformelike exanthem, which is followed by general exfoliation beginning at the edge of the fingernails and toenails. In 1 or 2 percent of cases, death has resulted from cardiac failure, and the cutaneous lesions have features of polyarteritis nodosa histologically. Rickettsiae have been demonstrated in blood vessel walls.

EMBOLISM, THROMBOSIS, AND INFARCTION

Embolism

Other froms of vasculitis are due to, or at least are associated with, embolism or thrombosis. To the first type belong skin lesions in certain cases of chronic sepsis, such as *gonococcemia*[14] or *meningococcemia*.[15] They involve capillaries and small vessels below the epidermis and around adnexa with acute inflammation and lead to extravasation of red blood cells. Fat embolism into small cutaneous vessels and resulting purpura are encountered after fracture of long bones.[16] Embolism of tubercle bacilli into the small vessels may cause *miliary tuberculosis* of the skin and is the supposed origin of *lichen scrofulosorum* and *papulonecrotic tuberculids* (Chap. 20).

Thrombosis

Thrombotic phenomena often involve larger vessels and produce several different manifestations. The most impressive one histologically is *thromboangiitis obliterans*, in which a large artery or vein at the subcutaneous border is occluded by an organizing thrombus, while the wall is frayed and occupied by chronic inflammatory infiltrate. This disorder, together with polyarteritis nodosa must be taken into consideration in the differential diagnosis of deep nodose lesions (Chap. 16).

Two special cases are *Mondor's disease* and *nonvenereal sclerosing lymphangiitis* of the penis. Mondor's disease, whether spontaneous or induced by trauma, involves superficial veins of the anterior thorax with a thrombophlebitis that goes through the classic three stages: formation of an intraluminal thrombus, organization of the thrombus with fibroblasts, and recanalization.[17] The same is true for the (to the uninitiated) somewhat frightening firm cord in the postcoronal area of the penis, which has usually been interpreted as lymphangiitis but probably also is a phlebitis which dissolves spontaneously.[18]

Livedo

A peculiar clinical manifestation is *livedo reticularis* or *racemosa*, which must be differentiated from the purely functional *cutis marmorata* seen mainly in children. The cause of the chronic and permanent types of livedo is subtotal occlusion of larger vessels deep in the dermis or subcutaneous tissue, and this may have a variety of histologic substrates. In years past, tuberculous or syphilitic arteritis leading to partial obstruction of vessels was a frequent cause. Recently, cholesterol embolism and the resulting chronic granulomatous vasculitis has been reported[19] in several cases. Vascular occlusion with deposition of fibrinoid and hyalinization of more superficial vessels (Fig. 15-6) is seen in cases of *cryoglobulinemia* and other forms of *dysproteinemic purpura* and ulceration, often corresponding to the clinical picture of *livedo* with ulceration.[20,21] The histologic changes usually include necrosis of epidermis and upper dermis and severe polymorphonuclear and round cell infiltrate. Acute and chronic *pernio*, on the other hand (Fig. 15-7), exhibits obliteration of deeper dermal vessels by intimal proliferation and, at times, adherent thrombi. There is associated mixed inflammatory infiltrate of varying degree.[22]

Infarction

Purpuric and necrotic lesions of various types and subcutaneous hematomas may be manifestations of *disseminated intravascular coagulation.*[23] Skin biopsy may lead to early diagnosis and shows involvement of the subpapillary plexus, with fibrin thrombi located centrally in the lumen. While many of these lesions have features of infarction, true anemic infarcts of the entire thickness of the skin are extremely rare, so rich and interconnected is cutaneous blood supply. The one disease that fulfills the clinical and histologic criteria of anemic infarct is *malignant atrophic papulosis* of Degos.[24] At the tip of the conical area of sclerotic connective tissue, which corresponds to the sunken porcelain-white clinical lesion, one may find the occluded vessel (Fig. 15-8). Inflammatory reaction is minimal.

Infarction of small vessels with *Mucor* has been seen in immunosuppressed patients.[25]

CHRONIC X-RAY DERMATITIS

Another not uncommon dermatosis, in which severe vascular damage plays a role in addition to damage affecting all other constituents of the skin, is *chronic X-ray dermatitis* (Fig. 15-9). Epidermal changes include hypertrophy or atrophy and spotty pigmentation and may progress to dysplasia and neoplasia (see poikiloderma, Chap. 44). The epidermis, however, does not exhibit the focal basal cell liquefaction of poikilodermas to which the clinical picture has great similarity. All layers of the dermis show severe sclerosis, uneven distribution and clumping of elastic fibers, and obliteration of large

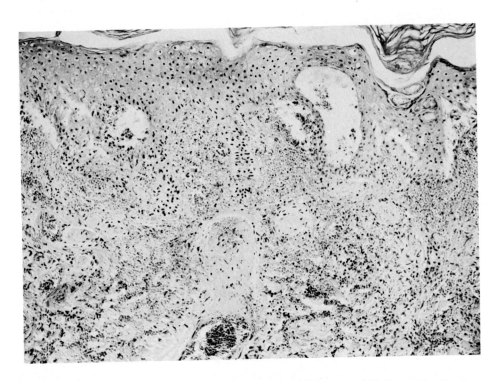

FIGURE 15–6.
Vascular occlusion with fibrinoid change, hemorrhage, dermal and epidermal necrosis in a case of livedo with summer ulcerations. Similar changes are encountered in atrophie blanche and lesions associated with dysproteinemia of various types. H&E. X135.

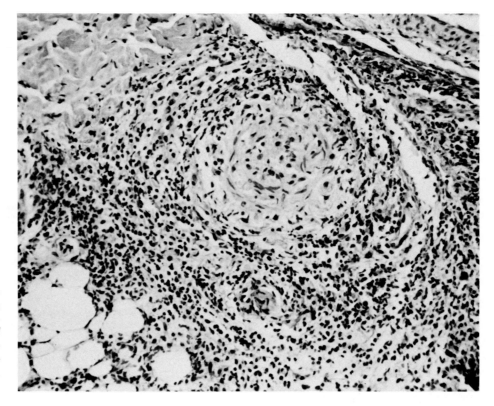

FIGURE 15–7.
Acute pernio (shoe boot pernio). Thrombotic occlusion of a small vessel at deep cutaneous border. Structure of wall obliterated by subacute inflammatory infiltrate, which also extends into surrounding tissue. H&E. X225.

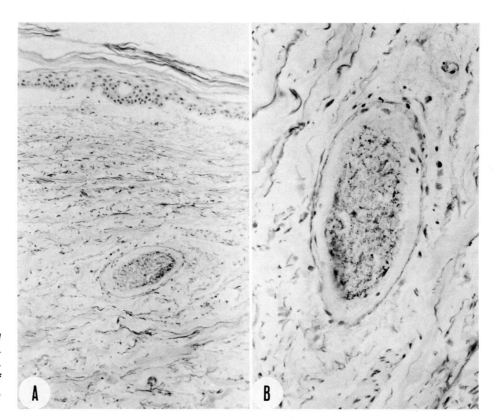

FIGURE 15–8.
Degos' disease. Infarction and necrosis of a medium-sized artery in deep dermis without inflammation. Elastica interna of artery well shown. O&G. **A.** *X125.* **B.** *X400.*

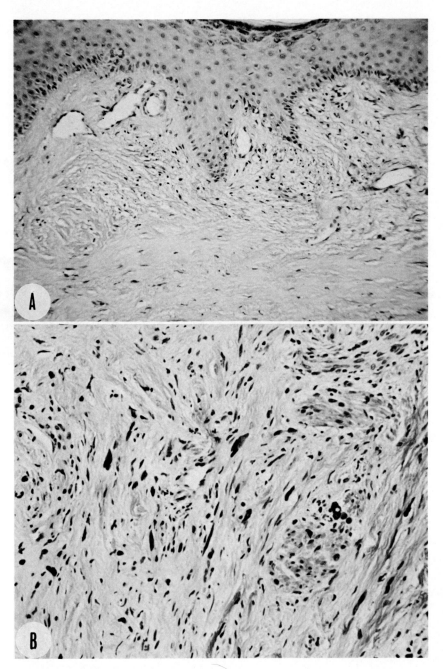

FIGURE 15–9.
Chronic X-ray damage. **A.** *While the epidermis is somewhat hypertrophic and hyperplastic, the dermis shows paucity of cells in the sclerotic pars reticularis and telangiectasia and distortion of collagen fibers in the pars papillaris. H&E. X135.* **B.** *Higher magnification shows damaged smooth muscle bundles in right half of picture, nuclei of giant fibroblasts in center, and unevenly sized collagen bundles in left half. H&E. X375.*

vessels with some new formation of ectatic, thin-walled vessels. A peculiar and almost pathognomonic feature is the presence of giant fibroblasts (Fig. 15-9B) similar to those seen in poorly growing tissue cultures. They seem to compensate for their inability to multiply by hypertrophy of nucleus and cytoplasm.

ERYTHEMA ELEVATUM DIUTINUM

An unusual type of leukocytoclastic vasculitis is encountered in erythema elevatum diutinum (Fig. 15-10). The disease[26] is characterized by the paradox that the cellular infiltrate consists almost entirely of neutrophils and eosinophils in spite of the chronic course.[27] The substance called "toxic hyalin" by Weidman is similar to fibrinoid in its staining reactions. It occupies a zone broader than the actual vessel wall and is seen as a coarse trabeculation of the connective tissue, similar to that found in granuloma faciale (Fig. 15-11). Cases formerly described as *extracellular cholesterosis* seem to be a variant of erythema elevatum diutinum in which cholesterol is deposited in the tissue.[28] The histologic differential diagnosis includes Sweet's

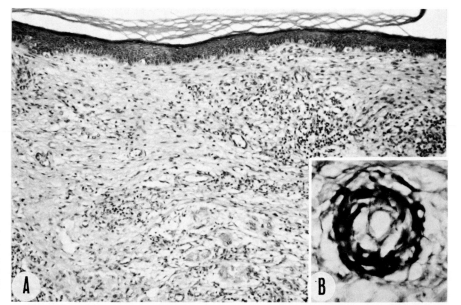

FIGURE 15–10.
*Erythema elevatum diutinum. **A.** Several of the involved vessels are surrounded by hyaline material. H&E. X135. **B.** Trabeculation of PAS-positive material surrounding a small vessel. Alcian blue-PAS. X400.*

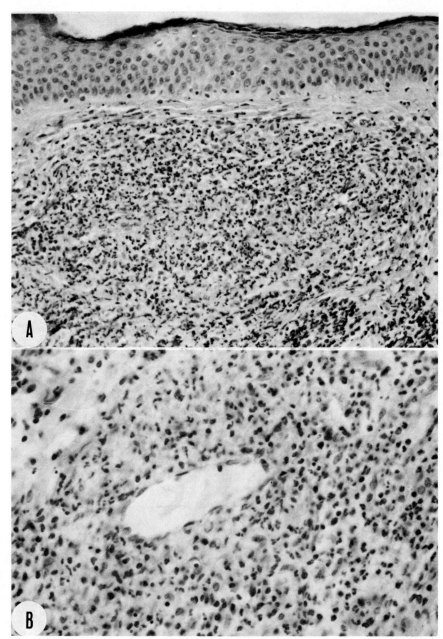

FIGURE 15–11.
*Granuloma faciale. **A.** Superficial portion, illustrating the grenz zone between epidermis and a mixed granulomatous infiltrate. H&E. X225. **B.** Dilated thin-walled vessel surrounded by disintegrating leukocytes in a zone of degenerating connective tissue. Mixed granulomatous infiltrate. H&E. X600.*

183

syndrome (Chap. 10), in which the peculiar perivascular changes are absent, and granuloma faciale, in which many histiocytes are present as proof of a granulomatous response.

GRANULOMA FACIALE

Granuloma faciale derives its name from the fact that it occurs almost exclusively on the face,[29,30] although a few disseminated cases have been recorded.[31] Once considered a member of the group of eosinophilic granulomas,[32] this peculiarly indolent disease[33] has highly characteristic histologic features (Fig. 15-11B), the most prominent of which is presence of neutrophilic leukocytes in a clinically chronic affection. Eosinophilic leukocytes are also usually present,[34] sometimes in large numbers, but are not absolutely necessary for diagnosis. Other features are the presence of histiocytes, lymphocytes, and plasma cells, a peculiar trabeculation of connective tissue (fibrinoid?) around thin-walled wide vessels, often associated with leukocytoclasia, and a free subepidermal zone (grenz zone). Multinucleated giant cells are rare, a few foam cells may occur, but phagocytosis of hemosiderin and melanin is more common. The epidermis usually shows no particular changes, and ulceration is most uncommon. Hair follicles and sweat glands slowly undergo atrophy. The granulomatous infiltrate may extend into the subcutaneous tissue.

The picture thus combines prominent granulomatous inflammation with leukocytoclastic vasculitis, a unique experience. There is some similarity to the Arthus phenomenon.[35] Granuloma faciale differs from erythema elevatum diutinum, in which there may be considerable fibrosis but rarely much histiocyte or plasma cell reaction.

STASIS DERMATITIS

Finally, we have to discuss common cutaneous changes of the lower extremities that are often called "stasis dermatitis" in the widest sense. It was recommended in Chapter 3 to avoid biopsy of lesions below the knee, if there is a choice. Even relatively young persons without obviously diseased skin may exhibit dilatation, tortuosity, and tufting of capillaries and thickening of the walls of deeper vessels as early signs of stasis. These changes lead to excessive fragility of capillary walls and diapedesis of red cells with advanced age, and it is a common experience that a generalized maculopapular drug eruption will become purpuric below the knees and heal with residual hemosiderin pigmentation. Vascular changes of this type, mild round cell infiltrate, and a moderate quantity of hemosiderin in dermal macrophages should be discounted in the diagnosis of other dermatoses if the specimen was obtained from the lower extremities. More definite vascular alterations are needed for a diagnosis of pigmented purpuric eruption (Chap. 13). Heavier deposits of hemosiderin that extend into the deeper layers are the substrate of *dermite ocre* of Favre-Chaix,[36] which is associated with ve-

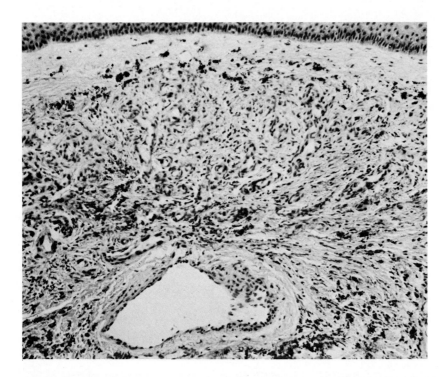

FIGURE 15–12.
Hypertrophic stasis dermatitis. Diffuse proliferation of superficial blood vessels, while the large deeper vessel is intact. Hemosiderotic macrophages are found in this condition and in Kaposi's sarcoma (Fig. 42-9). H&E. X100.

nous insufficiency. Variable degrees of dermal fibrosis, loss of elastic fibers, and atrophy of epidermis and adnexal structures (hair muscles, however,
usually survive and actually increase in size) are
additional nonspecific changes in leg skin that may
be quite disturbing in the interpretation of biopsy
specimens.

In cases that show clinical evidence of stasis dermatitis, one should, of course, expect evidence of
subacute or chronic eczematous tissue reaction
(Chap. 7) in addition to the changes just described.
Two variants need special mention. Peculiar localized forms of proliferation of superficial vessels
with heavy accumulation of hemosiderotic macrophages may produce nodes and plaques that arouse
the clinician's fear of Kaposi's sarcoma (Chap. 42).
The diffuse character and superficial location of the
vascular proliferation are the differentiating signs
of this *hypertrophic stasis dermatitis* (Fig. 15-12).

Atrophie Blanche

White atrophy (atrophie blanche) is at the other end
of the clinical spectrum. The chalky white skin is
sclerotic, with occasional telangiectasias and frequent painful ulcers. Biopsies are rarely taken in
this type of case because of the poor healing tendency, and we, therefore, must rely on published reports,[37-40] one of which[38] was based on 22 cases.
Occlusion of vessels by intimal thickening or fibrin
thrombi (Fig. 15-6) are mentioned in addition to fibrosis, but there is no unanimity as to whether the
clinically so characteristic disease is primarily a
vasculitis. In any case, it often precedes ulceration
and is not just due to fibrotic scarring.

REFERENCES

1. Weibel ER, Palade GE: New cytoplasmic components in arterial endothelia. J Cell Biol 23:101, 1964
2. Winkelmann RK, Ditto WB: Cutaneous and visceral
   syndromes of necrotizing or "allergic" angiitis. Medicine 43:59, 1964
3. Soter N: Clinical presentations and mechanisms of
   necrotizing angiitis of the skin. J Invest Dermatol
   17:354, 1976
4. Callen JP, Chanda JJ, Voorhees JJ: Cutaneous angiitis
   (vasculitis). Int J Dermatol 17:105, 1978
5. Ruiter M, Molenaar I: Ultrastructural changes in arteriolitis (vasculitis) allergica cutis superficialis. Br J
   Dermatol 85:14, 1970
6. Duperrat B: A propos des "angéites leucocytocla-
   siques." Ann Derm Siphiligr 99:391, 1972
7. Pierini LE, Abulafia J, Wainfeld S: Vascularitis
   alérgicas. Dermatol Ibero Lat Am 12 [Suppl 1], 1970
8. Diaz-Perez JL, Winkelmann RK: Cutaneous periarteritis nodosa. Arch Dermatol 110:407, 1974
9. Reed WB, Jensen AK, Konwaler BE, et al.: The cutaneous manifestations in Wegener's granulomatosis.
   Acta Derm Venereol (Stockh) 43:250, 1963
10. Churg J, Strauss L: Allergic granulomatosis, allergic
    angiitis, and periarteritis nodosa. Am J Pathol 27:277,
    1951
11. Burton JL, Burton PA: Pulmonary eosinophilia asso-
    ciated with vasculitis and extravascular granulomata.
    A case report and review of the literature. Br J Der-
    matol 87:412, 1972
12. Diaz L, Provost T, Tomasi T: Pustular necrotizing
    angiitis. Arch Dermatol 108:114, 1973
13. Kahn G: Mucocutaneous lymph node syndrome (Ka-
    wasaki's disease). A new disease remaking its debut.
    Arch Dermatol 114:948, 1978
14. Shapiro L, Taisch JA, Brownstein MH: Dermatohis-
    topathology of chronic gonococcal sepsis. Arch Der-
    matol 107:403, 1973
15. Sotto MN, Langer B, Hoshino-Shimizu S, DeBrito T:
    Pathogenesis of cutaneous lesions in acute meningo-
    coccemia in humans. J Infect Dis 133:506, 1976
16. Cole WG, Oakes BW: Skin petechiae and fat embo-
    lism. Aust NZ J Surg 42:401, 1973
17. Johnson WC, Walbrich R, Helwig EB: Superficial
    thrombophlebitis of the chest wall. JAMA 180:103,
    1962
18. Findlay GH, Whiting DA: Mondor's phlebitis of the
    penis. A condition miscalled 'non-venereal sclerosing
    lymphangitis.' Clin Exp Dermatol 2:45, 1977
19. Deschamps P, LeRoy D, Mandard JC, et al.: Livedo
    reticularis and nodules due to cholesterol embolism
    in the lower extremities. Br J Dermatol 97:93, 1977
20. Klüken N, Gerl R: Ätiopathogenetische und klin-
    ische Beziehungen der Livedo racemosa und der Vas-
    kulitiden zum Syndrom von O'Leary, Montgomery
    and Brunsting. Z Haut Geschlechtskr 47:807, 1972
21. Posternak F, Orusco M, Olmos L, Laugier P: Livedoid
    vasculitis (vascularite hyalinisante segmentaire) Étude
    immunohistopathologique. Ann Derm Venereol
    104:50, 1978
22. Coskey RJ, Mehregan AH: Shoe boot pernio. Arch
    Dermatol 109:56, 1974
23. Colman RW, Minna JD, Robboy SJ: Disseminated in-
    travascular coagulation: a dermatologic disease. Int J
    Dermatol 16:47, 1977
24. Degos R: Malignant atrophic papulosis. Br J Derma-
    tol 100:21, 1979
25. Kramer BS, Hernandez AD, Reddick RL, Levine A:
    Cutaneous infarction: manifestation of disseminated
    mucormycosis. Arch Dermatol 113:1075, 1977
26. Haber H: Erythema elevatum diutinum. Br J Derma-
    tol 67:121, 1955
27. Katz SI, Gallin JI, Hertz KC, et al.: Erythema eleva-
    tum diutinum: Skin and systemic manifestations,
    immunologic studies and successful treatment with
    dapsone. Medicine (Baltimore) 56:433, 1977
28. Wolff HH, Maciewski W, Scherer R: Erythema ele-
    vatum diutinum. I. Elektronenmikroskopie eines
    Falles mit extracellulärer Cholinesterose. Arch Der-
    matol Res 261:7, 1978
29. Pinkus H: Granulomas with eosinophilia ("eosino-
    philic granulomas"). Med Clin North Am 35:463,
    1951
30. Cobane JH, Straith CL, Pinkus H: Facial granulomas
    with eosinophilia. Their relation to other eosino-
    philic granulomas of the skin and to reticulogranu-
    loma. Arch Dermatol 61:442, 1950

31. Rusin LJ, Dubin HV, Taylor WB: Disseminated granuloma faciale. Arch Dermatol 112:1575, 1976
32. Lever W: Eosinophilic granuloma of the skin. Arch Dermatol 55:194, 1947
33. Pinkus H: Granuloma faciale. Dermatologica 105:85, 1952
34. Schwitzler L, Verret JL, Schubert B: Granuloma faciale. Ultrastructural study of three cases. J Cutan Pathol 4:123, 1977
35. Nieboer C, Kalsbeek GL: Immunofluorescence studies in granuloma eosinophilicum faciale. J Cutan Pathol 5:68, 1978
36. Odeh F, Goos M: Zur Histopathologie der Dermite ocre Favre-Chaix. Z Haut Geschlechtskr 47:147, 1972
37. Gray HR, Graham JH, Johnson W, et al.: Atrophie blanche: periodic painful ulcers of lower extremities: a clinical and histopathologic entity. Arch Dermatol 93:187, 1966
38. Kresbach M: Die Capillaritis alba. Fortschr Prakt Dermatol Venerol 7:135, 1973
39. Gilliam JN, Herndon JH, Prystowsky SD: Fibrinolytic therapy for vasculitis in atrophie blanche. Arch Dermatol 109:664, 1974
40. Stevanovic DV: Atrophie blanche: a sign of dermal blood occlusion. Arch Dermatol 109:858, 1974

16

Subcutaneous Inflammations: Panniculitis

Inflammatory processes involving the deepest layers of the dermis and the subcutaneous fat tissue are not rare in a dermatopathologist's material and constitute one of the major diagnostic headaches. There are several reasons for the difficulties encountered in differential diagnosis. Excisional biopsy of ample size by the use of a sharp knife is the ideal way of obtaining an adequate specimen. Punch biopsies may provide adequate samples in many other dermatoses but often produce inadequate material in these large and deep-seated plaques. The plug of tissue is obtained rather blindly and may or may not include pathognomonic portions of the tissue, even if the operator used a 6 or 8 mm punch and went as deeply as he should go—that is, more than halfway through the subcutaneous panniculus (Fig. 3-9). Only too often, the specimen contains either skin only or skin and a minimal amount of fat tissue.

If an ample specimen is supplied, the technician must be instructed to cut a considerable number of sections. One of the important points in diagnosis is the presence or absence of a pathologic larger blood vessel, and a conclusion cannot be reached on only a few sections. Another difficulty is the biologic propensity of fat tissue to react in a stereotyped manner to any insult. The response is known by the German term *Wucheratrophie* or *proliferating atrophy*. It means that normal fat tissue disappears and is replaced by fibroblasts and macrophages (Fig. 16-1) associated with a greater or lesser number of inflammatory cells. Once this proliferating atrophy is well established, it is impossible to recognize its cause and origin. It is also obvious that inflammation of the subcutaneous tissue has granulomatous features, so we will not be able to separate simple and granulomatous inflammation in this field.

The border between dermis and subcutis is not sharp. Fat lobes may be found in the dermis, especially around sweat coils, and the large vessels of the deep cutaneous plexus are partly within the dermis, partly below it. The subcutaneous panniculus consists of fat lobes separated by connective tissue septa, which usually contain larger vessels, while the fat lobes are richly supplied with tiny vessels. All these features must be kept in mind when one analyzes a deep nodose lesion. Since most of these occur on the legs, one should additionally consider the almost invariable presence of some stasis changes even in young persons (Chap. 15).

DIFFERENTIAL DIAGNOSIS

A practical approach to differential diagnosis would appear to be the following. First one should decide whether the principal seat of pathologic change, the center of gravity of the lesion, is in the mid-dermis, the cutaneous–subcutaneous border zone, the interlobular septa, or the fat lobes. Inflammatory

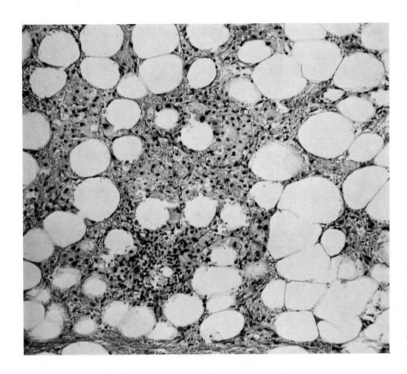

FIGURE 16–1.
Proliferating atrophy of fat tissue. The relatively large cells having gray-appearing cytoplasm are macrophages containing numerous small lipid droplets. H&E. X135.

changes usually involve all of these areas, but a representative section often permits a decision. A center of gravity in the mid-dermis automatically eliminates the lesion from our present consideration: it might be granuloma annulare, folliculitis, or something else. Center of gravity at the subcutaneous junction strongly suggests primary involvement of a larger vessel, because inflammation of sweat coils is very rare (Chap. 19). Primary seat in the interlobar septa is fairly common, and the infiltrate then invades the fat lobes from the periphery. True panniculitis (Fig. 16-2), on the other hand, will show a whole lobe of fat tissue involved with infiltrate and possibly necrosis or liquefaction. Small vessels in the center of the lobe are the primary site of disturbance. An instructive monograph was published by Niemi et al.[1]

The next point to be considered is the general character of the infiltrate. Well-developed epithelioid cell nodules, associated with round cells, in the absence of granulocytes are almost diagnostic of tuberculosis in the form of erythema induratum or of sarcoidosis or syphilis. The presence of polymorphonuclear leukocytes in a nonulcerated lesion points away from these three granulomatous diseases but may be found in deep fungous infections. Erythema nodosum often shows a peculiar mixture of more acute inflammation around small blood vessels and giant cell reaction of foreign-body type in the interlobar septa. Pure round cell infiltrate suggests lymphoma, and pure polymorphonuclear infiltrate suggests acute infection or allergic reaction.

After ascertaining these parameters, one should

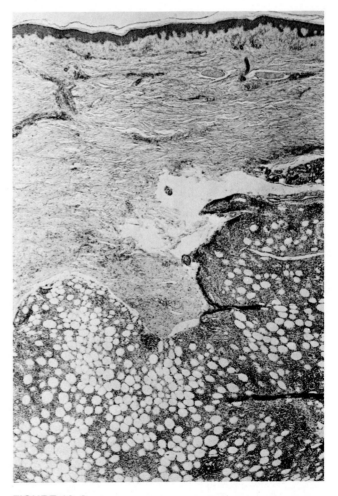

FIGURE 16–2.
Panniculitis. Entire fat lobes are involved with little change of surrounding connective tissue. H&E. X60.

institute a careful search for involvement of larger vessels and should remember, as was pointed out in the previous chapter, that vascular structure may be so completely obscured that even a sizable artery or vein resembles a fibrotic or granulomatous nodule in H&E sections. The O&G stain often brings surprises because elastic fibers are usually preserved, at least in part. Immunofluorescent studies may be helpful. A search for microorganisms using PAS and acid-fast methods should be made in doubtful cases.

INDIVIDUAL ENTITIES

Nodular Vasculitis

If a large artery or vein seems to be the center of the process, the diagnosis of nodular vasculitis is appropriate unless a more specific diagnosis suggests itself. One should remember that a relatively small biopsy may not include that vessel or that partial sectioning of a large specimen may miss it. In many cases, the diagnosis of nodular vasculitis is an admission of etiologic ignorance, but only too often, it is the best that can be made. Special manifestations of deep vasculitis are *Mondor's disease*, consisting of painful induration of a thrombosed deep chest vein (Chap. 15), *temporal arteritis (giant cell arteritis)*, a presumably allergic granulomatous vasculitis (Fig. 15-5) that may cause large and deep ulcerations of cranial skin,[2] and *nodular migratory panniculitis* (thrombophlebitis) of the legs,[3,4] which is remarkable for its prompt response to potassium iodide therapy.

Erythema Nodosum

The clinical term *erythema nodosum* lends itself to wide interpretation and has been used indiscriminately for any red or dusky nodosity of the lower legs. The etiology may vary from the classic tuberculosis to streptococcal infection or sarcoidosis and many other causes, among which *Yersinia* has been stressed.[5] We agree that there is not only the classic subacute form, which runs its course in a few weeks, but that more chronic forms exist.[6] We insist, however, on certain criteria for histologic diagnosis. Erythema nodosum (Fig. 3-9) involves small blood vessels and interlobar septa preferentially. The latter often show multinucleated giant cells (Fig. 16-3) even in early and relatively acute cases. Inflammatory cells include lymphocytes and usually at least some polymorphonuclears. Fat lobes are invaded by the infiltrate from the periph-

ery. The small granulomatous foci of Miescher are considered pathognomonic, but they are often not present. Definite areas of tissue necrosis rule out erythema nodosum, and so do typical epithelioid tubercles or many plasma cells or numerous eosinophils.

Erythema Induratum and Gummatous Syphilis

In fully developed lesions of *Bazin's disease*, the combination of tissue necrosis and well-organized tubercles makes a diagnosis of *erythema induratum* (Chap. 20) easy. However, the tuberculoid structure may be aped by proliferating atrophy of fat tissue, and, on the other hand, cases of proven tuberculous etiology may show nothing but nonspecific alterations. The theoretically present, deep tuberculous phlebitis is difficult to demonstrate. Clinically, ulcerated lesions may, of course, show polymorphonuclear infiltrate and other evidence of secondary infection. Presence of many plasma cells makes *gummatous syphilis* the more likely diagnosis.

Panniculitis

Panniculitis in the strict sense applies to inflammation of fat lobes rather than of interlobular septa or of large subcutaneous vessels. The fetal development (Chap. 2) makes each fat lobe a separate organ with a nourishing artery and two draining veins and explains the sharp limitation of panicular inflammation (Fig. 16-2). Once fat cells in a lobe are damaged, macrophages are attracted and, by phagocytosis, become foam cells. The mixture of fat atrophy and proliferation of inflammatory cells is called *Wucheratrophie* (Fig. 16-1) and is such a stereotyped response that it soon overshadows all specific processes and makes histopathologic diagnosis difficult.

The prototype of acute or subacute panniculitis was Weber–Christian's *febrile nonsuppurative nodular panniculitis*, but the diagnosis is made less and less frequently as diagnostic acumen increases.[7] While suppuration is ruled out by definition, many cases of the clinical Weber–Christian type undergo liquefaction necrosis and are called *liquefying panniculitis* (Fig. 16-4) on histologic examination. Any acute panniculitis contains polymorphonuclears, and the eventual outcome depends on many circumstances. We are usually content to diagnose panniculitis in the sense just defined.

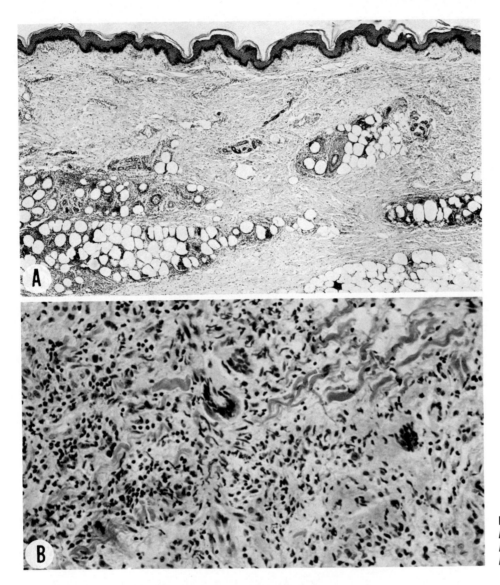

FIGURE 16–3.
Erythema nodosum (see also Fig. 3-9). **A.** *H&E. X90.* **B.** *H&E. X270.*

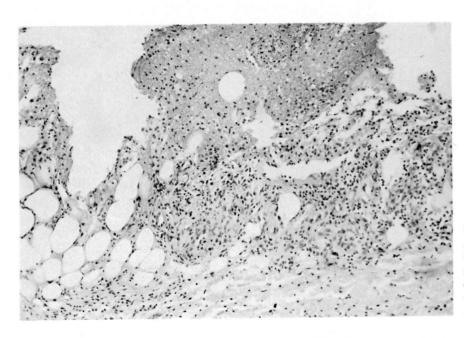

FIGURE 16–4.
Liquefying panniculitis. The center of the involved fat lobule has undergone necrosis, which is secondarily invaded by relatively small numbers of polymorphonuclear leukocytes. H&E. X125.

However, the presence of clefts in paraffin sections as evidence of fatty acid formation during life separates out several entities. *Nodular infantile fat necrosis* (Fig. 16-5)[8] and the generalized *sclerema neonatorum*[9] are diseases of infancy, while *pancreatitis* and *enzymemia* may produce similar changes in later life.[10] Rare, but potentially fatal, *necrotizing fasciitis* is usually caused by streptococci and affects the superficial fascia deep to subcutaneous fat tissue with acute necrotizing inflammation.[11]

Lupus Panniculitis

Chronic lupus erythematosus may manifest itself in rare instances as deep subcutaneous indurations (lupus profundus, Chap. 14) with or without the presence of discoid cutaneous lesions. Histologically (Fig. 14-5), there may be pure round cell infiltrate as in other forms, but the universal granulomatous reaction of damaged fat tissue (proliferating atrophy) may lead to mistakes in diagnosis, e.g., Darier-Roussy sarcoid (Chap. 20). Blood vessels of various sizes (Fig. 14-6) may be severely involved, and lymphoid follicles may form.[12]

Deep Fungous Infections

All the granulomatous mycoses, especially sporotrichosis, may have their center of gravity in subcutaneous tissue. They will be discussed in Section IV.

Eruptions Due to Hypersensitivity

Various drugs, particularly aspirin, can cause deep painful nodules simulating erythema nodosum or nodular vasculitis clinically as well as histologically. Unless one of these diagnoses can be made with assurance, it is wise to suggest aspirin or other drugs as a possible cause to the often unsuspecting clinician.

In spite of its rarity, we like to devote a few sentences to DNA autosensitivity[13,14] because the sequence of histologic events is so characteristic and because the first discovered case of this entity remained undiagnosed for over four years in spite of repeated biopsies, which led to such diagnoses as erythema nodosum, Weber–Christian panniculitis, and nodular vasculitis. The characteristic features were not seen until a very early lesion, 18 hours old, was obtained (Chap. 15). They consisted of profuse polymorphonuclear infiltrate, hyaline thrombi, and hemorrhage, as illustrated in Figure 15-1. As the patient was sensitive to her own white cells, their breakdown in the deep tissue caused a vicious cycle. Later, however, granulocytes were overshadowed by round cell infiltrate and macrophage reaction. Similar tissue reaction has been seen in somewhat more common cases of *autoerythrocyte sensitivity.*[15]

Other Inflammatory Entities

The Darier–Roussy type of *sarcoid* (Fig. 20-14) may cause deep-seated cutaneous–subcutaneous plaques

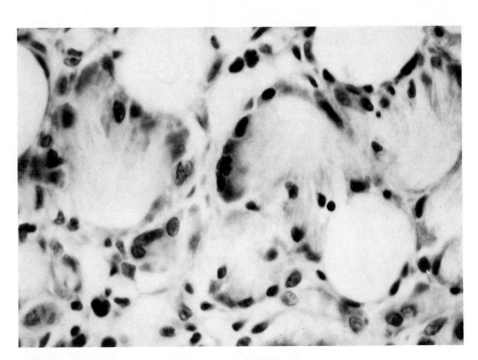

FIGURE 16–5.
Subcutaneous fat necrosis of newborn shows formation of multinucleated cells and clefts left by fatty acid crystals. H&E. X600.

characterized by typical epithelioid cell tubercles. *Spiegler-Fendt sarcoid*, on the other hand, is characterized by pure round cell nodes and belongs in the lymphoma group (Sec. VII). Deep-seated neoplasm, such as eccrine spiradenoma, glomus tumor, and Kaposi's sarcoma, should be easily ruled out by microscopic examination. Infestation with worms occurs mainly in tropical countries (Chap. 21).

One should not forget that the introduction of foreign matter of various types may produce subcutaneous nodes which range all the way from infected or sterile abscesses to indolent lipogranulomas.[15] In many cases, only a high rate of suspicion can solve puzzling cases by identifying morphologically or chemically mineral oil, silica, starch, and other substances, to which most recently impure preparations of silicone have been added. Some of these substances may produce subcutaneous calcifications. For additional data, see Chapter 20 (sarcoid granulomas), Chapter 21 (foreign-body granuloma), and Chapter 27 (foreign bodies).

Noninflammatory Entities

Piezogenic Papules. Under the name piezogenic pedal papules, painful herniations of fat tissue on the soles of the feet have been described, which seem to be provoked by pressure and exhibit degenerative changes of fat tissue, interlobar septa, and overlying dermis.[16] Nonpainful small herniations in similar location are not uncommon[17] and consist of normal fat tissue.

Cellulite. Another, and quite obscure, condition of fat tissue has caused considerable comment in Europe, more in lay circles than in the medical literature. Braun-Falco and Scherwitz,[18] however, felt compelled to investigate the tissue basis of the so-called *cellulite*, which refers to the slight puckering of the skin of the thighs of adipose women and has become a lucrative reason for therapy. They came to the conclusion that this "disease" is a normal phenomenon related to the fibrous retinacula that connect skin and fascia between the fat lobes.[19]

REFERENCES

1. Niemi K, Förström L, Haunukiela M, et al.: Nodules on the legs. A clinical, histological and immunohistological study of 82 patients representing different types of nodular panniculitis. Acta Derm Venereol (Stockh) 57:145, 1977
2. Hitch JM: Dermatologic manifestations of giant cell arteritis (temporal, cranial). Arch Dermatol 101:409, 1970
3. Vilanova X, Piñol Aguadé J: Subacute nodular migratory panniculitis. Br J Dermatol 71:45, 1959
4. Perry HO, Winkelmann RK: Subacute nodular migratory panniculitis. Arch Dermatol 89:170, 1964
5. Debois J, Vandepitte J, Degreef H: *Yersinia enterocolitica* as a cause of erythema nodosum. Deramtologica 156:65, 1978
6. Winkelmann RK, Förström L: New observations in the histopathology of erythema nodosum. J Invest Dermatol 65:441, 1975
7. Förström L, Winkelmann RK: Acute panniculitis. A clinical and histopathologic study of 34 cases. Arch Dermatol 113:909, 1977
8. Tsuji T: Subcutaneous fat necrosis of the newborn. Light and electron microscopic studies. Br J Dermatol 95:407, 1976
9. Oswalt GC Jr, Montes LF, Cassady G: Subcutaneous fat necrosis of the newborn. J Cutan Pathol 5:193, 1978
10. Hughes PSH, Apisarnthanarax P, Mullins JF: Subcutaneous fat necrosis associated with pancreatic disease. Arch Dermatol 111:506, 1975
11. Koehn GS: Necrotizing fasciitis. Arch Dermatol 114:581, 1978
12. Harris AB, Duncan SC, Ecker RI, Winkelmann RK: Lymphoid follicles in subcutaneous inflammatory disease. Arch Dermatol 115:442, 1979
13. Levin MB, Pinkus H: Autosensitivity to desoxyribonucleic acid (DNA). Report of a case with inflammatory skin lesions controlled by chloroquine. N Engl J Med 264:533, 1961
14. Pinnas JL, Tan EM, Teplitz RL, Boyer JT: Autosensitization to DNA: evidence for an immunologic basis. J Invest Dermatol 72:151, 1979
15. Hersle K, Mobacken H: Autoerythrocyte sensitization syndrome. Br J Dermatol 81:574, 1969
16. Harman RRM, Matthews CNA: Painful piezogenic pedal papules. Br J Dermatol 90:573, 1974
17. Schlappner OLA, Wood MG, Gerstein W, et al.: Painful and nonpainful piezogenic pedal papules. Arch Dermatol 106:729, 1972
18. Braun-Falco O, Scherwitz C: Zur Histopathologie der sogenannten Cellulitis. Hautarzt 23:71, 1972
19. Nürnberger F, Müller G: So-called cellulite: an invented disease. J Dermatol Surg Oncol 4:221, 1978

CHAPTER

17

Ulcers

Cutaneous ulceration is counted among the secondary manifestations which complicate primary lesions. Ulcers may result from infection, local lack of nutrition, neoplasia, and other causes. It would seem that they need no separate discussion. It was deemed advisable, however, to devote a chapter to ulcers because their clinical diagnosis is difficult and biopsy specimens have certain nonspecific features in common and have some differentiating signs not encountered in nonulcerated lesions.

An ulcer is defined as a loss of tissue that includes at least the epidermis and some superficial dermis. It may imply loss of the entire dermis. If only epidermis or some of its layers are absent, the microscopist speaks of erosion or denudation, but experience proves that the difference may be difficult to tell clinically. Thus, the acantholytic process of pemphigus and even the subepidermal bullae of other blistering diseases (Chap. 11) lead to denudation, not to ulceration. The uncomplicated syphilitic chancre (Chap. 2) and the primary lesion of granuloma inguinale (Chap. 21) may appear ulcerated to the clinician, but they usually retain enough of an epidermal covering to consider them only denuded histologically. Denudations are apt to be reepithelized rapidly without leaving permanent scars. Ulceration will lead to scarring regardless of whether only the papillary layer or the entire dermis was lost.

Biopsy of an ulcer needs special care and may lead to unsatisfactory specimens, even by the hands of experts, because the deep tissue often is friable and the presence of hard crust on the surface may require undue pressure. The specimen should include healthy skin at one margin and extend across the border an adequate distance into the bottom of the ulcer. Punch biopsy, therefore, is rarely adequate. A slice of tissue should be obtained by making two vertical incisions, 2 to 3 mm apart, through the thickness of the skin and into subcutaneous tissue deep enough to secure a coherent block of tissue. The slice is freed by connecting the two long parallel incisions by short cross incisions at either end and carefully undercutting the specimen in the subcutis. When biopsy of an ulcer is indicated, there is no use skimping with tissue. The pathologist then should not cut the specimen into smaller pieces but should carefully orient it so that sections are obtained of the entire block.

ULCERS, WOUNDS, AND GRANULATION TISSUE

An ulcer resulting from a pathologic process in or below the skin is different from a tissue defect (wound) resulting from sharp trauma, be it incidental or surgical. A clean wound will exhibit only minor amounts of devitalized tissue in the earliest stages and will show evidence of healing by granulation at later stages. An ulcer often will show a combination of the pathologic process that caused it with evidence of a healing effort similar to the granulation tissue of a wound. If the cause of the ulcer has been removed either spontaneously or by therapy, the healing ulcer may become very similar to a healing wound, and no specific diagnosis may be possible.

Granulation tissue (Fig. 17-1) is the simultaneous proliferation of fibroblasts forming young connective tissue and of endothelial sprouts forming capillary blood vessels, which may later acquire the attributes of arteries and veins. Inflammatory cells ranging from neutrophils to lymphocytes to phagocytic histiocytes also are present and may be very numerous if there is infection (Sec. IV). The granulations gradually fill the defect, sprouting blood vessels being arranged vertical to the skin surface. Scar formation is discussed in more detail in Chapter 41. In some healing wounds or ulcers, granulation tissue may become excessive (proud flesh) and may simulate granuloma pyogenicum clinically. The histologic differences (Figs. 41-1 and 42-7) are clear-cut.

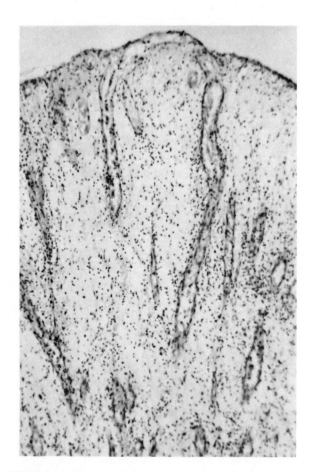

FIGURE 17-1.
Granulation tissue. Somewhat exuberant granulations fill the wound left by curettage of a basal cell epithelioma a few weeks earlier. Most of the tissue consists of vertical vascular sprouts embedded in loose edematous matrix containing inflammatory cells. Compare with the very different picture of granuloma pyogenicum (Fig. 42-7). H&E. X70.

Generic Features of Ulcers

The fact that epidermis and more or less dermis are lost in any ulcer implies that the epidermis ends at its edge. Generally, epidermis has a great propensity for coating defects, and it often descends down the rim of an ulcer. Exceptions to this rule have diagnostic significance in some infectious lesions, e.g., ecthyma and chancroid, and in some other lesions, e.g., pyoderma gangrenosum. Excessive epidermal proliferation at an ulcer's edge, on the other hand, can assume the features of pseudoepitheliomatous hyperplasia (Chap. 34), and it may take careful examination to differentiate it from squamous cell carcinoma.

The bottom of the ulcer may be covered with relatively healthy granulations or with debris and inflammatory cells due to secondary infection. It may also present a peculiar lining that combines necrotic material with acute inflammatory and granulomatous features, which is found typically in syphilitic (Fig. 20-11) and sporotrichotic (Fig. 21-8) gummas. It is proof that we are looking at the wall of a granulomatous cavity, the contents of which have disintegrated and have been lost. It is, as such, a nonspecific feature and may similarly be found in disintegrating epithelial cysts, around mucoceles, and in other conditions.

Because of the possibility that considerable portions of the pathologic substrate may have become necrotic, may have been completely lost before biopsy was taken, or may have been detached during transport and handling, the technician must embed all fragments that are found in the bottle, and the pathologist must look carefully for small foci of the specific pathologic process, be it inflammatory or neoplastic.

SPECIFIC ENTITIES

Many ulcers will be discussed in other chapters, especially under granulomatous inflammation (Sec. IV) and neoplasia (Sec. VII). Even the superficial dermatoses discussed in Section II may cause ulceration occasionally, either by themselves, e.g., ulcerating lichen planus,[1] or because of secondary infection or mechanical trauma to a denuded area. Pityriasis lichenoides et varioliformis acuta (Chap. 13), which typically presents superficial dermal necrosis, may ulcerate in some cases, and herpes zoster, especially in its severe gangrenous form (Chap. 12) may cause superficial or deeper ulcers. Ulceration was mentioned several times in the chapters on vasculitides and panniculitis. In all these instances, careful examination for signs of the underlying disease is necessary, although it may not always lead to success. There are, however, some diseases to be considered specifically in this chapter.

Bacterial Infections

Those bacterial infections that produce ulceration as a primary feature exert at least part of their influence through toxins and have certain unifying characteristics, such as absence of epidermal proliferation in the edge of the active lesion and vascular damage expressed either in thrombosis or in disintegration of vascular walls in the bottom of the ulcer. Inflammatory response varies from minimal in the so-called *Buruli ulcer*,[2] caused by *Mycobacterium ulcerans*, to more or less noncharacteristic mixed infiltrate in *anthrax*[3] and *ecthyma*, to granulomatous response in *tularemia* (Chap. 20) and others. Among the differentiating features is presence of identifiable microorganisms, which may be very numerous (anthrax), scarce (chancroid), or demonstrable only by special stains (mycobacteria). The amount of necrosis may vary from extensive (*M. ulcerans*) to moderate with formation of a pseudomembrane (diphtheria) to slight. Some examples follow.

Chancroid. Ducrey's streptobacillus of chancroid (*Haemophilus ducreyi*) always produces an ulcer. The epidermis stops abruptly at its edge (Fig. 17-2), giving the appearance of being dissolved. It slightly overhangs a recess in which the gram-negative microorganisms can be demonstrated among necrotic dermal tissue and polymorphonuclear cells. The floor of the rather shallow ulcer is similarly composed of necrotic tissue and a mixture of inflammatory cells exhibiting proliferation and thrombosis of vessels[4] and a deep zone of plasma cells and lymphocytes among which chains of bacilli may be demonstrable.[5] In practice, diagnosis of chancroid is better secured by using a chalazion curette to obtain a small amount of necrotic tissue from below the overhanging edge of the ulcer, using part of this material for culture and spreading some of it thinly on glass slides for Gram stain. The microorganisms can be seen as gram-negative thin rods forming "schools of fish" (Fig. 17-3).[6]

Ecthyma. Penetration of virulent cocci deeper into the skin than is found in impetigo (Chap. 11) causes dermal necrosis and severe inflammatory reaction with neutrophils and round cells. The surface of the ecthyma ulcer usually is covered with a heavy crust consisting of tissue ingredients bound together by dried serum. Colonies of cocci often are present. Ecthyma is apt to heal with irregular scars, which may present pseudoepitheliomatous proliferation of epidermis and adnexal epithelium in the early stages, before the process flattens out. Thus, there may be a temporary resemblance to bromoderma, North American blastomycosis, and other dermatoses producing fibrosis and epithelial hyperplasia.

Diphtheria. Diphtheria of the skin is rare and may produce either noncharacteristic eczematous changes (Chap. 7) or punched-out ulcers covered with a so-called pseudomembrane of necrotic material, fibrin, and neutrophils.[7] Numerous gram-positive bacilli may be present, but cultures are necessary for identification.

FIGURE 17–2.
Edge of penile ulcer diagnosed clinically as chancroid and excised as therapeutic measure in preantibiotic era. The sharp border and partial dissolution of the epidermis are characteristic of chancroid, but the presence of multinucleated epidermal giant cells strongly suggests the coexistence of herpes virus, a not uncommon experience. The nuclei of these cells showed inclusions at higher magnification. Coccobacilli highly suggestive of Ducrey bacilli were demonstrated in a similar section by O&G stain on the surface and in the necrotic base of the ulcer but not deeper in the tissue. H&E. X135.

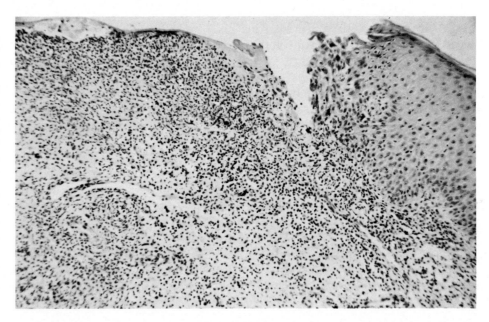

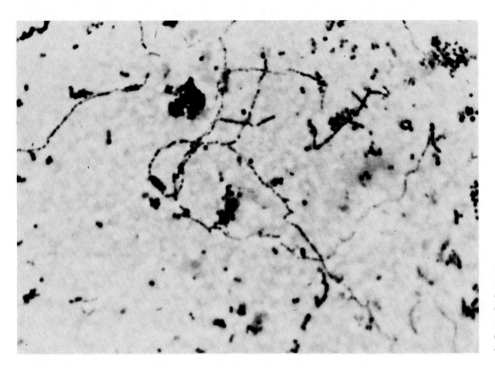

FIGURE 17–3.
Haemophilus ducreyi. Gram stain. X1100. (Smear of pure culture supplied by Dr. Thomas Chapel, Department of Dermatology, Wayne State University School of Medicine.)

Disturbances of Immunity

It has long been known that patients in the last stages of tuberculosis who exhibit weak or no immune reaction to tuberculin might develop ulcerating lesions (*tuberculosis orificialis*) that are teeming with bacilli but exhibit only a noncharacteristic subacute inflammatory response (Chap. 20). Along somewhat similar lines, malnourished and debilitated individuals may develop destructive ulcerative lesions of secondary syphilis containing numerous treponemes. Now that these old infectious diseases have been more or less controlled, we see iatrogenic immunodepression giving rise to infection by weak pathogens or saprophytes which may cause ulcers.[8] Histoplasmotic skin ulcers are seen in endemic areas in Asia and North America and may simulate carcinoma.[9] Mucormycosis may become very destructive.[10] The list could be prolonged. The tissue reaction usually is noncharacteristic and may be minor. While the infecting organisms generally are plentiful, it takes a certain degree of alertness to search for them.

Pyoderma Gangrenosum. Although the pathomechanism of the chronic and intractable ulcers associated with *ulcerative colitis* and also *Crohn's disease* is not completely elucidated,[11,12] pyoderma gangrenosum (Fig. 17-4) may be inserted here because it seems definitely related to disturbed immunity. The histologic picture is noncharacteristic and varies with the frequent changes between progression and partial healing seen in this condition. The epidermis may stop abruptly in the overhanging edge of an advancing ulcer, or it may show pseudoepitheliomatous hyperplasia simulating bromoderma, even to the presence of intraepithelial abscesses. There are no specific vascular alterations, and the inflammatory infiltrate consists of a mixture of cells. Eosinophils may or may not be prominent. The greatest value of histologic examination lies in ruling out specific infections, malignancy, or other diagnosable processes.

Other Entities

Leg Ulcers. Similarly, noncharacteristic features are encountered in the numerous leg ulcers due to stasis (Chap. 15) and arteriosclerosis. *Sickle cell ulcer* also has no characteristic tissue response, but an alert observer can often find the pathognomonic deformed red cells inside or outside of blood vessels. It almost seems that the osmotic changes accompanying tissue fixation provoke sickling (Fig. 17-5). Atrophie blanche and its ulcers were discussed in Chapter 15.

Necrotic Spider Bite. The bite of the brown recluse spider (*Loxosceles reclusa*) produces extensive tissue necrosis followed by ulceration in some individuals,[13] while it probably causes only minor reactions in others. The histomechanism has been suggested to be intravascular coagulation.[14]

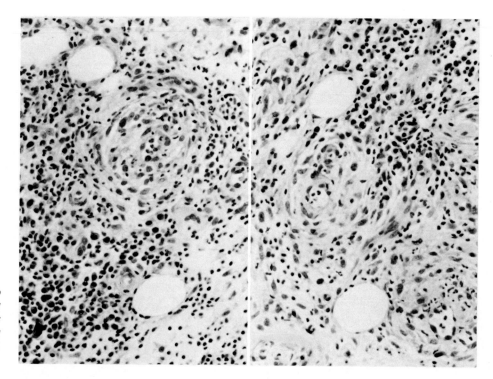

FIGURE 17–4.
Pyoderma gangrenosum. No necrosis shown in advancing edge of ulcer. Mild vasculitis and mixed cellular infiltrate in subcutaneous fat tissue. H&E. X250.

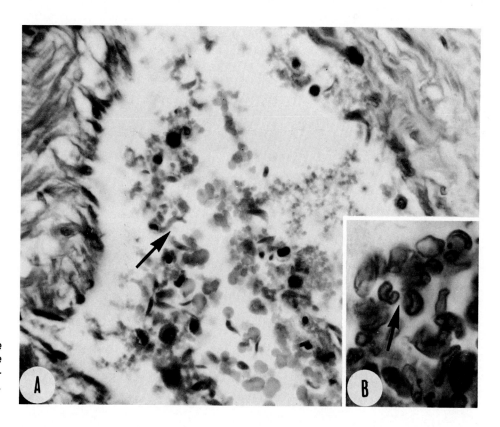

FIGURE 17–5.
Sickle cells in vessel at base of a leg ulcer. Some of the characteristic cells are indicated by arrows. **A.** *H&E. X475.* **B.** *H&E. X1000.*

Coumarin Necrosis. Coumarin and related drugs may cause extensive and deep necrosis, mainly around the buttocks. Histologically, subcutaneous veins contain fibrin thrombi,[15] possibly due to direct damage to the endothelium. There is no evidence of immune reaction, and the process may be related to a Shwartzman phenomenon.[16]

Chondrodermatitis Nodularis Chronica Helicis. One characteristic disorder, which is often biopsied to rule out skin cancer, is related to cartilage underlying the skin. Chronic nodular chondrodermatitis (Fig. 17-6) of the helix, more rarely of the antihelix, may easily be mistaken for squamous cell carcinoma in a superficial biopsy. While it is true that damaged cartilage is found also in clinically normal ears, there seems to be a definite association between the breaking down of cartilage and the nonhealing painful ulcer. With some experience, one can make the histologic diagnosis without seeing cartilage if one finds chronic vascular inflammation of the ordinarily thin subcutaneous tissue of the ear, associated with verrucous or pseudoepitheliomatous epidermal hyperplasia around a small ulcer.

Granuloma Fissuratum. An unusual lesion, granuloma fissuratum, probably caused by mechanical irritation in the upper labioalveolar junction of the mouth, has been described by Sutton, Jr.[17] Recently, similar lesions have been seen more commonly behind the ears or on the side of the nose, where they are evidently due to ill-fitting spectacle frames. The essential features, already pointed out by Sutton, seem to be the development of hypertrophic granulation tissue in a deep recess and the atypical proliferation of epidermis at either side, which is prevented from meeting the other side by the granulations. The lesion may be mistaken for a carcinoma, and its histologic resemblance to chondrodermatitis nodularis is striking. For these reasons, the term *acanthoma fissuratum* has been advocated lately.[18] The lesions heal spontaneously on removal of the pressure or do not recur after conservative excision.

Trophic Ulcers and Artifacts. A poorly defined term, trophic ulcer is applied to any nonhealing ulcer, especially on the lower extremities, which is thought to be caused and maintained by impaired tissue nutrition with or without disturbances of innervation. *Decubitus ulcers,* ulcers in diabetics, and the fingertip ulcers of *acrosclerosis* may be included here. None of them have histologic features that permit diagnosis, and examination usually is requested to rule out malignancy or other disorders.

Finally, if no specific diagnosis presents itself, the possibility of the patient's producing ulcers by mechanical or chemical means must be considered. Artifactual ulcerations usually show a disproportionately small amount of inflammatory reaction and sometimes have evidence of tissue destruction by heat or chemical necrosis, as mentioned in Chapter 3.

REFERENCES

1. Mahrle G, Gartmann M, Orfanos EC: Ulcerierender Lichen ruber der Füsse. Arch Dermatol Forsch 243:292, 1972
2. Connor DH, Lunn HF: Buruli ulceration. Arch Pathol 81:183, 1966
3. Loborich RJ, MacKillip BG, Conboy JR: Cutaneous anthrax. Am J Clin Pathol 13:505, 1943
4. Sheldon WH, Heyman A: Studies on chancroid. Am J Pathol 22:415, 1946

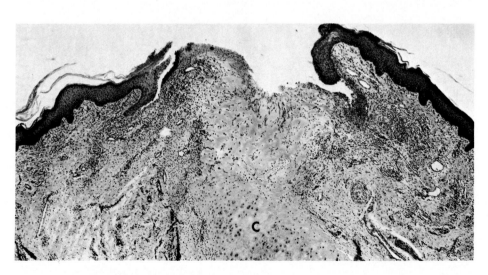

FIGURE 17–6.
Chondrodermatitis nodularis chronica helicis. Regenerating epidermis creeps down the sides of the ulcer, but there is no atypical hyperplasia. The central plug is necrotic connective tissue and cartilage (c). H&E. X60.

5. Unna PG: The Histopathology of the Diseases of the Skin. New York, Macmillan, 1896
6. Chapel TA, Brown WJ, Jeffries C, Stewart JA: How reliable is the morphological diagnosis of penile ulcerations? Sex Transmitted Dis 4:150, 1977
7. Allen AC: Survey of pathologic studies of cutaneous diseases during World War II. Arch Dermatol 57:19, 1948
8. Lomvardias S, Madge GE: Chaetoconidium and atypical acid-fast bacilli in skin ulcers. Arch Dermatol 106:875, 1972
9. Talvalkar GV: Histoplasmosis simulating carcinoma: a report of 3 cases. Indian J Cancer 9:149, 1972
10. Rabin ER, Lundberg GD, Mitchell ET: Mucormycosis in severely burned patients. N Engl J Med 264:1286, 1961
11. Jablonska S: Zur Pathogenese des Pyoderma gangraenosum. Hautarzt 15:584, 1964
12. Samitz MH: Skin complications of ulcerative colitis and Crohn's disease (with special reference to pyoderma gangrenosum). Cutis 12:533, 1973
13. Dillaha CJ, Jansen GT, Honeycutt WM, et al.: North American loxoscelism. JAMA 188:33, 1964
14. Berger RS, Adelstein EH, Anderson RC: Intravascular coagulation: the cause of necrotic arachidism. J Invest Dermatol 61:142, 1973
15. Nalbandian RM, Mader JJ, Barrett JL, et al.: Petechiae, ecchymoses, and necrosis of skin induced by coumarin congeners. JAMA 142:603, 1965
16. Altmeyer P, Welke S, Reuger A, Hufnagel D: Zur Pathogenese der sogenannten Cumarin-Nekrose. Akt Dermatol 2:65, 1976
17. Sutton RL, Jr: A fissured granulomatous lesion of the upper labio-alveolar fold. Arch Dermatol Syph 26:425, 1932
18. Tennstedt D, Lachapelle JM: Acanthome fissuré. Revue de la littérature et diagnostic histopathologique differentiel avec le nodule douloureux de l'oreille. Ann Derm Venereol 106:219, 1979

18

Inflammation Involving the Pilosebaceous Complex

Follicular inflammations are discussed here because they are located in the pars reticularis of the dermis—with the exception of the acrotrichial pustules of impetigo Bockhart, the superficial lesions of erythema toxicum neonatorum, and the recently described disseminate and recurrent infundibulofolliculitis. Inflammatory products may be found inside or outside the follicle, and often in both locations. If inflammatory infiltrate is present in perifollicular arrangement only, one has to decide whether it is a response to something present within the follicle, as in certain types of tinea, or results from concentration of small capillaries around follicles as in follicular exanthems and lichen scrofulosorum (Chap. 20). Follicular keratoses will be discussed here because they are often accompanied by inflammation. The decision to include alopecias, except pattern alopecia, may seem arbitrary, but in most biopsies of this type, examination of the hair itself is less important than that of the hair follicle, and most alopecias have associated inflammation.

STAPHYLOCOCCIC INFECTIONS

The extent and severity of *staphylococcic folliculitis* depend on the localization of the cocci, the size of the hair, and the immunologic situation of the host. While it is not easy to discern these determining factors in histologic sections, there is little doubt that *impetigo Bockhart* (Fig. 18-1) is a superficial infection of a small follicle, and *furuncle* is a deep infection, usually of a larger hair root. On the other hand, in a patient with furunculosis, the development of a small folliculitis, a medium-sized or large furuncle, or even a carbuncle, probably depends more on the immunologic defensive ability at the particular time than on the exact localization of the cocci.

In most types of staphylococcic folliculitis, polymorphonuclear infiltrates prevail to the point of abscess formation (Fig. 18-2). In a fully developed furuncle, a fairly broad column of perifollicular connective tissue becomes necrotic and densely infiltrated with neutrophils to form the clinically characteristic tough green plug. Below the lower end of the follicle, often in the subcutaneous tissue, an abscess containing demonstrable staphylococci develops, which is finally evacuated when the plug has been sequestered. On the other hand, in *sycosis vulgaris* of the beard, it is often only the upper part of the follicle that is involved, and the hair root survives and remains susceptible to the next attack.[1]

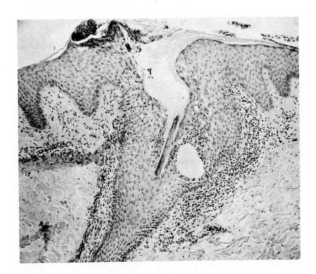

FIGURE 18–1.
Superficial folliculitis of impetigo Bockhart type. There is eczematous spongiosis and vesiculation of the upper portion of the follicular sheath, in contrast to the mucinous edema of sebaceous gland and sheath in alopecia mucinosa (see Figs. 18-20 and 18-21). H&E. X90.

ACNE VULGARIS AND RELATED CONDITIONS

In contrast to the hot folliculitis caused by virulent staphylococci and their toxins, the milder, less painful, but more protracted inflammation of an *acne pustule* or *abscess* probably is in great part caused by chemically irritating sebum in combination with less virulent microorganisms, especially *Corynebacterium acnes*.[2]

Histologically, the comedonic plug can be recognized in relatively early lesions. It may have a wide opening or a very narrow one (closed comedo). While open comedones may persist for several years,[3] the closed ones are likely to rupture (Fig. 18-3), releasing sebaceous and horny material into the dermis.[4] The initial acute inflammation may be followed by foreign-body granulomatous reaction and epithelial proliferation that grows around the abscess. In a deep cystic acne lesion, all the features of a mixed granulomatous infiltrate may be present (Fig. 18-4), and differential diagnosis from specific granulomatous disease may be difficult (Chap. 21). In such cases, the demonstration of a few keratin flakes or fragments of hair in the granuloma is helpful. Clinical information as to age of patient, location of lesion, and other characteristics often helps to confirm the impression that one is dealing with a nonspecific granuloma. In the rare cases of *acne fulminans*, the follicular reaction develops into an extensive, spreading, liquefying necrosis engulfing close-by follicles but shows no evidence of vasculitis or immune processes.[5] Comedonic plugs are also seen in sun-exposed aged skin,[6] especially in the condition outlined by Favre and Racouchot (Chap. 26) and after application of coal tar[4] and various other substances.

DERMATOPHYTIC FOLLICULITIS

As is well known from superficial fungous infection (Chap. 13), dermatophytes usually do not invade living tissues. They produce an inflammatory

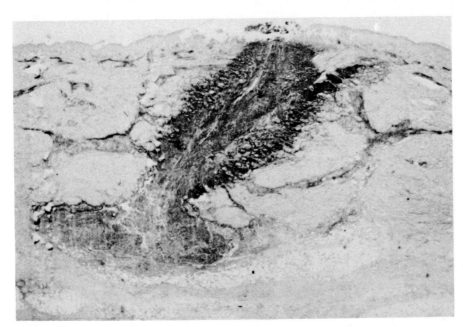

FIGURE 18–2.
Furuncle. The fully developed lesion was completely excised and healed per primam. The affected follicle slants downward and abuts in the fat tissue on a subcutaneous abscess, in the center of which gram-positive cocci were demonstrated. The epidermis is destroyed on top. The hair is visible in the center of the thick plug consisting of fibrin and massive numbers of neutrophilic leukocytes. Peripheral perivascular inflammatory infiltrate. H&E. ×4. (From Pinkus. J Cutan Pathol 6:517, 1979. Copyright © 1979 Munksgaard International Publishers, Copenhagen.

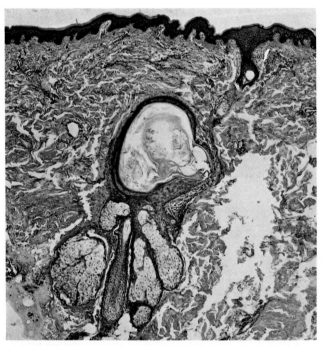

FIGURE 18–3.
Cystic dilatation of suprasebaceous portion of a follicle and rupture of wall in a relatively noninflammatory lesion of acne vulgaris. H&E. X45.

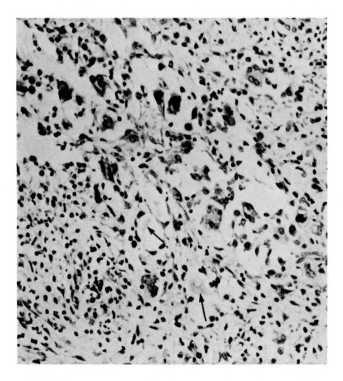

FIGURE 18–4.
Foreign-body type of granulomatous inflammation after rupture of a keratinous cyst. Arrows point to keratin flakes. H&E. X225.

reaction indirectly. The same holds true when a trichophyton or microsporon invades the follicle and possibly the hair. The finer details of *macrospore, microsporum, ectothrix,* and *endothrix* infection will not be discussed here. For a thorough discussion see Graham and Barroso-Tobila.[7] With the exception of *Trichophyton rubrum,* which may enter living tissue in the granulomatous lesions found usually on the legs of women (Fig. 18-5), fungal elements are found almost exclusively in or around the hair (Fig. 18-6), even in highly inflammatory *kerion* of the scalp or the *Majocchi granuloma.* It is, therefore, necessary to examine a sufficiently large number of sections in suspected cases, and one cannot be content until a hair-containing follicle or remnants of a hair shaft are found within the inflamed zone. Often, only one hair in a specimen is manifestly infected. Follicles quite close to but outside the lesion may be normal, and in the center of the inflammation, hairs and follicles may be completely destroyed. On the other hand, even in a rather superficial tinea, it may be impossible to find mycelia in the scale, while close inspection of vellus hair follicles shows hyphae and spores in the infundibulum. One must also realize that the infundibulum is often populated with nonpathogenic spores, and that demonstration of spores in a given section is not proof that they are responsible for the disease. Presence of hyphae is more convincing.

The inflammatory infiltrate may vary from minor accumulations of round cells, as in *Microsporum audouini* infections, to purulent and mixed granulomatous types in *M. canis* and *Trichophyton* infections.

OTHER DEEP FOLLICULAR INFLAMMATIONS

Perforating Folliculitis

In recent years, a peculiar type of *perforating folliculitis* (Fig. 18-7) has been seen with increasing frequency.[8] It has some clinical and superficial histologic similarity to Kyrle's extremely rare *hyperkeratosis follicularis et parafollicularis in cutem penetrans,* and some of the cases recently published under that name (see below) in fact were perforating folliculitis. Biopsy at various stages indicates that the spring action of a rolled-up thin hair produces a break of the follicular wall and causes reactive inflammation and some tissue necrosis lateral to the follicle. The small granulomatous abscess is secondarily surrounded by proliferating follicular epithelium. The sequestered mass consisting

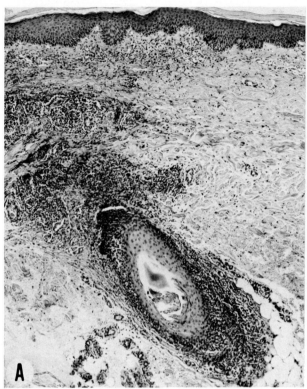

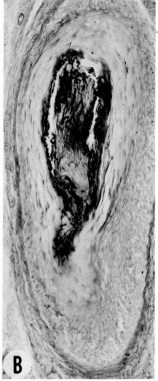

FIGURE 18–5.
*Granulomatous folliculitis due to Trichophyton rubrum. **A.** H&E. X75. **B.** Mycelia and spores in and around the hair. Alcian blue-PAS. X135.*

of pyknotic inflammatory cells, peculiar eosinophilic elastic fibers, and keratinous debris is then evacuated toward the surface within the follicle, a process quite different biologically from that envisioned by Kyrle.

The best histologic criterion is the presence of devitalized elastic fibers which, being eosinophilic, are easily recognized in O&G sections but not with other elastic fiber stains. Follicles obstructed from other causes and associated with granulomatous inflammation (Fig. 21-14) may come into differential diagnosis.

Necrotizing Folliculitis and Pityrosporum Folliculitis

A different clinical and histologic picture has been observed[9] in a number of patients, who presented very pruritic scattered papules not obviously related to hairs. Histologically (Fig. 18-8), a relatively small and sharply defined round cell infiltrate is seen that has destroyed a portion of the middle or deeper part of a vellus follicle without affecting the upper part. The hair root also may survive. *Necrotizing folliculitis* has proved intractable and contin-

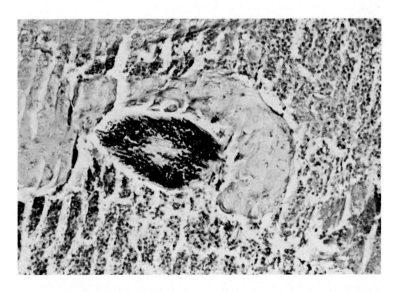

FIGURE 18–6.
Trichophyton violaceum (endothrix) infection of scalp hair with violent inflammatory reaction which has led to rupture of follicle. PAS-hematoxylin. X185.

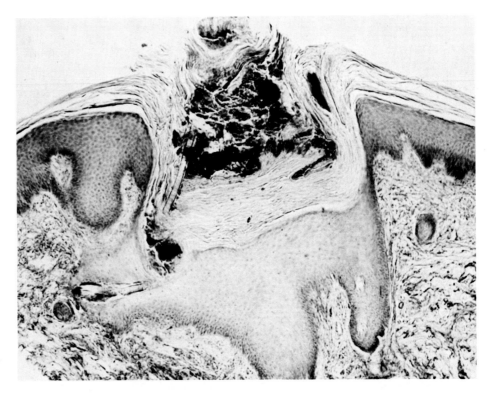

FIGURE 18–7.
Perforating folliculitis. Note the thin hair in the epithelial channel at left and mixture of keratin, leukocytes, and degenerated dermal fibers in the plug. H&E. X75. (From Mehregan and Coskey. Arch Dermatol 97:394, 1967.)

ues to recur after occasional spontaneous remissions. The histologic picture is similar to those described by Potter et al.[10] as *pityrosporum folliculitis* and by Kaidbey and Kligman[11] in *topical steroid acne,* but the clinical aspects are different inasmuch as there are obvious follicular papules and pustules in pityrosporum folliculitis and comedones in steroid acne.

Disorders Associated with Negroid Hair

Strongly curved hair brings with it peculiar hazards due to its tendency to be retained in the dermis as an irritating foreign body when the inflamed follicle breaks down or to grow back into the skin when it is shaved. Disorders based on these mechanisms, therefore, are most common in blacks.

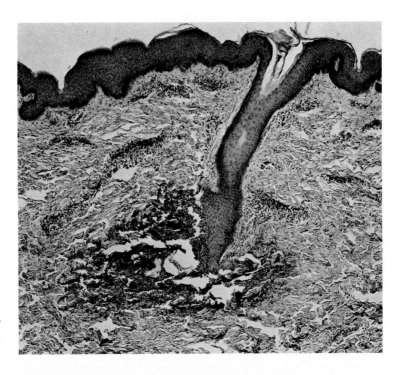

FIGURE 18–8.
Necrotizing folliculitis. The inflammatory process has destroyed a portion of follicular wall at level of bulge but does not involve entire follicle as in a furuncle. H&E. X75.

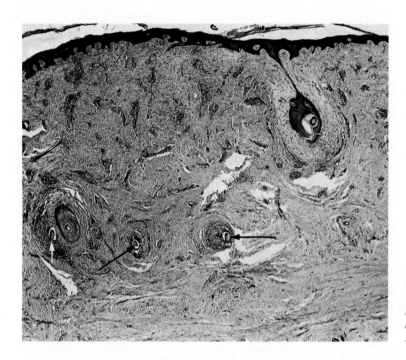

FIGURE 18–9.
Dermatitis papillaris capillitii. Three dead hairs (arrows) buried deep in skin by keloidal fibrous hyperplasia. Inflammatory reaction is relatively minor, chronic, and partly granulomatous. H&E. X35.

There are three such disorders: *folliculitis et perifolliculitis suffodiens et abscedens* (Hoffmann's disease), *acne keloid,* and *pseudofolliculitis* of the beard.

Hoffmann's Disease. We have not been impressed with the role of apocrine glands or the association with acne conglobata in Hoffmann's disease, and the simpler name *dissecting cellulitis of the scalp* does not do it justice. The course of the disease is best explained by, and treatment is based on, the assumption that Hoffmann's disease is primarily acute folliculitis and that its progression and chronicity are due to buried dead hairs which produce foreign-body inflammation in and below the skin, complicated by recurrent virulent infection. The histologic features bear out this concept and show extensive intradermal formation of sinuses lined with smooth stratified epithelium derived from disrupted follicles. The contents of the sinuses are remnants of hairs, flakes of keratin, and (in an acute attack) inflammatory cells. Cure can be achieved by thorough marsupialization of the burrowing sinuses after antibiotic therapy.

Acne Keloid. Buried dead hairs also are largely responsible for *dermatitis papillaris capillitii,* but infection plays a minor role. The patient's tendency to keloid formation contributes the characteristic features (Fig. 18-9).

Scarring Pseudofolliculitis. Chronic scarring pseudofolliculitis of the beard is primarily foreign-body reaction around the sharp, shaved ends of curved hairs which grow back into the skin (Fig. 18-10). It is encountered mainly in the beards of black men but may be seen in the pubic region and on the scalp.[12] Later stages are characterized by scarring and atrophy of hair.[13,14]

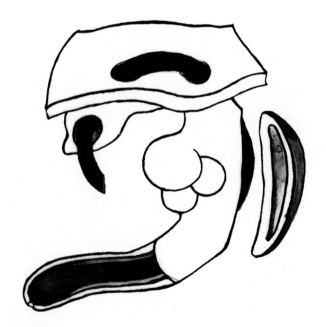

FIGURE 18–10.
Ingrowing hair in pseudofolliculitis of the beard. Negroid curved follicle is cut away to expose hair, sharp shaved end of which has reentered skin and is partly surrounded by an epithelial cuff (pseudofollicle). (Drawing by Dr. Felix Pinkus from a three-dimensional model reconstructed from serial sections, 1943.)

Pilonidal Sinus

A pilonidal sinus is a fistulous tract containing hairs surrounded by granulation tissue or sometimes sheathed in stratified epithelium, suggesting a follicle (Fig. 18-11). They are most commonly encountered in the coccygeal area of overweight young men, where it is assumed that dead hairs of this body region have penetrated the epidermis of the fossa coccygea. Basically similar sinuses are encountered in the interdigital webs of barbers and dairymen, where they contain trimmed human hair fragments and cattle hairs, respectively.

SUPERFICIAL LESIONS

The follicular infundibulum, including the acrotrichium and the intradermal portion down to the level of the sebaceous duct, may be involved, with spongiosis and inflammatory infiltrate in some cases of eczematous and atopic dermatitis.[15] This is commonly seen in perioral dermatitis (Chap. 8) and

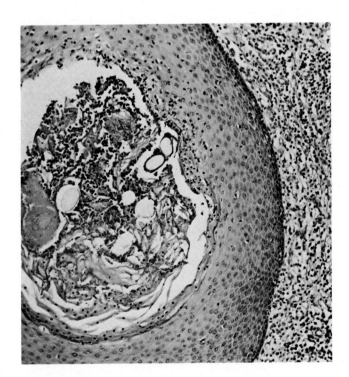

FIGURE 18–11.
Pilonidal sinus of sacral area. Cross section of a cavity surrounded by stratified epithelium and containing keratinous flakes, debris, leukocytes, and several small hairs. The original hypothesis that the hairs grow from matrices within the sinus as a congenital malformation has been replaced by the concept that dead hairs are sucked into the sinus from surrounding skin. H&E. X100.

in the follicular forms of seborrheic dermatitis. Mucinous edema may extend upward into this portion in follicular mucinosis (see below). There are, however, several clinical entities which specifically localize in the infundibulum. Of these, impetigo Bockhart was mentioned earlier (pg. 201–2).

Transient Erythema Toxicum and Melanosis of the Newborn

A rather harmless but sometimes alarming affection is *erythema toxicum neonatorum*, seen especially in warm climates and usually restricted to the folds of the neck. It consists of red spots and superficial follicular pustules, which typically contain eosinophils rather than neutrophils.[16] The acrosyringium may be similarly affected (Chap. 19).

Under the name *transient neonatal pustular melanosis* was described a similar eruption which leaves behind hyperpigmentation. Here the pustules contain neutrophils.[17]

Eosinophilic Pustular Folliculitis

This rare affection was reported exclusively from Japan[18] until a case was observed in Sweden.[19] It consists of follicular, tiny red papules with the formation of pustules on fairly well defined erythematous plaques that have a tendency to central involution and ring-shaped extension. Histologic examination shows subcorneal and intraepidermal pustules containing mainly eosinophils and involving follicles down to the level of the sebaceous gland. Blood eosinophilia is common. The differential diagnosis includes subcorneal pustular dermatosis, follicular mucinosis, and impetigo herpetiformis.

Disseminate and Recurrent Infundibulofolliculitis

A recently described entity[20,21] produces widespread and only slightly pruritic tiny papules which impress the observer as a goosefleshlike accentuation of all hair follicles on large areas of the trunk and extremities. The histologic picture (Fig. 18-12) of this disseminated eruption includes spongiotic edema of the infundibular portion of the follicle and mild surrounding mononuclear infiltrate. The cause is unknown, and the course is indefinite, but cases seen by us in Detroit leave little doubt that infundibulofolliculitis is a distinctive dermatosis.

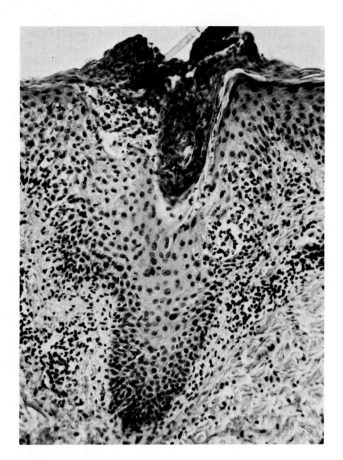

FIGURE 18–12.
Disseminated and recurrent infundibulofolliculitis. H&E. X180.

Folliculitis Decalvans

This term has been used somewhat loosely by various authors for progressive lesions on arms, legs, and other areas with relatively small hairs. It also has been applied to sycosis vulgaris, a chronic staphylococcic infection of the beard (see above). In the stricter sense, the term applies to a condition of the scalp in which polymorphonuclear cells are found inside the hair follicle, usually the upper portion, and in which chronic perifollicular inflammation leads to hair loss. It must be differentiated from pseudopelade of Brocq (see below).

FOLLICULAR KERATOSES

We encountered keratotic plugging of hair follicles as a more or less characteristic by-product of lupus erythematosus (Chap. 14) and lichen planus (Chap. 9). We shall also find it in lichen sclerosus et atro-

phicus (Chap. 25), lichen scrofulosorum (Chap. 20), and Darier's disease (Chap. 28). Comedones of acne vulgaris were mentioned earlier in this chapter. We shall now describe some conditions in which keratotic plugs are the outstanding characteristic.

Keratosis Pilaris and Related Conditions

These disorders come to the attention of the pathologist mainly in differential diagnosis from more significant dermatoses. If there is no other disturbance of the skin except a horny plug in the infundibulum (Fig. 18-13), we render a diagnosis of *keratosis pilaris*. There is some associated round cell infiltrate and telangiectasia in keratosis pilaris rubra. An acne comedo extends deeper into the sebaceous duct region and is more massive.

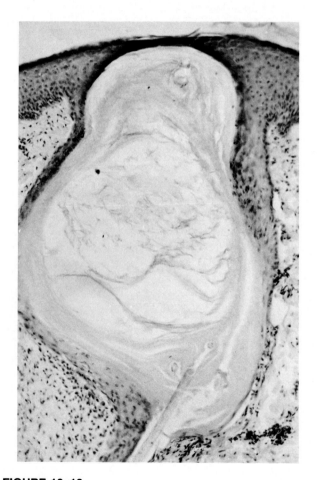

FIGURE 18–13.
Keratosis pilaris. Infundibular portion of small hair follicle greatly distended by a keratinous plug into which it enters from the bottom. The wall of the follicle is so thin, it is almost ready to rupture, but there is as yet practically no inflammatory reaction. H&E. X125.

Lichen spinulosus is most common in black children and resembles lichen scrofulosorum clinically. Histologically, we see a solid infundibular plug (Fig. 18-14), which projects above the skin surface and encases a hair shaft. The follicular wall is apt to be somewhat atrophic and the sebaceous gland tiny or absent, and there is a certain amount of perifollicular fibrosis and perivascular round cell infiltrate. The granulomatous reaction of lichen scrofulosorum (Fig. 20-2) is absent. The affection responds to high doses of vitamin A, and similar histologic pictures in adults are seen in vitamin A deficiency (*phrynoderma*). *Pellagra*, on the other hand, may be associated with the combination of follicular horny spines and large sebaceous glands in the central face, a long-known sign reemphasized by Pons et al.[22]

An inherited condition characterized by follicular plugging, redness, and atrophy is *ulerythema ophryogenes*, which may begin already in childhood in the lateral portions of the eyebrows and is gradually progressive. The histologic features bear out the clinical appearance and consist of absence of sebaceous glands, keratotic plugs in hair follicles, dermal fibrosis, and mild chronic inflammatory infiltrate.[23]

Kyrle's Disease

The nature of *hyperkeratosis follicularis et parafollicularis in cutem penetrans* has never been explained satisfactorily. Epidermal biology makes it difficult to consider active penetration of a horny plug into the dermis. Even in a *clavus* (Fig. 33-18B), where pressure from the outside forces the hyperkeratotic material downward, and in other instances of keratotic plugs associated with mechanical pressure,[24] there is always a thin epidermal covering around the tip of the conical plug. The only known instances where the living envelope wears away around keratinous material are in the confines of a cystically dilated hair follicle (Fig. 8-13) or other keratinizing cyst. It is noteworthy that some recent authors do not insist on complete penetration as a pathognomonic feature.[25] Kyrle's disease (Fig. 18-15) has always been extremely rare. The only case diagnosed by the senior author on clinical evidence had histologic features of Darier's disease, which also has been found in some published cases. This observation introduces one reasonable explanation because the acantholytically weakened basal layer of keratosis follicularis could give way to pressure of a large horny plug. The

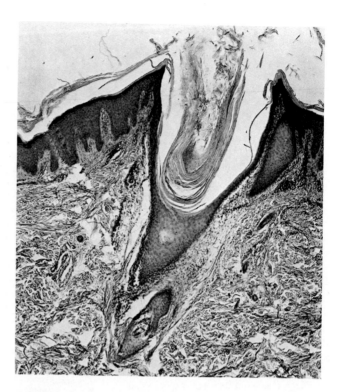

FIGURE 18–14.
Lichen spinulosus. H&E. X70. Compare with different picture of lichen scrofulosorum in Figure 20-2.

flood of observations some years ago of many cases of so-called Kyrle's disease[26] all over the country has been explained as being quite a different disorder, namely, *perforating folliculitis* (see above). Another disorder, hyperkeratosis lenticularis perstans (Sec. VI, Chap. 29), may have strong clinical similarity to Kyrle's disease but is an inherited disorder of keratinization.

Pityriasis Rubra Pilaris

Perhaps related to disturbed metabolism of vitamin A is pityriasis rubra pilaris (PRP), which has characteristic features in later stages, when keratotic plugs are well developed, but is easily confused with psoriasis in the early erythrodermic phase (Fig. 18-16), when the mitotic rate is also very high.[27] Points for differentiation are the more continuous parakeratosis and the absence of squirting papillae in PRP. The photomicrograph illustrates sebaceous atrophy and hypertrophy of the arrector muscle already in this early stage, but these features are better and more regularly developed in advanced cases. One may say that the skin is in a state of constant cutis anserina. The hypertrophic

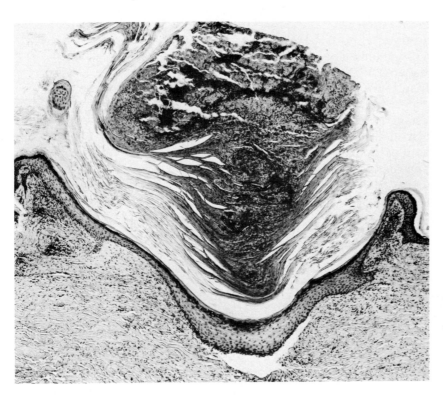

FIGURE 18–15.
Kyrle's disease. The illustration is taken from a case of perforating folliculitis with a keratotic plug that contains parakeratotic nuclei and pyknotic leukocytes. The epidermis is complete in the picture but is regenerated above scarlike dermis to which it does not closely adhere. Serial sections confirmed the diagnosis. H&E. X70. (From Mehregan. Curr Probl Dermatol 3:144, 1970.)

arrector pili pulls on the follicle, producing an angulation in the bulge region and often eliciting an epithelial tendon (Fig. 2-29) from the follicular wall. These features may have to be reconstructed

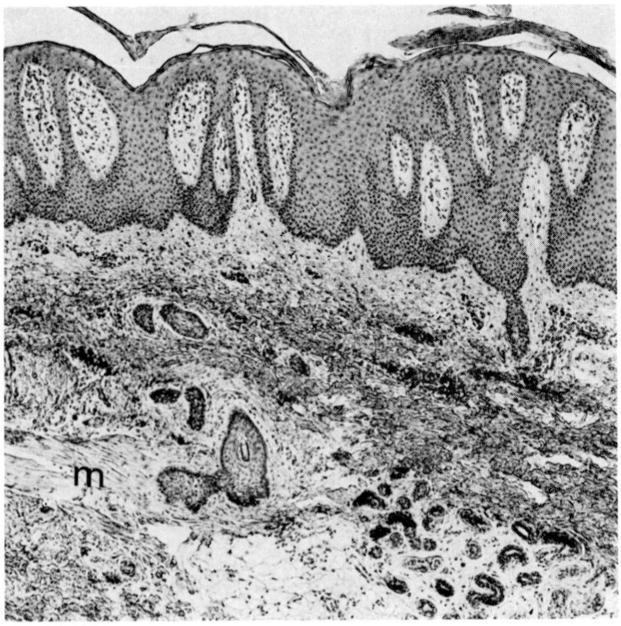

FIGURE 18–16.
Pityriasis rubra pilaris, early psoriasiform stage in a child. Note absence of suprapapillary exudate in epidermis and hyperplasia of arrector pili muscle (m), for which proliferation of bulge forms an epithelial tendon. H&E. X70.

from serial sections if the follicles are sectioned obliquely. The fully developed picture (Fig. 18-17) includes conical keratotic plugs in follicular openings and a thick, evenly acanthotic epidermis with accentuated ridges and papillae. The granular layer is thick and the horny layer orthokeratotic, except that, paradoxically, the shoulders of hair follicles show loss of keratohyalin and some parakeratosis.[28] The rete malpighi may show spongiosis in this limited area. Inflammatory infiltrate is moderate or minimal in all stages of PRP. Keratoderma palmare et plantare are common. A peculiar type of dermatomyositis (*type Wong*) has been reported (Chap. 14) in which PRP-like horny plugs form extensively in hair follicles, due to myositis of the arrector muscles.

ALOPECIAS

Here we will consider as a group all more or less inflammatory processes regularly associated with loss of hair. In most cases, biopsies of this type will have been taken from the scalp, and the most common question asked by the clinician is: What is the prognosis for restoration of hair? Histologic examination pays more attention to the hair follicle and the surrounding dermis than to the hair itself.

Under the microscope we can separate cases into two large groups: those in which hair follicles become smaller but do not disappear and those in

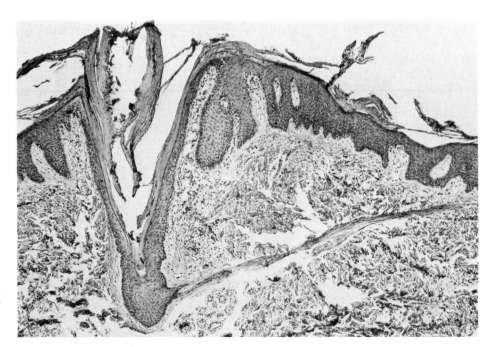

FIGURE 18–17.
Later stage of pityriasis rubra pilaris. Keratotic plug in a hair follicle which has formed an epithelial tendon for strong arrector muscle. Epidermis is orthokeratotic above a granular layer, except at shoulders of follicle where there is parakeratosis. H&E. X60.

which follicles are completely destroyed. The first group comprises patterned alopecia in both sexes, *alcopecia areata* and *alopecia mucinosa*. The second comprises the scarring alopecias related to pseudopelade. We shall defer discussion of pattern alopecia to Chapter 46 because there is little or no inflammation, and examination of the hair itself enters the diagnosis. Trichotillomania and other disturbances due to external causes also will be discussed there.

Alopecia Areata

In alopecia areata (Fig. 18-18), depending on the site from which the biopsy was obtained, one may find a larger or smaller number of strong follicles. Some of these will be empty, while others will show catagen-stage hair roots representing hairs soon to be lost. In between, there are smaller anagen follicles, the so-called miniature type which show signs of trichogenic activity, but have a rudimentary pa-

FIGURE 18–18.
*Alopecia areata. **A.** Some relatively normal hair follicles and a miniature follicle often found in alopecia areata. This follicle also has the configuration of a cloaked hair due to sebaceous atrophy. This not too uncommon abnormality has no pathologic significance in itself (see Epstein and Kligman. J Invest Dermatol 26:1, 1956). H&E. X75. **B.** Inflammatory infiltrate associated with follicles of reduced size containing remnants of inner root sheath but no hairs. H&E. X135.*

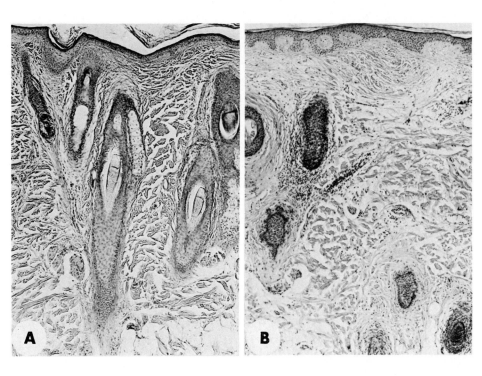

pilla and matrix and produce a minuscule hair or just inner root sheath.[29] Sebaceous glands usually are reduced in size along with the follicles. Perivascular infiltrate may be mild, moderate, or even pronounced (Fig. 18-19).[30]

Alopecia Mucinosa

Loss of hair is actually an incidental but quite regular phenomenon in the disease (Fig. 18-20) characterized by *follicular mucinosis*.[31] While in many cases the histologic picture is dominated by inflammatory infiltrate around hair roots, the primary lesion (*mucinosis follicularis*) is a perversion of metabolism in the sebaceous gland (Fig. 18-21) and the outer root sheath,[32] which leads to the accumulation of much mucinous material while the cells become stellate or rounded. In the earlier stages, the resemblance to a nest of mucinous basal cell epithelioma may be striking. Later, the entire hair follicle may be converted into a bag lined by compressed epithelial cells and filled with a plug of inspissated mucin mixed with less or more horny material. The mucin stains slightly bluish in not too highly decolorized H&E sections. It usually is metachromatic and PAS-negative. It stains brilliantly with the Hale procedure or alcian blue and

can be digested by hyaluronidase. The outer root sheath usually contains much glycogen which may suggest PAS-positivity of the mucin unless diastase digestion is used. The hair, whether large or small, eventually falls out, but the hair root usually survives, and new hair often is formed once the lesion heals. Inflammatory infiltrate may be almost absent, especially in those cases in which the clinical picture is that of follicular papules. In the inflammatory plaques of alopecia mucinosa, infiltrate may be moderate or heavy and often is a mixture of lymphocytes, eosinophils, plasma cells, and some histiocytes.

Once follicular mucinosis has been recognized in a biopsy, one has to decide whether one is dealing with a case of benign *alopecia mucinosa* or with a case of *mycosis fungoides* or other lymphoma, in which the mucinosis persists.[33,34] The occasional transformation of the benign form into lymphoblastoma has been well documented. For diagnostic features of the lymphoma see Chapter 44. The possibility that mucinous edema of the outer root sheath may occur symptomatically in *staphylococcic follicular keratosis*[35] cannot be denied. It is essential for the diagnosis of alopecia mucinosa to prove the presence of acid mucopolysaccharides in order to differentiate follicular mucinosis from occasional eczematous spongiosis of the root sheath in which mucinous substances are absent.

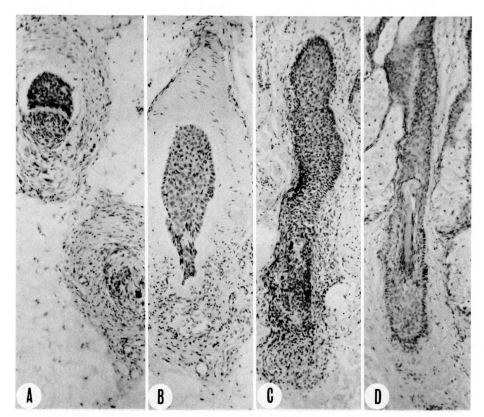

FIGURE 18–19.
Alopecia areata. Four hair follicles showing variable degrees of inflammatory infiltrate, reduction of epithelial root sheath, and thick fibrous root sheath. At left, a dermal papilla below the greatly reduced epithelial matrix (catagen). At right, small hair shaft in follicle at level of sebaceous gland. H&E. X125.

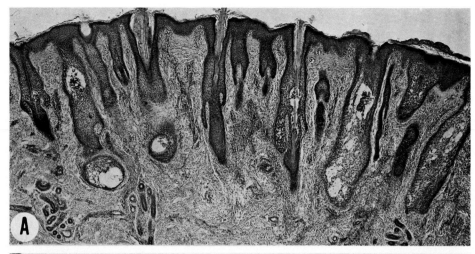

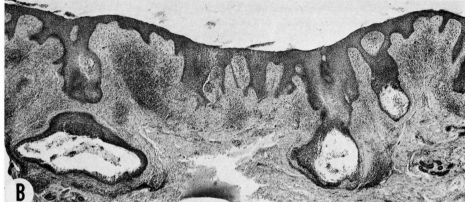

FIGURE 18–20.
Alopecia mucinosa. Two cases showing varying degrees of inflammatory reaction and cyst formation. H&E. X90.

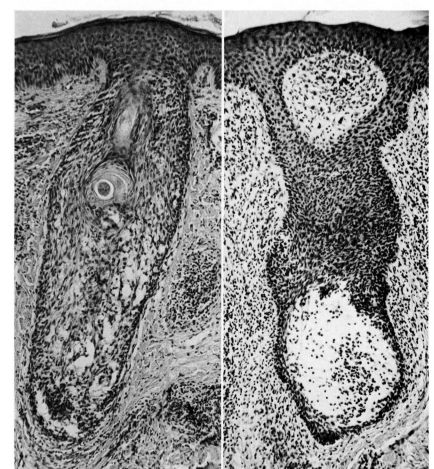

FIGURE 18–21.
Alopecia mucinosa. The follicle at left shows mucinous degeneration of outer root sheath and a small hair in the center. The follicle at right contains mucin in a cyst filled otherwise with degenerating epithelial and inflammatory cells. Moderately heavy mixed infiltrate in dermis. H&E. X250.

Alopecia Atrophicans

An extensive review of biopsy material from cases of *scarring alopecia*[36] convinced us that there is little true scar formation in pseudopelade of Brocq and other cases of idiopathic permanent alopecia. We, therefore, revert to the name *atrophying alopecia*, used by Brocq and other French authors, and reserve the scarring application to those cases of lupus erythematosus and lichen planopilaris of the scalp in which considerable inflammation leads to widespread loss of normal dermis and hair follicles and their replacement by a true scar (Chap. 41).

A biopsy of a suspected case of atrophying alopecia raises two questions of theoretical and practical significance: Is the loss of hair temporary or permanent? In the latter case, is there evidence of associated nonfollicular disease; or is it strictly an atrophying follicular process? Cases of folliculitis decalvans are ruled out by the presence of intrafollicular neutrophils. It will be seen that these questions are answered with greater ease if a good elastic fiber stain is used in the differential diagnosis.

Pseudopelade of Brocq. The epidermis usually preserves normal thickness with rete ridges and normal keratinization. There may be some keratotic plugging of hair follicles. The striking abnormality at scanning examination is a total absence of sebaceous glands. The number of hair follicles is diminished in proportion to the stage of the disease. There is moderate perifollicular infiltrate, mainly by small round cells, and the epithelial follicular wall is thinned and eventually disappears (Fig. 18-22). The inflammation is restricted to the upper permanent portion of the follicle, down to the bulge. The lower cyclic portion often is relatively well preserved but perishes, as is shown by one's ability to pull out anagen hairs (cheveux pseudopeladiques[37]). Occasionally, an affected hair may survive and grow back. The space left by the disappearing hair follicle is taken up by the thickened fibrous root sheath on which the surviving hair muscle inserts. There is diffuse loss of the subepidermal fine elastic fibers (Fig. 18-23) without much evidence of inflammation. The thickened fibrous root sheath, which extends into the subcutaneous tissue, is outlined by elastic fibers only in the dermis but not in the subcutis (Fig. 18-23). A peculiar feature is the formation of some fairly superficial small eccrine cysts, probably resulting from obstruction of the duct.

Fibrosing Alopecia. Until our recent review of almost 180 cases of atrophying alopecia, the condi-

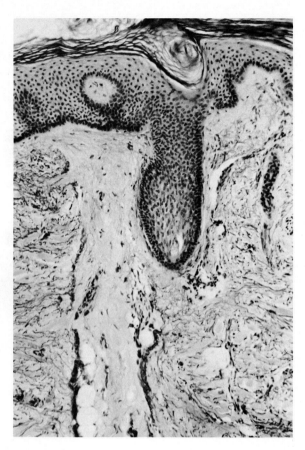

FIGURE 18–22.
Pseudopelade of Brocq. A reduced hair follicle containing a tiny hair next to the remnant of a completely lost follicle represented by a cord of fibrotic fibrous root sheath. H&E. X250.

tion of the elastic fibers in this disease had not been given much attention. It became obvious, however, that more than 100 cases presented strong hyperplasia of elastic fibers in the cyclic portion of the fibrous root sheath, where they are normally absent.[38] This condition is so striking that it was mentioned in the second edition of this book as a characteristic of pseudopelade. That statement must be corrected. All other changes are the same, but the development of strong elastic fibers in the lower portion of the fibrous root sheath is a striking dissimilarity (Fig. 18-24), which forces us to call these cases *fibrosing alopecia*. Preliminary impression suggests that these are cases of diffuse alopecia mainly in women (93 females to 13 males).

Alopecia Carcinomatosa. In rare cases, a metastasis from carinoma of the breast may cause a patch of alopecia without forming a nodule. Hair follicles become atrophic within a dense fibrous stroma surrounding individual large carcinomatous cells or small nests of cells.[39]

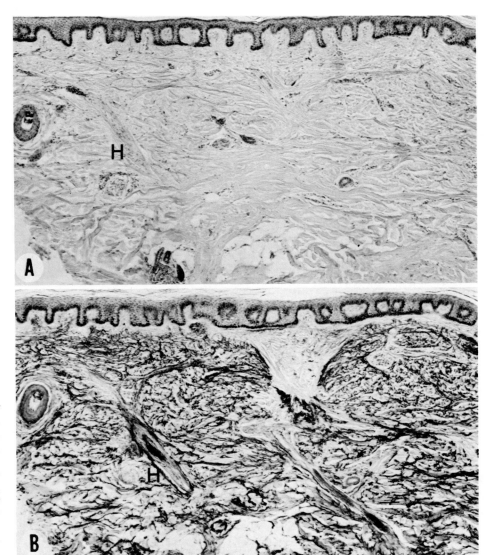

FIGURE 18–23.
*Pseudopelade. Comparison of
H&E (A) and O&G (B) stains
shows how much more informative the latter is in this disease. The atrophic follicle (H)
is barely discernible in A but
well outlined by elastic fibers
in B, which also shows loss of
superficial elastic fibers and
nail head appearance of the fibrous remnant of a completely
lost follicle. X70.*

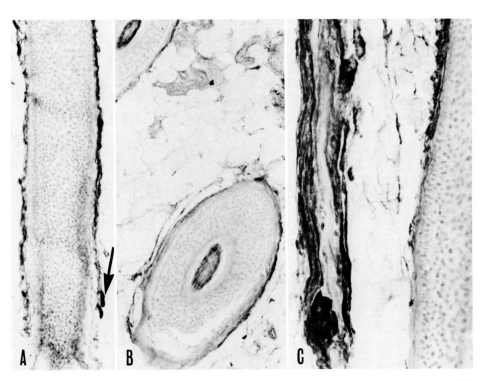

FIGURE 18–24.
*Fibrosing alopecia. A and B.
Relatively normal hair follicles
in longitudinal and oblique
section surrounded by strong
elastic fibers in their transient
(cyclic portion). In A, an arrow
points to two clumped Arao-
Perkins elastic bodies (Chap.
2) displaced sideways at a
spot just above the bulb of the
follicle. C. A similar follicle at
right, and fibrous remnant of a
lost follicle with thick elastic fibers at left. This is the mark of
fibrosing alopecia. H&E. A,
X100. B and C, X400. (From
Pinkus H. J Cutan Pathol 5:93,
1978. Copyright © 1978 Munksgaard International, Copenhagen.)*

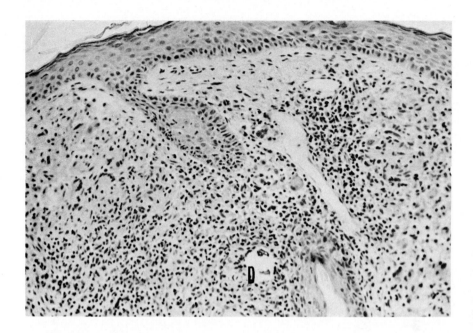

FIGURE 18–25.
Granulomatous rosacea. Mixed infiltrate with several multinucleated giant cells, telangiectasia, and remnants of hair follicles. Near bottom, a vacuole containing remnants of Demodex (D). H&E. X250.

ROSACEA, RHINOPHYMA, AND LEWANDOWSKY'S DISEASE

The histologic picture of *rosacea* varies along with its clinical forms.[40] The epidermis and upper dermis usually show features of seborrheic dermatitis in florid cases. Hair follicles may contain keratotic plugs and/or pus cells. The sebaceous glands tend to be large. There are variable amounts of interfollicular inflammatory infiltrate, which is mainly lymphocytic but may include neutrophils and some eosinophils and plasma cells. Marks[41] dis-

counts the primary role of the pilosebaceous apparatus and emphasizes damage to small vessels. Severe cases may show granulomatous reaction (Fig. 18-25), which often has the features of foreign-body granuloma, but may be of tuberculoid structure.[42] Variable amounts of fibrosis can be expected in the more chronic cases. This is especially true in patients whose condition approaches *rhinophyma* (Fig. 18-26). In these cases, the sebaceous glands may be tremendous and usually consist of many deep-seated lobes opening into a common sinus that is lined by stratified, keratinizing epithelium.

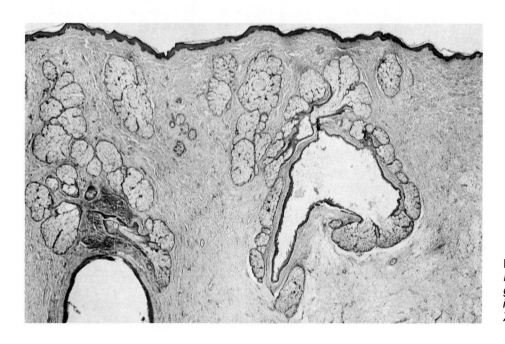

FIGURE 18–26.
Rhinophyma. Huge sebaceous glands and fibrosis with minor inflammatory infiltrate. H&E. X28.

Connective tissue, usually containing wide, thin-walled vessels, fills the spaces in between and may form the greatest volume of the hyperplastic masses. Inflammatory infiltrate may be minor or heavy and often includes features of foreign-body granulation tissue.

With some attention, one usually can find *Demodex* (Fig. 18-27) in the follicular channels and even deep in the sebaceous glands of rosacea.[43] However, they are similarly present in normal facial skin in many instances.[44] It is only when each follicle contains several *Demodex* that one begins to suspect an etiologic role. We are convinced that *demodicosis* exists as a disease simulating or complicating rosacea. One may hypothesize that some persons acquire allergy to *Demodex* as others do to a variety of other mites. We also have found dead *Demodex* or its fragments in the center of granulomatous nodules in rosacea (Fig. 18-28), a feature confirmed by Grosshans et al.[45] It appears irrefutable that *Demodex* can cause granulomatous reaction when it gets outside the follicle or gland, as may happen when these structures are destroyed by inflammation.

The peculiar papular affection of the face described by Lewandowsky as *rosacealike tuberculid*, but now thought to be rather *tuberculoid rosacea*, is difficult to differentiate from true micropapular tuberculid (Chap. 20). One needs serial sections because one has to decide whether the little granulomas are related to follicles or are truly interfollicular, as they ought to be in a tuberculid.

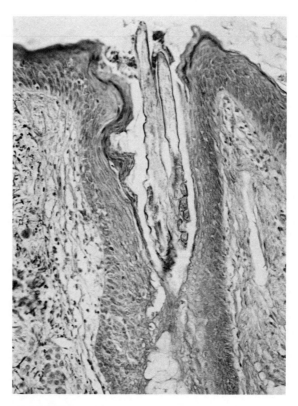

FIGURE 18–27.
Demodex folliculorum. *Two specimens lying head down in a follicular opening. O&G. X180.*

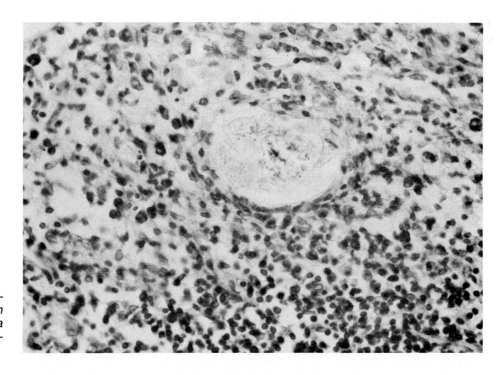

FIGURE 18–28.
Cross section of dead Demodex folliculorum *embedded in dense inflammatory tissue in a case of granulomatous rosacea. O&G. X465.*

REFERENCES

1. Pinkus H, Rudner E: Sycosis vulgaris agminata (Lutz). Dermat Monatsschr 151:628, 1965
2. Montagna W, Bell M, Strauss JS (eds): Sebaceous glands and acne vulgaris. J Invest Dermatol 62:117, 1974
3. Leyden JL, Kligman AM: Hairs in acne comedones. Arch Dermatol 106:851, 1972
4. Kaidbey KH, Kligman AM: A human model of coal tar acne. Arch Dermatol 109:212, 1974
5. Goldschmidt H, Leyden JL, Stein KH: Acne fulminans. Investigation of acute febrile ulcerative acne. Arch Dermatol 113:444, 1978
6. Izumi AK, Marples RR, Kligman AM: Senile (solar) comedones. J Invest Dermatol 61:46, 1973
7. Graham JH, Barroso-Tobila C: Dermal pathology of superficial fungus infections. In Baker RD (ed): The Pathologic Anatomy of Mycoses. Handbuch der speziellen pathologischen Anatomie und Histologie, vol. 3. pt 5. Berlin, New York, Springer-Verlag, 1971
8. Mehregan AH, Coskey RJ: Perforating folliculitis. Arch Dermatol 97:394, 1968
9. Heidelberg RP, Pinkus H: Necrotizing folliculitis. Presented at 1974 Annual Meeting of the National Medical Association
10. Potter BS, Burgoon CF, Johnson WC: Pityrosporum folliculitis. Arch Dermatol 107:388, 1973
11. Kaidbey KH, Kligman AM: The pathogenesis of topical steroid acne. J Invest Dermatol 62:31, 1974
12. Smith JD, Odom RB: Pseudofolliculitis capitis. Arch Dermatol 113:328, 1977
13. Pinkus H: Chronic scarring pseudofolliculitis of the Negro beard. Arch Dermatol 47:782, 1943
14. Strauss JS, Kligman AM: Pseudofolliculitis of the beard. Arch Dermatol 74:533, 1956
15. Ofuji S, Uehara M: Follicular eruptions of atopic dermatitis. Arch Dermatol 107:54, 1973
16. Freeman RG, Spiller R, Knox JM: Histopathology of erythema toxicum neonatorum. Arch Dermatol 82:586, 1960
17. Reveri M, Esterly NB, Fretzin DF, Pildes RS: Transient neonatal pustular melanosis. J Pediatr 88:831, 1976
18. Ishibashi A, Nishiyama Y, Miyata C, Chujo T: Eosinophilic pustular folliculitis. Dermatologica 149:240, 1974
19. Holst R. Eosinophilic pustular folliculitis. Report of a European case. Br J Dermatol 95:661, 1976
20. Kaidbey KH, Farah FS, Matta MT: Disseminate and recurrent infundibulo-folliculitis. Dermatologica 143:29, 1971
21. Hitch JM, Lund HZ: Disseminate and recurrent infundibulofolliculitis. Arch Dermatol 105:580, 1972
22. Pons S, Ortiz Medina A, Torrez Cortijo A: Disebacéa. Med Cutan Ibero Lat Am 7:313, 1973
23. Davenport DO: Ulerythema ophryogenes. Arch Dermatol 89:74, 1964
24. Tapernoux B, Delacrétaz J: Hyperkératose "en bouchons" d'origine mécanique. Dermatologica 143:201, 1971
25. Fajarre R, Alavaikko M: Kyrle's disease. Acta Derm Venereol (Stockh) 53:505, 1973
26. Constantine VS, Carter VH: Kyrle's disease II. Histopathologic findings in five cases and review of the literature. Arch Dermatol 97:633, 1968
27. Marks R, Griffiths A: The epidermis in pityriasis rubra pilaris. Br J Dermatol 89 [Suppl 9]: 19, 1973
28. Niemi KM, Kousa M, Storgårds K, Karvonen J: Pityriasis rubra pilaris. A clinico-pathological study with a special reference to autoradiography and histocompatibility antigens. Dermatologica 152:109, 1976
29. Pierard GE, de la Brassinne M: Cellular activity in the dermis surrounding the hair bulb in alopecia areata. J Cutan Pathol 2:240, 1975
30. Goos M: Zur Histopathologie der Alopecia areata mit besonderer Berücksichtigung ihrer Beziehungen zur Dauer, Lokalisation und Progression des Haarausfalls. Arch Dermatol Forsch 240:160, 1971
31. Pinkus H: Alopecia mucinosa. Inflammatory plaques with alopecia characterized by root-sheath mucinosis. Arch Dermatol 76:419, 1957
32. Ishibashi A: Histogenesis of mucin in follicular mucinosis. An electron microscopic study. Acta Derm Venereol (Stockh) 56:163, 1976
33. Coskey RJ, Mehregan AH: Alopecia mucinosa. Arch Dermatol 102:193, 1970
34. Civatte J, Laterza AM, Degos R: L'hypertrophie des follicules pilo-sébacés est-elle spéciale à la forme idiopathique de la mucinose folliculaire? Ann Dermatol Siphiligr 99:47, 1972
35. Borda J, Bianchi C, Carvalho A: Vinculaciones entre queratosis folicular estafilogena y mucinosis folicular. Arch Argent Dermatol 13:91, 1963
36. Pinkus H: Alopecia: clinicopathologic correlations. Int J Dermatol 19:245, 1980
37. Photinos PB: La Pseudo-Pelade de Brocq. Paris, N. Maloine, 1930
38. Pinkus H: Differential pattern of elastic fibers in scarring and non-scarring alopecias. J Cutan Pathol 5:93, 1978
39. Schultz-Ehrenburg U, Thies W: Alopecia scleroatrophicans carcinomatosa bei metastasierendem Mamma Karzinom. Z Hautkr 50:141, 1975
40. Marks R, Harcourt-Webster JN: Histopathology of rosacea. Arch Dermatol 100:683, 1969
41. Marks R: Histogenesis of the inflammatory component in rosacea. Proc R Soc Med 66:742, 1973
42. Mullanax MG, Kierland RR: Granulomatous rosacea. Arch Dermatol 101:206, 1970
43. Nutting WB: Hair follicle mites (acari demodicidae) of man. Int J Dermatol 15:79, 1976
44. Norm MS: *Demodex folliculorum:* incidence, regional distribution, pathogenicity. Dan Med Bull 18:14, 1971
45. Grosshans E, Kremer M, Maleville J, et al.: Le rôle des *Demodex folliculorum* dans l'histogenèse de la rosacéa granulomateuse. Bull Soc Fr Derm Syphiligr 79:639, 1972
46. Michelson HE: Does the rosacea-like tuberculid exist? Arch Dermatol 78:681, 1958

CHAPTER

19

Inflammations Involving Eccrine and Apocrine Glands

Eccrine and apocrine glands are much more rarely the seat of inflammation than is the pilosebaceous complex.[1]

ECCRINE GLANDS

Periporitis, a superficial pustular eruption around sweat pores and analogous to impetigo Bockhart, is almost exclusively found in young babies. Just as with the various types of *miliaria* of the adult, these lesions will rarely be biopsied. Either dermatosis is easily recognized under the microscope if one is aware of the typical corkscrew shape of the intraepidermal sweat duct unit (the acrosyringium) and keeps in mind that this structure persists uninvolved in most inflammatory dermatoses even in the presence of severe epidermal edema. Disruption of the acrosyringeal wall and presence of leukocytes in the lumen indicate involvement of the unit.[2] In *miliaria crystallina*, as it is often observed a few hours after acute defervescence in bedridden patients, fluid accumulates in the horny layer due to very superficial obstruction of the acrosyringium, and there is little inflammatory reaction. In *miliaria rubra*, a PAS-positive plug is present in the acrosyringium, and inflammation follows the great increase of resident cocci within a few days[3] (Fig. 19-1). We pointed out in Chapter 6 that the *dyshidrosiform* eruptions are of eczematous character and that the sweat ducts usually pass intact between the intraepidermal vesicles. Erythema toxicum neonatorum (Chap. 18), which may involve eccrine ducts[4] as well as hair follicles, and the toxic erythema with pustules following drug ingestion[5] are characterized by numerous eosinophils in the infiltrate.

Inflammatory involvement of the intradermal duct and the coil are even less frequent, except for the fact that there are numerous small blood vessels associated with these structures, and a more generalized perivascular infiltrate will also involve these vessels. Deep *eccrine gland abscesses*, formerly a severe and sometimes fatal disease of malnourished infants, have practically disappeared in the United States. The occasional case[6] seems to be associated with immunologic defects in the child. Histologically, a heavy mixed infiltrate of polymorphs and lymphocytes is found deep in the dermis around degenerating sweat coils. Careful examination of multiple sections is needed to rule out primary deep vasculitis. On the other hand, differentiation from a furuncle (Chap. 18) is simple because the thin eccrine duct never becomes the center of a necrotic plug, as is typical of deep follicular inflammation.

Sweat gland necrosis has been described in a case of bullous eruption induced by medicaments[7] and perhaps is more frequent than suspected. Sweat coil necrosis is observed after local injection of diphenhydramine.[8]

It may be mentioned here that localized scler-

219

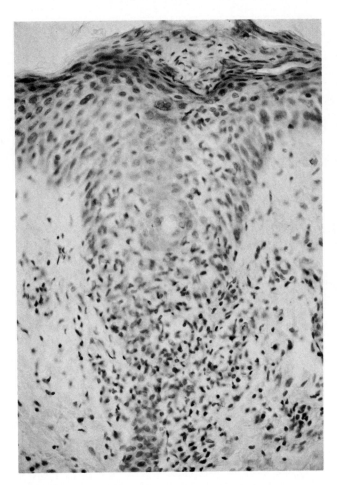

FIGURE 19–1.
Miliaria rubra. Edema and exocytosis in the sweat duct ridge surrounding the acrosyringium. The lesion is topped by a parakeratotic scale-crust, and there is edema and inflammatory infiltrate in the papillary dermis. That the acrosyringium is, in fact, ruptured in its lower part can be ascertained only in careful serial sections. H&E. X285.

oderma (*morphea*) often is characterized by atrophy of sweat coils and deep-seated focal perivascular round cell infiltrate. However, these two processes usually are not topically related.

APOCRINE GLANDS

Inasmuch as apocrine glands reach their full development only in puberty, they are rarely diseased in childhood. *Fox–Fordyce disease* and *hidradenitis suppurativa* are the outstanding examples of inflammation associated with the apocrine apparatus. The histologic basis of Fox–Fordyce disease has been demonstrated to be an obstruction of the apocrine duct (Fig. 19-2) where it enters the follicular wall. Serial sections usually are required to demonstrate this *apocrine miliaria*.[9,10] In routine diagnostic examination, it is sufficient to show inflammatory infiltrate encircling the upper one third of axillary hair follicles in order to corroborate a diagnosis of Fox–Fordyce disease.

Histologic confirmation of the diagnosis *hidradenitis suppurativa* is rarely required. Examination of surgical material usually reveals pockets of pus cells between heavy and often granulomatous inflammatory infiltrate in the subcutaneous and deep cutaneous tissue. Sweat glands (Fig. 19-3) may be encountered in various stages of disintegration, and

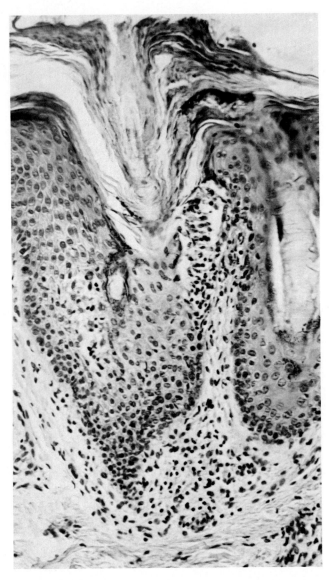

FIGURE 19–2.
Apocrine miliaria with relatively mild inflammatory infiltrate in Fox–Fordyce disease in a prepubertal girl. Two hair follicles side by side. The left one shows a longitudinal break in the right wall filled with degenerating and inflammatory cells. Some inflammatory cells also in left wall. H&E. X185. (From Mevorah et al. Dermatologica 136:43, 1968.)

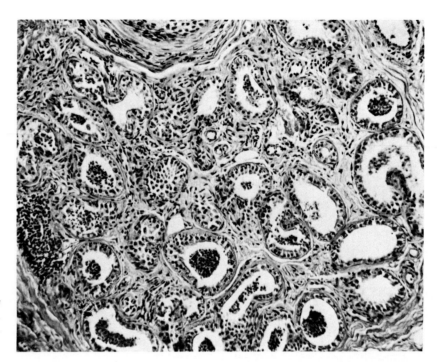

FIGURE 19–3.
Hidradenitis suppurativa. Well-preserved gland at periphery of lesion shows leukocytes in lumina and mild interstitial inflammation. H&E. X135.

few remain in the late stages of the disease. The solid necrotic plug of the furuncle is absent, just as it is absent in eccrine coil abscesses. The changes are those of a deep cellulitis with abscess formation. This explains the clinical features of a slowly enlarging deep swelling, which becomes fluctuant and eventually discharges liquid pus from a relatively small opening at the top of a dome. The process is quite distinct from the pointing of a furuncle and the elimination of a solid plug followed by thick pus. Thus, clinical and histologic knowledge combine in the differential diagnosis of follicular and apocrine abscesses.

We feel that apocrine glands play a minor role in the pathomechanisms of *acne conglobata* and *Hoffmann's disease (folliculitis et perifolliculitis suffodiens et abscedens).* These entities, therefore, were discussed in Chapter 18.

REFERENCES

1. Montagna W, Ellis RA, Silver AE (eds): Eccrine Glands and Eccrine Sweating. Advances in Biology of Skin, vol 3. New York, London, Pergamon, 1962
2. Dobson RL, Lobitz WC Jr: Some histochemical observations on the human eccrine sweat glands. II. The pathogenesis of miliaria. Arch Dermatol 75:653, 1957
3. Hölzle E, Kligman AM: The pathogenesis of miliaria rubra. Role of the resident microflora. Br J Dermatol 99:117, 1978
4. Duperrat B, Bret AJ: Erythema neonatorum allergicum. Br J Dermatol 73:300, 1961
5. Ogino A, Tagumi H, Takahashi C, Higuchi T: Generalized pustular toxic erythema: pathogenetic relationship between pustule and epidermal appendage (hair follicle or sweat duct). Acta Derm Venereol (Stockh) 58:257, 1978
6. Mopper C, Pinkus H, Iacobell P: Multiple sweat gland abscesses of infants. Arch Dermatol 71:177, 1955
7. Herschtal D, Robinson ML: Blisters of the skin in coma induced by amitryptidine and clorazepate dipotassium. Report of a case with underlying sweat gland necrosis. Arch Dermatol 115:499, 1979
8. Pinkus H: Personal observation
9. Shelley WB, Levy EJ: Apocrine sweat retention in man. II. Fox-Fordyce disease (apocrine miliaria). Arch Dermatol 73:38, 1958
10. Mevorah B, Duboff GS, Wass RW: Fox-Fordyce disease in prepubescent girls. Dermatologica 136:43, 1968

IV

GRANULOMATOUS INFLAMMATION AND PROLIFERATION

The derivation of the term *granulomatous inflammation* is complicated. It is related to granulation tissue, which was given that name originally on the macroscopic clinical basis that a healing wound looks granular. These granulations, of course, correspond to newly formed capillaries and surrounding fibroblasts, histiocytes, and fibrous connective tissue (Chap. 17). Always associated are the usual types of inflammatory cells, that is, polymorphonuclear leukocytes, small round cells (lymphocytes), and perhaps some plasma cells and eosinophils. Masses of microscopically similar tissue in various organs were then called "granulomas" by the use of the suffix meaning a tumor. Similar but now obsolete terms with more specific meaning were "tuberculoma" or "syphiloma," and even today we speak of "lepromatous leprosy." Eventually, when the suffix *-oma* was more specifically reserved for true neoplasms and when the reactive nature of tuberculous and other infiltrates had been recognized, the term *granulomatous inflammation* was preferred. However, *granuloma* persists in several dermatologic diagnoses (granuloma annulare) and, in fact, has been used recently for the very purpose of emphasizing the nonneoplastic nature of certain lesions, Thus "reticulohistiocytoma" has been replaced by *reticulohistiocytic granuloma*.

The simplest definition[1] for the microscopic picture of granulomatous inflammation is *an inflammatory process that contains histiocytes (reticuloendothelial cells)*. The word *histiocyte* is used here in the classic sense of a tissue cell capable of phagocytosis. There is no relation to neoplastic disease. As a matter of fact, disease processes containing histiocytes are stamped thereby as being inflammatory and not malignant. For a discussion of modern concepts of histiocytes as neoplastic cells see Chapter 44.

The cellular infiltrate of all simple inflammatory dermatoses consists predominantly of those cells that come into the skin from the bloodstream or of their modifications: neutrophilic and eosinophilic leukocytes, lymphocytes, and possibly plasma cells. They can disappear again without leaving a trace, either through cell death and absorption or by migration to other parts, such as lymph nodes. Histiocytes present in the tissue may be stimulated to become macrophages and may remain as evidence of past inflammation, e.g., the melanophages of postinflammatory pigmentation. If any appreciable number of histiocytes or their various derivatives, especially macrophages and epithelioid cells, are found in an inflammatory infiltrate, it is assumed that they are derived from reticuloendothelial cells by multiplication at the site of the lesion. This is what the old term "productive inflammation" (in contrast to exudative inflammation) implied, and it is a good concept to remember. Although there is recent experimental evidence[2] that mononuclear cells in chronic inflammation in small laboratory animals continuously come from the circulation, there is also evidence of cell proliferation in simple inflammatory infiltrates in man,[3,4] and one is entitled to reserve judgment on the cellular dynamics of granulomas in human skin (for reviews see Warren[5] and Epstein[6]). In any case, development of granulomatous inflammation appears to be a manifestation of cellular rather than humoral immunity. This is exemplified by the development of large epithelioid cell granulomas in patients deficient in circulating antibodies.[7]

It seems preferable to amplify and support the simple criterion of the presence of histiocytes by a few other statements when we are dealing with granulomatous dermatoses. There is production of new blood capillaries and their supporting mesenchymal cells. In addition, and this is important, the formation of granulomatous tissue practically always is associated with destruction of preexisting tissue in the skin. This is easily demonstrated by an elastic fiber stain, which shows absence of elastic fibers in the granulomatous zone. Closer inspection shows that collagenous fibers also are absent, digested, or absorbed. From this statement follows logically the last one: Granulomatous inflammation cannot heal without leaving some trace, either in the form of a defect or, more commonly, in the form of fibrosis and scar formation. These sequelae do not presuppose gross tissue necrosis such as we see in caseation, gummatous liquefaction, or abscess formation. The granulomatous infiltrate itself destroys tissue. The loss is temporarily hidden by the productive inflammation, which actually makes an excess of tissue. The loss becomes obvious only when the granulomatous process heals, either spontaneously or under treatment. Clinical and histologic features of granulomatous dermatoses become more meaningful if these facts are kept in mind.

The details of granulomatous tissue reaction vary widely, and that enables the histopathologist in many cases to make a fairly accurate diagnosis of specific disease even if he cannot demonstrate the responsible agent, be it a microorganism or some nonliving substance. However, there is considerable overlap between tissue reactions in various diseases, and one should always attempt to demonstrate a specific organism or other causative agent in the tissue for definite diagnosis. On the other hand, in some cases, the very absence of a demonstrable agent aids in the classification.

Once one has recognized the histologic picture in a section as being granulomatous inflammation, it is convenient to put it into one of two broad classes. One of these comprises processes which consist almost exclusively of round cells, epithelioid cells, and multinucleated giant cells. In this group are the major three old diseases: syphilis, tuberculosis, and leprosy. To these one must add less common and more recently recognized entities such as sarcoidosis, leishmaniasis, histoplasmosis, and some foreign-body granulomas. The other class is characterized by a mixed infiltrate in which neutrophilic leukocytes and eosinophils are added to round cells and histiocytic elements. In this group are most of the deep fungous infections, granulomatous halogen eruptions, and quite a few foreign-body granulomas. Granulomatous lesions associated with large vessels have some special characteristics, and these were touched on in Chapter 15.

In the title of this section, we included *granulomatous proliferation*: this refers to lesions of almost purely histiocytic character to which the concept of inflammation does not really apply. They comprise xanthomas and other processes that are not considered true neoplasms precisely because they consist of histiocytes and are reversible in many cases. From this group has been split off "histiocytosis X."

REFERENCES

1. Forbus WD: Granulomatous Inflammation. Springfield, Ill, Thomas, 1949
2. Spector WG: The cellular dynamics of granulomas. Proc R Soc Med 64:941, 1971
3. Lachapelle JM: Comparative study of ^{3}H-thymidine labelling of the dermal infiltrate of skin allergic and irritant patch test reactions in man. Br J Dermatol 87:460, 1972
4. Meuret G, Schmitt E, Hagedorn M: Monocytopoiesis in chronic eczematous diseases, psoriasis vulgaris, and mycosis fungoides. J Invest Dermatol 66:22, 1976
5. Warren KS: A functional classification of granulomatous inflammation. Ann NY Acad Sci 278:7, 1976
6. Epstein WL: Cutaneous granulomas. Int J Dermatol 16:574, 1977
7. Orfanos C, Meiers HG: Ulzerierende epitheloidzellige Granulomatose der Haut bei Antikörpermangelsyndrom. Differentialdiagnose und Literaturübersicht. Dermatologica 136:65, 1968

20

Predominantly Mononuclear Granulomas

When the senior author first learned dermatopathology in Germany, the diagnosis of granulomatous inflammation was simple and satisfactory. If a granulomatous lesion was not tuberculosis, it had to be syphilis, with the exception of pure epithelioid cell tubercles, which represented sarcoid. Leprosy was practically nonexistent, and other granulomatous diseases either were exotic or had not yet been identified. Today, in the United States, one has to take into consideration a much greater variety of possible causes, and in many instances, the histopathologist has to defer diagnosis pending the outcome of cultures and other laboratory tests, or he must leave the final decision to the clinician who may do a therapeutic test.

It has been pointed out in the preceding two pages that, as a rule of thumb, one may limit one's diagnostic deliberations to certain entities if the infiltrate consists entirely of mononuclear cells, and to others if appreciable numbers of neutrophilic and/or eosinophilic leukocytes are present.

In this chapter we discuss the first group, which includes the diagnoses listed in Table 20-1. Of these, tuberculosis remains didactically most important in spite of the fact that cutaneous tuberculosis is quite rare in the United States.

TUBERCULOSIS

Biology

The significance of tuberculosis for biologically based teaching of histopathology rests on several facts. The disease is due to a well-defined organism, which can be cultured and to which a number of animal species are susceptible. It was a very common disease in the days when bacteriology and immunology developed and was intensively studied. Thus, the results of many animal experiments are available in addition to wide clinical experience.

It soon became clear that the result of infection of man or animal with the tubercle bacillus depended on six interacting factors: number and virulence of the bacilli, mode and site of inoculation, and native resistance and immunologic response of the host. Their multifarious combination produces a variety of clinical and histologic pictures.

That the number of bacilli matters can be shown easily in the guinea pig, which is so highly susceptible to human bacilli. More or less virulent strains have been identified by microbiologists, and there is little doubt that the result of an intradermal inoculation will differ from that of an intravenous in-

TABLE 20–1.
Mononuclear Granulomas

	Histiocytes	Lymphocytes	Plasma Cells	Layering	Caseation	Seat	Identifiable Causative Agents
Infectious Diseases							
Tuberculosis	(+) to +++	+ to +++	−	++	0 to (+)	Superficial to deep	Acid-fast bacilli + to 0
Leprosy, lepromatous	++	+	(+)	(+)	0	Variable, perineural	Acid-fast bacilli ++ to ++++
Leprosy, tuberculoid	+++	+	(+)	+	0	Variable, perineural	Acid-fast bacilli (+) to 0
Late syphilis	++	++	++	(+)	+ to +++	Deep	None
Sarcoidosis	++++	0 to +	−	+	(+)	Superficial and deep	None
Histoplasmosis	+++	+	−	−	0	Medium	Intracellular bodies
Leishmaniasis, early	+++	++	+	+	0	Superficial	Intracellular bodies (Donovan)
Leishmaniasis, late	+++	+	−	++	0	Superficial to mid-dermis	None
Tularemia	+++	+	+	+	+	Variable	None
Rhinoscleroma	+	+	++	−	−	Variable	Frisch bacilli
Foreign-body Granulomas							
Paraffinoma	++++	(+)	−	−	0	Deep	Empty spaces
Silica granuloma	++++	+	−	−	0	Variable	Polarizing crystals
Zirconium granuloma	++	++	−	+	0 to (+)	Superficial	None
Beryllium granuloma	+++	+	−	+	+++	Variable	None

jection in the animal. The significance of mode and site for cutaneous disease of man will be discussed later. It is also well known that animal species vary greatly in their native resistance, and within the human species, individual susceptibility is obviously different even in the same family. However, where histopathologic examination is concerned, we find again, as in many previous chapters, that tissue response is the basis of our diagnosis, and while tissue response is the product of all the variables mentioned, it depends mainly on the immunologic state of the individual at the time the presenting lesion developed.

The tubercle bacillus does not produce a toxin. Large quantities of dead bacilli can be inoculated into a virgin organism without inflammatory response. However, a few living bacilli are apt to provoke a response. The response develops slowly and depends on the initiation of an immune reaction, usually one of hypersensitivity.

In order to understand this thoroughly, it is pertinent to be aware of Koch's original experiment. If living bacilli are inoculated into a scratch in the

skin of an animal that has never been exposed, a barely noticeable traumatic reaction will take place. Otherwise, nothing obvious happens for one to two weeks. Then, a subacute type of inflammation sets in, and an ulcer develops, which usually persists until the death of the animal. Local lymph nodes will become infected, and generalization of the disease into various organs leads to death. If, however, the inoculation is repeated at a different site in an already diseased but not yet marasmic animal, there will be a stormy local reaction with tissue necrosis and acute inflammatory response. This wound will heal in spite of the fact that the animal succumbs to its general infection.

Histologically, after the first few days, the slowly developing primary inflammatory response consists of lymphocytes and increasing numbers of histiocytic macrophages, which engulf the numerous and proliferating bacilli. The histiocytic, granulomatous response to the primary inoculation is never enough to destroy all bacilli, and in the undermining ulcer of the dying animal, bacilli multiply again and may be found in masses among a nonspecific inflammatory infiltrate. Quite in contrast, the second inoculation provokes a massive polymorphonuclear exudate within 24 hours which is associated with tissue necrosis and leads to the mechanical elimination of most of the inoculum. The remaining bacilli are gradually destroyed in tuberculoid granulomatous infiltrate.

This basic experiment of Robert Koch, which was repeated, examined histologically, and interpreted in immunologic terms by Lewandowsky,[1] provides the biologic basis for analysis not only of the many clinical and histologic variants of cutaneous tuberculosis but of other chronic granulomatous infections as well. It plainly shows that the tubercle bacillus is but a bland foreign body to the not previously exposed host. The living bacillus, however, has the power to provoke an immunologic response which may take many forms, from polymorphonuclear exudate to round cell infiltrate, to epithelioid cell response, and to acute tissue necrosis. Jadassohn–Lewandowsky's law was formulated on this basis: Where microorganisms proliferate in the tissues unchecked by immunologic processes, only nonspecific inflammatory infiltrate will be found. Where immunologic power is strong, development of histiocytic, and particularly of epithelioid, cell response leads to reduction and disappearance of the bacilli. To this may be added that unusually high sensitivity to bacterial products may lead to primary tissue necrosis with secondary tuberculoid response. It also should be emphasized that anergic nonspecific inflammation is found at the beginning and at the end. It characterizes the tissue reaction before immunity develops in the virgin host and after it has been exhausted in the marasmic host.

TUBERCULODERMAS

On the basis of this discussion, we can tabulate tuberculodermas by correlating their histologic features with the immunologic state of the patient and the site of inoculation, as shown in Table 20-2.

Primary Tuberculosis

Just as in the animal, inoculation of the skin of a noninfected human being results in a chain of events quite different from any caused by superinfection. A primary complex of local lesion and satellite lymphadenopathy develops similar to that in the lung. There is little doubt that the first histo-

TABLE 20–2.
Tuberculodermas

A. Primary tuberculosis
B. Chronic lesions in host with relatively high immunity
  1. Lupus vulgaris
  2. Lupus tumidus
  3. Tuberculosis verrucosa cutis
  4. Scrofuloderma
C. Spontaneously involuting lesions in hypersensitive host (tuberculids)
  1. Lichen scrofulosorum
  2. Papulonecrotic tuberculid
  3. Erythema induratum
  4. Facial tuberculids
D. Progressive lesions in host with low immunity
  1. Acute miliary tuberculosis
  2. Tuberculosis orificialis

Adapted from Michelson and Laymon. Classification of tuberculosis of the skin. Arch Dermatol 52:108, 1945

logic stages are just as nonspecific as those in the guinea pig's skin, but biopsies of this type of lesion are usually not taken until lack of healing and swelling of lymph nodes arouse suspicion.[2,3] At that time, several weeks after inoculation, a more or less well developed epithelioid cell and lymphocyte response is found similar to that in lupus vulgaris. However, the tuberculoid response often is associated with ulceration, and acid-fast bacilli may be demonstrable. In very young infants with poor immunologic ability, the ulcer may develop progressively, and death from generalized infection may result just as in the guinea pig. In older individuals the primary site may heal with fibrosis and scarring, or it may turn into and persist as *lupus vulgaris*.

Tuberculodermas in Infected Hosts

Lupus Vulgaris. *Tuberculosis luposa* (Fig. 20-1) is the prototype of chronic tuberculoderma in a previously infected individual. The patient usually has a fair relative immunity, and it is rare to find *lupus vulgaris* in tuberculosis sanitaria. The histologic picture is characterized by epithelioid cell nodules embedded in shells of lymphocytes (tubercles). Multinucleated giant cells (Fig. 5-16A) may be sparse or more numerous and usually are typical Langhans cells. Plasma cells, eosinophils, and neutrophilic polymorphonuclears are absent or rare. The quantitative relation of epithelioid cells and lymphocytes varies. In some cases, one sees only a few histiocytic nodules in the sea of small round cells. In other cases, there are thin rims of lymphocytes around conglomerate tubercles, a picture very

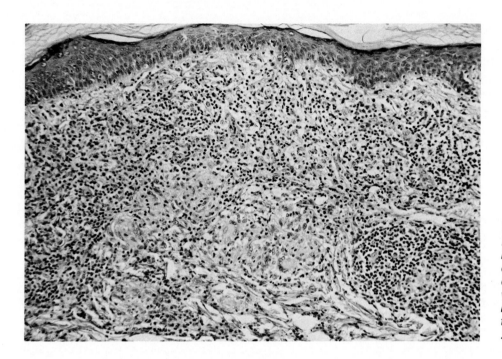

FIGURE 20–1.
Lupus vulgaris. Nodules of epithelioid cells and small round cells furnish approximately equal portions of the infiltrate which borders on the epidermis. At least one Langhans type giant cell is seen. H&E. X135.

similar to *sarcoidosis*. Concentric layering of the tubercles is better developed in tuberculosis than in any of the other granulomatous diseases, but one may encounter a more diffuse scattering of round cells in the nodes. The notorious avascularity of tuberculous infiltrate is difficult to judge in the skin because the mass of tuberculous tissue is not very great, and the rich cutaneous vasculature persists between the nodes. Caseation is practically unheard of in tuberculodermas, except in *lupus miliaris disseminatus faciei* (which probably has no relation to tuberculosis—see below). Microscopic foci of central necrosis are rarely seen.

The specific infiltrate usually occupies the upper part of the dermis in lupus vulgaris, but larger or smaller masses may be found deeper. The infiltrate borders on the epidermis from below, thinning it often, but rarely producing ulceration. The superficial seat of the granuloma, which differentiates tuberculosis from syphilis, is the basis of the clinical probe test. Firm pressure will make a blunt probe break through the epidermis and penetrate the soft granulomatous tissue. This test also makes obvious that the normal dermis has been destroyed and replaced by the infiltrate. When lupus vulgaris heals, either spontaneously or under treatment, it leaves a void that is replaced by fibrosis or leads to atrophic scars. Histologically, just as clinically, it is characteristic for the disease to show persistent or recurrent tubercles in the fibrotic areas. It is a thankless task to look for acid-fast bacilli in sections of lupus vulgaris, although modern staining methods may lead to success.[4] Culture and animal

inoculation must be used to demonstrate the microorganism, which may be of the bovine type.[5] Differential diagnosis includes the late stage of Oriental leishmaniasis.

Lupus Tumidus and Other Variants. In contrast to the classic atrophying form leading to the peaked nose, the shrunken lips, and the everted eyelids of the lupus patient's face, there is another form of tuberculosis luposa, which is particularly common in the American black. This *lupus tumidus* produces large circumscribed swellings which look like keloids but are peculiarly soft to the touch. Histologically, there are masses of well-layered tubercles. In this form, plasma cells are commonly found between the lymphocytes around and between the epithelioid nodes.

If lupus vulgaris involves the distal parts of the extremities, it may be associated with verrucous epidermal hyperplasia and must be differentiated from *tuberculosis verrucosa cutis*.

Tuberculosis Verrucosa Cutis. This form is usually due to the exogenous superinfection in individuals with a high degree of immunity. Butchers' and pathologists' warts are classic examples. Partly due to the immunologic background, partly to the specific terrain of the acral skin, there is a strong tendency to verrucous epidermal hyperplasia and to fibrosis in these lesions. Tuberculoid tissue may have to be searched for and is usually found just below the epidermis. Presence of bacilli must be demonstrated by culture or animal test.

Scrofuloderma. The histologic picture of *scrofuloderma* is influenced by its peculiar pathomechanism of massive infection by contiguity from underlying lymph nodes. Tuberculoid reaction usually is mixed with nonspecific inflammation in an open and deep sinus. Acid-fast bacilli are more apt to be demonstrable in this *tuberculosis cutis colliquativa* than in other members of the group.

Tuberculids

The concept of tuberculids was introduced by Darier almost 80 years ago and, in somewhat modified form, was supported by vast clinical evidence over many years, although the clinching postulate of demonstration of the causative agent in the lesion could not be fulfilled. This was attributed to the basic concept that tuberculids are due to the hematogenous lodging of small numbers of bacilli in cutaneous vessels of a highly tuberculin-sensitive individual. According to the hypothesis, the embolus of bacilli which either are dead on arrival or are quickly overcome by tissue immunity acts like a tuberculin injection, and the details of the tissue response depend on the site and size of the vessel involved and the balance between sensitivity and immunity of the individual. The entire concept of the existence of tuberculids has been attacked in recent years[6] on modern, but similarly speculative, immunologic grounds. In an age in which tuberculosis has become extremely rare in developed countries, it will be very difficult to accumulate sufficient clinical, pathologic, and factual immunologic evidence in the United States to decide this controversy one way or the other.[7] Dermatologists in less developed countries, however, encounter tuberculids not infrequently.[8,9] Tissue reactions, as we have pointed out repeatedly, are often characteristic but rarely specific for one disease. Erythema nodosum often was a symptom of tuberculous infection at a time when tuberculosis was common, and it may at present be due to coccidioidomycosis in places in which this disease is endemic, but it is more often based on streptococcic infection in other areas. Similarly, skin lesions resembling tuberculids may have other etiology. Lichen trichophyticus (lichenoid trichophytid) is well known to observant dermatologists in children in the acute stages of *Microsporum* infection. Lichen spinulosus (Chap. 18) closely resembles lichen scrofulosorum clinically. Granuloma annulare, especially the perforating type (Chap. 22), must be differentiated from papulonecrotic tuberculid. The existence of these dermatoses, however, is no reason to deny the existence of a lichenoid tuberculid. This guide is not the place to delve deeper into nosologic questions. The senior author, however, remains convinced, on the basis of personal experience and conversation with experienced dermatologists practicing in countries where tuberculosis is more prevalent than in the United States, that tuberculids exist, and we shall discuss them on the basis that the histologic picture is best understood if we accept the classic concept.

Lichen Scrofulosorum. The lichenoid tuberculid (Fig. 20-2), according to this hypothesis, results if small perifollicular vessels are involved and the number of bacilli or degree of sensitivity is not

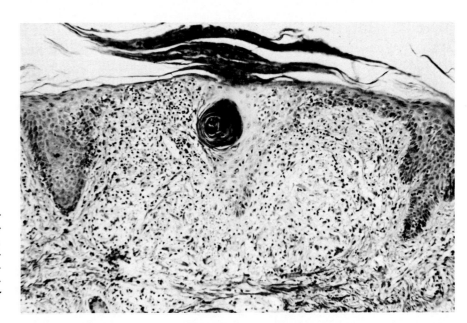

FIGURE 20–2.
Lichen scrofulosorum. Note destruction of elastic fibers by relatively mild granulomatous infiltrate. The epithelial structures are affected secondarily and have reacted with parakeratosis on the epidermal surface and in the follicular infundibulum. O&G. X135.

large enough to produce tissue necrosis. It has been seen after BCG inoculation[10] in response to the depot of tuberculin that a more or less pronounced tuberculoid granulomatous reaction will develop in perifollicular localization. Early stages may show mainly lymphocytes, fully developed lesions, epithelioid cells, and giant cells, and late stages will show fibrosis. The lesion heals spontaneously in a few weeks, and a biopsy site must be chosen judiciously for best results. Too young a lesion may show noncharacteristic inflammatory infiltrate. Several illustrative cases associated with active tuberculosis and well responding to antituberculous treatment were published recently by Smith et al.[11] and by Hudson from England.[12]

Differential diagnosis from papular lesions of late secondary syphilis may not always be possible. Somewhat deeper localization and presence of plasma cells speak for syphilis. The granulomas of papular sarcoidosis usually are more massive and better defined than those produced by the fleeting process of lichen scrofulosorum.

Papulonecrotic Tuberculid. If the involved vessel or the number of bacilli is larger and the sensitivity high, the bacillary embolus will produce primary tissue necrosis similar to that produced by an overdose of intradermal tuberculin. The necrotic tissue becomes surrounded by histiocytes and lymphocytes, which usually assume tuberculoid configuration (Fig. 20-3) Eventually, the necrotic plug is sequestered and eliminated to the outside, and the characteristic punched-out scar results. It is

important to realize that the necrosis in this case is not caseation but is primary necrosis of healthy tissue. The granuloma develops secondarily.[9] Therefore, an elastic fiber stain will show persistence of elastic fibers in the central necrosis, while these are destroyed in the peripheral granuloma. A comparison of Figure 20-3 and Figure 13-6 shows the fundamental difference of the histomechanisms of papulonecrotic tuberculid and acute pityriasis lichenoides, which may come into clinical differential diagnosis, although the random distribution of lesions is quite different from the localization of the tuberculid on the extensor surfaces near the joints of the extremities. If necrosis is less complete and granulomatous response less severe, clinical sloughing may be absent, and the histologic picture may be remarkably similar to granuloma annulare (Chap. 22).

Erythema Induratum. *Bazin's disease* has become extremely rare, not only because the prevalence of tuberculosis has decreased but also because better nutrition and change of living habits have almost eliminated the flabby and anemic, pasty young girl who was its principal victim. It is, however, by no means extinct.[8,13] The term *erythema induratum* is now often used loosely for chronic nodose lesions of the lower extremities, which histologically belong to the group of nodular vasculitis (Chap. 15). The tuberculous form (Bazin's disease) supposedly results from involvement of a subcutaneous vein with a hyperergic tuberculous inflammation. The tissue reaction in erythema in-

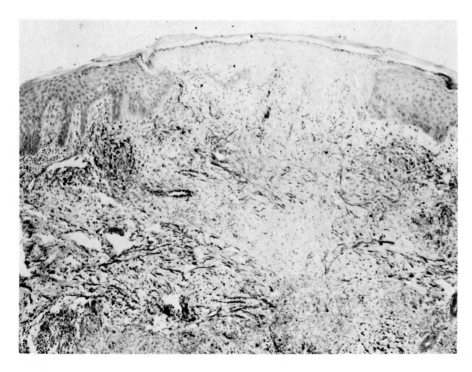

FIGURE 20–3.
Papulonecrotic tuberculid. Necrosis of epidermis and dermis with preservation of elastic fibers. The latter are partly destroyed in granulomatous infiltrate surrounding primary necrosis. O&G. X75.

duratum is modified by the reaction to damaged fat tissue, the proliferating atrophy discussed in Chapter 16. This stereotyped response of the damaged panniculus often overshadows the typical tuberculoid response. Furthermore, as pointed out in the discussion on panniculitis, it is difficult to find the initial focus in a large and often ulcerated lesion. Unless the pathologist is lucky enough to find typical tubercles, he must be content with calling the changes compatible with erythema induratum and must ask the clinician to validate the diagnosis by the results of other examinations. According to Bolgert,[13] a second biopsy done after the patient has been started on antituberculous therapy may be more conclusive.

Facial Tuberculids. Also insecure, but for other reasons, is the histologic diagnosis of the tuberculodermas occurring on the face. Already the nomenclature is bewildering, starting with the old *folliclis* and *acnitis* and progressing to Lewandowsky's *rosacealike tuberculid,* Michelson's *micropapular tuberculid,* and *lupus miliaris disseminatus faciei.* We will not even consider *lupus pernio, angiolupoid,* and Boeck's *lupoid* because they are manifestations of sarcoidosis. Because of the constant absence of bacilli and the frequent absence of evidence of systemic tuberculosis, there is strong doubt of the tuberculous nature of some of these lesions.

Histologically, diagnosis is problematic because of the frequent occurrence of foreign-body granulomas on the face. These are reactions either to follicular contents, such as keratin, sebum, and *De-modex,* or to breakdown of follicular cysts. If one wants to make a diagnosis of facial tuberculid, one has to exclude these factors in every individual case, and that can be done only by examining a fair number of serial sections. What looks like a splendid tubercle in the interfollicular skin in one section often turns out to be a foreign-body granuloma related to a hair follicle or cyst or containing *Demodex* when serial sections are examined (Chap. 18).

A highly conservative approach is justified in the diagnosis of tuberculids of the face. One must require well-layered tubercles situated between hair follicles and not related to them. If such are found, one may suggest a diagnosis of *micropapular tuberculid,* but verification is the task of the clinician. In all doubtful cases, a final diagnosis of *tuberculidlike (granulomatous) rosacea* (Chap. 18) is probably the correct one. Lesions showing variable amounts of granulomatous and acute inflammation associated with necrosis remain very doubtful, and the diagnoses acnitis and folliclis are practically obsolete.

There is, however, one highly characteristic histologic picture. A combination of a well-developed conglomerate tubercle with central caseation necrosis permits the histologic diagnosis of *lupus miliaris disseminatus faciei* (Fig. 20-4), and this diagnosis should be made only in the presence of caseation. O&G stain usually will show a neat ring of elastic fibers in the center of the caseous material. It is more likely that this ring is part of the isthmus of a hair follicle than of an occluded artery. The eruption of small facial papules having a

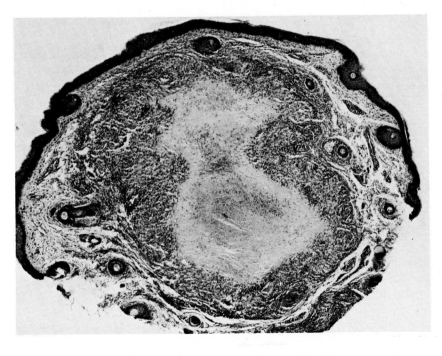

FIGURE 20–4.
Lupus miliaris disseminatus faciei. H&E.
X45.

yellow center, which corresponds to the caseous material but is often mistaken for a pustule, is most likely not related to tuberculosis,[14] but the awkward name is well established, and the histomorphologic expression of whatever the underlying process is is among the most characteristic ones in dermatopathology.

Progressive Lesions in a Host With Low Immunity

A patient who is anergic as a result of never having been exposed to tubercle bacilli will respond with nonspecific inflammation to proliferating organisms, and a similar response may be all a patient can produce whose immunologic powers have been overwhelmed or exhausted (secondary anergy). A situation of this type develops in miliary tuberculosis or in far-progressed involvement of lungs or bowels when large numbers of bacilli reach the skin through hematogenous dissemination or direct inoculation from infected discharges.

Miliary tuberculosis of the skin does not differ much from that of other organs in its histologic expression. Numerous bacilli can be demonstrated in an infiltrate of lymphocytes with the barest indication of granulomatous reaction.

Tuberculosis orificialis also often presents only polymorphonuclear and round cell infiltrate in the bottom of the ulcers which develop in oral mucosa or anal skin. However, depending on the degree of immunologic resistance left in the patient, a variable amount of epithelioid cell response may be found. The number of demonstrable bacilli varies in inverse relation.

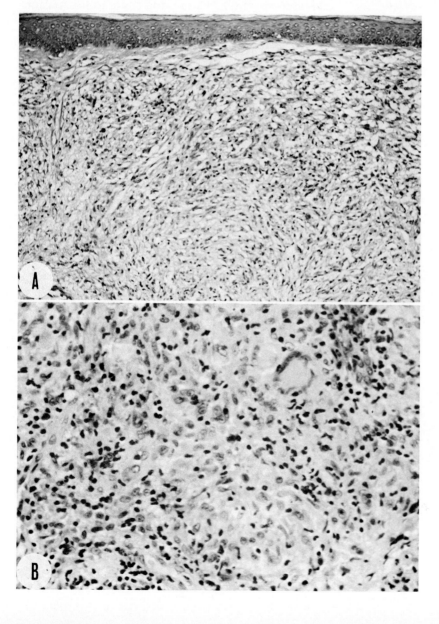

FIGURE 20–5.
*Hansen's disease. **A.** Histoid form consisting of histiocytes between collagenous fibers. **B.** Tuberculoid type. H&E. X250.*

LEPROSY (HANSEN'S DISEASE)

Leprosy, the other disease associated with an acid-fast bacillus, is remarkable for the similarities and the differences of the tissue reactions encountered. So-called *tuberculoid leprosy* follows Lewandowsky's law and exhibits a strong epithelioid cell tissue reaction (Fig. 20-5B), in which few or no bacilli can be demonstrated. The picture of this type of Hansen's disease may be so similar to that of sarcoidosis that it offers diagnostic difficulties. On the other hand, the *lepromatous type*, in which bacilli are numerous and tissue immunity is low, far from having nonspecific inflammatory infiltrate, also shows a highly characteristic picture (Fig. 20-6A) in which nodular accumulations of histiocytes predominate. These, however, do not have the character of epitheloid cells but look foamy (Table 20-3) because they contain large quantities of bacilli (Fig. 20-6B) and also nonpolarizing lipids.[15,16] Lepra cells, also called *Virchow cells,* may be considered a special type of foreign-body reaction rather than an expression of immunity.

The pathogenesis and etiology of the various forms of leprosy are much less clear than those of tuberculosis because of our inability to culture the bacillus in vitro and because of the unavailability of experimental animals. Both of these hindrances seem to be overcome by reports of cultivation of leprosy bacilli on hyaluronic acid-containing media[17] and by inoculation of mouse foot pads[18] and production of the disease in armadillos.[19] These results suggest that the last of Koch's postulates is going to be fulfilled to prove Hansen's bacillus as the etiologic agent of the disease.

The various classifications of lepromatous lesions also seem to have come to a consensus in recent years[20] in the division of the disease into two polar forms, the *lepromatous* and the *tuberculoid,* and having these bridged by *borderline* lesions, which vary from BL (borderline lepromatous) to BT (borderline tuberculoid). That leaves early *indeterminate* cases and the various puzzling manifestations of *reactional states.*

Histologically, one can understand the findings better by remembering that the bacillus primarily involves nerves and, in the nerves, Schwann cells, which phagocytize it and harbor it. The rest seems to depend on the ability of the host to react. If cell-mediated immunity remains low and no positive Mitsuda reaction develops in the lepromatous form, tissue macrophages will take up the proliferating rods and will become filled with clusters and globes of bacilli. On the other hand, if tissue immunity develops, histiocytes will destroy bacilli and will form epithelioid tubercles. The aim of the pathologist will have to be to prove or disprove involvement of nerves, and that requires a sizable

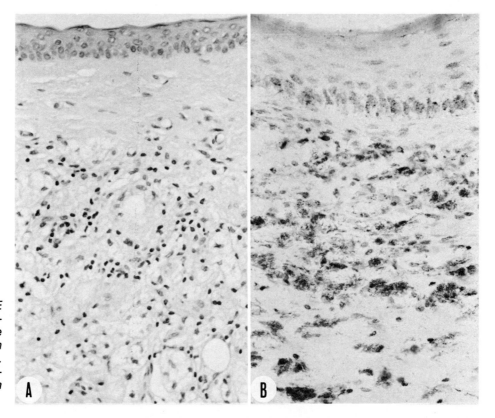

FIGURE 20–6.
Lepromatous leprosy. **A.** *H&E stain shows large foamy histiocytes (Virchow cells) and some lymphocytes. Compare with Figure 23-2, xanthoma cells.* **B.** *Fite stain shows innumerable acid-fast bacilli clumped in the histiocytes. X800.*

TABLE 20–3.
Microorganisms Found in Mononuclear Cells in Granulomas

Disease	Clinical Type	Organisms	Stain	Size
Leprosy	Lepromatous	*Mycobacterium leprae* Hansen bacilli in Virchow (foam) cells	Fite modification of acid-fast stain	2–8 μ by 0.2–0.5 μ
Tuberculosis	Scrofuloderma and anergic types	*Mycobacterium tuberculosis*	Acid-fast	1–4 μ by 0.3–0.6 μ
Rhinoscleroma	Granulomatous ulcer	*Klebsiella rhinoscleromatis* (Frisch bacilli in Mikulicz cells)	Giemsa, PAS, gram-negative	2–5 μ by 0.5 μ
Granuloma inguinale	Semidenuded granulomas	*Donovania granulomatis* (Donovan bodies)	H&E, Giemsa, gram-negative	1–2 μ
Histoplasmosis	Granulomatous ulcer	*Histoplasma capsulatum*	H&E, Giemsa, PAS	2–4 μ encapsulated
Histoplasmosis African	Lymphatic involvement	*Histoplasma capsulatum duboisii*	H&E, PAS	8–15 μ
Leishmaniasis, oriental	Early granuloma (oriental sore, Aleppo boil, etc.)	*Leishmania tropica* (Donovan bodies)	H&E, Giemsa	2–4 μ
Leishmaniasis, American	Granulomatous ulcer	*Leishmania braziliensis*	H&E, Giemsa	2–4 μ
Leishmaniasis, post–kala-azar	Macular, erythematous, nodular	*Leishmania donovani*	H&E, Giemsa	2–4 μ
Malakoplakia	Granuloma	Michaelis-Gutmann body	H&E, von Kossa iron stain	10–16 μ

and deep-reaching biopsy specimen that must include subcutaneous tissue or biopsy of a palpably affected nerve. In lepromatous leprosy, there usually remains a narrow, free, subepidermal grenz zone, while the infiltrate presses against the epidermis in tuberculoid cases.

In borderline lesions, all shadings from the lepromatous to the tuberculoid form are represented, and scattered lymphocytic infiltrates prevail in early indeterminate cases. It is, of course, often advisable to search for bacilli by scraping incised skin and doing acid-fast stain on the smears.

A technical note must be added: to stain for tubercle bacilli by any one of the modifications of the Ziehl–Neelsen method is easy. However, Hansen's bacilli (Fig. 20-6B) are much less acid-fast, and great care must be taken not to decolorize the bacilli in the acid-alcohol bath (Chap. 3). Otherwise, false negative results will be obtained. Many modifications and different stains have been developed because of this difficulty. In laboratories which do not have much experience in this field, one must insist that the technician use lepromatous tissue rather than tuberculous tissue as the positive control.

Reactional states seem to be related to shifts of tissue immunity, sometimes in the course of treatment, and involve fairly acute flare-ups of lesions. Exacerbation of the disease process is the so-called *lepra reaction* in lepromatous leprosy. Another manifestation is *erythema nodosum leprosum*, which leads to painful nodular lesions in which many bacilli are granular and degenerating. The histologic picture differs decisively from ordinary erythema nodosum.

The *Lucio phenomenon*, encountered mainly in Central America,[21] represents a necrotizing vasculitis with many bacilli in cases of diffuse leprosy in which the entire skin is affected. It leads to superficial ulcers. *Histoid leprosy* (Fig. 20-5A) has been described as showing tumorous collections of histiocytes separated by dense collagen fibers deep in the dermis. The histiocytes range from unmodified to foamy cells containing many bacilli. The clinical lesions are protuberant nodules, often constricted at the base. This variant, found mainly in Northern India,[22] is probably not a distinct entity but must be considered in differential diagnosis from neurofibromas.

ATYPICAL MYCOBACTERIA

An every increasing number of atypical acid-fast bacilli have been described. They may produce a great variety of inflammatory, purulent, or granulomatous tissue reactions, depending on their antigenicity and the individual immune reaction of the host. One must keep these microorganisms in mind whenever history or atypical clinical and histologic pictures are suggestive.[23,24] Infection by *Mycobacterium ulcerans* was mentioned in Chapter

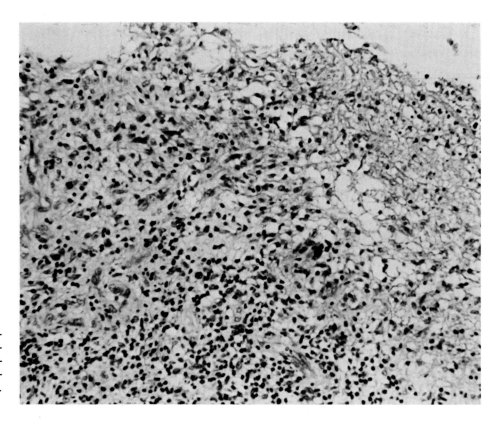

FIGURE 20–7.
Mycobacterium marinum infection (swimming-pool or fish-tank granuloma). Ulcerated surface and rather noncharacteristic granulomatous infiltrate H&E. X225.

17. In the United States, the most commonly encountered lesions (Fig. 20-7) are swimming-pool and fish-tank granulomas,[25] caused by *M. balnei* or *M. marinum*. Histologic examination for acid-fast organisms should be supplemented by culture on appropriate media and at different temperatures.

SYPHILIS

The third of the large granulomatous diseases, syphilis, offers its own intriguing peculiarities, in part due to the very different nature of the infectious agent. It is well recognized that the motile *Treponema pallidum* is widely distributed in the body long before any inflammatory tissue reaction sets in. This fact, along with the fairly lawful sequence of primary, secondary, and tertiary manifestations are eloquent proof of the preeminent role of tissue immunity in the histologic reaction.

The hallmark of the syphilitic tissue reaction is the plasma cell. Otherwise, there is little similarity between the massive inflammatory reaction of the chancre, the relatively mild vasculitis of the secondary exanthem, and the gummatous or tuberculoid granuloma of the tertiary stage. Plasma cells may be practically absent in some cases or may not be impressive in number. If, however, a skin lesion contains many plasma cells, the thought of syphilis

should enter the examiner's mind and should be dismissed only if a different diagnosis can be established with certainty. At the present time, when the incidence of syphilis is on the rise, and the level of suspicion of many clinicians is low, it is preferable to consider syphilis too often rather than to overlook it.

Primary

The primary lesion, the *chancre*, is not an ulcer but an induration. Correspondingly (Fig. 20-8), the epidermis is present and often is acanthotic. It usually is highly edematous, invaded by inflammatory cells, and covered by a parakeratotic crust. This explains the clinical features of oozing and apparent denudation, but true erosion or an ulcer occurs only secondary to trauma or nonspecific infection. The underlying dermis is densely infiltrated with a mixture of lymphocytes and plasma cells. Other cell types may be present. The endothelial and peripheral cells of blood vessels are swollen and increased, and the lesion may assume features of both vasculitis and of granulomatous inflammation. Silver stains will reveal treponemes in variable number, more commonly in the epidermis than in the dermis. Organisms, of course, will be absent if antibiotic therapy has been given before biopsy.

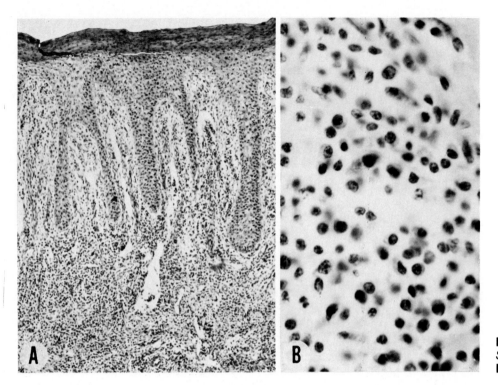

FIGURE 20–8.
Syphilitic chancre. **A.** *H&E. X70.*
B. *H&E. X600.*

Secondary

The *secondary exanthem* (Fig. 20-9), depending on the clinical severity of the lesion, may show nothing but perivascular round cell infiltrate, resembling that of a drug eruption, or may present evidence of plasmocytic vasculitis. Invasion of the epidermis by round cells is common, as are edema and acanthosis. A peculiar washed-out appearance

of the epidermis due to pale-staining nuclei and cytoplasm is fairly characteristic. Differential diagnosis[26,27] among a drug eruption, psoriasis, pityriasis lichenoides chronica, reticulosis, and a papule of secondary syphilis may be difficult. A sarcoid tissue reaction[28] and a perifollicular reaction mimicking lichen scrofulosorum may be observed. The presence of plasma cells speaks strongly for syphilis. Treponemes are difficult to demonstrate ex-

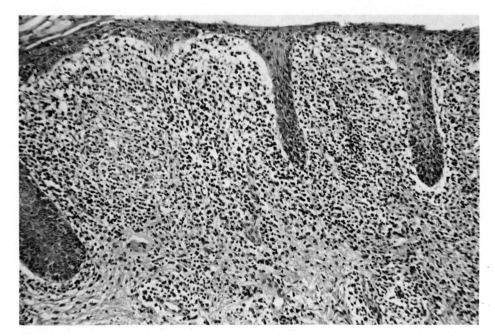

FIGURE 20–9.
Secondary syphilitic papule. This lesion presents heavier and more diffuse infiltrate than one would find in an early roseola. The large number of plasma cells speaks for syphilis. Note that the epidermis presents general hypoplasia combined with ridge hyperplasia and is invaded by round cells. H&E. X135.

cept in *condylomata lata*, in which histologic reaction in dermis and epidermis exceeds that of the glabrous skin papule.

Malignant ulcerative lesions develop in the secondary stage in malnourished, alcoholic individuals[29] and also in diabetics and sometimes in a seemingly healthy person.[30] Deep ulcers may develop, and in a personally observed case, the vomer in the nose became necrotic and was expelled. Histologic examination usually reveals severe vasculitis and otherwise the usual plasmocytic infiltrate, modified by tissue necrosis and ulceration (Chap. 17).

Tertiary

Later, secondary lesions may show pictures between that of early secondary and granulomatous *tertiary syphilis*. As far as the latter is concerned, the student must remember that the syphilitic *gumma* is only one, and not the most common, cutaneous manifestation. *Superficial nodular* and *noduloulcerative* lesions are encountered more frequently and are histologically characterized by a tuberculoid picture (Fig. 20-10) rather than by that of the gumma. Recognition of the latter under the microscope (Fig. 20-11) actually is not easy because the necrotic center usually has fallen out during biopsy or tissue preparation, and the sections present only part of the granulomatous wall (Chap. 17), which may resemble the granulomatous wall around a mucocele or a degenerated epithelial cyst. Again, presence of plasma cells and evidence of vasculitis speak for syphilis. One should also remember that other infections, especially sporotrichosis, produce gummatous lesions, and in differentiation from the latter, even the presence of plasma cells and vascular changes are not helpful (Chap. 21).

Tuberculoid tissue reaction is frequently encountered in tertiary cutaneous syphilis. Differentiation from tuberculosis is assisted by several factors. The center of gravity, high in the dermis in lupus vulgaris, is in the deep dermis even in clinically superficial-looking syphilids. The neat layering of the tuberculous granuloma usually is absent. Giant cells, epithelioid cells, and round cells are mixed, or may occur separated from each other. Plasma cells, common in syphilis, are rare in tuberculosis, except lupus tumidus. Areas of necrosis are much more frequent in syphilis. Perivascular arrangement of granulomatous nodes is of less significance. Epidermal hyperplasia, sometimes of pseudoepitheliomatous character, is often encountered in syphilis and is rare in tuberculosis.

Fibrosis as evidence of scar formation is almost

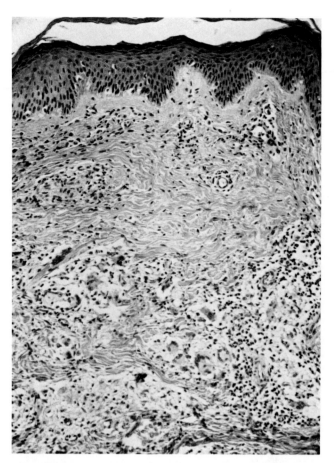

FIGURE 20–10.
Nodular tertiary syphilis. Disorganized tuberculoid infiltrate, predominantly in deep dermis. H&E. X135.

always found in tertiary syphilis and is more evident in O&G stains because of absence of elastic fibers in the granulomatous as well as in fibrotic parts. This stain is helpful in syphilis also because it makes plasma cells stand out much more plainly and assures one of the absence of eosinophils, which are more common in fungous granulomas.

Another cutaneous manifestation of late syphilis, the *juxta-articular node*, will be discussed together with other palisading granulomas in Chapter 22.

OTHER TREPONEMATOSES

Some unusual clinical forms of treponemal infection appear to be due to unfavorable socioeconomic circumstances rather than to different species of treponemes. These nonvenereal endemic types of syphilis are known as *bejel* and by other names.[31] *Yaws (frambesia)* and *pinta*, however, are caused by *T. pertenue* and *T. carateum*, respectively. Al-

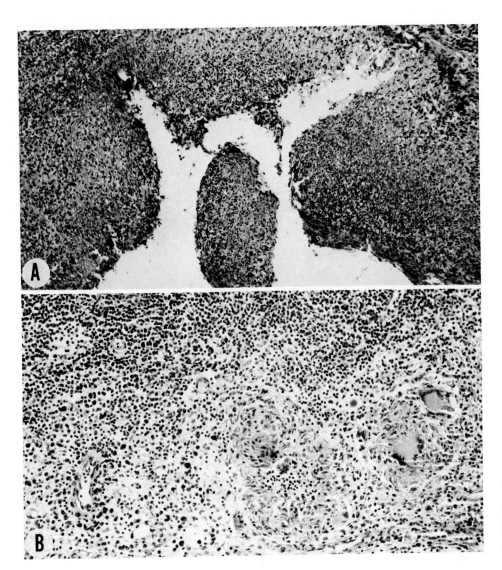

FIGURE 20–11.
Syphilitic gumma. **A.** *Necrotic wall with surrounding granulomatous infiltrate. H&E. X135.* **B.** *Tuberculoid and plasma cell reaction. H&E. X185.*

though morphologically indistinguishable from *T. pallidum*, these organisms are acknowledged as separate species, and tissue reactions present certain differences from syphilis. Lesions of yaws[32] exhibit more excessive epidermal and less definite vascular involvement. Pinta shows peculiar disturbances of melanization associated with basal cell liquefaction and macrophage pigmentation in the primary and secondary stages (Fig. 20-12) and epidermal atrophy in the late stages, thus having features of the poikilodermatous tissue reaction (Chap. 9). A mixed infiltrate with a high percentage of plasma cells is found in all these affections.[33]

SARCOIDOSIS AND SARCOID REACTIONS

The word *sarcoid* means sarcomalike and was used originally for a variety of lesions resembling malignant mesodermal disease. Boeck applied the term to lesions which we now consider the cutaneous

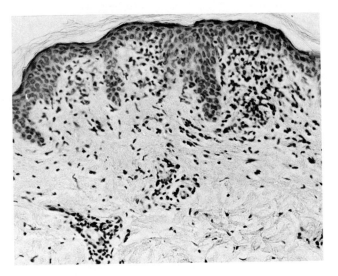

FIGURE 20–12.
Pinta. Secondary stage showing mild round cell and plasma cell infiltrate invading the epidermis and causing basal cell and melanocyte degeneration. Note resemblance to a lichenoid reaction. H&E. X250.

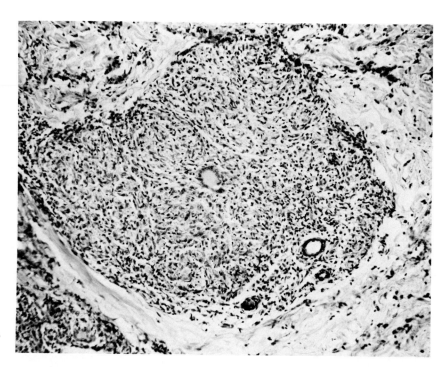

FIGURE 20–13.
Naked epithelioid cell tubercle representing sarcoid reaction. H&E. X135.

manifestations of the generalized disease called *sarcoidosis.*[34] Although there is no doubt that sarcoidosis is a distinct disease, it is true that the tissue reaction, which we see under the microscope and which seems to be highly specific, may actually be due to many different exciting agents ranging from microorganisms to nonliving organic and inorganic substances. The cautious pathologist, therefore, will usually make a diagnosis of *sarcoid reaction* or *noncaseating granuloma* unless a specific exciting agent is found in the tissue. It also seems that in this field,[35] the specific immunologic or quasi-immunologic status of the host is of utmost importance.

Sarcoid reaction (Fig. 20-13) is characterized by well-defined epithelioid cell nodes which may or may not have multinucleated giant cells of Langhans type. In the purest form, these tubercles lie naked in the tissue, but they may have thin shells of round cells, or round cells may be scattered between the epitheloid cells. Elastic fiber stain makes it obvious that these granulomatous masses have destroyed and replaced normal tissue.

Sarcoid reaction in the skin, if combined with clinical information, can be interpreted as sarcoidosis with reasonable confidence. However, one must be aware of pitfalls. The histologic pictures of lupus vulgaris and Boeck's sarcoid can merge. If one examines a series containing cases of both diseases, one can find almost any quantitative combination of epithelioid and round cells, and some cases may remain in doubt. Similarly, tuberculoid leprosy and sarcoidosis may look much alike. In-

volvement of nerves and hair muscles speaks for leprosy, involvement of the epidermis for sarcoidosis. Even syphilis may mimic sarcoidosis.[36]

In order to rule out *silica granuloma,* one should examine every case of sarcoid reaction under polarized light. However, we have two cases on file in which the first biopsy specimen showed double refractile bodies, but the patient had proven sarcoidosis. It was ascertained that old scars had been biopsied, in one case on the chin, in the other on the knee, and that embedded silica from dirt probably had acted as a localizing factor. Later specimens did not contain the foreign material. Similar experiences have been reported in tattoos.[37] It must be remembered that other granuloma-producing substances are not birefringent and are less easily ruled out. The most common ones in recent years are beryllium and zirconium.

Cutaneous Sarcoidosis

The clinical picture of sarcoidosis of the skin is so variable that it is taking the place of syphilis in mimicking almost any other skin disease. It ranges from lichenoid lesions to large nodules and may be erythrodermatous[38] and ichthyosiform.[39] It may rarely ulcerate. Hypopigmented lesions in dark skin[40] can be sources of error.

Boeck's sarcoid shows epithelioid cell nodules or sausage-shaped masses mainly in the upper dermis. They usually do not approach the epidermis as massively as the tubercles of lupus vulgaris and, on

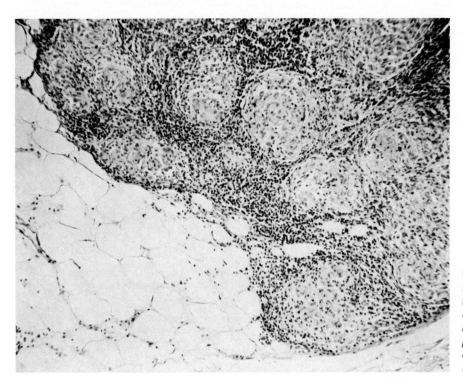

FIGURE 20–14.
Darier–Roussy sarcoid. Note the difference between this specific granulomatous reaction in the subcutaneous tissue and the nonspecific proliferating atrophy of fat tissue shown in Figures 16-1 and 16-2. H&E. X135.

the other hand, extend often somewhat deeper. While lymphocytic shells often are present around the superficial nodules, the deeper ones tend to be naked epithelioid cell tubercles. Although in other organs, sarcoidosis is the prototype of noncaseating granuloma formation, in the skin, microscopic foci of central necrosis actually favor a diagnosis of sarcoidosis over lupus vulgaris.

In *Darier–Roussy's sarcoid* (Fig. 20-14), similar granulomas are found deep in the skin and often involve the subcutaneous tissue. *Spiegler–Fendt sarcoid* does not belong here and will be mentioned under lymphomas. Variants of sarcoid, rarely seen in the United States, are *lupus pernio* and *angiolupoid*, which combine epithelioid cell response with increased vascularity. One should remember that lupus erythematosus profundus (Chap. 16) may produce lipogranulomatous reactions similating Darier–Roussy sarcoid.

The *Kveim test*, the intradermal injection of sterilized sarcoid tissue, should reproduce the histologic sarcoid reaction faithfully (Fig. 20-15) in order to be considered positive. Granulomas formed in the subcutis are not convincing.

Sarcoid Foreign-Body Granulomas

Metallic compounds containing silicon, beryllium, or zirconium are well known to produce sarcoid reaction. It seems likely that specific sensitization is

necessary for this to happen, although truly allergic reaction has been ruled out for silica granuloma.[35] Silicates *(silica)*, and especially talc crystals, sometimes are visible as colorless spicules in giant cells. However, polarized light (Fig. 20-16B) is much more apt to show them, and this simple type of examination (Chap. 3), which requires only two pieces of Polaroid film, should be used in every case of sarcoid reaction, although more elaborate methods are available.[41] Beryllium and zirconium compounds do not polarize light and are not demonstrable in histologic sections. *Beryllium* granulomas (Fig. 20-17) are characterized by massive infiltrates, usually showing central caseation necrosis, and fibrosis. *Zirconium* is more apt to cause tiny superficial tubercles without necrosis,[42] and allergic sensitization is involved in their formation.[43]

If *paraffin* is deposited in or under the skin, it is apt to be broken up into even tinier particles which become embedded in diffuse masses of epithelioid and giant cells. In paraffin-embedded and paraffin-processed sections, only the clefts left by the foreign material remain, but the picture is so characteristic that the diagnosis (paraffinoma) usually can be suspected. Other forms of lipogranulomatous reaction caused by foreign substances were mentioned in Chapter 16. The peculiar sclerosis following parenteral administration of *pentazocine* will be considered in Chapter 25. Hard indurations characterized by fibrosis and histiocytic granulomatous reaction also have been described after

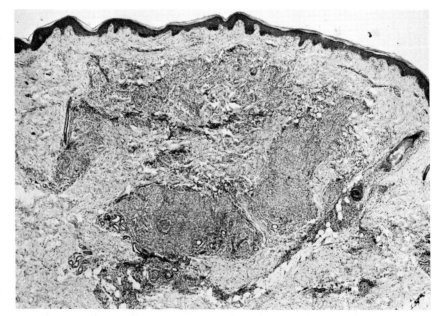

FIGURE 20–15.
Positive Kveim test. The picture illustrates specific sarcoid reaction to Kveim antigen properly placed in the dermis. If the antigen is deposited too deep (in subcutaneous tissue), proliferating atrophy of fat tissue may cast doubt on histologic interpretation. H&E. X75.

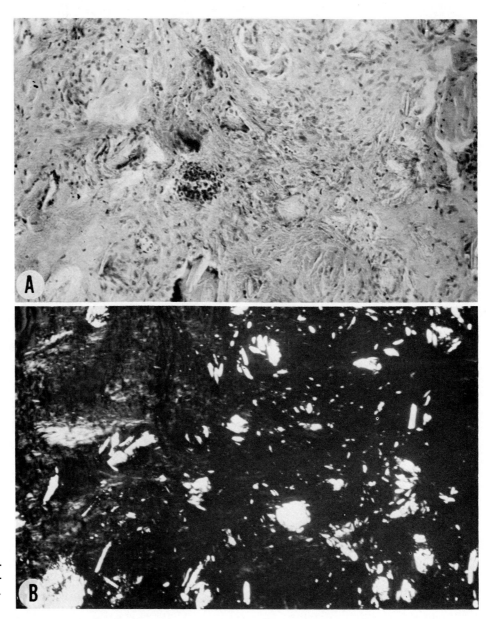

FIGURE 20–16.
*Silica granuloma. **A.** Photographed in bright light. **B.** Photographed in polarized lignt. H&E. X135.*

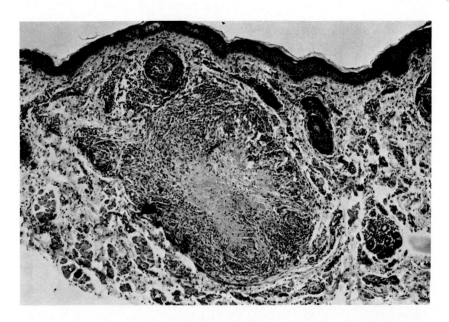

FIGURE 20–17.
Beryllium granuloma. A relatively small nodule was chosen to show striking similarity to lupus miliaris disseminatus faciei (Fig. 20-4) owing to central caseation necrosis of a sarcoidal infiltrate. H&E. X60.

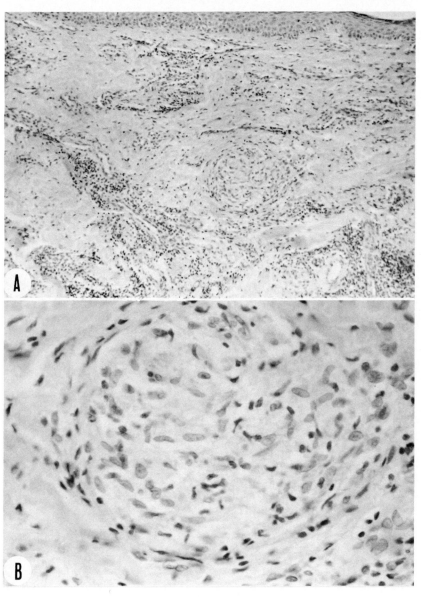

FIGURE 20–18.
*Cheilitis granulomatosa. Fibrosis and infiltrate of epithelioid nodes and small round cells. H&E. **A.** X125. **B.** X400.*

the injection of *polyvinyl pyrrolidone*,[44] used as an excipient for medications of impure *silicones*[45] for cosmetic purposes, and after accidental inoculation of acrylic and nylon fibers.[46]

Sarcoid Reactions of Unknown Etiology

Sarcoidosis being a disease of undetermined cause, it might seem incongruous to separate from it other noncaseating granulomas of unknown etiology. It is, in fact, one of the most frustrating tasks of the dermatopathologist to arrive at such a distinction, and it must be made in cooperation with the clinician and radiologist. There are occasional lesions in the skin, often histologically not quite typical of the classic sarcoid granuloma but definitely in the mononuclear group and not exhibiting caseation, gummatous necrosis, or even necrobiosis, in which no evidence of systemic sarcoidosis or other systemic disease or local infection can be demonstrated, and a foreign-body granuloma can be ruled out with reasonable certainty. Some of these cases remain undiagnosable and irretrievably lost in the files. Occasionally, however, a clinicohistologic pattern develops through prolonged observation of a number of patients and eventually leads to rubrication under a new name.

One of these patterns was described by Miescher as *granulomatosis disciformis*, and similar lesions have been identified as "Miescher's granuloma of the face." Their discussion will be deferred to Chapter 22 because of probable relation to necrobiosis lipoidica.

Another pattern is the *Melkersson–Rosenthal syndrome*, presenting a combination of transitory facial paralysis and lingua plicata (scrotal tongue) with fluctuating swelling of the upper lip or, sometimes, other parts of the face.[47] Histologically, the indurated tissues of the lip exhibit sarcoid granulomas (Fig. 20-18), associated with smaller or larger numbers of lymphocytes and plasma cells (*Miescher's cheilitis granulomatosa*). The cause is unknown.

MALAKOPLAKIA

The occurrence of malakoplakia (derived from the Greek term for "soft") in the skin has been reported recently.[48,49] Ordinarily, it is a benign inflammation of the urinary tract presenting distinct inclusion bodies in large histiocytes. These *Michaelis–Gutman bodies* have been recognized as bacterial in origin and are encrusted with calcium

and iron (Chap. 27). Most commonly, *Escherichia coli* is associated with the lesions, but *Staphylococcus aureus* and *Pseudomonas* have been found, and in two cases, *Leishmania tropica* seemed to be involved.[50] The lesions consist of accumulations of large histiocytes mixed with some other inflammatory cells.

HISTOPLASMOSIS

The cutaneous reaction to *Histoplasma capsulatum* is characterized by large numbers of histiocytes, often in epithelioid arrangement but usually larger than ordinary epithelioid cells because they contain the fungus, which is fairly well demonstrated by Giemsa stain but may require methenamine silver for identification.[51] PAS stains the fungal cell wall but not the capsule (Table 20-3).

It takes a high level of suspicion to think of histoplasmosis and to institute a search for the inconspicuous organism. Although mucocutaneous ulcers are the most common manifestation in persons who may be otherwise healthy or may have pulmonary lesions, erythrodermatic forms[52] (Chap. 44) and skin ulcerations resembling carcinomas[53] may be seen, and other unusual manifestations may occur in immunosuppressed patients.

African histoplasmosis is caused by a much more conspicuous fungus, *Histoplasma duboisii*.[54]

CUTANEOUS LEISHMANIASIS

There are three species of protozoan leishmaniae causing cutaneous disease. *Leishmania tropica* causes self-limited nodular lesions, known as *Oriental sores* or by other local names, and in some cases late chronic granulomas resembling lupus vulgaris. It is endemic in the Eastern Mediterranean and Western Asiatic countries. *Leishmania donovani*, the cause of kala-azar in Eastern Asia, may produce post–kala-azar granulomas in the skin, and *Leishmania braziliensis* is responsible for slowly extending chronic ulcerations in South and Central America.

The primary lesion of Oriental leishmaniasis (Fig. 20-19A) usually shows a combination of histiocytic nodules and lymphocytes closely associated with acanthotic epidermis.[55] The organisms (Fig. 20-19B) are easily demonstrated by Giemsa stain in the florid lesion (Table 20-3). The much rarer late recurrences have a histologic picture so similar to lupus vulgaris that differential diagnosis is impossible. In accordance with Lewandowsky's

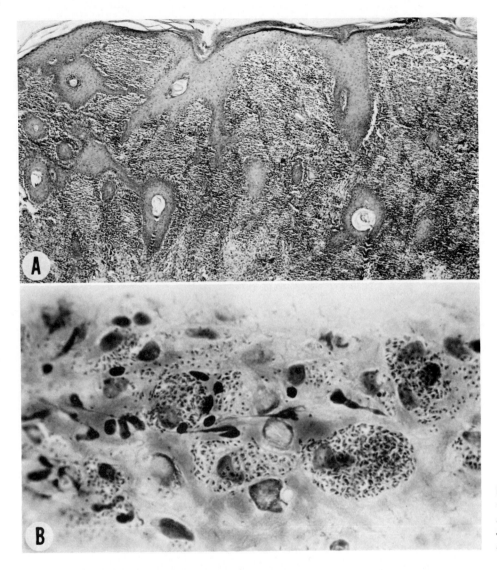

FIGURE 20–19.
Cutaneous leishmaniasis. **A.**
H&E. X75. **B.** *Giemsa-stained smear, to show tissue form of Leishmania tropica. X1100.*

rule, no or a few leishmaniae are visible in the tuberculoid tissue.[56] The tissue reactions in *post–kala-azar dermal leishmaniasis*[57,58] and *American leishmaniasis*[59] vary in many histologic details and in the number of demonstrable organisms, in reciprocal relation to the formation of tuberculoid granulomas. The three leishmaniae are morphologically indistinguishable but can be cultured and differentiated immunologically.

The American form, which is now seen occasionally in the United States in military personnel[60] and travelers, can also occur in a disseminated anergic form,[61] in which the accumulation of numerous histiocytes filled with leishmania organisms may simulate lepromatous leprosy at low-power examination. Exanthematic spread of lichenoid or nodular lesions may also occur by hematogenous dissemination,[62] and these leishmanids may or may not contain demonstrable organisms.

TULAREMIA AND RHINOSCLEROMA

Two other bacterial diseases may occasionally involve the skin with granulomatous ulcers, tularemia and rhinoscleroma. *Tularemia*, caused by *Francisella tularensis*, may have an ulcerative primary lesion[63] exhibiting a central necrotic zone, an intermediate tuberculoid zone, and an outer zone containing lymphocytes, histiocytes, and plasma cells. Blood vessels of the outer zone show endothelial proliferation and infiltration of the wall by inflammatory cells. Extravasated erythrocytes often are seen in all zones. Later stages may exhibit a sarcoid reaction. Bacilli are not recognizable in tissue sections but may be identified by immunofluorescence.[64] Histologic differentiation from a syphilitic or sporotrichotic gumma may be difficult.

The tissue reaction of *rhinoscleroma*[65] is characterized by the great number of plasma cells in a granulomatous mononuclear infiltrate and by two specific features: the *Mikulicz cell*, which is a very large (up to 100 μ), roundish cell containing numerous Frisch bacilli *(Klebsiella rhinoscleromatis)*, and the *Russel bodies* (Fig. 5-15), which are hyaline bodies formed in plasma cells. The latter may also occur in other diseases.

REFERENCES

1. Lewandowsky F: Die Tuberkulose der Haut. Berlin, Springer-Verlag, 1916
2. Mahlberg FA, Rodermund OE, Müller RW: Ein Fall von Zirkumzisionstuberkulose. Hautarzt 28:424, 1977
3. Goette DK, Jacobson KW, Doty RD: Primary inoculation tuberculosis of the skin. Prosector's paronychia. Arch Dermatol 114:567, 1978
4. Mihan R, Ayres S Jr: Lupus vulgaris. Arch Dermatol 107:620, 1973
5. Hart V, Weedon D: Lupus vulgaris and *Mycobacterium bovis*. Aust J Dermatol 18:86, 1977
6. Lever WF, Schaumburg-Lever G: Histopathology of the Skin, 5th ed. Philadelphia, Lippincott, 1975, p 382
7. Iden DL, Rogers RS III, Schroeter AL: Papulonecrotic tuberculid secondary to *Mycobacterium bovis*. Arch Dermatol 114:564, 1978
8. Wong KC: Erythema induratum: follow-up study of 46 patients. Dermatol Dig 10:51, 1971
9. Morrison JGL, Fourie FD: The papulonecrotic tuberculide: from Arthus reaction to lupus vulgaris. Br J Dermatol 91:263, 1974
10. Nagy E, Mézsáros C, Somyói I: Nach BCG-Vaccination aufgetretener Lichen scrofulosorum. Z Hautkr 47:859, 1972
11. Smith NP, Ryan TJ, Sanderson KV, Sarkany I: Lichen scrofulosorum. A report of four cases. Br J Dermatol 94:319, 1976
12. Hudson PM: Tuberculide (lichen scrofolusorum) secondary to osseous tuberculosis. Clin Exp Dermatol 1:391, 1976
13. Bolgert M: Les hypodermites tuberculeuses ne sont pas des affections historiques. Arch Belg Dermatol 26:179, 1970
14. Simon N: Ist der Lupus miliaris disseminatus tuberkulöser Ätiologie? Hautarzt 26:625, 1975
15. Tilden IL: Lepromatous leprosy: a reticulo-endothelial disease. Am J Clin Pathol 15:165, 1945
16. Haensch R, Schmalbruch H: Zur Morphologie der Leprazelle. Arch Dermatol Forsch 241:179, 1971
17. Skinsnes OK, Matsuo E, Chang PHC, Anderson B: In vitro cultivation of leprosy bacilli on hyaluronic acid based medium. I. Preliminary report. Int J Lepr 43:193, 1975
18. Shephard CC: The experimental disease that follows the injection of human leprosy bacilli into foot pads of mice. J Exp Med 112:445, 1960
19. Storrs EE, Walsh GP, Burchfield HP, Binford CH: Leprosy in the armadillo: new model for biomedical research. Science 183:851, 1974.
20. Browne SG: Mycobacterial diseases: leprosy. In Fitzpatrick TB, et al. (eds): Dermatology in General Medicine. New York, McGraw-Hill, 1979
21. Rea TH, Levan NE: Lucio's phenomenon and diffuse non-nodular lepromatous leprosy. Arch Dermatol 114:1023, 1978
22. Kroll JJ, Shapiro L: The histoid variety of lepromatous leprosy. Int J Dermatol 12:74, 1973
23. Feldman RA, Hershfield E: Mycobacterial skin infection by unidentified species: report of 29 patients. Ann Intern Med 80:445, 1974
24. Even-Paz Z, Haas H, Sacks T, Rosenmann E: *Mycobacterium marinum* skin infections mimicking cutaneous leishmaniasis. Br J Dermatol 94:435, 1976
25. Zeligman I: *Mycobacterium marinum* granuloma. Arch Dermatol 106:26, 1972
26. Prakit J, Ackerman AB: Histologic patterns of secondary syphilis. Arch Dermatol 107:373, 1973
27. Abell E, Marks R, Wilson-Jones E: Secondary syphilis: a clinico-pathological review. Br J Dermatol 93:53, 1975
28. Izumi AK and Navin JJ: Sarcoidal secondary syphilis. Cutis 14:833, 1974
29. Fisher DA, Chang LW, Tuffanelli DL: Lues maligna. Presentation of a case and a review of the literature. Arch Dermatol 99:70, 1979
30. Mirande LM, Landolfi JM, Pedemonte LH, et al.: Lúes ulcerative precoz o maligna. Considereiziones a propósito de dos casos. Análisis bibliográfico. Med Cutan Iber Lat Am 5:171, 1977
31. Wajdi Kanan M, Kaudil E: Bejel or non-venereal endemic syphilis. Br J Dermatol 84:461, 1971
32. Hopkins DR: Yaws in the Americas 1950–1975. J Infect Dis 136:548, 1977
33. Hasselmann CM: Comparative studies on the histopathology of syphilis, yaws, and pinta. Br J Vener Dis 33:5, 1957
34. Siltzbach LE (ed): Seventh International Conference on Sarcoidosis and Other Granulomatous Diseases. Ann NY Acad Sci 278:1, 1976
35. Epstein WL: Granulomatous hypersensitivity. Prog Allergy 11:36, 1967
36. Kahn LB, Gordon W: Sarcoid-like granulomas in secondary syphilis: Clinical and histopathologic study of 5 cases. Arch Pathol 92:334, 1971
37. Erickson JG, Petko E: Sarcoidal reactions in multiple tattoos with systemic sarcoidosis. Cutis 11:163, 1973
38. Morrison JGL: Sarcoidosis in a child, presenting as an erythroderma with keratotic spines and palmar pits. Br J Dermatol 95:93, 1976
39. Karch JC, Goody HE, Luscombe HA: Ichthyosiform sarcoidosis. Arch Dermatol 114:100, 1978
40. Clayton R, Breathnach A, Martin B, Feiwel M: Hypopigmented sarcoidosis in the Negro. Br J Dermatol 96:119, 1977
41. Terzakis JA, Shustak SR, Stock EG: Talc granuloma identified by x-ray microanalysis. JAMA 239:2371, 1978
42. Kleinhaus D, Knoth W: Axilläre Granulome (Zirkonium?). Dermatologica 152:161, 1976
43. Shelley WB, Hurley HJ: The allergic origin of zirconium deodorant granulomas. Br J Dermatol 70:75, 1958
44. Thivolet J, Leung TK, Duverne J, et al.: Ultrastructural morphology and histochemistry (acid phosphatase) of cutaneous infiltration by polyvinyl-pyrrolidone. Br J Dermatol 83:661, 1970
45. Delage C, Shane JJ, Johnson FB: Mammary silicone granuloma. Arch Dermatol 108:104, 1973

46. Cortez Pimentel J: Sarcoid granulomas of the skin produced by acrylic and nylon fibers. Br J Dermatol 96:673, 1977
47. Laymon CW: Cheilitis granulomatosa and Melkerssohn-Rosenthal syndrome. Arch Dermatol 83:112, 1963
48. Moore WM III, Stokes TL, Cabanas VY: Malakoplakia of the skin. Am J Clin Pathol 60:218, 1973
49. Arul KJ, Emmerson RW: Malakoplakia of the skin. Clin Exp Dermatol 2:131, 1977
50. Sandbank M: Michaelis-Guttmann bodies in macrophages of cutaneous leishmaniasis. J Cutan Pathol 3:263, 1976
51. Schwarz J: Histoplasmosis. In Baker RD (ed): The Pathologic Anatomy of Mycoses. Handbuch der speziellen pathologischen Anatomie und Histologie, vol 3, pt 5. Berlin, New York, Springer-Verlag, 1971
52. Cramer HJ: Erythrodermatische Hauthistoplasmose. Deramtologica 146:249, 1973
53. Talvalkar GV: Histoplasmosis simulating carcinoma: a report of three cases. Indian J Cancer 9:149, 1972
54. Nethercott JR, Schachter K, Givan KF, Ryder DE: Histoplasmosis due to *Histoplasma capsulatum var duboisii* in a Canadian immigrant. Arch Dermatol 114:595, 1978
55. Rau RC, Dubin HV, Taylor WB: *Leishmania topica* infections in travellers. Arch Dermatol 112:197, 1976
56. Nicobis GD, Tosca AD, Stratigos JD, Capetanakis JA: A clinical and histological study of cutaneous leishmaniasis. Acta Derm Venereol (Stockh) 58:521, 1978
57. Munro DD: Post–kala-azar dermal leishmaniasis. Br J Dermatol 87:374, 1972
58. Girgla HS, Marsden RA, Singh GM, Ryan TJ: Post–kala-azar dermal leishmaniasis. Br J Dermatol 97:307, 1977
59. Kerdel-Vegas F: Leishmaniasis tegumentaris americana. Caracas, Biblioteka de la Academia de Ciencias Fiscas, Matèmaticas y Naturales de Venezuela, 1972
60. Kern F, Pedersen JK: Leishmaniasis in the United States. A report of ten cases in military personnel. JAMA 226:872, 1973
61. Convit J, Kerdel-Vegas F, Gordon B: Disseminated anergic American leishmaniasis. Br J Dermatol 74:132, 1962
62. Silva JR, Netto MP de O: Leishmanids. Int J Dermatol 12:104, 1973
63. Schuermann H, Reich H: Zur Klinik und Histologie des cutan lokalisierten tularämischen Primäraffekts. Arch Dermat Syph 190:579, 1950
64. White JD, McGavran MH: Identification of *Pasteurella tularensis* by immunofluorescence. JAMA 194:2940, 1965
65. Kerdel-Vegas F, Convit J, Gordon B, Goihman M: Rhinoscleroma. Springfield, Ill., Thomas, 1963

21

Mixed Cell Granulomas

With the exception of histoplasmosis, deep mycotic infections of the skin contain neutrophilic and eosinophilic leukocytes in addition to histiocytes and round cells. Thus, a mixture of all these cells in a granuloma strongly points to fungous infection. There are exceptions, however: halogen eruptions—especially bromoderma—arthropod bites, lesions caused by worms and larvae, and some foreign-body granulomas also are in this group. Ulcerated lesions of tuberculosis, leprosy, or syphilis will show neutrophils, but these are usually restricted to the surface layers. Of other chronic infections, granuloma inguinale and lymphogranuloma venereum belong to the mixed cell granulomas.

At this point, we must discuss the diagnostic value of eosinophilic cells in a granuloma. Their number may be large, and they may occur diffusely scattered, in groups, or in clumps. While they stand out much more strikingly in O&G preparations, they are apt to attract the pathologist's attention even in H&E sections. At one time, their diagnostic value was overrated to the point of creating the diagnostic term "eosinophilic granuloma." It became clear, however,[1] that eosinophils may occur in large numbers in such diverse entities as reactions to insect bite, foreign-body granulomas, and Hodgkin's disease. A diagnosis of eosinophilic granuloma is worse than meaningless because it misleads the clinician into believing that he is dealing with a specific disease. Historically, the term, if used at all, should be restricted to *eosinophilic*

granuloma of bone and should always be used with this specification. Related lesions in the skin are part of the spectrum of *histiocytosis X* (Langerhans cell granuloma) and will be discussed in Chapter 24. *Granuloma faciale*, once included in the pseudogroup of eosinophilic granulomas, was discussed in Chapter 15. As a general guiding principle, it is best to accept this rule: If a granulomatous lesion contains a striking number of eosinophils, discount them, and try to ascertain what the diagnosis would be in their absence. Only after this determination has been made should one take into account the knowledge that some diseases are more apt to have eosinophils in the infiltrate than others. Hodgkin's disease is perhaps the only one in which a complete lack of eosinophils raises grave doubt in the diagnosis (Chap. 44).

EOSINOPHILIC CELLULITIS

An extraordinary syndrome was described by Wells and elaborated by him[2] and by Spiegel and Winkelmann[3] as *eosinophilic cellulitis. Wells' syndrome* is the other exception where accumulation of eosinophils in the skin and phagocytosis of eosinophilic granules seem to be the starting point of the dermatosis.

Patients with eosinophilic cellulitis develop acute inflammation of the skin that becomes granulomatous and subsides. Histologic examination shows many degenerating eosinophils which collect around areas of necrotic collagen *(flame figures)* and are taken up by palisading histiocytes producing a picture similar to a palisading granuloma (Chap. 22). Somewhat similar pictures were described by Wells[2] in other diseases, such as bullous pemphigoid and various eruptions in the eczematous group, again confirming the rule that presence of many eosinophils in a skin lesion is a symptom and not the disease itself.

FUNGAL GRANULOMAS

In most instances, positive diagnosis of a fungal granuloma can be made by finding the characteristic organism in the section. The fungi of North American and South American *blastomycosis*, *coccidioidomycosis*, *chromomycosis*, and *actinomycosis* with its congeners usually can be identified in H&E sections and can be seen better in O&G sections. *Cryptococcus* and *Sporotrichum*, on

the other hand, are almost never recognized with these stains. Here, PAS stain after digestion of the tissue sections with amylase (diastase) has made it possible to demonstrate the organisms in many cases.

If organisms are not demonstrable, diagnosis becomes much less secure. Although there are characteristic tissue reactions to each one of these fungi, there is enough variation and overlap to be confusing. An encyclopedic discussion of all human fungous diseases was published under the editorship of Baker.[4] The following are short descriptions of the more typical features.

Coccidioidomycosis

Primary cutaneous infection is rare except in laboratory personnel. Dissemination into the skin may occur from the bloodstream.[5] Skin sections show massive granulomatous reaction, almost of foreign-body character (Fig. 21-1), with many giant cells

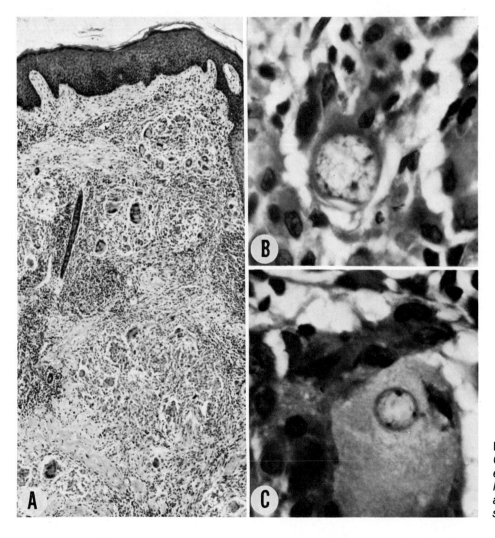

FIGURE 21–1.
Coccidioidomycosis. **A.** *Foreign-body type granuloma. H&E. X60.* **B** *and* **C.** *Larger and smaller cysts with endosporulation. H&E. X800.*

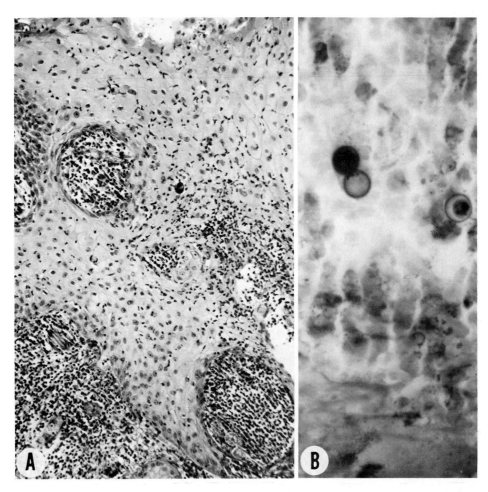

FIGURE 21–2.
North American blastomycosis. **A.** *Pseudoepitheliomatous hyperplasia with intraepidermal abscesses and granulomatous infiltrate. H&E. X135.* **B.** *Blastomyces dermatitidis. PAS-light green. X800.*

containing the characteristic cysts of *Coccidioides immitis,* measuring from 10 to 80 μ. Some epidermal hyperplasia often is present but rarely as pronounced as in blastomycosis.

North American Blastomycosis

The combination of a mixed granulomatous infiltrate with pseudoepitheliomatous hyperplasia is the outstanding histologic feature (Fig. 21-2). Intraepithelial abscesses and multinucleated giant cells complete the picture. The characteristic spores (Fig. 21-2B) are generally found in giant cells but may be free in the tissue, especially in intraepidermal abscesses (Fig. 5-12D). Search for them is assisted in H&E sections by closing the iris diaphragm of the microscope in order to bring out the refractile thick membrane. The membrane usually stains greenish blue in O&G sections and is dark magenta in PAS stain. *Blastomyces dermatitidis* measures from 8 to 15 μ in diameter. The most important differential diagnosis is bromoderma (see below), and this should be suspected if no multinucleated giant cells are present and careful search

reveals no fungi. Pyodermatous lesions also may mimic the pseudoepitheliomatous proliferation of blastomycosis[6] (Chap. 34).

South American Blastomycosis

The disease due to *Paracoccidioides braziliensis*[7] has histologic features somewhat similar to other fungous granulomas. Organisms are easily found, and measure 10 to 60 μ with one or multiple buds. A remarkable form of South American blastomycosis caused by a related fungus is Jorge Lobo's *keloidal type.*[8] The striking histologic picture is illustrated in Figure 21-3. The fungus *(Loboa loboi)* is difficult to culture. It probably persists in macrophages because of defective cellular immunity.

Chromomycosis (Chromoblastomycosis)

A mixed granulomatous infiltrate with verrucous epidermal hyperplasia is characteristic of this type of lesion.[9] The naturally brown, thick-walled organisms (Fig. 21-4) which belong to the genera *Phi-*

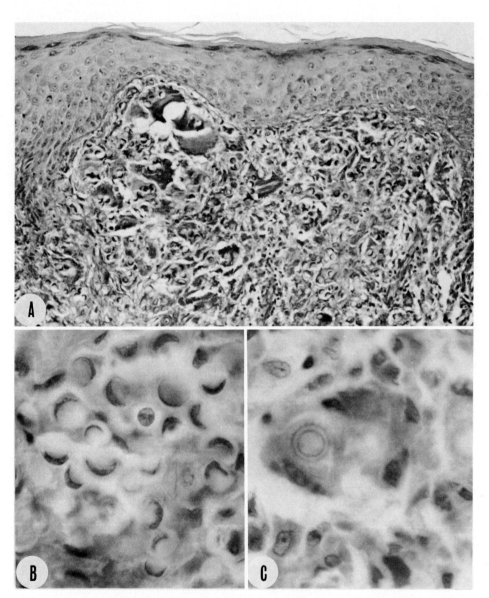

FIGURE 21–3.
Lobo's type of South American blastomycosis. Numerous organisms are present in large multinucleated giant cells. PAS-hematoxylin. A. X250. B. and C. X800.

lophora, Cladosporium, and *Fonsecaea* are usually sparse and show up better in a lightly stained section than in one overstained with eosin. The cell wall does not change color in either H&E or O&G sections but is tinged by PAS. According to Zaias and Rebell,[10] diagnosis is simplified by identifying in the clinical lesion black dots, which consist of inflammatory products and hemorrhage undergoing transepidermal elimination,[11] and scraping them off and softening them in potassium hydroxide. Round "Medlar bodies" as well as hyphal elements can be identified by this method.

Actinomycosis, Nocardiosis, Botryomycosis

Granulomatous lesions with sinuses discharging pus that contains macroscopically visible granules can be caused by true fungi or by actinomycetes. The former are known as *maduromycosis,* while the term *mycetoma* may be applied to all.[12] Similar lesions caused by bacteria are known as *botryomycosis.* Histologic distinction among the different types[13] is difficult, and one has to realize that, occasionally, *Trichophyton* and *Microsporum* species can cause mycetoma.[14] As a group they have characteristic features. The colonies of organisms are already visible under the scanning lens (Fig. 21-5A). The granules (Fig. 21-5B) usually are present within large accumulations of polymorphonuclear leukocytes (abscesses), surrounded by granulomatous and fibrotic reaction without any distinguishing characteristics. All common stains are suitable for their demonstration. The granules are gram-positive; only occasionally do they have to be differentiated from similar bacterial colonies found in *human bo-*

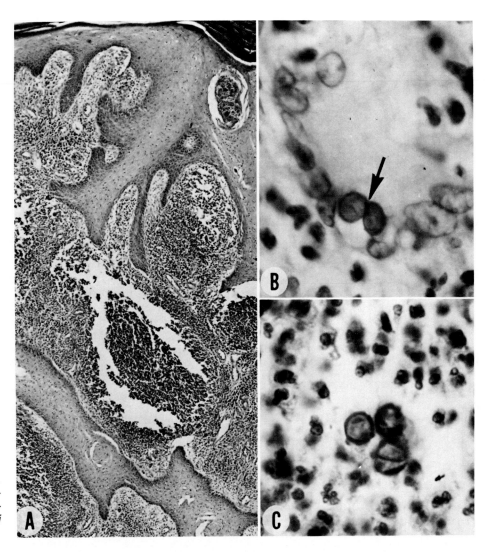

FIGURE 21–4.
Chromomycosis. **A.** *H&E. X135.* **B.** *Sclerotic cells (arrow) between nuclei of a multinucleated giant cell.* **C.** *Fungi free in tissue. H&E. X1100.*

tryomycosis. The latter, which usually are staphylococcal colonies (Fig. 21-6), do not exhibit filamentous and club-shaped structures, but cultural identification is necessary in every case.[15]

Cryptococcosis

Cryptococcus neoformans, the organism of *European blastomycosis* resembles a lymphocyte so much in sections and smears that it is difficult to identify by routine stains. One may begin to suspect *Cryptococcus* if one sees budding yeast forms. India ink preparations of smears or PAS stain are required for morphologic identification, but only a culture can really identify the fungus. The granulomatous infiltrate (Fig. 21-7) resembles that of the other deep mycoses. Primary cutaneous infection is rare,[16] but secondary skin lesions are becoming more common in immunosuppressed patients.[17]

Sporotrichosis

Sporotrichosis (Fig. 21-8) should be suspected when one sees a mixed granuloma, including multinucleated giant cells, and cannot find microorganisms even on thorough search. However, the sporotrichotic lesion has additional characteristics to support the suspicion. Just as the clinical lesion represents a gumma, so one finds necrotic liquefied tissue mixed with polymorphonuclear cells in the center, surrounded by a granulomatous wall. The latter consists of a tuberculoid inner zone with epithelioid nodules, multinucleated giant cells, and round cells and an outer syphiloid zone, in which plasma cells and small round cells prevail. Eosinophils are often scattered in considerable numbers or may form small clumps. It is only since we use PAS stain after thorough amylase digestion that we have been able to identify the fungus in the great majority of cases. The presence of glycogen in leu-

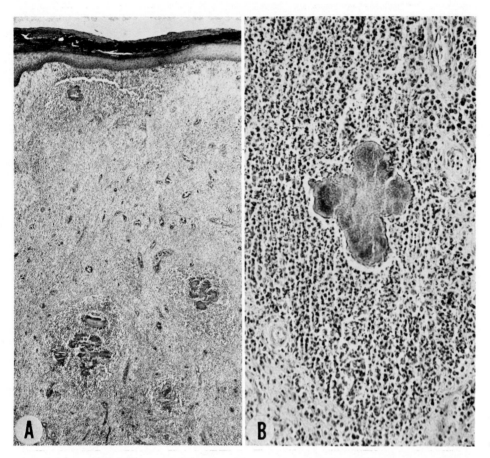

FIGURE 21–5.
Maduromycosis. **A.** *H&E. X30.* **B.** *Granule in abscess. H&E. X225.*

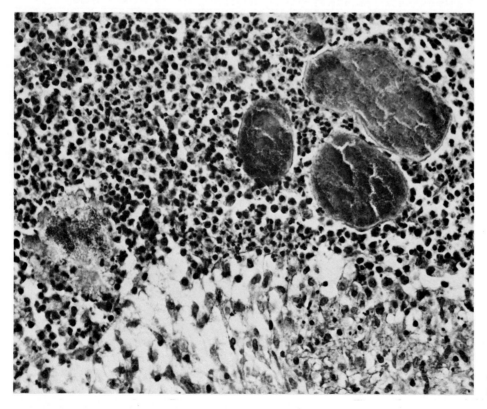

FIGURE 21–6.
Human botryomycosis. The "granules" are colonies of staphyloccocci embedded in hyaline material. H&E. X370.

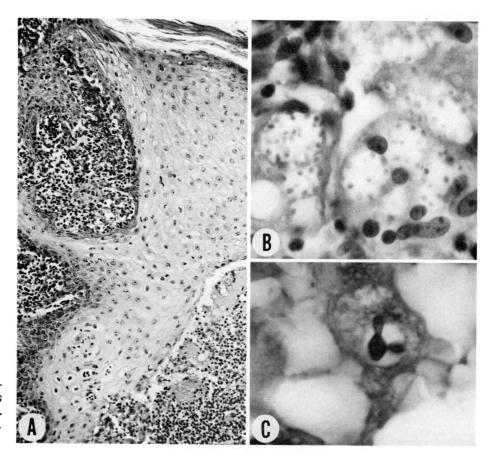

FIGURE 21–7.
*Cryptococcosis. **A.** Van Gieson. X135. **B.** Tiny organisms in tissue. Van Gieson. X800. **C.** Budding of yeastlike organism. PAS-picric acid. X2400.*

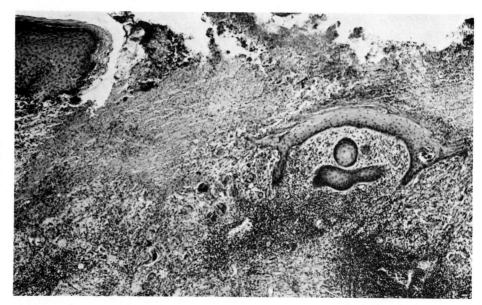

FIGURE 21–8.
Sporotrichosis. Acanthotic edge of epidermis in upper left corner. Necrotic tissue forms the floor of an ulcer. The granulomatous infiltrate has tuberculoid and syphiloid features. Proliferating epithelium in the tissue is probably derived from hair follicles or sweat glands. Observe similarity of tissue reaction to a syphilitic gumma (Fig. 20-11). H&E. X60.

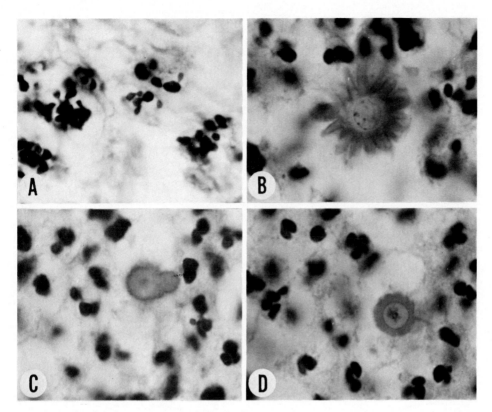

FIGURE 21–9.
Sporotrichum schenckii. **A.** *Oval and round budding spores in human tissue. PAS-light-green after amylase digestion. X1100.* **B, C,** *and* **D.** *Asteroid spores in small abscesses, a rare observation in a North American case. H&E. X1350. (From Pinkus and Grekin. Arch Dermatol 97:394, 1950.)*

kocytes and debris obscures it. In sections from which glycogen has been removed, one often finds surprising numbers of small oval spores, not infrequently budding (Fig. 21-9A). Elongated, cigar-shaped bodies may also be seen.

Peculiar large *asteroid spores* are commonly seen in tropical countries, especially in the southern hemisphere, but only in exceptional cases in the United States. Those observed by us[18] (Fig. 21-9B, C, and D) were lying free in microabscesses surrounded by a histiocytic wall. The wall of the spore takes the PAS stain, while the rays do not, in support of the view that the rays are material contributed by the host. Similar asteroid spores may occur in other fungous infections,[19] perhaps as a sign of an antibody–antigen reaction.

Opportunistic Fungi

Prolonged survival of immunodeficient individuals and therapeutic induction of immunodeficiency in many patients has produced cases of unusual infection, not a few due to fungi of low pathogenicity. Occasionally, susceptibility is confined to one microorganism, as in the case of *Serratia* granuloma reported by Epstein and Carson.[20] In this group may be counted the long-known victims of *chronic granulomatous candidiasis*, who are incapable of coping with this ordinarily not highly path-

ogenic yeast. Among the organisms found in immunodepressed patients are *Aspergillus, Alternaria,*[21] *Phycomycetes,* and others. Tissue reaction may be almost absent, of noncharacteristic inflammatory nature, or more or less granulomatous, depending on the immunologic circumstances (Jadassohn–Lewandowsky rule, see Chap. 20). Occasionally, mycetomalike granulomas may be found.[22] Fungous infection may also be induced by contaminated occlusive dressings.[23]

PROTOTHECOSIS

In the last several years, sporadic cases of localized granulomatous inflammation have been recorded in which round bodies forming internal septa were identified (Fig. 21-10). The responsible organisms are achloric algae *(Prototheca spp.).* They grow yeastlike on all common media.[24]

WORMS AND LARVAE

We also make short mention of cutaneous and subcutaneous reactions to parasitic worms and burrowing insect larvae. Most of these are restricted to tropical and subtropical countries.[25] In the United States, only hookworm infestation in the form of creeping eruption (larva migrans) is seen with any

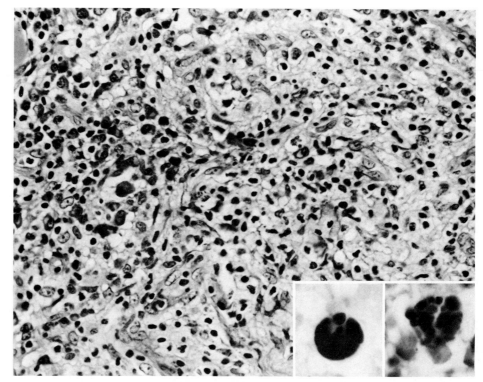

FIGURE 21–10.
Prototothecosis. Granulation tissue harboring large dark-staining cells. H&E. X400. Insets show algae with internal septa between nuclei. X1100. (From Nabai and Mehregan. J Cutan Pathol 1:180, 1974. Copyright © 1974 Munksgaard International, Copenhagen.)

frequency, but subcutaneous nodules due to *Cysticercus cellulosae* have been reported.[26] Odd cases of abscesses due to fly larvae[27] and sand fleas[28] have been seen. Among the tropical parasitoses, *filiariasis*,[29] *onchocerciasis*[30] *loaisis, dirofiliariasis*,[31] and *schistosomiasis*[32] may come to the dermato-

pathologists's attention. Recognition of unfamiliar structures in the tissue as sections of the responsible organism is the most important diagnostic point, as it was in finding the larva of *Gnathostoma spinigerum* (Fig. 21-11) in an excisional biopsy specimen of creeping eruption in a Chinese.[33]

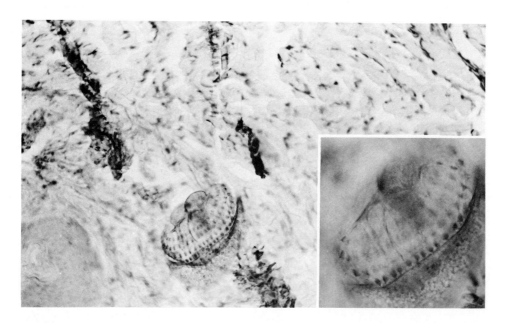

FIGURE 21–11.
Gnathostoma spinigerum. Head bulb of third stage larva in human skin. O&G. X250. Inset shows the larval head at higher magnification, exhibiting the diagnostic four rows of spines. (From Pinkus, Fan, and DeGiusti. Int J Dermatol, in press.)

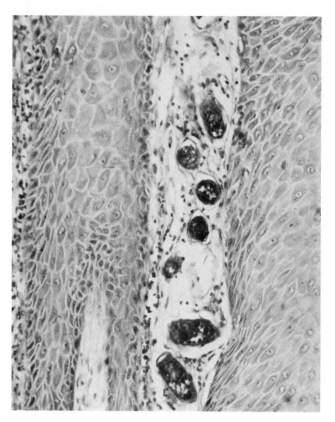

FIGURE 21–12.
Schistosomiasis. Encapsulated ova sectioned at various angles. H&E. X180. (Specimen supplied by Dr. H. Z. Lund, The Moses H. Cone Memorial Hospital, Greensboro, N.C.)

Tissue reaction may vary from lymphangitis to abscess formation and foreign-body granulomas. *Schistosoma* is illustrated in Figure 21-12.

HALOGEN ERUPTIONS

Ingestion of iodides, fluorides, or bromides will produce granulomatous lesions in predisposed patients. The more common side effect of iodide medication is development of small follicular pustules, but in some cases these become furunculoid clinically and granulomatous histologically. The infiltrate consists of a mixture of the cells mentioned earlier and is apt to include numerous polymorphonuclear leukocytes. Multinucleated giant cells are rare and are found as a response to disintegrating hair follicles. Papulonodular eruptions have been observed after intraoral application of fluoride containing gels.[34]

Bromoderma usually is a more chronic, often verrucous lesion, clinically resembling North American blastomycosis. Histologic resemblance (Fig. 21-13) also is striking, the main difference being the absence of multinucleated giant cells. This and the absence of demonstrable organisms in a lesion characterized by much epidermal hyperplasia, intraepithelial abscesses, and a mixed granulomatous infiltrate should arouse strong suspicion of bromoderma. The final diagnosis must be based on result of cultures, blood determination of bromides, and clinical history.

Granuloma Gluteale Infantum

In the bromodema group may belong vegetating granulomas on the buttocks of babies[35] described as *granuloma gluteale infantum*.[36] They exhibit epidermal acanthosis and hyperkeratosis with a mixed granulomatous infiltrate in the dermis and fibrinoid degeneration of vessel walls. They follow diaper dermatitis and involute spontaneously after several months. Similar eruptions may be found in the aged.[37]

FOREIGN-BODY GRANULOMAS

While lesions due to silica, zirconium, beryllium, and some other substances (Chap. 20) usually are in the sarcoid reaction group, there are many other in-

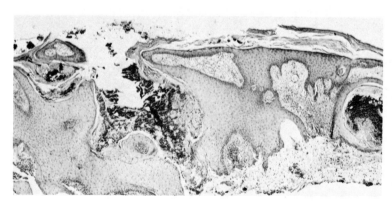

FIGURE 21–13.
Bromoderma. Pseudoepitheliomatous proliferation of epidermis enclosing necrotic tissue and inflammatory cells. H&E. X75.

stances in which a mixed cell granuloma results from reaction to a foreign body. To distinguish this type of granuloma from fungous and halogen-caused lesions is difficult. It is most commonly encountered on the face or other hairy regions because horny material (Fig. 18-4) and sebum are the most common causes. One outstanding example is the formation of large granulomas and abscesses (Fig. 21-14) under a benign intradermal nevus. The lesions form around obstructed and degenerating hair follicles or small follicular cysts and often cause anxiety for patient and physician because malignant melanoma is suspected (Chap. 32). Lesions containing all the ingredients of true granulomatous inflammation also develop if the wall of an epidermoid or trichilemmal cyst breaks down. In such instances, the large number of foreign-body type giant cells often gives a clue. The diagnosis can be made if flakes of keratinous material are recognized or foam cells have developed in response to lipids. Keratinous material sometimes polarizes light. Otherwise, it can be identified by structure and staining reaction.

In other cases, granulomas develop around foreign bodies penetrating the skin from the outside. Wood splinters, thorns, cactus spines,[38] and other vegetable matter may be identified by their birefringence, which reveals even tiny particles and their structural characteristics. Arthropods, stinging and biting insects, and ticks may produce long-last-

ing mixed cell granulomas, presumably due to the retention of chitinous material, which, however, is not usually demonstrable. Because of their peculiar features, they will be discussed under pseudolymphomas (Chap. 44). Granulomatous reactions may develop in tattoos containing mercury or other chemicals to which an occasional person may become sensitized.

GRANULOMA INGUINALE

This bacillary disease, assumed to be caused by *Donovania granulomatis*, produces superficial granulomatous lesions, although it may become destructive and mutilating.[39] It shares with the

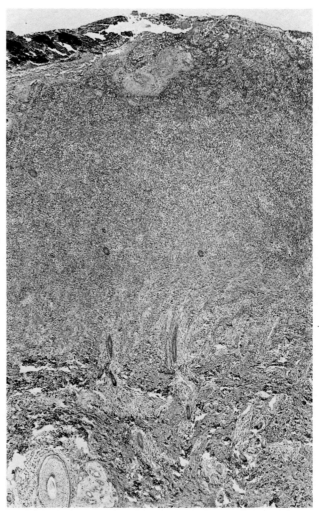

FIGURE 21–15.
Granuloma inguinale. Diffuse granulomatous infiltrate extends from epidermis into middermis and has a fairly sharp lower border. Note persistence of epidermis below surface crust. H&E. X30.

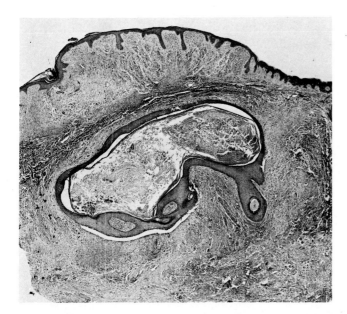

FIGURE 21–14.
Intradermal nevus cell nevus with underlying follicular cyst which is surrounded by granulomatous reaction (nevus of Duperrat). H&E. X28. (See Duperrat. Ann Dermatol Syphiligr 81:251, 1954.)

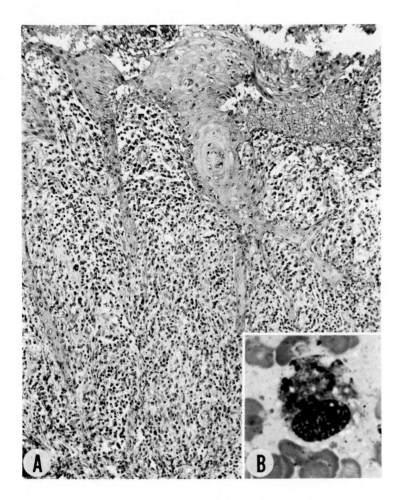

FIGURE 21–16.
Granuloma inguinale. **A.** *Epidermis persists and shows some pseudoepitheliomatous proliferation above a diffuse mixed granulomatous infiltrate. H&E. X135.* **B.** *Donovania granulomatis in a large mononuclear cell. Smear, Wright's blood stain. X1100.*

syphilitic chancre the peculiarity that it looks ulcerated clinically, while histologically the epidermis persists for long periods. In fact, the epidermis often is acanthotic (Figs. 21-15 and 21-16) and almost verrucous even though denuded of its surface layers. The granulomatous infiltrate (Fig. 21-15) at low power is dense and amorphous and hugs the epidermis. It usually has a very sharp lower edge in the middermis. Higher power reveals a colorful mixture of cells with little or no organization except around blood vessels. Lymphocytes, plasma cells, neutrophils, and eosinophils are present, in addition to scattered histiocytes. Multinucleated cells are rare. The characteristic cell is a pale-staining macrophage, which contains the diagnostic *Donovan bodies* (Fig. 21-16B and Table 20-3). These cells are more common in the superficial parts of the granuloma.[40] If one prepares smears for diagnosis, one must scrape the lesions, not just wipe superficial purulent matter on the slide.

LYMPHOGRANULOMA VENEREUM

Lymphogranuloma inguinale is mentioned here mainly for the purpose of pointing out that it is not a skin disease but a disorder of lymph nodes. The primary lesion in the skin is so small and fleeting that it is rarely biopsied. The late cutaneous changes, called *ésthiomène*, are lymphedematous masses with superimposed infection and ulceration and have no diagnostic features histologically. The lymphadenopathy is granulomatous with star-shaped abscesses.

REFERENCES

1. Pinkus H: Granulomas with eosinophilia ("eosinophilic granulomas"). Med Clin North Am 35:463, 1951
2. Wells GC, Smith NP: Eosinophilic cellulitis. Br J Dermatol 100:101, 1979
3. Spiegel GT, Winkelmann RK: Wells' syndrome. Recurrent granulomatous dermatitis with eosinophilia. Arch Dermatol 115:611, 1979
4. Baker RD (ed): The Pathologic Anatomy of Mycoses: Human Infection with Fungi, Actinomycetes, and Algae. Handbuch der speziellen pathologischen Anatomie und Histologie, vol 3, pt 5. Berlin, New York, Springer-Verlag, 1971
5. Basler RSW, Lagomarsino SL: Coccidioidomycosis: Clinical review and treatment update. Int J Dermatol 18:104, 1979

6. Su D, Duncan SC, Perry HO: Blastomycosis-like pyoderma. Arch Dermatol 115:170, 1979
7. Kroll JJ, Walzer, RA: Paracoccidioidomycosis in the United States. Arch Dermatol 106:543, 1972
8. Bhawan J, Walker Bain R, Purtilo DT, et al.: Lobomycosis. An electron microscopic, histochemical and immunologic study. J Cutan Pathol 3:5, 1976
9. Zaias N: Chromomycosis. J Cutan Pathol 5:155, 1978
10. Zaias N, Rebell G: A simple and accurate diagnostic method in chromoblastomycosis. Arch Dermatol 108:545, 1973
11. Batres E, Wolf JE, Rudolph AH, Knox JM: Transepithelial elimination of cutaneous chromomycosis. Arch Dermatol 114:1231, 1978
12. Mahgoub ES, Murray IG: Mycetoma. London, Heinemann, 1973
13. Weese WC, Smith IM: Study of 57 cases of actinomycosis over a 36 year period: diagnostic "failure" with good prognosis after treatment. Arch Intern Med 135:1562, 1975
14. Burgoon CF Jr, Bland F, Johnson WC, et al.: Mycetoma formation in *Trichophyton rubrum* infection. Br J Dermatol 90:155, 1974
15. Picon K, Batres E, Jarratt M: Botryomycosis. A bacterial cause of mycetoma. Arch Dermatol 115:609, 1979
16. Miura T, Akiba H, Saito N, et al.: Primary cutaneous cryptococcosis. Dermatologica 142:374, 1971
17. Schupbach CW, Wheeler CE Jr, Briggaman RA, et al.: Cutaneous manifestations of disseminated cryptococcosis. Arch Dermatol 112:1734, 1976
18. Pinkus H, Grekin JN: Sporotrichosis with asteroid tissue forms. Arch Dermatol 61:813, 1950
19. Prokš C, Vitovec J, Vladík P: Asteroide Körperchen bei Aspergillose. Mykosen 15:427, 1972
20. Epstein E, Carson TE: Serratia granuloma. JAMA 223:670, 1973
21. Pedersen NB, Mårahi P-A, Hallberg T, Jonsson N: Cutaneous alternariosis. Br J Dermatol 94:201, 1976
22. Jonquieres EDL, Castello CA, Negroni R, et al.: Seudomicetoma cutaneo ficomicotico con acentuade hepato-splenomegalia. Int J Dermatol 11:89, 1972
23. Hammond DE, Winkelmann RK: Cutaneous phycomycosis. Report of three cases with identification of *Rhizopus.* Arch Dermatol 115:990, 1979
24. Nabai H, Mehregan AH: Cutaneous protothecosis. Report of a case from Iran. J Cutan Pathol 1:180, 1974
25. Simons RDGP (ed): Handbook of Tropical Dermatology. Amsterdam, New York, Elsevier, 1953
26. King DT, Gilbert DJ, Gurevitch AW, et al.: Subcutaneous cysticercosis. Arch Dermatol 115:236, 1979
27. DeGiusti DL, Zackheim H: A first report of *Wohlfartia vigil* (Walker) myiasis in man in Michigan. JAMA 184:782, 1963
28. Goldman L: Tungiasis in travelers from tropical Africa. JAMA 236:1386, 1976
29. Jung RC, Harris FH: Human filiarial infection in Louisiana. Arch Pathol 69:371, 1960
30. Kpodzro K, Menning G, Bitho M, Vovor M: Onchocercomes. A propos de 41 cas au C.H.U. de Lomé. Castellania (Berlin) 4:187, 1976
31. Payan HM: Human infection with dirofilaria. Arch Dermatol 114:593, 1978
32. Torres VM: Dermatological manifestations of schistosomiasis mansoni. Arch Dermatol 112:1539, 1976
33. Degiusti DL, Fan J, Pinkus H: Creeping eruption due to *Gnathostoma spinigerum* in Taiwan. Int J Dermatol. In press
34. Blasik LG, Spencer SK: Fluoroderma. Arch Dermatol 115:1334, 1979
35. Basex A, Dupré A, Christol B, et al.: Le granulome glutéal infantile (Tappeiner-Pfleger). Faut-il le concevoir comme des "fluorides végétantes de contact" ou des "halogénides du nourrisson?" Ann Dermatol Syphiligr 99:121, 1972
36. Uyeda K, Nakayasu K, Takeishi Y, et al.: Kaposi sarcoma-like granuloma on diaper dermatitis. Arch Dermatol 107:605, 1973
37. Maekawa Y, Sakazaki Y, Hagashibara T: Diaper area granuloma of the aged. Arch Dermatol 114:382, 1978
38. Schreiber MM, Shapiro SI, Berry CZ: Cactus granuloma of the skin. Arch Dermatol 104:374, 1971
39. Davis CM: Granuloma inguinale, a clinical, histological, and ultrastructural study. JAMA 211:632, 1970
40. Khan KP, Bhattacharya SK, Datta AK: Donovanosis: a histological study. Indian J Dermatol 41:4, 1975

CHAPTER

22

Palisading Granulomas

A palisading granuloma exhibits a primary focus of localized damage to the dermis which affects the cells more than the fibers and is accompanied by deposits of abnormal substances. This area of *necrobiosis* is surrounded by a granulomatous reaction in which rather loosely arranged histiocytes have a tendency to point radially toward the center of degeneration. Lymphocytes and altered blood vessels usually are found more peripherally. Recent immunologic studies have shown evidence of vasculitis, suggesting that the central area of necrobiosis may be related to vascular occlusion. This finding reminds us of the concept of papulonecrotic tuberculid, in which primary tissue necrosis is supposed to be due to an embolus of bacteria occluding small vessels, with resulting toxic necrosis of the surrounding tissue in a host with high immune reaction to tuberculin. The histologic changes of papulonecrotic tuberculid are indeed very similar to those of granuloma annulare.[1]

The primary cause of the vascular occlusion may vary and in some cases remains unknown. *Granuloma annulare, necrobiosis lipoidica, rheumatic* and *rheumatoid nodules,* and the *juxta-articular nodes* of syphilis are in this group. The latest addition is cat-scratch disease. The lesions of this group must be sharply differentiated from lesions in which a granulomatous wall surrounds a central area of necrosis, which is secondary to the granuloma. Outstanding examples of the latter category are lupus miliaris faciei (Fig. 20-4), gummatous syphilis (Fig. 20-11), and sporotrichotic gumma (Fig. 21-8) (Chaps. 20 and 21). Beryllium granuloma (Fig. 20-17) exemplifies a somewhat different proc-

ess in which tissue has probably been damaged by the presence of foreign material. Deposition of urates in a gouty tophus (Chap. 27) produces a palisading granuloma, and so does degeneration of eosinophils in eosinophilic cellulitis (Chap. 21) and perhaps in the Churg-Strauss syndrome (Chap. 15), in which the involvement of blood vessels is likely.

Miescher's *granulomatosis disciformis* will be discussed in this chapter in the differential diagnosis of necrobiosis lipoidica, although it does not exhibit necrobiosis.

GRANULOMA ANNULARE

The most characteristic representative of the palisading granuloma is *granuloma annulare.* Just as the clinical lesion usually is a ring, so does the annular shape dominate the histologic picture. Each of the small papules that often compose the clinical ring-shaped rim is made up of one or several palisading granulomas. These are more often ovoid (Fig. 22-1) than round and are commonly located in the upper half of the pars reticularis. They may sit higher or lower, however, and usually are small and are either single or multiple. Occasionally, a large lesion may occupy almost the entire width of the dermis.

The histologic diagnosis of granuloma annulare is best made under low power because it is the peculiar configuration that counts rather than details of the lesion. An ovoid infiltrate in the mid-dermis should arouse suspicion. If the necrobiotic center is

261

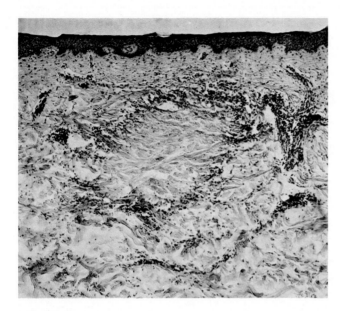

FIGURE 22–1.
Granuloma annulare. Note absence of nuclei in central zone. H&E. X75.

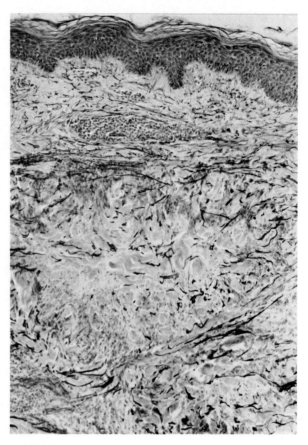

FIGURE 22–2.
Granuloma annulare showing persistence of many elastic fibers in central necrobiotic zone, their absence in granulomatous wall. O&G. X135.

small, it may be missed in some sections, and multiple sections must be examined. The size and degree of degenerative change vary widely. It ranges from a small focus of stringy hematoxylinophilic material between well-preserved connective tissue bundles to sizable areas of complete necrosis. The most typical expression is an ovoid area in which one sees only traces of nuclear dust between normal-appearing collagen bundles and some amorphous mucoid material which stains bluish in H&E sections and metachromatic with toluidine blue but is not obvious in O&G stain. The latter, however, reveals persistence of elastic fibers and thus testifies to primary tissue damage. Elastic fibers persist even if the center is more definitely necrotic (Fig. 22-2) and the collagen bundles assume a washed-out or ground-glass appearance. In such cases, small vessels and sweat ducts running through the area will also undergo necrosis.

The granulomatous wall varies considerably in quantity and composition. Typical is a loose, almost reticular arrangement of fusiform or stellate fixed-tissue-type cells that fill the interfascicular spaces and more or less point their ends toward the center. Epithelioid cell nodes and multinucleated giant cells (Fig. 22-3) are found if the infiltrate is more massive. Lymphocytes surround blood vessels in the periphery. While they are not numerous in typical cases, they may occasionally overshadow the histiocytic ovals and their necrobiotic centers. O&G sections show considerable destruction of elastic fibers in the granulomatous wall, but in gen-

eral this stain is not favorable for diagnosis because presence of elastic fibers in the center is more impressive than their lack in the thin wall. Dahl et al.[2] have brought evidence by immunofluorescent studies that IgM, complement, and fibrinogen are deposited on blood vessels of the granulomatous wall and fibrinogen in the necrobiotic center. This suggests an immunologic process in granuloma annulare, which is protracted rather than acute as in the vasculitides we described in Chapter 15. The deposition of fibrin is the hallmark of delayed hypersensitivity.[3] Perhaps additional work will show a cause for granuloma annulare, which at present is completely unknown after tuberculosis has been ruled out, and the association with sarcoidosis is extremely rare.[4]

The great variability in the details of the lesion is the reason for the advice to train one's eye for diagnosis of granuloma annulare under the low-power lens by recognizing its general configuration and location in the pars reticularis.

Major deviations from this localization occur in

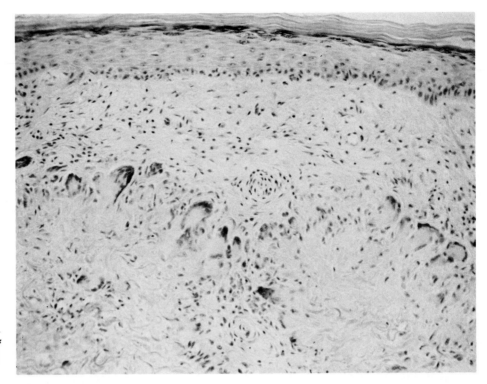

FIGURE 22–3.
Granuloma annulare containing an unusual number of multinucleated giant cells. H&E. X180.

two directions and give rise to interesting diagnostic deliberations. In rare cases, granuloma annulare may develop in the subcutaneous fat tissue. Because of the lack of tough collagen in this area, central necrosis is apt to be more complete, and the granulomatous wall is heavier (Fig. 22-4). In these lesions, large numbers of eosinophils may be found, often disintegrating and leaving eosinophilic dust in the center. It is important to know of this variant, because it is indistinguishable histologically from rheumatic or rheumatoid nodes.[5] The diagnosis becomes obvious if the patient, usually a child,

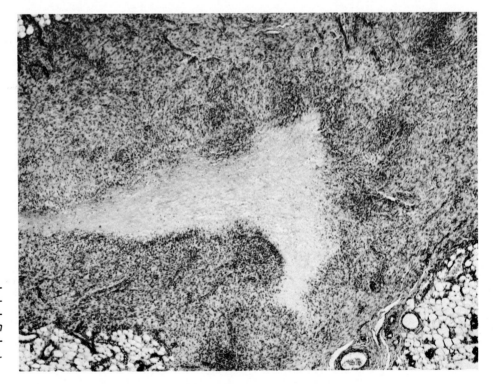

FIGURE 22–4.
Subcutaneous granuloma annulare. Complete central necrosis and heavy granulomatous wall make lesion morphologically indistinguishable from a rheumatic node. H&E. X45.

also has typical cutaneous lesions, but cases are on record where a diagnosis of rheumatic fever was made mistakenly on the strength of histologic examination, and the child was kept on a rheumatic prevention regimen for a prolonged time. Cases of this type should be examined thoroughly for any other evidence of rheumatic fever. If none is found, the isolated subcutaneous nodules can be accepted as harmless granuloma annulare. The occasional association of granuloma annulare, rheumatic nodes, and necrobiosis lipoidica in one patient with a family history of diabetes mellitus and rheumatoid arthritis has been reported[6] and speaks for some underlying personal predisposition.

On the other hand, the necrobiotic center may develop unusually high in the dermis, especially on the fingers. It may then involve the epidermis in the necrosis, and the similarity to papulonecrotic tuberculid may be striking clinically and histologically (Fig. 22-5). This phenomenon was observed as a rare event by Pinkus in 1934,[1] but in recent years it has been described more frequently, and cases of generalized *perforating granuloma annulare* have been seen[7] (Chap. 5). It seems possible that such cases would have been diagnosed as papulonecrotic tuberculids (Chap. 20) in years past when tuberculosis was common in many countries.

A histologic picture similar to granuloma annulare, but with heavier granulomatous infiltrate, is encountered in an African disease called *granuloma multiforme*[8] and in an occasional case of cutaneous *schistosomiasis*.[9]

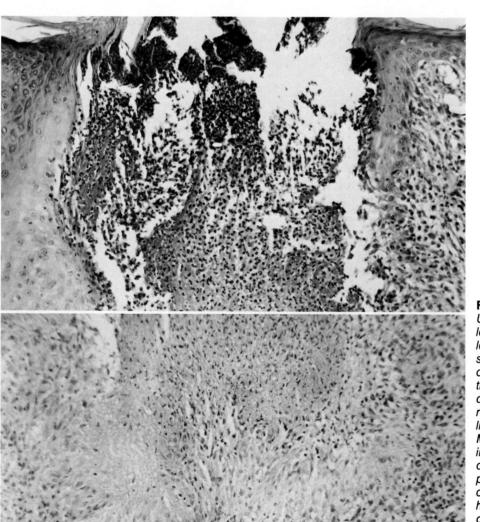

FIGURE 22–5.
Ulcerating (perforating) granuloma annulare. Upper and lower portions are shown. Lesion of finger where the necrobiotic focus lies close to thick epidermis. Epidermis has disintegrated above the necrobiosis and shows some proliferative activity at the sides. Many polymorphs are present in the necrotic tissue being discharged to the surface. The picture has some similarity to chondrodermatitis nodularis helicis (Fig. 17-6), and both diseases may be classified as transepithelial elimination (Chap. 5) or as chronic ulceration (Chap. 17). H&E. X135. (From Mehregan A. Curr Prob Dermatol 3:144, 1970.)

Actinic Granuloma

Ring-shaped, slowly expanding papular plaques are seen occasionally on the neck of severely sun-exposed persons and are submitted under the provisional clinical diagnosis of granuloma annulare. The histologic picture is compatible, with the provision that there is heavier granulomatous infiltrate with numerous multinucleated giant cells which engulf and digest the actinically damaged elastotic fibers of the region (Chap. 26). In 1975, O'Brien suggested[10] that this picture is not related to granuloma annulare but signifies destruction and repair of actinically damaged connective tissue, and he enlarged on that view in a recent article.[11] The opposite view was sponsored by Ragaz and Ackerman,[12] that actinic granuloma is granuloma annulare changed by the presence of elastotic material. There are two points that may give an answer to this controversy. It was pointed out above that the primary focus of necrobiosis of granuloma annulare retains its normal elastic fibers but that these are destroyed by the granulomatous inflammation. It is unknown what happens in the very beginning of actinic granuloma. The second point is absence or destruction of cutaneous adnexa in the lesion. They often are necrotic in granuloma annulare, a feature that speaks for a necrotizing primary event. O'Brien[10] says that hair follicles are preserved in actinic granuloma. The affection is certainly distinct from the macular facial lesions of Miescher's granuloma.

NECROBIOSIS LIPOIDICA

We purposely list necrobiosis lipoidica without the addition of *diabeticorum*. Although there is much evidence for an association of the skin disease with diabetes,[13] there is no definite difference in the histologic picture between patients having overt diabetes mellitus and those who do not have even laboratory evidence at the time the biopsy is taken.

In routine histologic sections, the features of necrobiosis lipoidica (Fig. 22-6) are similar in principle to granuloma annulare, the main difference being that the areas of necrobiosis are less focal. Instead of closed rings, one finds more often a sandwiching effect of alternating zones of tissue degeneration and infiltrate. Usually, the latter is heavier and more definitely granulomatous. Multinucleated giant cells and epithelioid nodules are frequently found. Immunofluorescence shows globulins in vascular walls and fibrinogen in the necrotic areas,[14] very similar to granuloma annulare. The crucial differentiating test is demonstration of extracellular lipids in the necrotic areas. This, however, requires frozen sections of fresh tissue, and

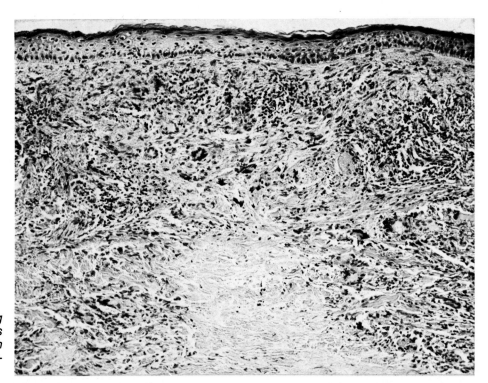

FIGURE 22-6.
Necrobiosis lipoidica, showing the upper rim of necrobiosis and granuloma, both of which extend downward into the dermis. H&E. X135.

the clinician must alert the laboratory to do these before the specimen is embedded in paraffin. Actually, fat stain is not necessary for diagnosis in most cases. Metachromatic substances may be present in necrobiosis lipoidica and are not an exclusive feature of granuloma annulare.

Granulomatosis Disciformis (Miescher)

When Miescher coined the term *granulomatosis disciformis chronica et progressiva* for lesions resembling the clinical violet-red plaques of necrobiosis lipoidica in nondiabetic patients, the histologic criteria included the absence of necrobiosis. There has been increasing doubt of the value of clinical or histologic distinction between these two manifestations[15] as they affect lower extremities and possibly the trunk. On the other hand, rare cases have been collected by several authors[16,17] of a quite distinctive dermatosis producing slowly progressive gray-brown rings on forehead and scalp, which leave slightly atrophic skin in the center. The histologic picture (Fig. 22-7) shows a mixed cell granuloma in the dermis without presence of necrobiosis. We believe that this distinctive clinicohistologic combination may well be given the name *Miescher's granuloma of the face* in distinction from widespread lesions of necrobiosis lipoidica in diabetics, which may involve the scalp

and exhibit severe necrosis, accumulation of extracellular lipids, and extensive sarcoidal granulomatous infiltrate.[18,19] We repeat that there is neither necrobiosis nor palisading in these lesions, and they are discussed here rather than in Chapter 21 only because of historical associations.

RHEUMATIC AND RHEUMATOID NODES

Palisading granulomas associated with rheumatic fever or rheumatoid arthritis usually develop in the subcutaneous tissue but may be found in the skin. They often exhibit more complete necrosis of the center and heavier granulomatous walls than granuloma annulare and may reach considerable size. The principles of differential diagnosis from granuloma annulare were discussed under that heading. To sum it up once more: location is not important, but association with systemic disease is. *Gouty tophi* will be discussed in Chapter 27.

Juxta-articular Nodes of Syphilis

While the nodes of rheumatoid arthritis may be found close to joints but may occur elsewhere, similar lesions in old syphilitics are practically always situated near elbows and knees and may reach large size. Histologically, *syphilitic juxta-articular nodes*

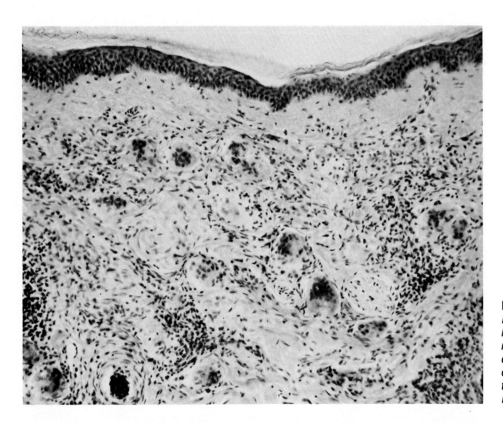

FIGURE 22–7.
Miescher's granuloma of forehead. Disorganized granulomatous infiltrate without areas of necrobiosis. Note similarity of histologic picture to nodular tertiary syphilis (Fig. 20-10). H&E. X180.

resemble the other palisading granulomas and are differentiated from gummas by their hard fibrotic centers. These centers grow by deposition of fibrous tissue and contain only remnants of elastic fibers. The granulomatous wall may be relatively thin and often contains plasma cells as a clue to syphilitic origin.

CAT-SCRATCH DISEASE

The primary inoculation site,[20] as well as the reaction to Hangor-Rose's skin test,[21] shows a palisading granuloma that may lead to necrosis of the overlying epidermis. It is similar to the granulomas formed in lymph nodes and exhibits necrosis of cells without deposition of acid mucous substances in the center and histiocytes, giant cells, and a mantle of lymphocytes in the periphery. Eosinophils often are scattered in the surroundings.

REFERENCES

1. Pinkus H: Über atypische Tuberkulide: zugleich ein Beitrag zur Ätiologie des Granuloma annulare. Arch Dermat Syph (Berlin) 170:194, 1934
2. Dahl MV, Ullman S, Goltz RW: Vasculitis in granuloma annulare. Histopathology and direct immunofluorescence. Arch Dermatol 113:463, 1977
3. Winkelmann RK: New insights into granuloma annulare. J Am Acad Dermatol 1:83, 1979
4. Umbert P, Winkelmann RK: Granuloma annulare and sarcoidosis. Br J Dermatol 97:481, 1977
5. Elliott GB, Hill RM, Kliman MR, et al.: Deep granuloma annulare and "non-rheumatoid rheumatoid nodule." Cutis 11:76, 1973
6. Burton JL: Granuloma annulare, rheumatoid nodules and necrobiosis lipoidica. Br J Dermatol 97 [Suppl]:52, 1977
7. Ågren-Jonsson S, Holst R, Dahlquist I: Perforating granuloma annulare: report of three cases from Scandinavia. Acta Derm Venereol (Stockh) 57:543, 1977
8. Meyers WM, Connor DH, Shannon R: Histologic characteristics of granuloma multiforme (Mkar disease); including a comparison with leprosy and granuloma annulare; report of first cases from Congo (Kinshasa). Int J Lepr 38:241, 1970
9. Findlay GH, Whiting DA: Disseminated and zosteriform cutaneous schistosomiasis. Br J Dermatol 85 [Suppl 7]:98, 1971
10. O'Brien JP: Actinic granuloma. Arch Dermatol 111:460, 1975
11. O'Brien JP: Is actinic granuloma a specific condition? Another view: Perhaps the concept should be extended. Am J Dermatopathol 1:51, 1979
12. Ragaz A, Ackerman AB: Is actinic granuloma a specific condition? Am J Dermatopathol 1:43, 1979
13. Muller SA, Winkelmann RK: Necrobiosis lipoidica diabeticorum. A clinical and pathological investigation of 171 cases. Arch Dermatol 93:272, 1966
14. Ullman S, Dahl MV: Necrobiosis lipoidica. An immunofluorescence study. Arch Dermatol 113:1671, 1977
15. Muller SA, Winkelmann RK: Necrobiosis lipoidica diabeticorum. Histopathologic study of 98 cases. Arch Dermatol 94:1, 1966
16. Wilson-Jones E: Necrobiosis lipoidica presenting on the face and scalp. Trans St Johns Hosp Dermatol Soc 57:202, 1971
17. Mehregan AH, Altman J: Miescher's granuloma of the face. A variant of the necrobiosis lipoidica-granuloma annulare spectrum. Arch Dermatol 107:62, 1973
18. Mehregan AH, Pinkus H: Necrobiosis lipoidica with sarcoid reaction. Arch Dermatol 83:143, 1961
19. Gaethe G: Necrobiosis lipoidica diabeticorum of the scalp. Arch Dermatol 89:865, 1964
20. Johnson WT, Helwig EB: Cat-scratch disease. Histopathologic changes in the skin. Arch Dermatol 100:148, 1969
21. Czarnetzki BM, Pomeranz JR, Khanderka PK, et al.: Cat-scratch disease skin test. Studies of specificity and histopathologic features. Arch Dermatol 111:736, 1975

CHAPTER

23

Predominantly Histiocytic Lesions

The presence of histiocytes being the essential feature of granulomatous inflammation, a lesion consisting entirely of histiocytes should be the prototype of this form of tissue reaction. However, simple inspection makes one feel that pure accumulations of histiocytes belong rather in the field of tumors, of neoplastic lesions. And thus they were classified by the old authors. *Xanthoma* is the outstanding example and *histiocytoma* is another. Xanthomas, histiocytomas, and others now are considered reactive lesions, and some xanthomas regress without a trace and others through fibrosis and scarring. A recent change in the usage of the word *histiocyte* has led to a reclassification of malignant reticuloendothelial lesions, and the term *malignant histiocytoma* is now frequently encountered in pathology literature. This situation will be discussed in Chapter 44.

While histiocytes predominate in the lesions to be discussed here, other cells may be present. The histiocytes may occur in a nonphagocytic state or may appear as foam cells (lipophages) or macrophages containing hemosiderin and other substances. Differentiation from epithelioid tubercles of sarcoid reactions and from lepromatous leprosy sometimes is based more on configuration of the entire lesion than on cytologic characteristics. Carrington and Winkelmann[1] reviewed electron microscopic characteristics and differences of various histiocytic diseases. In rare instances, one may be hard pressed to tell a benign histiocytic lesion from

a malignant epithelial tumor. Discussion of the lesion *atypical fibroxanthoma* will be found in Chapter 41.

XANTHOMA

A more or less pure accumulation of large cells with pale foamy cytoplasm[2] is characteristic of all clinical forms of xanthoma. If fresh tissue is available, frozen sections stained with scarlet red or other lipid stains (Fig. 23-1) will confirm the diagnosis, but this is neither feasible nor necessary in routine diagnosis. The clinician, however, must realize that one cannot ask the pathologist to demonstrate lipids in a paraffin section and thus must specify frozen sections in a doubtful case when the specimen is submitted. Experience leads to the advice that such a request should be made in red letters on the request blank and also on the bottle containing the specimen lest a technician inadvertently process it for paraffin embedding.

The metabolic and genetic disorders leading to xanthoma formation have been clarified in past years.[3] They must be investigated in every case, whether we recognize clinically tuberous, eruptive, or plane xanthomas. Various types of lipids are taken up from the bloodstream by primitive dermal mesenchymal cells that become macrophages.[4,5] An outstanding characteristic of all xanthoma cells is that they contain birefringent substances.

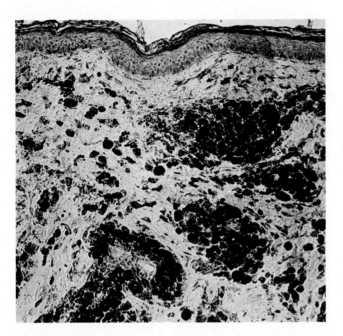

FIGURE 23–1.
Xanthoma, frozen section stained with Sudan IV and hematoxylin. Foam cells appear black in photograph. X135.

Histologic differentiation of the various clinical types of xanthoma is difficult and is based on ancillary features. For instance, if the foam cells are distributed in small nests near to and in between striated muscle bundles, one is entitled to make a diagnosis of xanthelasma (Fig. 23-2) of the eyelid. Large accumulations of foam cells (Fig. 23-1) suggest tuberous xanthoma rather than the eruptive type. The former may become quite fibrotic, and

the latter is apt to show evidence of cellular disintegration so that some lipid may be free in the tissue. Paraffin sections show empty spaces in addition to foam cells. In normolipemic plane xanthomatosis, foam cells are present in large areas of skin, and there may be associated paraproteinemia.[6] Verruciform xanthomas occur in the oral mucosa and on the vulva (Chap. 45). The characteristic Touton giant cell (Fig. 5-17B) may be found in all forms of xanthoma, but usually in small numbers.

Although other disturbances of lipid metabolism (Gaucher's disease, Niemann–Pick's disease) may produce foam cells in other organs, the skin is spared in these disorders.

JUVENILE XANTHOGRANULOMA

This lesion,[7] formerly called *nevoxanthoendothelioma* and also found in adults,[8] usually can be differentiated histologically from other xanthomas. It often presents (Fig. 23-3) a relatively large number of multinucleated cells, some of which may be of the Touton type, but good foam cells are relatively rare, and in many cases the lesion consists of compact histiocytes. Only high-power study reveals vacuolation of the cytoplasm. Small round cells and a variable number of eosinophils are often present. The picture may closely resemble that of *xanthoma disseminatum*, one of the manifestations of *histiocytosis X (Langerhans cell granuloma)*, which will be discussed in Chapter 24. An important dif-

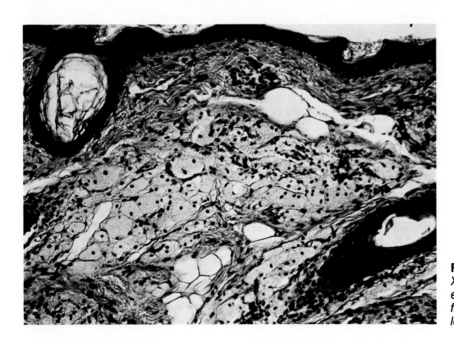

FIGURE 23–2.
Xanthelasma of eyelid. Note the difference between foam cells of lesion and fat cells (F) which are present near lower border. H&E. X135.

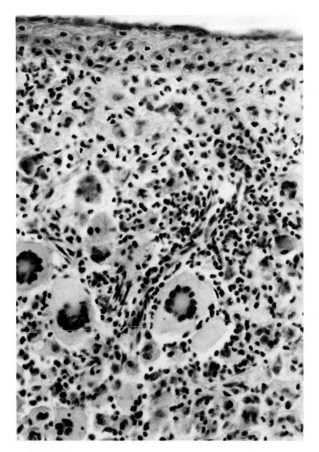

FIGURE 23–3.
*Juvenile xanthogranuloma. Touton giant cells and histio-
cytes with rather solid cytoplasm mixed with small round
cells. No invasion of epidermis. H&E. X90.*

ference is the absence of epidermal invasion by
mononuclear cells in the juvenile xanthogranuloma. Under the electron microscope, the cytoplasmic granules of Birbeck are absent.[9]

HISTIOCYTOMA

Nature

There is fairly general agreement that *histiocytomas* are not true tumors but reactive accumulations of cells. However, the nature of the predomi-
nant cell is debated, and this doubt is expressed in
the designations *fibroma durum, histiocytoma,
subepidermal nodular fibrosis,* and others. The entirely noncommittal term *nodulus cutaneus* is not
the worst. It seems likely that many of these lesions start as reactions to mosquito bites or other
minor trauma. Keeping in mind the pluripotentiality of mesenchymal cells, one might rationalize the

histologic features by the assumption that histiocytes accumulate in response to injury, that some
may become macrophages, and that later many become fibroblasts. Or fibroblasts may be of perivascular origin. A variable degree of vascular proliferation, one of the common features of productive
inflammation (Sec. IV), adds to the colorful spectrum of histologic findings. However, there is little
to support the contention that histiocytomas are
sclerosing hemangiomas. A last feature, which will
be discussed in some detail below, is the pronounced tendency of the epidermis and pilar complexes to undergo reactive changes.

Histology

The histologic picture (Fig. 23-4) of a typical histiocytoma has two components. There is a roughly
lenticular accumulation of fixed-tissue-type cells in
the midcorium, and there is perivascular round cell
infiltrate around the periphery of the quasitumor.
The latter feature is quite constant and serves in
the differentiation from *dermatofibrosarcoma protuberans* (Chap. 41). Sudan-stained frozen sections
are apt to reveal fine lipid droplets in the perivascular cells. The main lesion has no sharp border
and certainly has no capsule, and fusiform or stellate cells are present between the collagen bundles
of the periphery. In this respect, the lesion differs
from *keloid.* On the other hand, there is no shelf
effect such as we shall encounter with dermatofibrosarcoma protuberans.

The cells of the main lesion are fusiform or stellate and usually are arranged in whorls or bending
streams rather than in straight intersecting bundles
such as are seen in *leiomyomas.* Variable amounts
of collagen fibers and bundles are present. Some of
these are old dermal tissue with associated remnants of elastic fibers. Others are new fibers formed
by fibroblasts in the lesion and are free of elastic fibers. In these respects, histiocytoma also differs
from leiomyoma, in which new elastic fibers frequently are formed. Blood vessels usually are small
in number and size, but they may become prominent and then often are the source of small hemorrhages followed by macrophage formation.

The view that most of the constituent cells are
histiocytes is based mainly on experiments[12] which
showed that locally injected colloidal iron is taken
up by the tumor cells, thereby revealing their phagocytic nature. In routine histologic examination,
one may find single or clustered foam cells and
other cells containing hemosiderin.

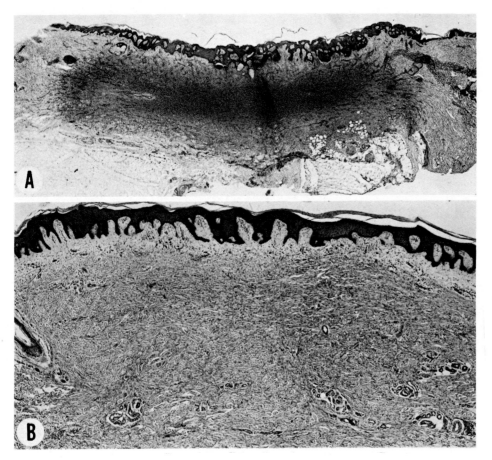

FIGURE 23–4.
Histiocytoma. **A.** *Low-power view shows seat of roughly lenticular lesion in mid-dermis, absence of a distinct border, and reactive epidermal proliferation which is papillomatous in some areas, while other areas simulate superficial basal cell epithelioma. H&E. X9.* **B.** *Less cellular lesion at higher magnification. Shows whorled arrangement of fibrous bundles. Note persistence of sweat coils below benign lesion and cross section of a duct traversing the lesion. H&E. X60.*

Variants

Variants of the typical picture are in four main directions. Old lesions may become very fibrotic, and they then really deserve the title *subepidermal nodular fibrosis.* Other lesions are more cellular than average, may grow to considerable size, and

may involve subcutaneous fat tissue. These often have a more pronounced cartwheel pattern (Figs. 23-5 and 41-10), and the differentiation from dermatofibrosarcoma protuberans may become difficult. Attention should be paid to the presence of perivascular round cell infiltrate in the periphery, characteristic of histiocytoma, and absence of the

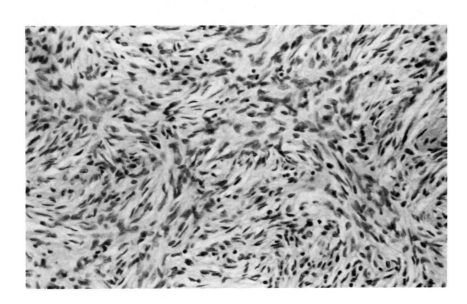

FIGURE 23–5.
Cartwheel pattern approximated in a histiocytoma. Compare with Figure 41-10 (dermatofibrosarcoma protuberans). H&E. X250.

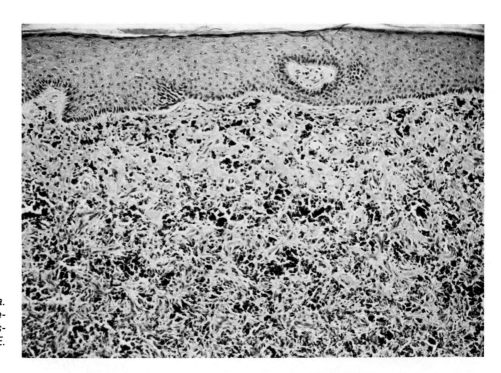

FIGURE 23–6.
Hemosiderotic histiocytoma. Dark masses are clumps of hemosiderin in histiocytes transformed into macrophages. H&E. X135.

deep fibroblastic shelf, which we shall find as a feature of dermatofibrosarcoma. The third variant is the *hemosiderotic histiocytoma.* These are lesions, more vascular than usual, which may grow to large size due to a vicious cycle of repeated small hemorrhage and reactive proliferation of histiocytes which engulf blood pigment and lipid. Thus, macrophages, multinucleated giant cells, and thin-walled blood vessels dominate the picture. These lesions may look almost black and clinically arouse suspicion of malignant melanoma. H&E sections (Fig. 23-6) may at first sight support this suspicion due to the presence of large quantities of brown pigment. O&G sections reveal the nonmelanin nature of the pigment, thus making stain for hemosiderin unnecessary, especially when the foamy cytoplasm of many cells is appreciated. A fourth modification is the *xanthomatized histiocytoma,* in which most of the cells contain lipid. These lesions may reach a size of several centimeters, are often located on the legs, and may be sessile or pedunculated. Many look yellow on gross section, but true foam cells may be surprisingly few because the lipid is present as very fine droplets. A malignant fibrous histiocytoma will be discussed in Chapter 41.

Associated Epithelial Changes

Of great practical and theoretical significance are epithelial changes associated with histiocytomas. They are present in more than half of the cases[13]

and take three principal forms. The simplest is general acanthosis and hyperkeratosis of the epidermis, resembling that of lichenification. It may be mentioned that epidermal atrophy can be encountered, especially after trauma and scarring. More complicated and interesting are two other changes, one of which simulates seborrheic verruca, the other one basal cell epithelioma. Papillomatous hyperplasia of the epidermis exhibiting horny pearls and retarded maturation of prickle cells, and thus resembling seborrheic verruca (Chap. 33), are not uncommon. The question of whether such changes constitute a true seborrheic verruca associated with the histiocytoma is theoretically intriguing but of no great practical importance. However, considerable theoretical and practical importance attaches to the question of whether basal cell epithelioma is associated with the benign mesodermal pseudotumor in as high as 8 percent of cases.[14]

Thorough examination of serial sections of well over a thousand histiocytomas has convinced the senior author[15] that pictures as illustrated in Figure 23-7 mimic superficial basal cell epithelioma and are the result of peculiar regressive and proliferative changes of hair follicles (Fig. 23-8) but are not true neoplasia. True basalioma may be found in rare cases.[16,17] Attentive study of histiocytomas reveals that hair follicles and eccrine glands are affected in a different manner by the slow accumulation of cells and fibers in the middermis. The sweat coil is fixed deep to the tumor. The duct continues to make its way through the tumor to the

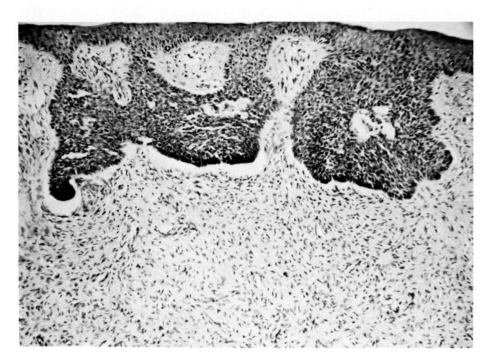

FIGURE 23–7.
Basaliomalike epithelial proliferation above a histiocytoma. H&E. X135.

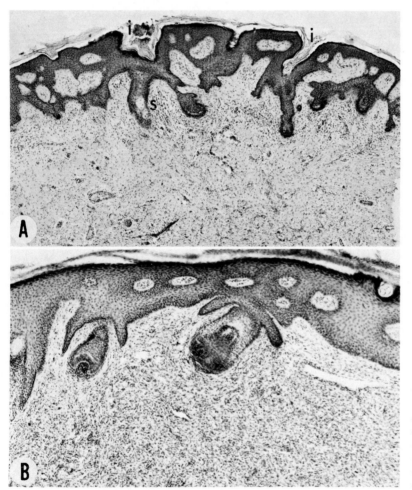

FIGURE 23–8.
*Regressive changes of pilary complexes above histiocytoma. **A.** Tiny sebaceous gland (s) associated with rudimentary hair root and infundibulum (i). Three other rudimentary hair roots, one connected with infundibulum (i), at right. Note similarity to Figure 23-7. H&E. X90. **B.** Two foreshortened hair follicles resembling cloaked hairs. (See legend for Fig. 18-18.) H&E. X135.*

surface unless it is eventually choked off and disappears. In that case, the entire eccrine unit atrophies. The roots of vellus or terminal hairs, on the other hand, are mobile. With each hair change, about twice a year, the lower follicle disintegrates (Chap. 2), and the dermal papilla moves upward close to the sebaceous gland, which usually is situated above or in the upper portion of the histiocytoma. With the onset of the next anagen, the hair root tries to grow down but finds its path blocked. The entire follicle is foreshortened and will form a new hair above the tumor. As the latter expands and presses closer to the epidermis, hair matrices, often still associated with sebaceous glands, can be found almost immediately below the epidermis. The final step seems to be a diffuse spreading of the material of epithelial matrix and mesodermal papilla along the lower surface of the epidermis. This process gives rise to multiple foci (Fig. 23-8) strongly resembling fetal hair germs or the rudimentary matrix–papilla complexes found in organoid nevi and trichoepitheliomas. That they still represent a pilar complex often is documented by the presence of a keratinizing channel in the epidermis and the occasional presence of a tiny but mature sebaceous gland. Whether a picture as shown in Figure 23-7 is the final stage of this process or now truly represents neoplasia is a question one cannot decide in the histologic section. The overwhelming biologic evidence seems to be in favor of pseudoneoplasia.

RETICULOHISTIOCYTOMA

Lesions of a type perhaps better called *reticulohistiocytic granuloma* are encountered as small single papules or in multiple form. In the latter case, they may be associated with telescoping fingers and other evidence of multisystem disease.[18-20] Histologically (Fig. 23-9), they are composed of histiocytes and multinucleated cells, which may be bizarre. If one is cognizant of this lesion, one will not be misled into a diagnosis of sarcoma (Chap. 41).

REFERENCES

1. Carrington SG, Winkelmann RK: Electron microscopy of histiocytic diseases of the skin. Acta Derm Venereol (Stockh) 52:161, 1972
2. Braun-Falco O: Origin, structure, and function of the xanthoma cell. Nutr Metab 15:68, 1973
3. Fredrickson DS: Plasma lipid abnormalities and cutaneous and subcutaneous xanthomas. In Fitzpatrick TB, et al. (eds): Dermatology in General Medicine, 2nd ed. New York, McGraw-Hill, 1979, pp 1112–1125
4. Bulkley BH, Buja LM, Ferrans VJ, et al.: Tuberous xanthoma in homozygous type II hyperlipoproteinemia: histologic, histochemical and electron microscopic study. Arch Pathol 99:293, 1975
5. Braun-Falco O: Struktur und Morphogenese von Xanthomen by Hyperlipoproteinämie von Type III. Eine morphologische, histochemische und elektronenmikroskopische Untersuchung. Hautarzt 27:122, 1976
6. Weber G, Pilgrim M: Contribution to the knowledge of normolipemic plane xanthomatosis. Br J Dermatol 90:465, 1974
7. Helwig EB, Hackney VC: Juvenile xanthogranuloma (nevoxanthoendothelioma). Am J Pathol 30:625, 1954
8. Rodriguez J, Ackerman AB: Xanthogranuloma in adults. Arch Dermatol 112:43, 1976
9. Esterly NB, Sahihi T, Medenica M: Juvenile xanthogranuloma. An atypical case with study of ultrastructure. Arch Dermatol 105:99, 1972
10. Niemi KN: The benign fibrohistiocytic tumors of the skin. Acta Derm Venereol [Suppl] (Stockh) 63:1, 1970
11. Vilanova JR, Flint A: The morphological variations of fibrous histiocytomas. J Cutan Pathol 1:155, 1974

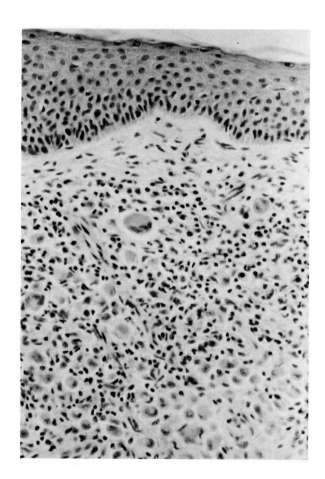

FIGURE 23–9.
Multicentric reticulohistiocytoma. Histiocytes and small multinucleated giant cells are mixed with small round cells. H&E. X250.

12. Senear FE, Caro MR: Histiocytoma cutis. Arch Dermatol 33:209, 1936
13. Schoenfeld RJ: Epidermal proliferation overlying histiocytomas. Arch Dermatol 90:266, 1964
14. Bryant J: Basal cell carcinoma overlying long-standing dermatofibromas. Arch Dermatol 113:1445, 1977
15. Pinkus H: Pathobiology of the pilary complex. Jpn J Dermatol [B] 77:304, 1967
16. Thies W, Hennies T: Über die Assoziation eines Histiocytoms mit einem Basaliom. Hautarzt 19:163, 1968
17. Goette DK, Helwig EB: Basal cell carcinomas and basal cell carcinoma-like changes overlying dermatofibromas. Arch Dermatol 111:589, 1975
18. Haustein UF, Thormann T, Klug H, et al.: Histologische und elektronenmikroskopische Befunde bei Histiocytosis gigantocellularis. Dermatologica 146:177, 1973
19. Rendall JRS, Vanhegan RI, Robb-Smith AHT, et al.: Atypical reticulohistiocytosis with paraproteinemia. Arch Dermatol 113:1576, 1977
20. Chevrant-Breton J: La réticulo-histiocytose multicentrique. Revue de la littérature récente (depuis 1969). Ann Derm Venereol 104:745, 1977

24

Langerhans Cell Granulomas

It is to Lichtenstein's credit that he pulled together three manifestations of a "peculiar inflammatory histiocytosis" and integrated them into a single nosologic entity.[1] The name he gave the entity, *histiocytosis X*, appears to be a sign of desperation. Much has been written taking all sides in the discussion of this disease,[2] which Pinkus et al.[3] had previously called *reticulogranuloma*, pointing out that the specific cell seemed to be of reticuloendothelial nature—being capable of phagocytosis—and that the lesions were neither simple inflammatory proliferations nor were they truly malignant sarcomas. They possessed the essential features of a granuloma consisting of histiocytes invading and destroying tissue but eventually healing by fibrosis (Sec. IV).

Introduction of electron microscopy cast an unexpected light on the matter, when it was found that the large cells, which together with eosinophils are the substrate of the granuloma, contain the specific Birbeck granules found in epidermal Langerhans cells.[4,5] Since this discovery, Langerhans cells have been demonstrated in a great variety of dermal and extradermal tissues, and it has become clear that they derive from a mononuclear stem cell in the bone marrow but that they are a specialized subpopulation of the mononuclear phagocyte system, different from histiocytes[6] and macrophages.[7]

Just as metachromatic or acidophilic granules make a cell a mast cell or an eosinophil, so the Birbeck granule stamps a cell as a Langerhans cell. We recognize this fact by calling lesions consisting of these cells *Langerhans cell granulomas*. We obviously need an electron microscope to prove the nature of the cell, but, fortunately, other histologic properties of the lesions make this requirement unnecessary for diagnosis in most instances (pp. 270–71).

SKIN MANIFESTATIONS

The skin manifestations of Langerhans cell granuloma are manifold.[7] They range from disseminated tiny papules to plaques of oozing, crusting dermatitis of the scalp to deep granulomatous ulcerations of the genitoanal area or the oral mucosa (Chap. 45). The histologic feature common to all of them is the presence of Langerhans cells and the more or less proliferative and destructive character that is the hallmark of all granulomatous inflammation. The lesions do destroy tissue, but they may regress and heal with fibrosis (exemplified by *eosinophilic granuloma of bone*).

The Langerhans cells (L-cells) may assume various forms, which are the substrate of the different clinical manifestations. They may be found (Fig. 24-1) as solid, fairly large cells with pale-staining ovoid nuclei in the *nonlipid forms (Letterer-Siwe type)*, or they may take up lipid and hemosiderin in Hand-Schüller-Christian disease and become foam

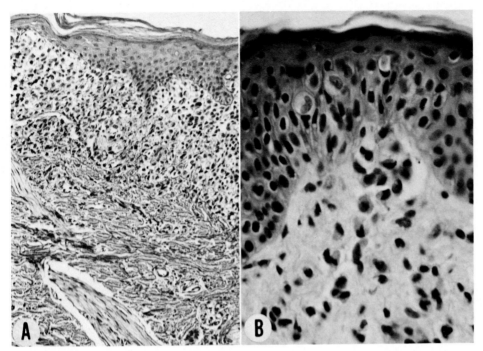

FIGURE 24–1.
A. *Nonlipid L-cell granuloma. H&E. X180.* **B.** *Invasion of epidermis by large mononuclear cells, one of which has kidney-shaped nucleus of the monocyte. H&E. X370. (From Pinkus et al. Am J Dis Child 77:503, 1949.)*

cells. L-cells are a specific type of mesodermal cell that (like many others) have phagocytic properties and were called "histiocytes" for superficial reasons of resemblance in the days before the electron microscope.[7]

If we consider Langerhans cells as a specialized subpopulation of the mononuclear phagocytic system, some of the difficulties that plagued earlier authors disappear. Their specific affinity for antigenic substances (e.g., contact allergens, ferritin) and their function in allergic dermatoses may be explained.[8] Their occurrence in great numbers in L-cell granuloma, which many pathologists still consider a malignant disease, can be understood, as can occasional cases of truly malignant transformation.[9] We know that histiocytes without L-granules are the substrate of juvenile xanthogranuloma and that these cells behave differently.

The cells of L-cell granulomas often are not true foam cells even in lesions that look yellow clinically because the lipid occurs in a more finely divided form. On the other hand, macrophages containing both lipid and hemosiderin may be prominent in the ulcerative lesions. One outstanding feature of the disease (Fig. 24-1B) is the tendency for mononuclear cells to invade, and often destroy, the epidermis. This feature is a fairly good differentiating sign from juvenile xanthogranuloma in the papular form and leads to the oozing, crusting (pseudoseborrheic) scalp involvement in Letterer-Siwe cases. Multinucleated giant cells may or may not be present and are apt to be of foreign-body type just as often as of the Touton type. Eo-

sinophils may be completely absent in the papular forms of *xanthoma disseminatum* and are often present in large numbers in the ulcerating granulomatous lesions of the genitoanal area and in the mouth. Neutrophils usually are absent or rare. The contrast between clinical oozing and seeming pustulation and the histologic picture of granulomatous chronic inflammation is one of the clues leading to correct diagnosis.

L-CELL GRANULOMAS IN ADULTS

The group of L-cell granulomas includes the nonlipid Letterer-Siwe disease, the lipid granulomas of Hand-Schüller-Christian disease, and the solitary eosinophilic granuloma of bone. While it is a disease of the young, cases have been seen in old age.[10,11] Attention should be paid to papular eruptions[12] and to the occurrence[13] of ulcerative granulomatous lesions of the mouth and the genitoanal area in adults, which have all the histologic features of Hand-Schüller-Christian disease (Chap. 45). These quite destructive lesions are often treated as infections or malignancy until properly classified.

BENIGN RETICULOHISTIOCYTOSIS OF NEWBORNS

Another peculiar group of cases is the Hashimoto-Pritzker type of reticulohistiocytoma in newborns, which heal spontaneously within some months.

Electron microscopy reveals large cells, some of which have typical L-granules, while most of them contain dense bodies with myelin configuration.[14,15]

REFERENCES

1. Lichtenstein L: Histiocytosis X: integration of eosinophilic granuloma of bone, "Letterer-Siwe disease," and "Schüller-Christian disease" as related manifestations of a single nosologic entity. Arch Pathol 56:84, 1953
2. Lieberman PH, Jones CR, Dargeon HWK, et al.: A reappraisal of eosinophilic granuloma of bone, Hand-Schüller-Christian syndrome and Letterer-Siwe syndrome. Medicine 48:375, 1969
3. Pinkus H, Copps LA, Custer C, et al.: Reticulogranuloma: report of a case of eosinophilic granuloma of bone associated with nonlipid reticulosis of skin and oral mucosa under the clinical picture of Hand-Schüller-Christian disease. Am J Dis Child 77:503, 1949
4. Basset F, Turiaf J: Identification par la microscope électronique de particules de nature probablement virale dans les lésions granulomateuses d'une histiocytose X pulmonaire. C R Acad Sci (Paris) 261:3701, 1965
5. Kobayasi T, Asboe-Hansen G: Granules of Langerhans cell in Letterer-Siwe's disease. Acta Derm Venereol (Stockh) 52:257, 1972
6. Katz SI, Tamaki K, Sachs DH: Epidermal Langerhans cells are derived from cells originating in bone marrow. Nature 282:324, 1979
7. Nezelof C, Basset F, Rouseau MF: Histiocytosis X. Histiogenetic arguments for a Langerhans cell origin. Biomedicine 18:365, 1973
8. Juhlin L (ed): The Langerhans' cell and contact dermatitis. Symposium. Acta Derm Venereol [Suppl] (Stockh) 79, 1978
9. Fülop E, Vessei E: Malignant transformation of Hand-Schüller-Christian type of histiocytosis X. Börgyóvy Vener Szle 50:34, 1974
10. Dalezal JF, Thomson ST: Hand-Schüller-Christian disease in a septuagenarian. Arch Dermatol 114:85, 1978
11. Chevrant-Breton J: La maladie de Letterer-Siwe de l'adulte. Revue de la littérature. Ann Derm Venereol 105:301, 1978
12. Vollum DI: Letterer-Siwe disease in the adult. Clin Exp Dermatol 4:395, 1979
13. Vallet C: Granulome éosinophile péri-vulvaire et péri-anal (histiocytosis X). A propos d'un cas, revue de 44 cas de la littérature. Thèse de Paris. 1974
14. Hashimoto K, Pritzker MS: Electron microscopic study of reticulohistiocytoma. An unusual case of congenital, self-healing reticulohistiocytosis. Arch Dermatol 107:263, 1973
15. Mascaro JM, Aliaga A, Mascaro-Galy C: Réticulose congénitale auto-involutive (type Hashimoto-Pritzker). Ann Derm Venereol 105:223, 1978

SECTION

V

METABOLIC AND OTHER NONINFLAMMATORY DERMAL DISEASES

Obviously, there can be no strict division between inflammatory and noninflammatory dermatoses. Just as obviously, all skin diseases are accompanied by changed metabolism, and in some of those discussed in this section we only presume that metabolic derangement is the primary cause. Yet there are a number of nonneoplastic skin diseases in which inflammatory changes are minor or are overshadowed by alterations of the fibrous constituents and ground substance. In others, deposition of various abnormal substances is the diagnostic feature. In these groups, we encounter even greater diagnostic difficulties if we rely merely on H&E stains. The O&G procedure, especially when its results are compared with H&E-stained sections, is informative in many cases, but special stains are needed in some instances, and a high level of suspicion is advisable so that the proper stains will be employed.

A table published by W.B. Reed[1] lists a wide variety of skin disturbances ranging from hair loss to tumors and includes many noninflammatory cutaneous disorders. A new book on genetic diseases of the skin[2] also discusses many of the abnormalities that are included in this section. An excellent review of many facets of normal and pathologic structure and biochemistry of connective tissue was recently published in France with most papers in English.[3]

REFERENCES

1. Reed WB: Congenital and genetic disorders associated with malignant and nonmalignant tumors. Arch Dermatol 111:525, 1975
2. Der Kaloustian VM, Kurban AK: Genetic Diseases of the Skin. New York, Springer-Verlag, 1979
3. Biochemistry of Normal and Pathologic Connective Tissues. Paris, Editions au Centre National de la Recherche Scientifique (no. 287), 1978

25

Changes of Collagen and Ground Substance

Destruction, new formation, and other changes of the collagen fibers and bundles were encountered in granulomatous inflammatory diseases. Changes in ground substance are to be assumed in any skin section exhibiting edema. In this chapter we deal mainly with scleroderma in the localized and general forms, sclerodermoid processes, scleredema, various forms of myxedema, and lymphedema. Lichen sclerosus et atrophicus and atrophodermas and lipodystrophies are put here for convenience and differential diagnosis. Reactive perforating collagenosis and the Ehlers–Danlos syndrome also find their legitimate place in this chapter.

SCLERODERMA

Generalized

Generalized scleroderma has a variable but well-defined clinical symptomatology.[1] The histologic diagnosis of generalized scleroderma (systemic sclerosis) is unsatisfactory in the early stages and not too secure in late stages. Whatever it is that gives the skin the hidebound consistency and the glistening aspect is poorly expressed in stained paraffin sections. In any case, one has to have a fairly large and deep biopsy extending well into the subcutaneous tissue in order to evaluate all changes completely. Some of the features that must be weighed in differential diagnosis from clinically similar conditions are indeed negative ones: the epidermis preserves its normal configuration for a long time, the elastic fibers are preserved, and there is no or little inflammatory infiltrate. The most impressive changes in a well-developed case (Fig. 25-1) are that the collagen bundles of the pars reticularis are thick and the interfascicular spaces are narrow or almost absent. Structural differences between pars reticularis and papillaris are blurred because the latter also looks dense. Fixed-tissue-type cells are few, giving a desert look to the dermis. It has been suggested that sclerodermatous fibroblasts in tissue culture produce more collagen than normal ones.[2]

Small blood vessels, especially those of the papillary and subpapillary layers, generally are few and narrow, although excessive telangiectasia may be a prominent clinical feature. The width of the dermis is increased, not only because the collagen bundles are thicker but also because new dermal tissue replaces part of the subcutaneous fat tissue.[3] All these points are subject to individual judgment and may be influenced by technical differences in tissue preparation (Chap. 3). This is particularly true for the width of interfascicular spaces. If inflammatory infiltrate is present, it is usually of small round cell type with plasma cells[4] and is located in the deep dermis. Special attention should be given to the eccrine coils, which are apt to show signs of atrophy earlier than hair follicles and often seem to be situated in the mid-dermis, owing to the forma-

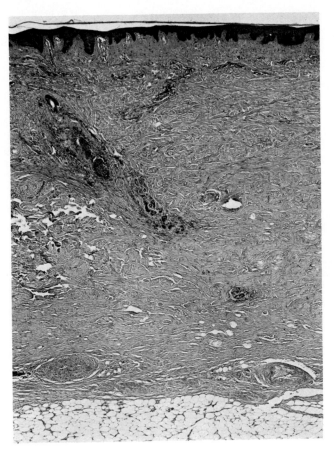

FIGURE 25–1.
Diffuse, generalized scleroderma. H&E. X45.

tion of dermal bundles below them. However, one has to realize that there are deeper and more superficial coils in normal skin and that the coils are apt to lie within the dermis in thick-skinned areas, such as the back of the trunk. To judge the size of sweat coils is impossible unless one examines a considerable number of sections. A somewhat more reliable feature is flattening of secretory cells and corresponding widening of the lumen.

In rare cases of systemic sclerosis as well as widespread morphea, the development of vesicles and bullae has been observed. They seem to be due to obstruction of superficial lymphatics by the sclerodermatous process[5,6] and are different from the subepidermal bullae encountered in lichen sclerosus et atrophicus (see below).

The internist often seeks help from a skin biopsy in early and questionable cases of systemic sclerosis. He must be told that microscopic examination of a skin specimen, usually obtained from a finger or the wrist, is apt to be less informative than clinical judgment. Its main value is in ruling out other skin disease and in establishing a record for comparison with later biopsies.

Morphea and Linear Scleroderma

Histologic diagnosis is more satisfactory[7] in *localized scleroderma* or *morphea* (Fig. 25-2), which

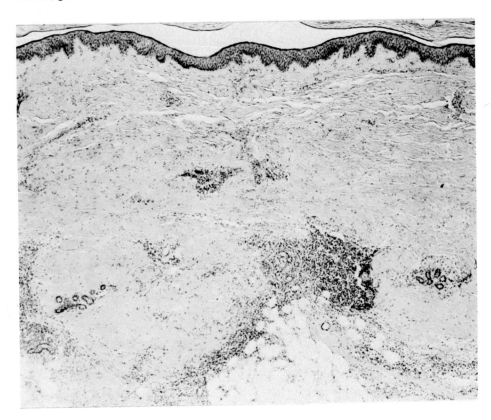

FIGURE 25–2.
Morphea. Lesion shows somewhat more inflammatory infiltrate than average case. Note obliteration of differences between pars papillaris and pars reticularis of dermis and extension of dense fibrous tissue below sweat coils, which seem atrophic. H&E. X60.

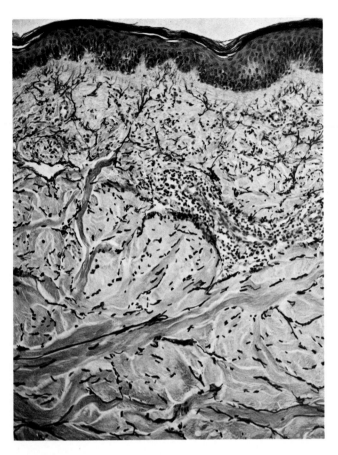

FIGURE 25–3.
Morphea at higher magnification. Structure of epidermis and distribution of connective tissue fibers are quite normal. Elastic fibers are chopped into pieces of different lengths by microtome knife. There is no fragmentation of elastic fibers. The collagen bundles are thick and dense, interfascicular spaces narrow. O&G. X135.

usually has to be differentiated from lichen sclerosus, atrophoderma, and other dermatoses with which it may be confused clinically. Most of the description given for generalized scleroderma is applicable. The epidermis usually is relatively normal, elastic fibers are preserved (Fig. 25-3), the dermis looks dense, and fibrocytes are sparse. While pars papillaris and reticularis are involved equally in some cases and the structural differences between them are obliterated, there are cases in which the subpapillary layer looks more sclerotic than the deeper portions, or the sclerosis may spare the upper dermis and involve mainly the deep dermis and even the subcutaneous tissue. Inflammatory infiltrate is more regularly found (Fig. 25-2) than in generalized scleroderma. It usually involves deep dermal vessels and may be spotty and mild or rather pronounced and almost continuous. In these cases the differentiation from lichen sclerosus et atrophicus may be difficult. Plasma cells are rare, and granulomatous infiltrate is not found, except secondary to calcification.

Nothing of special note can be said about the *linear type of scleroderma* except that it may involve the deeper tissue along with the skin. *Linear melorheostotic scleroderma* is a rare event encountered in association with, but probably not secondary to, specific bone lesions and also involving the subcutaneous tissue.[8] The calcifying form, so-called CRST syndrome, will be mentioned in Chapter 27.

Sclerodermoid Disorders

Attention is directed here to the prior discussion of pseudosclerodermatous artifact (Chap. 3, Fig. 3-5).

Sclerodermoid changes are encountered in the Winchester syndrome,[9,10] in which an abnormal function of fibroblasts is suspected. Scleroderma may be imitated by *pachydermoperiostosis*, which affects both skin and bones of extremities and face and exhibits thickened dermis and thick fibrous bands extending into the subcutis.[11] In contrast to scleroderma, however, there is an increase of fibroblasts and ground substance.[12] *Sclerodermoid* hardening of exposed skin occurs in porphyria cutanea tarda and is difficult to distinguish from scleroderma histologically, except that it usually does not involve subcutaneous tissue and is associated with actinic elastosis and possibly some evidence of scar formation from preceding blistering (Chap. 11). On the other hand, Fleischmajer and Nedwich[13] found the subcutaneous tissue replaced by hyalinized connective tissue in a sclerodermoid plaque of *Werner's syndrome*. Recently, a completely new type of severe and extensive sclerodermoid change of skin and subcutaneous tissue has been observed after *pentazocine* injections.[14] There is extensive collagenous fibrosis, and the elastic fibers are correspondingly reduced. *Acroosteolysis* may produce sclerodermoid histology in both its spontaneous[15] and occupational forms.[16] *Graft-versus-host reaction* may assume sclerodermoid aspects in the chronic stage both clinically and histologically. While the pathomechanism is speculative at present, investigation of more cases may throw light on the pathogenesis of scleroderma.[17]

Eosinophilic Fasciitis

Shulman[18] described a number of patients with onset of deep induration after physical exercise which subsided slowly under steroid therapy. Histologic

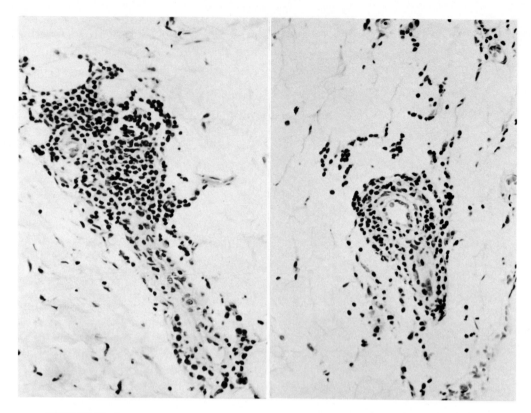

FIGURE 25–4.
Eosinophilic fasciitis. Perivascular infiltrate in fat tissue near deep fascia. H&E. X400.

examination showed sclerosing deep fasciitis with perivascular infiltrate (Fig. 25-4) and increased numbers of eosinophils in the blood count. Two dozen cases have been reported in the last few years. Fleischmajer et al.[19] suggest that there are transitions between *eosinophilic fasciitis* and systemic sclerosis, but the more acute onset and favorable outcome in many cases are remarkable and force one to demand large biopsy specimens, including deep fascia, in suspected cases.

ATROPHODERMAS AND LIPODYSTROPHIES

Atrophoderma of Pasini and Pierini

In pure cases of *idiopathic atrophoderma* of Pasini and Pierini,[20,21] none of the features of scleroderma or any other alteration are present except that epidermis and dermis are somewhat thinner than normal. This feature (Fig. 25-5) can be recognized only by comparison. Examination (Chap. 3) requires either a fairly long strip of skin extending from normal across the shoulder into the depressed area, or two 6-mm punch biopsies, one taken outside, the other inside the lesion. Both must include a considerable portion of the subcutaneous panniculus and

should be processed together and mounted side by side for comparison.

Senile Atrophy

In pure *senile atrophy* unrelated to climatic influences or disease, the thickness of the epidermis is reduced by one or two cell layers, and rete ridges and papillae tend to be effaced. The dermis exhibits progressive loss of papillary capillaries and some general thinning that does not strikingly alter the proportion of collagenous and elastic fibers, although aged skin probably contains relatively more elastin than does young adult skin. The lobes of the subcutaneous fat tissue may grow smaller because fat cells are reduced in size. Pilar and eccrine apparatuses may or may not be affected. In truth, the nonexposed integument of many old individuals does not exhibit any noticeable histologic changes.

Progeria

A generalized form of atrophy is *progeria*,[22,23] in which all elements of skin and subcutaneous tissue are atrophic. The deeper parts of the dermis may show hyalinization.

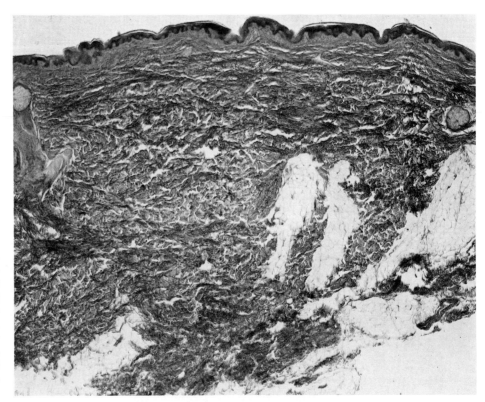

FIGURE 25–5.
Idiopathic atrophoderma (Pasini and Pierini). Normal dermis at left is almost twice as thick as atrophic dermis at right, as indicated by distribution of subcutaneous fat tissue. Skin presents no other structural or inflammatory changes. H&E. X45. (From Mehregan and Pinkus: Dermatol Dig 7:49, 1968.)

Diabetic Dermopathy

Localized *atrophic and pigmented macules* on the shins of diabetic men have been described as due to diabetic microangiopathy.[24] We have not been able to convince ourselves of how to distinguish them histologically from post-traumatic scars in a very vulnerable region of the skin also exhibiting angiopathy[25] in a diabetic patient. Anetoderma will be dealt with in Chapter 26.

Corticosteroid Atrophy

Atrophy caused by local application of corticosteroid preparations, whether fluorinated or not, can be most disturbing and must be considered in many skin biopsy specimens of chronic disease. The perioral dermatitis evidently caused by long-continued steroid applications to facial skin is a prominent example and was discussed in Chapter 8. Epidermal atrophy of varying degree occurs early.[26] The visible and palpable thinning of the skin is due mainly to a decrease of collagen, leading to a crowding together of elastic fibers, which, however, do not exhibit the changes of actinic elastosis. Sweat coils are found much closer to the epidermis than in normal skin. These changes were discussed in detail by Wilson-Jones and by others in a symposium on corticosteroid therapy.[27]

Acrodermatitis Chronica Atrophicans

Acrodermatitis chronica atrophicans can lead to extreme degrees of cutaneous and subcutaneous atrophy but is the end result of a characteristic inflammatory process, which probably is due to an infectious agent endemic in parts of the Old World.[28,29] In the early stages, the dermis is edematous and contains focal infiltrate of lymphocytes, plasma cells, and some histiocytes. Elastic fibers are destroyed early, and epidermis and pilosebaceous complexes undergo atrophy, while eccrine glands are apt to persist. In later stages, the inflammatory component disappears, but the extensive loss of elastic fibers differentiates the lesion from primary atrophies. Cases have been reported in which malignant lymphoma developed.[30]

Lipodystrophy

Several clinical forms of lipodystrophy exist. Congenital lipodystrophy,[31] localized atrophy after insulin injections, Gower's panatrophy, and lipodystrophia centrifugalis abdominalis[32,33] all are characterized by more or less complete disappearance of subcutaneous fat tissue without specific histologic characteristics, although the last-named rare condition is said to have inflammatory infiltrate and sclerosis in deep dermis and panniculus.

Aplasia Cutis Congenita

The most extreme instances of cutaneous atrophy or defective development are cases of aplasia cutis congenita.[34] These defects are most often seen on the scalp of newborn infants and gradually heal with an atrophic scar devoid of cutaneous adnexa. They have been interpreted as aplastic (minus) nevi (Sec. VII) by Schoenfeld and Mehregan.[35] Another type of congenital localized absence of skin with other associated abnormalities was described by Bart et al.[36] This particular lesion is often localized to the legs and has some features of epidermolysis bullosa. It is inherited in autosomal dominant fashion, although it may be encountered as a solitary case.[37]

LICHEN SCLEROSUS ET ATROPHICUS

In contrast to morphea, lichen sclerosus et atrophicus (Figs. 5-2 and 25-6) exhibits marked changes not only of collagen but of epidermis and elastic fibers as well. The rete malpighi is thinned, and ridges and papillae are flattened or lost. Basal cells are flat, often vacuolated. The horny and granular layers are thick and are partly responsible for the chalky white clinical appearance. Hair follicles and sweat glands undergo atrophy, and their ostia are dilated with keratin corresponding to the black comedolike plugs of the typical early case. Later, they may disappear completely. The most characteristic feature is a peculiar homogenization of the

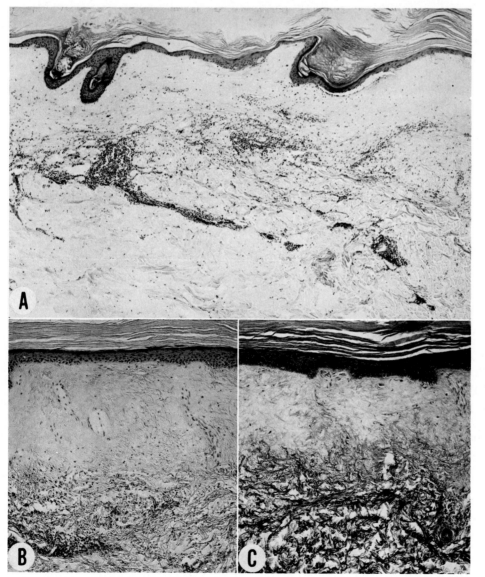

FIGURE 25–6.
*Lichen sclerosus et atrophicus. **A.** Dense hyperkeratosis, epidermal atrophy, and keratotic plugging of hair follicles and sweat ducts above a zone of edematous dermis and deep infiltrate. The subepidermal cleft is probably a technical artifact but indicates diminished adhesion between epidermis and dermis. H&E. X45. **B** and **C.** Sections of another specimen stained H&E and O&G, respectively, to show edematous homogenization and loss of elastic fibers of pars papillaris and upper pars reticularis. X75.*

upper dermis, which on closer analysis is quite different from sclerosis.[38] The collagen bundles seem to become diffused within the markedly increased ground substance, which gives the impression of edema in H&E and O&G sections, and stains positive for hyaluronic acid. In pronounced cases, especially in the genital area of children, this change leads to subepidermal bullae through rarefaction of the fibers. Within this zone, a few ectatic thin-walled vessels are seen which may rupture and produce hemorrhage. O&G stains (Fig. 25–6C) show interesting phenomena. Even though the homogenized zone may be narrow, it always involves the pars reticularis, the pars papillaris frequently being just as atrophic as the epidermis. Elastic fibers are diminished either in foci or diffusely. O&G stain also emphasizes loss of epidermal pigment and presence of melanin-filled macrophages in the upper dermis.

Below the involved zone, there is round cell infiltrate which may be focal or continuous. Below it, the dermis is normal. Sections through an entire small papule show the infiltrate beginning at either side just at the epidermis and curving below the homogenized zone. If the infiltrate is fairly heavy, the similarity to atrophying lichen planus (Fig. 9-8) may be striking in H&E sections. O&G sections, however, show that all the changes in lichen planus are in the widened pars papillaris, while they are in the pars reticularis in lichen sclerosus. If the infiltrate is minor, and one is dealing with a small portion of a larger plaque, differential diagnosis from morphea may be difficult. Epidermal atrophy and derangement of elastic fibers speak for lichen sclerosus.

Lichen sclerosus et atrophicus may affect any part of the skin surface, including palms and soles, but has a predilection for the female anogenital region, where it has been confused with leukoplakia and often is called *kraurosis vulvae*. Lesions on the glans penis were given the appellation *balanitis xerotica obliterans*. These localizations will be discussed in Chapter 45.

REACTIVE PERFORATING COLLAGENOSIS

A remarkable histobiologic process involving collagenous tissue was described a few years ago[39] and has since been recognized in at least 24 other cases. Autosomal dominance has been suggested, and the condition seems to be a congenital tendency of connective tissue of the upper dermis to become easily damaged by superficial scratches and possibly by cold.[40] The devitalized portion of dermis is then eliminated transepidermally amid some reactive inflammation (Fig. 25-7; see also Fig. 5-12B). Isolated instances of basophilic damaged collagen undergoing transepithelial elimination in the form of self-healing verrucous papules were repeatedly described in the French literature (*collagénome perforant verruciforme*[41]).

EHLERS–DANLOS SYNDROME

Cutis hyperelastica has traditionally been discussed in chapters on elastic tissue disturbances. It seems, however, likely that Ehlers-Danlos syndrome is due to a disturbance in collagen rather than in elastic fibers.[42–44] Based on clinical manifestations, mode of inheritance, and underlying biochemical defects, eight types of Ehlers-Danlos syndrome have been recognized (Table 25-1).[45] Histologic examination is peculiarly disappointing. If there is any alteration at all, it is a relative abundance of elastic tissue in relation to collagen. One should, however, keep in mind that specimens taken from afflicted patients contract more than normal skin and ought to be stretched to original size and fixed in this state before any quantitative estimate is attempted. The secondary lesions, hematomas and fibrotic scars, will of course show definite histologic changes.

SCLEREDEMA, LYMPHEDEMA, AND MYXEDEMA

The wooden hard indurations of *scleredema adultorum* are histologically disappointing because they are due to increased hyaluronic acid in the ground substance. Routine H&E and O&G sections show little, inasmuch as edema is difficult to judge. Mucopolysaccharide stains are needed. *Lymphedema* also is hard to recognize, but pronounced cases show such excessive fraying and separation of collagen bundles that a spectacular picture results. Dilated lymph vessels, so inconspicuous in H&E sections, often stand out nicely in O&G sections due to their elastic coat. Cases of *verrucous lymphedema* (Fig. 25-8) show an even more spectacular configuration. It is worth remembering that most cases clinically suspected to be *pyoderma vegetans* turn out to be verrucous lymphedema with some secondary inflammation.

Myxedema of the generalized and tuberous types show essentially similar features (Fig. 25-9), except that the changes are fairly sharply localized in the second form. H&E and O&G sections show wi-

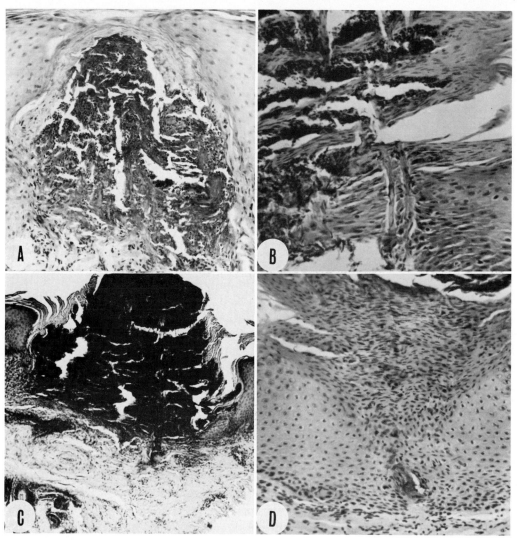

FIGURE 25–7.
*Reactive perforating collagenosis. **A** and **C**. Early and late stage of the process. H&E. **B** and **D**. Details of thin collagen bundles being eliminated transepidermally. H&E. **A**. X135. **B**. X135. **C**. X45. **D**. X90.*

TABLE 25–1.
Clinical, Genetic, and Biochemical Classification of Ehlers–Danlos Syndrome

Type	Inheritance	Clinical Manifestations	Biochemical Defects
Gravis	Autosomal dominant	Hyperextensibility of skin, marked fragility, atrophic scars, and molluscoid pseudotumors, hypermobility of joints	Unknown
Mitis	Autosomal dominant	Hyperextensibility of skin, hypermobility of joints, bleeding problems	Unknown
Benign hypermobile	Autosomal dominant	Marked joint hypermobility, minimal skin manifestations	Unknown
Ecchymotic	Autosomal recessive	Hypermobility limited to digits, skin fragility with ecchymoses, arterial rupture	Deficiency of type III collagen
X-linked	X-linked recessive	Minimal joint hypermobility, hyperextensibility of skin with bruising, skeletal disorders	Lysyl oxidase deficiency
Ocular	Autosomal recessive	Hyperextensibility of skin, hypermobility of joints, scleral and corneal fragility	Lysyl hydroxylase deficiency
Arthrocalasis multiplex congenita	Autosomal recessive	Hyperextensibility and fragility of skin, hypermobility of joints, short stature, multiple dislocations	Defective conversion of procollagen to collagen
Periodontitis	Autosomal dominant	Minimal skin hyperextensibility, hypermobility of joints, advanced periodontitis	Unknown

Adapted from Bauer and Uitto.[43]

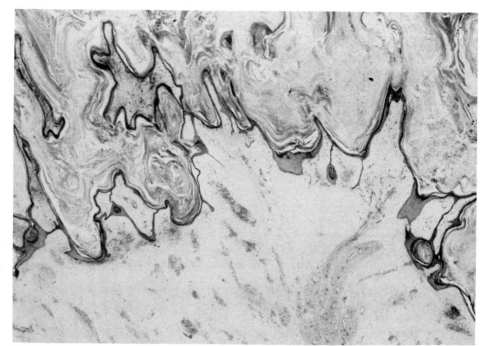

FIGURE 25–8.
Verrucous lymphedema. Extreme rarefication of collagenous substance of dermis, which, however, is rich in blood vessels. Voluminous papillae have elevated the thin and hyperkeratotic epidermis to produce a highly papillomatous pattern. H&E. X28.

dened interfascicular spaces as in simple edema but also show fraying of collagen bundles, which may become almost as extreme as in lymphedema. The mucin, being mainly hyaluronic acid, stains bright blue with Hale method or alcian blue stain and may entirely obscure the collagen in such sections. It is unusual, though, to find resemblance to myxomatous tissue because the fibrocytes do not assume stellate shape or form a network.

Mucopolysaccharidoses

We just mention here *Hurler's syndrome* and other mucopolysaccharidoses and mucolipidoses,[46] in which various unusual metachromatic substances are deposited in many types of cells, including dermal fibrocytes and epidermal cells. These deposits may appear as cytoplasmic vacuoles in routine sections and may require fixation in alcohol because

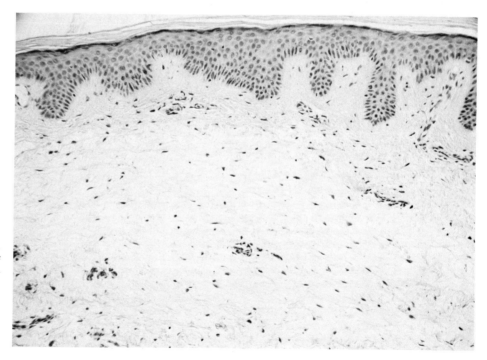

FIGURE 25–9.
Pretibial myxedema. The increased mucinous content of the ground substance is not evident in either H&E or O&G sections and must be confirmed by methods for demonstration of hyaluronic acid. H&E. X135.

of their water solubility. An electron microscopic study of the specific subscapular papulosis of *Hunter's syndrome* was offered by Larrègne et al.[47]

Lichen Myxedematosus: Papular Mucinosis and Scleromyxedema

Accumulation of mucin substances, especially hyaluronic acid, is characteristic of a number of clinical disease pictures not related to thyroid disease. In some of these, it is a helpful but secondary diagnostic feature, while in others, it is pathognomonic. To the first group belong *acute lupus erythematosus, dermatomyositis, lichen sclerosus et atrophicus, granuloma annulare,* and *Degos' malignant papulosis.* The second group includes localized lesions, such as *mucous papules* and *synovial lesions* (see below), and more widespread ones, such as *papular mucinosis* and *scleromyxedema.* The two latter have been lumped together in North American literature under the name *lichen myxedematosus* but deserve to be kept apart because there are considerable differences in clinical picture, prognosis, histologic changes, and pathogenesis.[48-50]

The clinical manifestations of papular mucinosis, grouped papules which come and go over a period of months or years, are represented by myxomatous histologic changes.[51] There is an ill-defined area in which collagen bundles are frayed,

and stellate fibrocytes are suspended in the meshes filled with hyaluronic acid (Fig. 25-10).

Scleromyxedema, on the other hand, clinically characterized by general thickening of the skin on which papules and nodules are superimposed, often gives the impression of a fibroma histologically because there is considerable increase of fixed tissue cells with relatively little increase in ground substance (Fig. 25-11), at least in young lesions. A specific paraprotein has been found in the serum in most cases.

REM Syndrome

An erythematous reticular maculopapular eruption encountered usually on the backs of women was described by Steigleder et al.[52] as *reticular erythematous mucinous syndrome*, because increased amounts of hyaluronic acid were found in addition to perivascular round cell infiltrates. The rash responds to chloroquine administration. Further investigation will be needed to establish it as a separate entity.[53]

SYNOVIAL LESIONS AND MUCOUS PAPULES

Isolated papules and nodules consisting of myxomatous tissue may occur anywhere on the skin,

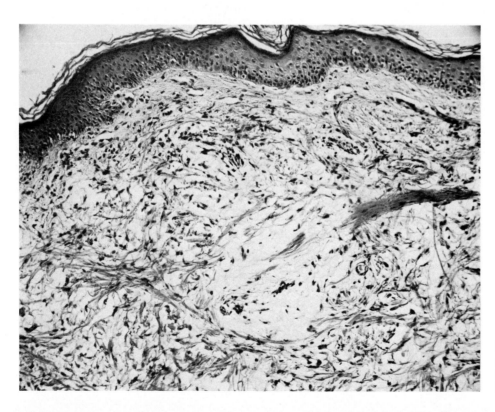

FIGURE 25–10.
Papular mucinosis. Note myxomatous aspect due to stellate fibroblasts. H&E. X135.

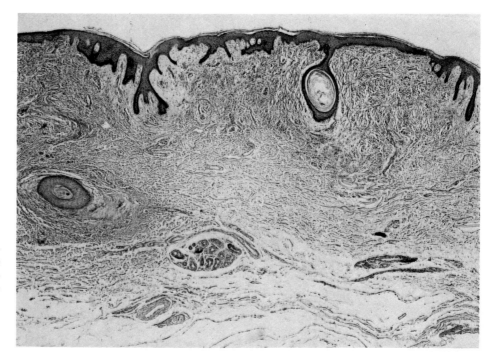

FIGURE 25–11.
Scleromyxedema. Overall impression is that of a fibroma. In some of these lesions it requires a high level of suspicion to recognize mucinous change. Note general thickening of skin. H&E. X30. (From Rudner et al. Arch Dermatol 93:3, 1966.)

but there is a typical localization on the distal phalanx of the finger, just proximal to the nail fold. These lesions clinically resemble cysts and are known as *synovial lesions* or *myxoid cysts*.[54] They discharge mucinous fluid or jelly periodically and then fill again. Histologically, no true cyst is found. The tissue (Fig. 25–12A, B) may vary from a fibromatous to a myxomatous aspect, depending on the stage. It is fairly characteristic that the epidermis is very thin though hyperkeratotic, and sometimes one finds layers of inspissated mucus alternating with keratinous lamellae. The connection which these lesions often have with joint[55] or tendon sheath usually cannot be demonstrated in sections.

Larger cutaneous plaques consisting of myxomatous tissue raise the question of a true myxoma (Chap. 41) versus a reactive process.

AFFECTIONS OF EAR CARTILAGE

The elastic cartilage of the ear is so close to the skin that lesions affecting it must be considered. The most common one, *chondrodermatitis nodularis chronica helicis* was discussed in Chapter 17.

Long-continued traumatic injury to the ears of professional boxers leads to the so-called cauliflower ear. A similar affection, without definite history of trauma, was investigated by Mendelson and Lund[56] under the name *pseudocyst of the auricle*. It was found to consist of eosinophilic hyalinized material deposited between the superficial and deep portions of the cartilage and including cystic

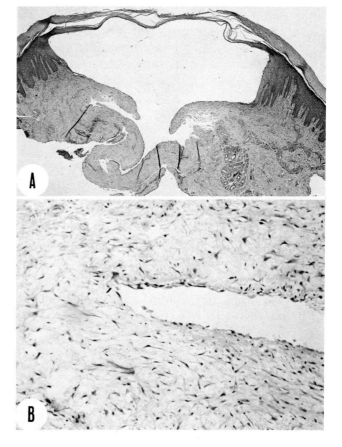

FIGURE 25–12.
Synovial lesion of finger. **A.** *Note extension into deep tissue, pressure atrophy of epidermis, and absence of cyst wall. H&E. X30.* **B.** *Myxomatous aspect of connective tissue. H&E. X250.*

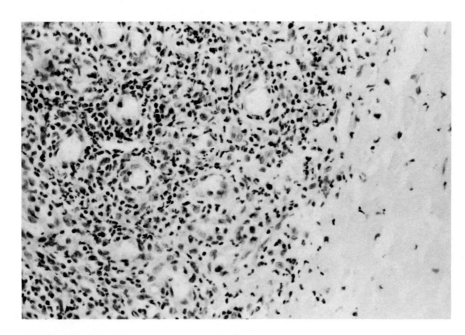

FIGURE 25–13.
Relapsing polychondritis. Devitalized cartilage on right. Vascular granulation tissue with infiltrate containing polymorphs, both neutrophilic and eosinophilic, on left. H&E. X250.

spaces and scattered chondroblasts and fibroblasts.

A potentially much more serious disease, *relapsing polychondritis,* often is manifested first on the ears. Histologically (Fig. 25-13), the cartilage shows diminished metachromasia and peripheral inflammatory infiltrate with round cells, plasma cells, eosinophils, and polymorphonuclears. An autoimmune reaction is the suspected cause.[57,58]

REFERENCES

1. Jablonska S (ed): Scleroderma and Pseudoscleroderma, 2nd ed. Warsaw, Polish Medical Publishers, 1975
2. Le Roy EC: Increased collagen synthesis by scleroderma skin fibroblasts in vitro: possible defect in regulation or activation of scleroderma fibroblasts. J Clin Invest 54:880, 1974
3. Fleischmajer R, Damiano V, Nedwich A: Alteration of subcutaneous tissue in systemic scleroderma. Arch Dermatol 105:59, 1972
4. Fleischmajer R, Perlish JS, West, WP: Ultrastructure of cutaneous cellular infiltrates in scleroderma. Arch Dermatol 113:1661, 1977
5. Garb J, Sims FC: Scleroderma with bullous lesions. Report of a case and review of the literature. Dermatologica 119:341, 1959
6. Tuffanelli DL: Lymphangiectasis due to scleroderma. Arch Dermatol 111:1216, 1975
7. Fleischmajer R, Nedwich A: Generalized morphea: histology of the dermis and subcutaneous tissue. Arch Dermatol 106:509, 1972
8. Miyashi Y, Horio T, Yamada A, et al.: Linear melorheostotic scleroderma with hypertrichosis. Arch Dermatol 115:1233, 1979
9. Cohen AH, Hollister DW, Reed WB: The skin in the Winchester syndrome. Histologic and ultrastructural studies. Arch Dermatol 111:230, 1975
10. Nabai H, Mehregan AH, Mortezai A, et al.: Winchester syndrome: report of a case from Iran. J Cutan Pathol 4:281, 1977
11. Vogl A, Goldfischer S: Pachydermoperiostosis. Am J Med 33:166, 1962
12. Hambrick GW, Carter DM: Pachydermoperiostosis. Arch Dermatol 94:504, 1966
13. Fleischmajer R, Nedwich A: Werner's syndrome. Am J Med 54:111, 1973
14. Parks DL, Perry HO, Muller SA: Cutaneous complications of pentazocine injections. Arch Dermatol 104:231, 1971
15. Meyerson, LB, Meier GC: Cutaneous lesions in acroosteolysis. Arch Dermatol 106:224, 1972
16. Markowitz SS, McDonald CJ, Fethiere W, et al.: Occupational acroosteolysis. Arch Dermatol 106:219, 1972
17. Spielvogel RL, Goltz RW, Kersey JH: Scleroderma-like changes in chronic graft vs host disease. Arch Dermatol 113:1424, 1977
18. Shulman LE: Diffuse fasciitis with eosinophilia: a new syndrome? Trans Assoc Am Physicians 88:70, 1975
19. Fleischmajer R, Jacotot AB, Shore S, et al.: Scleroderma, eosinophilia, and diffuse fasciitis. Arch Dermatol 114:1320, 1978
20. Canizares O, Sachs PM, Jaimovich L, et al.: Idiopathic atrophoderma of Pasini and Pierini. Arch Dermatol 77:42, 1958
21. Pierini LE, Abulafia J, Mosto SJ: Atrophodermie idiopathique progressive et états voisins. Ann Dermatol Syphiligr 97:391, 1970
22. DeBusk FL: The Hutchinson–Gilford progeria syndrome. J Pediatr 80:697, 1972
23. Fleischmajer R, Nedwich A: Progeria (Hutchinson-Gilford). Arch Dermatol 107:253, 1973b
24. Kerl H, Kresbach H: Prätibiale atrophische Pigmentflecke; ein mikrovaskulär bedingtes Hautsymptom des Diabetes mellitus. Hautarzt 23:59, 1972
25. Lisi P: La microangiopatia diabetica cutanea. Ann Ital Dermatol Clin Sper 32:111, 1978

26. Kelly EW Jr: The effects of triamcinolone on human skin. J Natl Med Assoc 55:510, 1963

27. Polano MK, et al. (eds): Advances in topical cortosteroid therapy. Dermatologica 152 [Suppl 1], 1976

28. Hauser W: Zur Klinik, Ätiologie und Pathogenese der Akrodermatitis chronica atrophicans. Hautarzt 6:77, 1955

29. Negosanti M, Varotti C, Cocchia D, et al.: Acrodermatite cronica atrofizzante. Osservazioni cliniche ed ultramicrospociche. Arch Ital Dermatol 40:15, 1975

30. Goos M: Acrodermatitis chronica atrophicans and malignant lymphoma. Acta Derm Venereol (Stockh) 51:457, 1971

31. Gordon H, Pimestone BL, Leary PM, et al.: Congenital generalized lipodystrophy with abnormal growth hormone homeostasis. Arch Dermatol 104:551, 1971

32. Cairns RJ: Lipodystrophia centrifugalis abdominalis infantilis. Br J Dermatol 95 [Suppl 14]:44, 1976

33. Imamura S, Yamada M: Lipodystrophia centrifugalis abdominalis infantilis. Br J Dermatol 96:96, 1977

34. Deekin JH, Caplan RM: Aplasia cutis congenita. Arch Dermatol 102:386, 1970

35. Schoenfeld RJ, Mehregan AH: Aplastic nevus—the "minus" nevus. Cutis 12:386, 1973

36. Bart BJ, Gorlin RJ, Anderson VE, et al.: Congential localized absence of skin and associated abnormalities resembling epidermolysis bullosa. Arch Dermatol 93:296, 1966

37. Smith SZ, Crain DL: A mechanobullous disease of the newborn. Bart's syndrome. Arch Dermatol 114:81, 1978

38. Mann PR, Cowan MA: Ultrastructural changes in four cases of lichen sclerosus et atrophicus. Br J Dermatol 89:223, 1973

39. Mehregan AH, Schwartz OD, Livingood CS: Reactive perforating collagenosis. Arch Dermatol 96:277, 1967

40. Kanan MW: Familial reactive perforating collagenosis and intolerance to cold. Br J Dermatol 91:405, 1974

41. Guilaine J, Molas G, Collonier C, et al.: Un nouveau cas de collagénome perforant verruciforme de Laugier et Woringer. Ann Dermatol Venereol 104:409, 1977

42. Pinnell SR, Krane SM, Kenzora JE, et al.: A heritable disorder of connective tissue: hydroxylysine-deficient collagen disease. N Engl J Med 286:1013, 1972

43. Bauer EA, Uitto J: Collagen in cutaneous diseases. Int J Dermatol 18:251, 1979

44. Bassière ML: Acrokérato-élastoidose. Bull Soc Fr Dermatol Syphiligr 81:27, 1974

45. Sulica VI, Cooper PH, Pope MF, et al.: Cutaneous histologic features in Ehlers-Danlos syndrome. Study of 21 patients. Arch Dermatol 115:40, 1979

46. Greaves MW, Inman PM: Cutaneous changes in the Morquio syndrome. Br J Dermatol 81:29, 1969

47. Larrègne M, Debray H, Père C, et al.: Papulose sous-scapulaire systématisée avec corps anhistes en microscopie électronique: signes cutanés spécifiques de la maladie de Hunter. Ann Dermatol Venereol 105:57, 1978

48. Rudner EJ, Mehregan AH, Pinkus H: Scleromyxedema, a variant of lichen myxedematosus. Arch Dermatol 93:3, 1966

49. Colomb D, Vittori F, Beyvin AJ, et al.: La mort d'une mucinose papuleuse de type scléro-myxoedème d'Arndt-Gottron. Nouveaux documents anatomo-cliniques, biologiques et ultra-structuraux. Ann Dermatol Syphiligr (Paris) 101:519, 1974

50. Piérard GE, Hermans JF, Lapière CM: Dynamics of the connective tissue remodeling and of its impaired mechanical properties in scleromyxedema. J Cutan Pathol 4:203, 1977

51. Coskey RJ, Mehregan AH: Papular mucinosis. Int J Dermatol 16:741, 1977

52. Steigleder GK, Gartmann H, Linker U: REM syndrome: reticular erythematous mucinosis (round-cell erythematosis), a new entity? Br J Dermatol 91:191, 1974

53. Morrison WL, Shea CR, Parrish JA: Reticular erythematous mucinosis syndrome. Report of two cases. Arch Dermatol 115:1340, 1979

54. Johnson WC, Graham JH, Helwig EB: Cutaneous myxoid cyst. JAMA 191:15, 1965

55. Newmeyer WL, Kilgore ES Jr, Graham WP III: Mucous cysts: the dorsal distal interphalangeal joint ganglion. Plast Reconstr Surg 53:313, 1974

56. Mendelson DS, Lund HZ: The history of pseudocyst of the auricle: resemblance and possible relation to cauliflower ear. Arch Dermatol 114:1831, 1978

57. Martin JM, Roenigk HH, Lynch W, et al.: Relapsing polychondritis treated with dapsone. Arch Dermatol 112:1272, 1976

58. Barranco VP, Minor DB, Solomon H: Treatment of relapsing polychondritis with dapsone. Arch Dermatol 112:1286, 1976

CHAPTER
26

Disorders of Elastic Fibers

NORMAL PROPERTIES

The elastic fibers of the skin form a three-dimensional network in the pars reticularis and around the subpapillary vascular plexus. They have a brushlike arrangement in the upper portion of the pars papillaris (Chap. 2). Their function is to prevent overstretching of the skin and to return the stretched skin to its normal configuration. Localized loss of superficial fibers leads to the wrinkled appearance seen in *superficial scars* or to the mild atrophy following *lichen planus* and some other conditions. Loss of fibers in the pars reticularis leads to bulging and buttonhole-type loss of resistance in the affected area (*stria, anetoderma*) unless the skin is at the same time hardened by collagenous fibrosis.

In electron microscopy, elastic fibers are made up of two distinct components, the fibrillar (elastic fibrils or microfibrils) portion and the homogeneous matrix.[1] The elastic fibrils range in diameter from 5 to 15 nm and are moderately electron dense. Their surfaces appear homogeneous or show a periodicity of 12 to 17 nm.[2] The matrix is electron transparent or shows slight density. In contrast the collagen fibers are made of bundles of tightly packed fibrils. The fibrils are 30 to 60 nm in diameter and are moderately electron dense, showing cross striation appearing at 64 to 78 nm intervals.[3]

It was pointed out in Chapters 5 and 6 that thorough knowledge of the normal configuration and distribution of elastic fibers and routine examination for elastic fiber pathology is of great value in a variety of dermatoses ranging from inflammation to neoplasia. We point out again that many elastic fibers are chopped into short pieces by the microtome knife and that these fragments should not be mistaken for pathologic fragmentation (Fig. 5-18). Tinctorial properties were discussed in Chapter 3. Here we recall that elastic fibers are practically unidentifiable in H&E-stained sections, while routine use of the O&G stain permits appraisal of this important constituent of the skin in every case. Acid orcein is the most satisfactory elastic fiber stain for pathologic skin because it stains practically no other tissue components, while the Verhoeff procedure stains nuclei, and Gomori's aldehyde fuchsin stains mucin. The Verhoeff method also does not stain young and thin elastic fibers, recently designated as elaunin fibers.[4]

DISTURBANCES

Diseases and conditions specifically characterized by alterations and disturbances of the elastic tissue are shown in Table 26-1. They were thoroughly discussed at a congress of French dermatologists in 1965[5] and by Reed et al.[6] in 1973.

TABLE 26–1.
Disturbances of Elastic Tissue

Congenital
  Circumscribed
    Nevus elasticus, Lewandowsky type (minus nevus)
    Juvenile elastoma; nevus elasticus, Staricco–
    Mehregan type (plus nevus)
  Generalized
    Cutis laxa (generalized elastolysis)
    Pseudoxanthoma elasticum
Acquired
  Idiopathic
    Elastosis perforans serpiginosa
    Anetoderma, primary
  Induced
    Actinic elastosis and related conditions
    Anetoderma, secondary
    Stria distensa

Congenitial

Nevus Elasticus. Nevoid disturbances of elastic tissue which manifest themselves clinically as papules or plaques of pale or yellowish color may be on the minus or plus side. Lewandowsky's *nevus elasticus regionis mammariae* actually is a collagenous nevus in which elastic fibers are distributed in an uneven manner. Other lesions, described as *juve-*

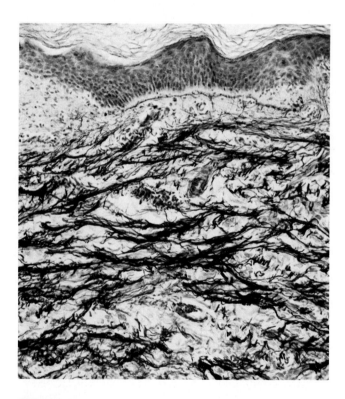

FIGURE 26–1.
Nevus elasticus (juvenile elastoma) shows hyperplasia of morphologically normal elastic fibers. O&G. X135.

nile elastoma or *nevus elasticus en tumeurs disséminés*, show a marked increase (Fig. 26-1) in number and diameter of elastic fibers. There may be increased vascularity.[7] In Buschke–Ollendorff syndrome (*dermatofibrosis lenticularis disseminata*), multiple papular and plaquelike skin lesions occur in association with osteopoikilosis. Skin lesions show localized elastic tissue hyperplasia that is indistinguishable from nevus elasticus.[8,9]

Pseudoxanthoma Elasticum. Although this disease is an inherited systemic disorder of connective tissue,[1] expression of the trait is peculiarly patchy even in the skin. The specific changes (Fig. 26-2) are seen in the middermis, while pars papillaris and deep dermis usually show normal elastic morphology.[10] In the affected foci, the fibers stain more strongly with hematoxylin because they contain more calcium, and thus they become more visible in H&E sections, having a tinge similar to basophilic degeneration seen in actinic elastosis (see below).

The peculiar morphology of the affected fibers has been described as broken, frayed, or curled. The best comparison seems to be that of raveled wool (Zola Cooper). The increased calcium content, which makes the Von Kossa stain a favorite means of identification, is very obvious in the quantitative studies of the affected areas.[11] Sometimes massive calcification and secondary foreign-body granuloma lead to the formation of intrafollicular or transepidermal perforating channels.[12,13] Acid mucopolysaccharides demonstrable by the Hale method or alcian blue stain also are increased. Electron microscopic studies show primary depositions of calcium salts in the homogeneous matrix of the elastic fibers in addition to minor abnormalities of the collagen fibrils.[1] Cutaneous changes clinically similar and histologically indistinguishable from pseudoxanthoma have been reported in farmers exposed to saltpeter during land fertilization.[14,15]

Cutis Laxa. *Generalized elastolysis* is a good term to describe the clinical and histologic features of this disease. The soft and inelastic skin, which hangs in thick folds and seems much too large for the infant's body (*dermatomegaly*), shows a breakdown of elastic fibers (Fig. 26-3) into small fibrous particles or dustlike granules.[16–18] The severity of the changes varies topographically, and some areas of skin may look quite normal. In association with the breakdown of elastic fibers, there may be marked deposition of acid mucopolysaccharides forming small lakes between the connective tissue fibers. Systemic manifestations of cutis laxa in-

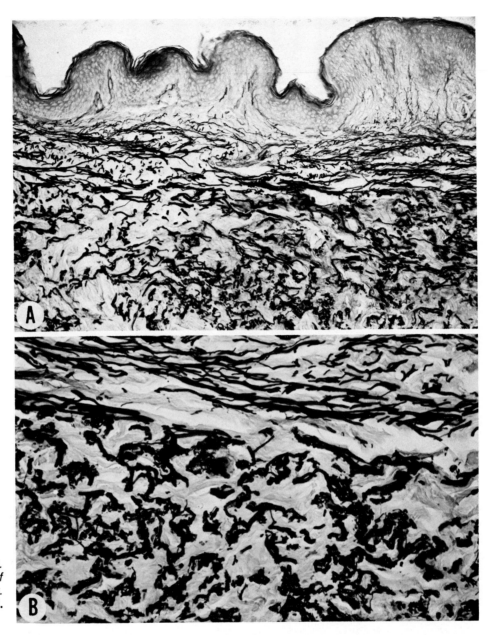

FIGURE 26–2.
Pseudoxanthoma elasticum. Raveled-wool appearance of elastic fibers in mid-dermis only. Aldehyde fuchsin. **A.** *X135.* **B.** *X225.*

clude pulmonary emphysema, cardiovascular abnormalities, various types of hernia, and multiple diverticula of the urinary bladder.[17]

The acquired form of cutis laxa appears later in life. Occasionally, a stage of generalized erythema or urticarial edema precedes the development of loose skin changes.[19] This form is not heritable but can be associated with emphysema and digestive tract abnormalities.[20]

Acquired

Elastosis Perforans Serpiginosa. The clinical picture of keratotic papules arranged in a ring or in serpiginous configuration around an atrophic center can be shown histologically (Figs. 26-4 and 26-5) to arise in a skin that has an overabundance of elastic fibers.[21] They may be otherwise normal or may be genetically defective, as in the cases associated with Ehlers–Danlos syndrome, osteogenesis imperfecta, or Marfan's syndrome.[22] Elastosis perforans serpiginosa may occur together with a generalized defective vascular system.[23,24] In another situation, elastosis perforans serpiginosa has appeared in patients with Down's syndrome under treatment with penicillamine. In these instances, abnormal elastic fibers exhibiting serrated outline can be demonstrated in the skin and respiratory system.[25,26] Outside the ring, the superficial elastic

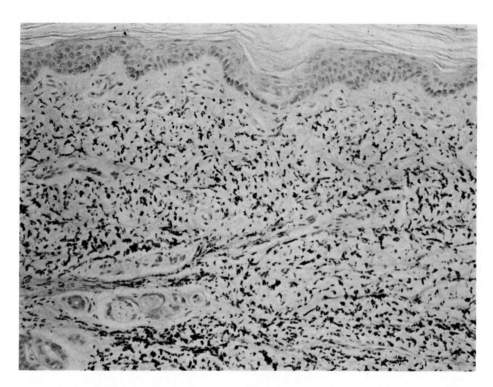

FIGURE 26–3.
Cutis laxa exhibits true fragmentation of elastic fibers (elastolysis). O&G. X225.

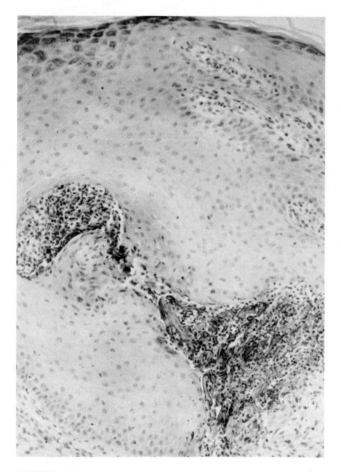

FIGURE 26–4.
Elastosis perforans serpiginosa. Perforating channel in proliferating epidermis contains connective tissue including refractile elastic fibers and leukocytes. H&E. X135.

fibers are coarser than normal and, in some areas, overlap with the lower border of the epidermal basal cells. In H&E sections, epithelial changes catch the eye (Fig. 26-4). There is epidermal thickening, sometimes resembling pseudoepitheliomatous proliferation, around single or multiple perforating channels. These canals extend from the corium to the skin surface either in a straight line or in wavy or corkscrew fashion.[22] They contain loose parakeratotic flakes peripherally and a central dense mass of bluish-staining necrobiotic material made up of exfoliating keratinocytes and degenerating inflammatory cells with which are mixed brightly eosinophilic fibers. The latter may resemble fungal mycelia if KOH preparations are examined. Small streams of connective tissue fibers mixed with degenerating leukocytic nuclei enter the perforating channels from below, and O&G stain shows that the elastic fibers lose their orceinophilia and become brightly eosinophilic. There may be foci of foreign-body granuloma, and the upper dermis inside the ring has lost its elastic fibers and resembles a fibrotic scar.

It is essential, then, to do elastic fiber stain whenever elastosis perforans is suggested by the clinical picture or when the histologic changes arouse suspicion. In H&E sections, it may be impossible to differentiate this disease from *reactive perforating collagenosis* (Chap. 25), *Kyrle's disease* (Chap. 18), or *perforating folliculitis* (Chap. 18). All of the latter lack the general elastic hyperplasia which is practically always associated with perfo-

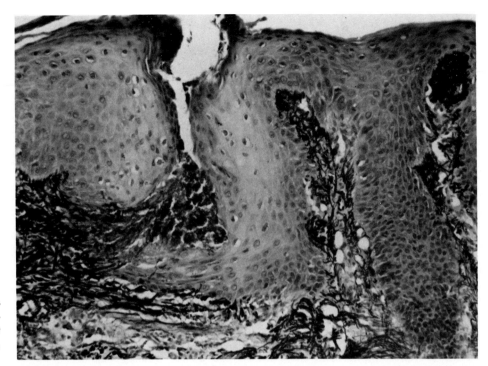

FIGURE 26–5.
Elastosis perforans serpiginosa. Note general hyperplasia of elastic fibers in dermis below perforating channels. O&G. X135.

rating elastosis. Collagenosis and Kyrle's disease do not contain either normal or eosinophilic elastic fibers in the perforating material. Although such fibers are often present in perforating folliculitis, the pathogenetic process is quite different in that affection, and the relation to a hair follicle is easily recognized.

Anetoderma. The three clinical types of *idiopathic macular atrophy*—that described by Jadassohn, the form named after Schweninger and Buzzi, and the Pelizzari type—share with each other and with secondary anetoderma one decisive histologic feature, that is, complete absence of elastic fibers (Fig. 26-6) in a skin otherwise practically normal.[27]

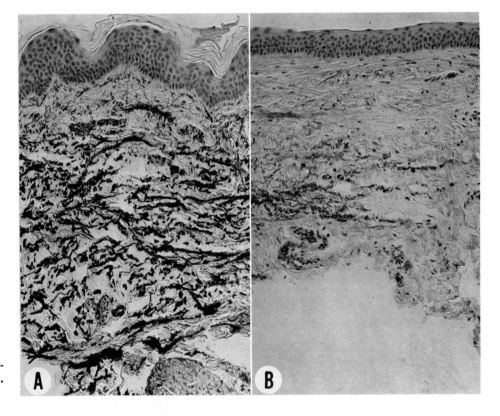

FIGURE 26–6.
*Anetoderma. Schweninger-Buzzi type. **A.** Normal skin. **B.** Lesion. O&G. X135.*

The early inflammatory stage of Jadassohn's disease will show some perivascular infiltrate, swollen and homogenized collagen bundles, and fragmentation of elastic fibers. The fully developed lesions, however, are undiagnosable in H&E sections, while O&G stain reveals a sharply limited area of elastic fiber defect. New formation of very thin elastic fibers may take place in a few cases. Some thinning of epidermis and dermis may be present, but this feature is difficult to judge in routine biopsy material and, in any case, is not diagnostic. Similar changes associated with hair follicles have been described as *perifollicular elastolysis*.[28] Patchy loss of dermal elastic fibers may produce a clinical appearance of superficial wrinkles and follicular prominence.[29,30] Blepharochalasis is another manifestation of loss of dermal elastic fibers in localized skin areas.[31]

Actinic Elastosis. Senile changes are mild in skin areas not ordinarily exposed to sunlight. On the other hand, aging skin habitually exposed to light shows characteristic alterations unless it is protected by heavy pigmentation. The facial skin of individuals with poor tanning ability who lead an outdoor life in the southern United States may show beginning "senile elastosis" or "basophilic degeneration" of the corium before the end of the second decade. These two terms are used here only to point out that they are inappropriate. The changes are characteristic not of old age but of sun-exposed skin,[32] and there is no good evidence that elastotic skin is functionally inferior. On the contrary, the replacement of collagen by elastin may well be adaptive, enabling the integument to survive under adverse conditions.

Early stages of actinic elastosis are characterized by a relative increase and thickening of elastic fibers. Later (Fig. 26-7), the fibers appear curled and conglomerated, and eventually amorphous masses may be formed. At the same time, orceinophilia gradually decreases, and in more advanced stages the fibers may stain a pale gray-brown. They also acquire affinity for hematoxylin and, thus, show gray or bluish in H&E sections. Only in severe cases do they become truly basophilic and stain blue in O&G sections. This feature may be due to an increase in acid mucopolysaccharides, which can be demonstrated by AB-PAS stain. Sudanophilic substances also are present and may be plentiful (*imbibitio lipoidica telae elasticae*[33]).

Characteristically, elastotic changes are confined to the upper third or half of the dermis and spare a narrow subepidermal grenz zone as an indication that we are dealing with a biologic process rather than with a simple physicochemical effect. The

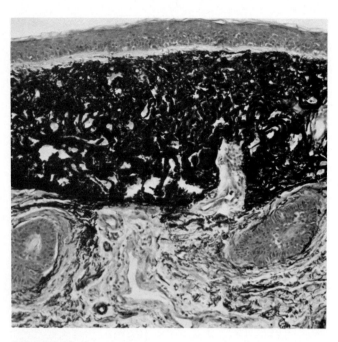

FIGURE 26–7.
Actinic elastosis of face. Degree of elastic hyperplasia and clumping is high, but orceinophilia is fully preserved. In other cases of similar degree, fibers may stain more with basic dye and less with orcein. Note narrow subepidermal grenz zone and relatively normal dermis below elastotic layer. O&G. X185.

grenz zone, being the immediate support of, and interacting constantly with, the epidermis, behaves differently from the deeper layers. The elastotic zone usually is well vascularized, and silver impregnation reveals a net of reticulum fibrils. Both features speak against considering actinic elastosis as a degenerative process. Electron microscopy of severely actinic, exposed skin areas shows depletion of collagen fibrils. The affected elastic fibers contain large masses of electron-dense grains or many large holes leading to widening of their diameter.[1]

In *erythema ab igne*, long exposure to radiant heat leads to depletion of collagen fibers and increased elastic tissue in addition to inflammatory changes.[34,35] Changes similar to severe actinic elastosis are also present in *degenerative collagenous plaques* of the palms (Fig. 26-8), also called kerato-elastoidosis marginalis, and in elastosis senilis hyperkeratotica striata.[36–38]

Special Forms Related to Personal Predisposition. The elastotic material is not always evenly distributed and may even form circumscribed tumorlike nodules, which arouse clinical suspicion of basalioma or other neoplasia.[39] *Nodular elastosis with cysts and comedones*, as described by Favre and Racouchot,[40] seems to affect predisposed indi-

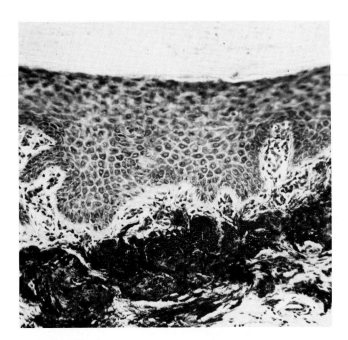

FIGURE 26–8.
Degenerative collagenous plaque of hand (Burks). This type of lesion, also called keratoelastoidosis marginalis (Kocsard), is characterized by acanthosis with hyperkeratosis and dermal changes, which may be due to a combination of mechanical trauma (tool handling) and actinic exposure (farming). O&G. X135. (From Mehregan. Arch Dermatol 93:633, 1966.)

viduals, especially elderly men, whose faces had considerable exposure to the sun. Histologically, it shows a combination of the features mentioned in the name with mild inflammatory changes.

Peculiarly localized to forearms and arms of el-

derly individuals, especially women, is the condition described as *stellate spontaneous pseudoscars.*[41] The clinical combination of atrophic skin with senile purpura, bizarre stellate scars, and possibly small ulcers and crusts often arouses suspicion of dermatitis factitia but seems to be due to a combination of factors leading to increased fragility of the skin.[42,43] Histologically (Fig. 26-9), there is a combination of actinic elastosis with spotty round cell infiltrate and focal loss of elastic fibers. Extravasation of red blood cells and epidermal and dermal atrophy complete the picture.

Another disorder that seems to require the combination of actinic influence and individual predisposition is *colloid milium.* The dome-shaped translucent papules seen clinically correspond to dilated and confluent papillae filled with chunks of an amorphous material (Fig. 26-10) which stains a pale gray with a tinge of blue in O&G sections but is PAS-positive and gives other staining reactions similar to amyloid. It may border directly on the epidermis, leaving no grenz zone. Below the colloid, the dermis shows a high degree of actinic elastosis. In electron microscopy, colloid milium is made up of tightly packed, filamentous bundles.[44] Individual filaments are 8 to 10 nm wide and form wavy and whorled fascicles. The presence of melanosomes, nuclear remnants, and desmosomelike structures suggests epidermal origin.[45]

Stria Distensa. While the topography and direction of striae are related to mechanical stress, their occurrence and severity depend on damage to elastic fibers under the influence of hormones related

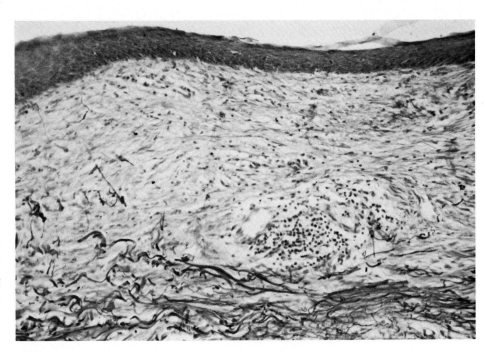

FIGURE 26–9.
Stellate spontaneous pseudoscar. Scarlike fibrosis and loss of elastic fibers in upper dermis, mild perivascular round cell infiltrate. Degenerating erythrocytes scattered between collagen fibers. O&G. X180.

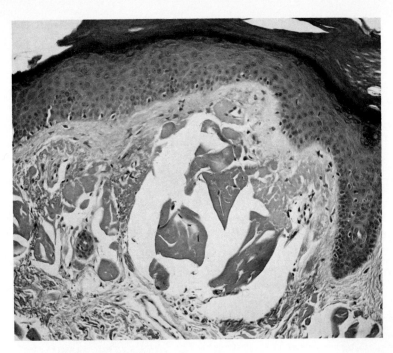

FIGURE 26–10.
Colloid milium. Fragmentation and retraction of brittle amorphous material is artifact. H&E. X135.

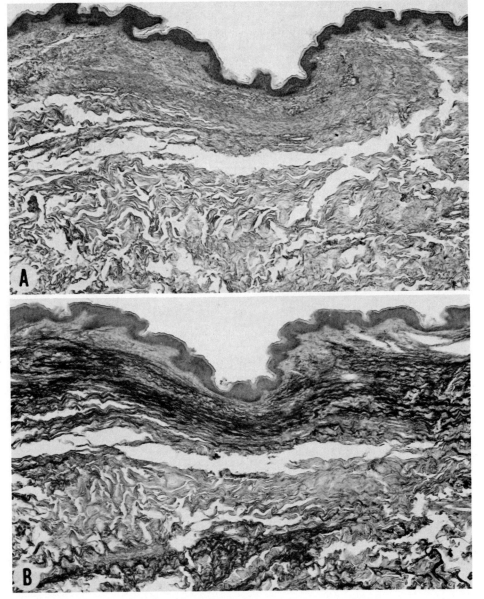

FIGURE 26–11.
*Stria distensa. This is a quiescent older lesion. Note retracted and truly fragmented original elastic fibers to both sides and below stria, while new thin fibers have been formed parallel to the collagen bundles but only in upper dermis. **A.** H&E. X60. **B.** O&G. X60.*

to physiologic stress. The fresh stria, which clinically may look red or bluish, exhibits actual breakage and retraction of the thick elastic fibers of the reticular portion of the dermis, while the collagen bundles appear stretched across the width of the stria parallel to the skin surface. The red or livid clinical color is due to engorgement of blood vessels and some inflammatory infiltrate. The ends of broken elastic fibers are curled up at both sides of the stria. Fibers of the pars papillaris retain normal configuration. Older, white, and sunken striae exhibit new formation of thin elastic fibers (Fig. 26-11) in the upper half of the dermis parallel to the stretched collagen bundles, a feature that gave rise to the inaccurate interpretation that elastic fibers are stretched and thinned in a stria.[46] Elastic tissue usually remains defective in the lower half of the dermis, and the entire skin, epidermis as well as corium, usually remains thinner.

REFERENCES

1. Danielsen L: Morphological changes in pseudoxanthoma elasticum and senile skin. Acta Derm Venereol [Suppl] (Stockh) 83, 1979.
2. Kobayasi T: Electron microscopy of the elastic fibers and the dermal membrane in normal human skin. Acta Derm Venereol (Stockh) 48:303, 1968
3. Montagna W, Parakkal PF: The Structure and Function of the Skin, 3rd ed. New York: Academic Press, 1974, pp 96–141
4. Cotta-Pereira G, Guerra Rodrigo F, Bittencourt-Sampaio S: Oxytalan, elaunin, and elastic fibers in the human skin. J Invest Dermatol 66:143, 1976
5. Maladies du Tissu Elastique Cutané. XII Congres de L'Association des Dermatologistes et Syphiligraphes de Langue Française. Juin 1965. Paris, Masson et Cie, 1968
6. Reed RJ, Clark WH, Mihm MC: The cutaneous elastoses. Hum Pathol 4:187, 1973
7. Staricco RG, Mehregan AH: Nevus elasticus and nevus elasticus vascularis. Arch Dermatol 84:943, 1961
8. Barriere H, Litoux P, Bureau B, Muscat G: Naevus elastique avec osteopoecilie. Bull Soc Fr Derm Syphiligr 81:387, 1974
9. Morrison JGL, Wilson-Jones E, MacDonald DM: Juvenile elastoma and osteopoikilosis (the Buschke-Ollendorff syndrome) Br J Dermatol 97:417, 1977
10. Eng AM, Bryant J: Clinical pathologic observations in pseudoxanthoma elasticum. Int J Dermatol 14:586, 1975
11. Reeve EB, Neldner KH, Subryan V, Gordon SG: Development of calcification of skin lesions in thirty-nine patients with pseudoxanthoma elasticum. Clin Exp Dermatol 4:291, 1979
12. Hicks J, Carpenter CL, Reed RJ: Periumbilical perforating pseudoxanthoma elasticum. Arch Dermatol 115:300, 1979
13. Mehregan AH: Perforating dermatoses: A clinicopathologic review. Int J Dermatol 16:19, 1977
14. Christensen OB: An exogenous variety of pseudoxanthoma elasticum in old farmers. Acta Derm Venereol (Stockh) 58:319, 1978
15. Nielsen AO, Christiansen OB, Hentzer B, et al.: Saltpeter-induced dermal changes electron microscopically indistinguishable from pseudoxanthoma elasticum. Acta Derm Venereol (Stockh) 58:323, 1978
16. Goltz RW, Hult A, Goldfarb M, et al.: Cutis laxa. A manifestation of generalized elastolysis. Arch Dermatol 92:373, 1965
17. Mehregan AH, Lee SC, Nabai H: Cutis laxa (generalized elastolysis). A report of four cases with autopsy findings. J Cutan Pathol 5:116, 1978
18. Hashimoto K, Kanzaki T: Cutis laxa, ultrastructural and biochemical studies. Arch Dermatol 111:861, 1975
19. Verhagen AR, Woerdeman MJ: Post-inflammatory elastolysis and cutis laxa. Br J Dermatol 92:183, 1975
20. Reed WB, Horowitz RE, Beighton P: Acquired cutis laxa: primary generalized elastolysis. Arch Dermatol 103:661, 1971
21. Volpin D, Pasquali-Ronchetti I, Castellani I, et al.: Ultrastructural and biochemical studies on a case of elastosis perforans serpiginosa. Dermatologica 156:209, 1978
22. Mehregan AH: Elastosis perforans serpiginosa, a review of the literature and report of eleven cases. Arch Dermatol 97:381, 1968
23. London ID, Givhan EG, Garrick J, Mehregan A: Elastosis perforans serpiginosa with systemic involvement. South Med J 67:225, 1974
24. Eide J: Elastosis perforans serpiginosa with widespread arterial lesions: a case report. Acta Derm Venereol (Stockh) 57:533, 1977
25. Kirsch N, Hukill PB: Elastosis perforans serpiginosa induced by penicillamine. Electron microscopic observations. Arch Dermatol 113:630, 1977
26. Bardach M, Gebhart W, Niebauer G: "Lumpy-bumpy" elastic fibers in the skin and lungs of a patient with a penicillamine-induced elastosis perforans serpiginosa. J Cutan Pathol 6:243, 1979
27. Chargin L, Silver J: Macular atrophy of the skin. Arch Derm Syphilgr 24:614, 1931
28. Varadi DP, Saqueton AC: Perifollicular elastolysis. Br J Dermatol 83:143, 1970
29. Shelley WB, Wood MG: Wrinkles due to idiopathic loss of dermal elastic tissue. Br J Dermatol 97:441, 1977
30. Brenner W, Gschnait F, Konrad K, et al.: Non-inflammatory dermal elastolysis. Br J Dermatol 99:335, 1978
31. Brazin SA, Stern LJ, Johnson TW: Unilateral blepharochalasis. Arch Dermatol 115:479, 1979
32. Braun-Falco O: Die Morphogenese der senil-aktinischen Elastose; eine elektronenmikroskopische Untersuchung. Arch Klin Exp Dermatol 235:138, 1969
33. Urbach E. Imbibitio lipoidica telae elasticae degeneratae. Acta Derm Venereol (Stockh) 15:69, 1934
34. Johnson WC, Butterworth T. Erythema ab igne elastosis. Arch Dermatol 104:128, 1971
35. Shahrad P, Marks R: The wages of warmth: changes in erythema ab igne. Br J Dermatol 97:179, 1977
36. Mehregan AH: Degenerative collagenous plaques of hands. Arch Dermatol 93:633, 1966
37. Massé R, Quillard A, Héry B, et al.: Acrokeratoelastoidose de Costa. Étude en microscope électronique.

Ann Derm Venereol 104:441, 1977

38. Korting GW, Hoede N: Elastosis senilis hyperkeratotica striata. Dermatologica 150:300, 1975

39. Degos R, Civatte J, Belaïch S: L'élastome en nappe du nez. Arch Belg Dermatol 26:247, 1970

40. Helm F. Nodular cutaneous elastosis with cysts and comedones (Favre–Racouchot syndrome). Arch Dermatol 84:666, 1961

41. Colomb D: Documents cliniques et histologiques sur les "pseudocicatrices stellaires spontanées"; étude de quelques facteurs étiologiques accessoires, endehors de la sénescence cutanée. Bull Soc Fr Derm Syphiligr 75:649, 1968

42. Colomb D: Stellate spontaneous pseudoscars: senile and presenile forms, especially those forms caused by prolonged corticoid therapy. Arch Dermatol 105:551, 1972

43. Björnberg A, Mobacken H: "Spontaneous stellate pseudoscars" of the arms caused by increased skin fragility. Acta Derm Venereol (Stockh) 52:151, 1972

44. Hashimoto K, Katzmann RL, Kang AH, Kanzaki T; Electron microscopical and biochemical analysis of colloid milium. Arch Dermatol 111:49, 1975

45. Ebner H, Gebhart W. Colloid milium: Light and electron microscopic investigations. Clin Exp Dermatol 2:217, 1977

46. Pinkus H, Keech MK, Mehregan AH: Histopathology of striae distensae, with special reference to striae and wound healing in the Marfan syndrome. J Invest Dermatol 46:283, 1966

CHAPTER

27

Various Extracellular Deposits

Having dealt with accumulations of excessive ground substance (mucin) in Chapter 25, we will consider here substances of a less physiologic nature: lipids, calcium, hyaline substances, amyloid, pigments, and foreign bodies.

LIPIDS

Extracellular deposits of lipid spring from four principal sources: disintegration of xanthomatous foam cells, disintegration of blood, disintegration of fat cells, and metabolic accumulation. Thus, in many cases lipid becomes extracellular secondarily. It was mentioned in Chapter 23 that the cells of eruptive xanthomas have a tendency to rupture, with release of lipids into the tissue. It also was mentioned that in vascular histiocytomas, foam cells result from the ingestion of blood lipids derived from repeated small hemorrhages. It is possible that foam cells in L-cell gramuloma (histiocytosis X) are due to similar mechanisms. Free lipid can be demonstrated in these and other cases of hemorrhage if proper stains are done. Of greater diagnostic significance is free lipid in various cases of fat necrosis. Here are to be mentioned sclerema neonatorum, fat necrosis in pancreatic disease, and various forms of panniculitis. The first two lead to the formation of crystals recognized in paraffin sections as clefts (Fig. 16-5), often fan shaped. The last,

whether they are of the purulent or liquefying type, usually do not have this feature.

While deranged metabolism does play a part in xanthomas and other accumulations of lipid in skin, there are some processes in which sudanophilic material is deposited without provoking an inflammatory or granulomatous reaction. One of these is actinic elastosis, especially the severe form seen as *cutis rhomboidalis nuchae.* The pronounced yellow tinge of this type of skin is partly due to the yellow color of elastic tissue and partly to lipids which can be demonstrated in frozen section (*imbibitio lipoidica telae elasticae,* Chap. 26). Lipoid proteinosis also may be mentioned (see below). Two other disorders exhibiting extracellular deposits of lupids are necrobiosis lipoidica (Chap. 22) and *extracellular cholesterosis,* the latter considered to be a variant of erythema elevatum diutinum (Chap. 15). Although there is inflammatory infiltrate present in both, this probably is not caused by the lipid material.

CALCIUM

The presence of insoluble calcium salts is easily seen in H&E sections because nothing except masses of pyknotic nuclei and keratohyalin is tinged in the same dark purple color. Confirmation is offered by O&G stain in a negative manner: The

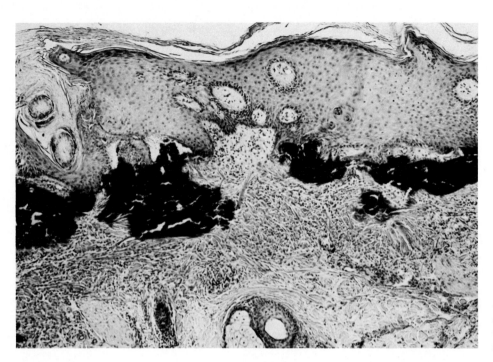

FIGURE 27–1.
Calcification of superficial dermis after electroencephalography due to the calcium chloride content of the electrode paste. H&E. X75.

deposits of calcium do not stain, while nuclei do. On the other hand, O&G stain permits one to analyze the matrix on which calcium was deposited, e.g., elastic fibers, shadow cells of pilomatricoma. Special stains (Von Kossa and others) were discussed in Chapter 3. That only insoluble forms of calcium are shown in sections is just as true as with many other substances, since all soluble salts are removed in processing. A vivid demonstration of this fact is found in *traumatic tissue necrosis* from application of strong calcium chloride solution to slightly abraded skin.[1,2] In this condition (Fig. 27-1), calcium is not seen in the epidermis, and it becomes stainable only after it has been precipitated as carbonate or phosphate in the dermis.

One must remember that calcium usually is deposited on a pathologic substrate, and it is important to identify this if possible. Calcium may be found in collagenous tissue in scleroderma (*CRST syndrome*) and juvenile dermatomyositis, in elastic fibers in *pseudoxanthoma elasticum,* in faded epithelium in *Malherbe's tumor,* and in keratinized material in *epidermoid* and *trichilemmal cysts.* Other clinical manifestations of calcinosis cutis include the solitary nodular calcinosis (Fig. 27-2) of Winer,[3,4] calcinosis cutis of scrotum,[5,6] auricular calcification,[7] and massive tumoral calcinosis.[8-10] Solitary calcified nodules in young children probably result from calcification of nests of nevus cells or hamartomatous structures.[3] Free calcium globes are not infrequently present in *trichoepitheliomas* and other benign *harmartomatous* conditions later

in life, and such globes may secondarily be transformed into bone. It seems likely that, in these cases, calcium was originally deposited on the horny matter of milia and other cysts. Admittedly, it is not always possible to demonstrate the primary substrate morphologically,[5] but even in cases of so-called *metastatic calcinosis,* where calcium probably is precipitated in the ground substance,[11] and in such metabolic disorders as Albright's *hereditary osteodystrophy,*[12,13] one may presuppose localizing factors in the connective tissue.[8]

Michaelis–Gutman bodies are lamellar calcified bodies found inside and outside of histiocytes in malakoplakia (Chap. 20). They measure 5 to 15 μ and also react to PAS and often to Perls' stain for ferric iron.

BONE

Small globes of bony tissue are found infrequently beneath old pigmented nevi or in adnexal tumors.[14] *Osteomas* are often secondary to inflamed and broken down hair follicles or epithelial cysts but may also be primary (Fig. 27-3). Calcification often precedes development of bony tissue. A distinctive variety appears as multiple skin color or bluish nodules in areas affected by long-standing acne vulgaris.[15] Subungual exocytoses are outgrowths of normal bony tissue or calcified cartilagenous remains.[16] These may be single or multiple and are usually asymptomatic unless traumatized or secondarily infected.

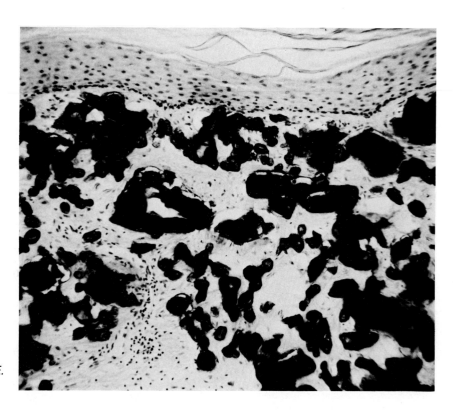

FIGURE 27–2.
Nodular calcinosis of children. H&E. X135.

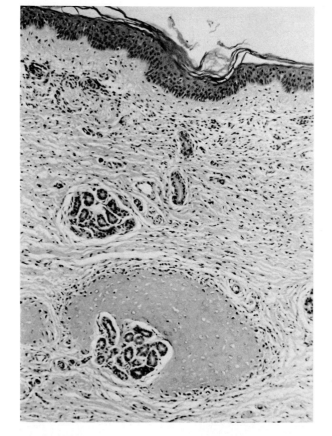

FIGURE 27–3.
Osteoma cutis in a child. The ossification involves the connective tissue associated with one sweat coil. There was no indication of any predisposing cause. H&E. X125.

URIC ACID

Gouty tophi are due to deposits of urates to which the tissues react with granulomatous inflammation. The histologic picture (Fig. 27-4) is that of a palisading granuloma (Chap. 22), especially when formalin fixation has converted the characteristic needlelike crystals into an amorphous mass. When urate crystals are preserved, they stain moderately with hematoxylin or appear gray in transmitted light, and they polarize light. Special stain is rarely needed for their identification, and one should remember that tophi calcify secondarily.

HYALIN

The term *hyalin* may be applied to an ill-defined variety of amorphous insoluble substances in the skin, probably of a proteinaceous nature. All *hyaline substances* stain pink in H&E and O&G sections, with the exception of amyloid, which will be discussed separately. All of them react with the PAS procedure. Some contain lipids, which can be demonstrated in frozen sections.

Hyaline bodies of epithelial origin are found in lichen planus (Chap. 9). Hyalinization of small vessel walls is seen in the pigmented purpuric eruptions (Chap. 13). So-called toxic hyalin characteristically surrounds vessels in erythema elevatum

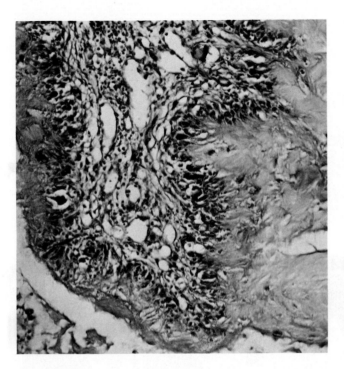

FIGURE 27–4.
Gouty tophus presenting features of a palisading granuloma. Most of crystalline structure of urates has been lost due to formalin fixation. H&E. X135.

diutinum (Chap. 15), and a similar picture of hyaline perivascular trabeculation is seen in granuloma faciale. Hyaline substances are also encountered in skin lesions associated with dysproteinemia (Fig. 15-6) and in atrophie blanche, Degos' malig-

nant papulosis, and other dermatoses. These substances probably are fibrinoid or related to it.

Extensive hyalinization, beginning as a coating of papillary vessels and progressing to large masses filling papillae and subpapillary layer, is seen equally in *lipoid proteinosis (hyalinosis cutis et mucosae)*[17,18] and *erythropoietic protoporphyria*[19,20] (Fig. 27-5). In lipoid proteinosis (hyalinosis cutis et mucosae), hyalin deposition occurs in the superficial network of capillary blood vessels, in eccrine sweat coils, and in hair muscles.[21,22] Hyalin is PAS positive and diastase resistant. It is argyrophilic, weakly reactive with colloidal iron, and stains positive with Sudan III for fat. It is most likely composed of neutral mucopolysaccharide with some hyaluronic acid, tryptophan, neutral fat, and cholesterol. In electron microscopy, it shows up as 8 to 10 nm fibrillar structures forming bundles and whorls.[23] Massive deposition of hyalin and fibroblasts occurs in juvenile hyalin fibromatosis in childhood[24] (Chap. 41). In erythropoietic protoporphyria, endothelial cells of superficial capillary blood vessels are primary targets of the photodynamic reaction.[25] Electron microscopy shows multiplication of the basement membrane surrounding small vessels in the upper dermis. Multilayered basement membrane reflects consecutive reparative processes which follow endothelial cell injuries and relate to the duration and severity of the skin lesions.[26] Foamy exudate of plasma and cell debris seen in early lesions provide the basic substrate for the formation of fibrillar material that

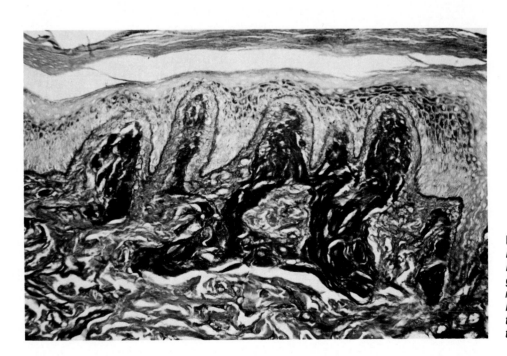

FIGURE 27–5.
Erythropoietic protoporphyria. Hyaline masses in dermis and glycogen in acanthotic epidermis appear dark in this alcian blue-PAS-stained section. Histologic picture is very similar to that of lipoid proteinosis. X135.

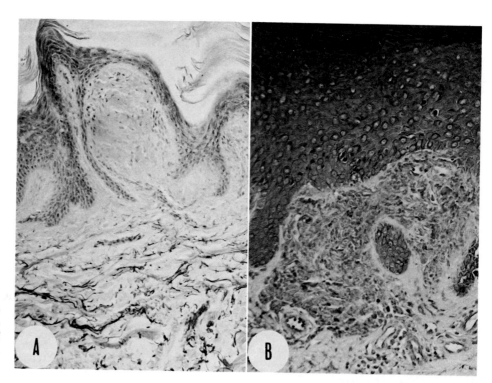

FIGURE 27–6.
Lichen amyloidosus. **A.** *Amyloid deposits in widened papillae. O&G. X135.* **B.** *Amyloid below acanthotic epidermis. Crystal violet. X180.*

characterized hyalin deposits in chronic lesions.[25] Final diagnosis of EPP is made by demonstration of fluorescent erythrocytes or excess protoporphyrin in blood or feces.[27]

AMYLOID

Amyloid occurs in the skin in *primary systemic amyloidosis*, as purely cutaneous *lichen amyloidosus (lichenoid amyloidosis)*, and as *macular amyloidosis*, which may be a variant of the lichenoid form.[28-30] In the diffuse biphasic variety, generalized macular eruption is associated with the lichenoid papular lesions of the pretibial area.[31] Macular and lichenoid lesions also occur together in the familial form of primary cutaneous amyloidosis.[32,33] Poikilodermalike eruptions[34] and nodular infiltrated lesions[35] are other morphologic variations of primary cutaneous amyloidosis. Cutaneous amyloidosis may be associated with urticarial exanthem and deafness as part of *Muckle–Wells syndrome*.[36] While the skin as a rule is spared in *secondary systemic amyloidosis*, deposits were found as rings around subcutaneous fat cells in each of eight cases.[37] Furthermore, amyloid is encountered once in a while in the stroma of basal cell epitheliomas, in Bowen's disease, and in benign cutaneous tumors.

While deposits may be massive in the systemic form, the lichenoid papules often contain only minute quantities of amyloid in individual papillae. It takes a high level of suspicion to suspect amyloid in H&E sections, because it either does not stain differently from collagen or may be slightly bluish to gray at best. A suspicion-arousing feature is the association of a few melanophages with pink-staining material in a wide papilla, epidermal lichenification, and the presence in the epidermis of globes of amorphous eosinophilic material. Many special stains have been recommended for amyloid. They become unnecessary in skin if the O&G stain is done. It stains amyloid (Fig. 27-6) a light sky blue (or grayish blue if the section was decolorized too much), a hue which no other substance will take. While no claim is made for the specificity of this staining reaction in other material, it has proved its value in skin sections. The only other amorphous substances that stain similarly are fibrin and some forms of fibrinoid, but the hue is a colder greenish blue as a rule. The hyaline substance of colloid milium, which reacts like amyloid in most stains, is clearly different in O&G sections because it is tinged with orcein. Electron microscopy shows amyloid in the form of short, straight, and nonbranching filaments measuring 6 to 9 nm[38,39] in diameter. Falsely programmed fibroblasts are responsible for deposition of amyloid filaments. Fibroblasts are found containing amorphous material and surrounded by aggregation of amyloid filamentous material.

BLOOD AND BLOOD PIGMENT

Extravasation of blood may be due to trauma or various pathologic conditions affecting vascular walls or the blood itself. With the exception of leukemia, where the number of white cells is relatively large, evidence of hemorrhage in the tissue sections exists in the presence of free erythrocytes in the tissue. It was pointed out in Chapter 5 that biopsy trauma must be suspected if only fresh red cells are seen. It takes, however, several days before appreciable numbers disintegrate, and fresh spontaneous *purpura* cannot be ruled out by this criterion. In many cases of purpura, an inflammatory reaction sets in soon, but it may be absent in some, such as *scurvy* or *senile purpura*. The formation of hemosiderin takes even longer, and it was mentioned in the discussion of pigmented purpuric eruptions (Chap. 13) that hemosiderin is rarely seen because biopsy usually is taken of fresh purpuric papules. On the other hand, hemosiderin may be present in a large quantity in specimens taken from the lower legs of older persons for a variety of reasons, especially if the characteristic yellow-brown to brown-black discoloration informs the clinician of long-standing stasis damage. These hemosiderin deposits may provoke the thought of Kaposi's sarcoma if they are associated with considerable vascular proliferation (Chap. 15). Stable hemosiderin, in contrast to melanin, does not change color in O&G sections (Chap. 3), but early products of hemoglobin disintegration, which still contain proteinaceous components, may take a light grass-green color, quite distinct from the dark green of melanin.

FOREIGN BODIES

Colored foreign matter will be discussed in Chapter 30. Of colorless materials, the easiest to recognize is *silica* (Fig. 20-16), owing to its birefringence. It was mentioned in Chapter 20 that any sarcoid granuloma should be examined in polarized light to rule out silica. On the other hand, it is practically impossible to identify small particles of glass, except in very special cases. We once found spicules of *fiberglass* in the epidermis in a case of self-inflicted injury. Greatest care must be exercised to make sure that the foreign body (Chap. 3) is within the section and not above or below it. This can usually be done by using the fine adjustment of the microscope and ascertaining that nuclei or other identifiable structures are visible in the same focal plane with the foreign body. It is helpful to have serial sections. If portions of the same particle are found in similar location in two or more consecutive sections, one is pretty sure it was in the tissue before embedding but not necessarily before surgery. *Dirt* tattooed into skin through an abrasion usually consists in part of silica and in part of nonpolarizing particles, which may be colored. Other substances, such as *plant fibers* (usually birefringent), *sutures*, and parts of *arthropods*, are found occasionally. Starch granules (Fig. 3-19) and silica needles (talc) were identified in a subcutaneous granuloma resulting from injection of face powder, the most common material containing a mixture of these two ingredients. The starch granules were seen in a PAS stain done to search for fungi and were first thought to be due to contamination. Then, the routine use of polarized light revealed talc crystals and permitted the examiner to solve the case which had gone undiagnosed for several years. A suspecting mind and knowledge of the morphology of foreign material are important for the unraveling of such cases.

REFERENCES

1. Zackheim, HS, Pinkus H: Calcium chloride necrosis of the skin. Report of two cases. Arch Dermatol 76:244, 1957
2. Schoenfeld RJ, Grekin JN, Mehregan AH: Calcium deposition in the skin. A report of four cases following electroencephalography. Neurology 15:477, 1965
3. Shmunes E, Wood MG: Subepidermal calcified nodules. Arch Dermatol 105:593, 1972
4. Weigand DA: Subepidermal calcified nodule. Report of a case with apparent hair follicle origin. J Cutan Pathol 3:109, 1976
5. Shapiro L, Platt N, Torres-Rodrigues VM: Idiopathic calcinosis of the scrotum. Arch Dermatol 102:199, 1970
6. Fisher BK, Dvoretzky I: Idiopathic calcinosis of the scrotum. Arch Dermatol 114:957, 1978
7. Chadwick JM, Downham TF: Auricular calcification. Int J Dermatol 17:799, 1978
8. Whiting DA, Simson IW, Kallmeyer JC, et al.: Unusual cutaneous lesions in tumoral calcinosis. Arch Dermatol 102:465, 1970
9. Pursley TV, Prince MJ, Chausmer AB, Raimer SS: Cutaneous manifestations of tumoral calcinosis. Arch Dermatol 115:1100, 1979
10. Barrière H, Welin J, Visset LJ, Vigier P: Lipo-calcinogranulomatose de Teutschlaender ou Calcinose tumorale de Inclan. Ann Derm Venereol 104:136, 1977
11. Putkonen T, Wangel GA: Renal hyperparathyroidism with metastatic calcification of the skin. Dermatologica 118:127, 1959
12. Brook CGD, Valman HB: Osteoma cutis and Albright's hereditary osteodystrophy. Br J Dermatol 85:471, 1971
13. Barranco VP: Cutaneous ossification in pseudohypoparathyroidism. Arch Dermatol 104:643, 1971

14. Coskey JR, Mehregan AH: Metaplastic bone formation in an organoid nevus. Arch Dermatol 102:233, 1970
15. Basler RSW: Calcifying acne lesions. Int J Dermatol 16:755, 1977
16. Lebowitz SS, Miller OF, Dickey RF: Subungual exostosis. Cutis 13:426, 1974
17. Hashimoto K, Klingmüller G, Rodermund OE: Hyalinosis cutis et mucosae. Acta Derm Venereol 52:179, 1972
18. Hofer PA: Urbach-Wiethe disease (lipoglycoproteinosis, lipoid proteinosis, hyalinosis cutis et mucosae). A review. Acta Derm Venereol 53 [Suppl 71]:1, 1973
19. VanderWalt JJ, Heyl T: Lipoid proteinosis and erythropoietic protoporphyria. Arch Dermatol 104:501, 1971
20. Sasai Y: Erythropoietic protoporphyria: histochemical study of hyaline material. Acta Derm Venereol (Stockh) 53:179, 1973
21. Caro I: Lipoid proteinosis. Int J Dermatol 17:388, 1978
22. Ishibashi A: Histogenesis of hyalinosis cutis et mucosae. Accumulation of basal lamina glycoprotein (Type III and/or Type IV Collagen?) from smooth muscle system. J Dermatol (Tokyo) 5:265, 1978
23. Ebner H, Gebhart W: Light and electron microscopic differentiation of amyloid or colloid or hyaline bodies. Br J Dermatol 92:637, 1975
24. Kitano Y, Horiki M, Aoki T, Sagami S: Two cases of juvenile hyalin fibromatosis. Some histological, electron microscopic and tissue culture observations. Arch Dermatol 106:877, 1972
25. Gschnait F, Wolff K, Konrad K: Erythropoietic protoporphyria: Submicroscopic events during the acute photosensitivity flare. Br J Dermatol 92:545, 1975
26. Nonaka S, Nishimoto K, Hirowatari T, et al.: Electron microscopic study of porphyrias. J Dermatol (Tokyo) 2:87, 1975
27. Poh-Fitzpatrick MB: Erythropoietic protoporphyria. Int J Dermatol 17:359, 1978
28. Black MM: The nature, pathogenesis and staining properties of amyloid. Br J Dermatol 87:280, 1972
29. Black MM, Wilson-Jones E: Macular amyloidosis; a study of 21 cases with special reference to the role of the epidermis in its histogenesis. Br J Dermatol 84:199, 1971
30. Brownstein MHL, Hashimoto K, Greenwald G: Biphasic amyloidosis: link between macular and lichenoid forms. Br J Dermatol 88:25, 1973
31. Piamphongsant T, Kullavanijaya P: Diffuse biphasic amyloidosis. Dermatologica 153: 243, 1976
32. Eng AM, Cogan L, Gunnar RM, Blekys I: Familial generalized dyschromic amyloidosis cutis. J Cutan Pathol 3:102, 1976
33. Vasily DB, Bhatia SG, Uhlin SR: Familial primary cutaneous amyloidosis. Clinical, genetic, and immunofluorescent studies. Arch Dermatol 114:1173, 1978
34. Ogino A, Tanaka S: Poikiloderma-like cutaneous amyloidosis. Report of a case and review of the literature. Dermatologica 115:301, 1977
35. Chapel TA, Birmingham DJ, Malinowski YE: Nodular primary localized cutaneous amyloidosis. Arch Dermatol 113:1248, 1977
36. Muckle TJ: The Muckle–Wells' syndrome. Br J Dermatol 100:87, 1979
37. Westermark P: Occurrence of amyloid deposits in the skin in secondary systemic amyloidosis. Acta Pathol Microbiol Scand [A] 80A: 718, 1972
38. Runne U, Orfanos CE: Amyloid production by dermal fibroblasts. Electron microscopic studies on the origin of amyloid in various dermatoses and skin tumors. Br J Dermatol 97:155, 1977
39. Kobayasi T, Asboe-Hansen G: Ultrastructure of skin in primary systemic amyloidosis. Acta Derm Venereol (Stockh) 59:407, 1979

SECTION

VI

NONNEOPLASTIC EPITHELIAL AND PIGMENTARY DISORDERS

We have discussed a great variety of changes of epidermis and adnexal epithelium associated with inflammatory disease in the widest sense. We will discuss epithelial nevi and neoplasms in Section VII. In between these large groups of disorders, there are some that seem to fit neither definition. The epidermis appears to be abnormal in itself, without depending on dermal stimuli. Thus, epidermis from cases of lamellar ichthyosis transplanted into athymic nude mice[1] retained its abnormal properties for long times. Removal of epidermis and superficial dermis in Darier's disease resulted in long-lasting remissions, an indication that the epidermis was inherently abnormal.[2] The changes tend to be generalized or at least widespread, are often inconstant in their expression, and seem to be due to inborn metabolic derangement rather than to inflammation, malformation, or neoplasia. Then there are the virus epidermoses, which are neither inflammatory nor neoplastic in the usual sense. And finally, it seems convenient to discuss here various disturbances of skin color which also are not definitely related to inflammation or neoplasia.

REFERENCES

1. Briggaman RA, Wheeler CE Jr: Lamellar ichthyosis: long-term graft studies on congenitally athymic nude mice. J Invest Dermatol 67:567, 1976
2. Dellon AL, Chretien PB, Peck GL: Successful treatment of Darier's disease by partial-thickness removal of skin. Plast Reconstr Surg 59:823, 1977

28

Darier's and Hailey-Hailey's Diseases

Keratosis follicularis and chronic *benign familial pemphigus* have in common the basic histologic feature of acantholysis leading to suprabasal cleft formation. They share this feature with the acantholytic diseases of the pemphigus group (Chap. 11). In this guide to histopathologic diagnosis, we cannot discuss electron microscopic or immunohistochemical differences. We should, however, as in other diseases, take into consideration all available clinical features, morphology as well as the general course of the disease. On that basis, pemphigus vulgaris and vegetans, Hailey–Hailey's disease, and Darier's disease are well definable. Difficulties of histologic differentiation, which do exist in some cases, should make us admit our diagnostic limitations rather than postulate the identity of diseases. While suprabasal acantholysis is the common feature, most cases present sufficiently diagnostic differences in other respects. These are listed in Table 28-1, which clearly shows variable, but rather characteristic, combinations for each disease.

KERATOSIS FOLLICULARIS (DARIER)

The histologic picture of the average case of Darier's disease (Fig. 28-1) presents relatively small foci of dry suprabasal clefting that give the impression of being largely due to retraction during tissue processing. The same areas usually show a minor degree of basal layer budding and exhibit individual cell keratinization, so that a smaller or larger number of dyskeratotic cells (benign dyskeratosis, Chap. 5) are mixed with normally keratinizing cells in the granular and horny layers. The clefting thus extends from the basal layer through the granular layer, and there is no coherent roof except the stratum corneum.

The dyskeratotic cells were morphologically divided into *corps ronds* and *grains* (Fig. 5-10) by Darier, and this division has been maintained and supported by recent electron microscopic work, which suggests a somewhat different cytogenesis for either form.[1,2] In routine histologic sections, corps ronds are large roundish cells with a central vesicular nucleus and are separated by an empty cleft from the surrounding prickle cells. They have a dense outer rim and may contain keratohyalin granules. Grains are smaller, eosinophilic, and presumably cornified bodies of round, elongated, or irregular shape and may or may not contain remnants of a nucleus. They are usually found in the stratum corneum, and there is no obvious reason for not assuming that corps ronds and grains are consecutive stages in the process of individual cell keratinization leading from a large prickle cell without prickles (Chap. 2) through a granular stage to a shrunken, nonnucleated, keratinized body.

TABLE 28–1.
Differential Features of Some Acantholytic Diseases

	Pemphigus Vulgaris	Pemphigus Vegetans	Hailey-Hailey	Darier
Suprabasal acantholysis	+	+	+	+
Dry cleft	−	+	−	+
Lake or bulla	+	+	+	−
Tombstone basal cells	+	+	−	−
Degeneration of acantholytic cells	+	+	−	−
Dyskeratosis	−	−	±	+
Basal layer budding	−	+	+ +	+ to + + +
Pseudoepitheliomatous proliferation	−	−	−	+
Acantholysis affecting follicular sheath	±	+	−	+
Inflammatory infiltrate	+	+ + +	± to +	± to + +

If the lesion is more severe, all these features increase in proportion, but variations may occur. For instance, in the moist creases of the skin, suprabasal clefting (Fig. 28-2) may become much more extensive, while individual cell keratinization decreases. These cases resemble Hailey–Hailey's disease, and differential diagnosis may require more than one biopsy. It should be remembered that benign familial pemphigus is a chronically recurrent disease in which vesicular or crusted lesions come and go and usually respond to antibiotic therapy, while keratosis follicularis is a progressive disease which, in typical cases, builds up over the years to more and more severe horny and verrucous foci responding, if at all, only to high doses of vitamin A and, in some cases, to lead oleate ointment or the modern retinoic acid applications.

All in all, the histologic features of Darier's disease are remarkably constant, while the clinical picture may vary from zosteriform arrangement,[3,4] resembling ichthyosis hystrix (Chap. 29), to papular or macroscopically inapparent single or multiple lesions,[5] in addition to the typical generalized form. Darier's disease may involve the mucous membranes (Chap. 45). The principal histologic variation is excessive downward budding of acantholytic epithelium (Fig. 28-3), which leads to convoluted masses. These structures, on cross section, consist of two rows of basal cells separated by a cleft.[6] However, in some cases, their thickness builds up,

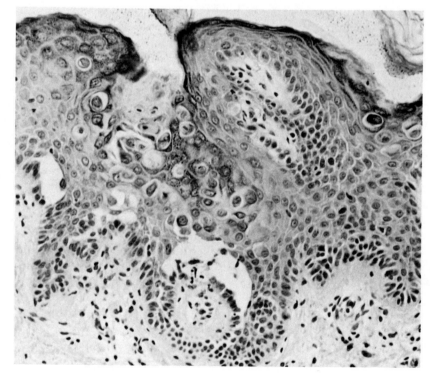

FIGURE 28–1.
Darier's keratosis follicularis. Suprabasal clefts and corps ronds are evident. Grains with or without pyknotic nuclei are discernible in the horny plug. H&E. X135. (From Sutton. Diseases of the Skin, 11th ed, 1956. Courtesy of Dr. R.L. Sutton, Jr. Contributed by H. Pinkus.)

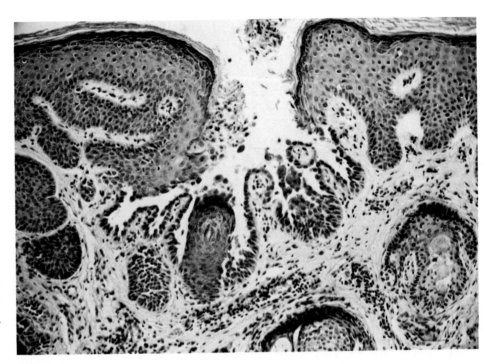

FIGURE 28–2.
Basal budding and extensive clefting due to acantholysis in Darier's disease. Eccrine keratinocytes in wall of sweat duct are not affected. H&E. X135.

and the central cells assume prickle cell character and may even form horn pearls. Such *pseudoepitheliomatous proliferation* should not be mistaken for squamous cell carcinoma. High degrees of proliferating clefting epidermis may mislead the casual observer to the assumption that he is dealing with a papilliferous cyst, as in *syringadenoma papilliferum*.[7] Figure 28-4 tries to elucidate the three-dimensional structural differences between the gyrated epithelial mass of Darier's disease, which our

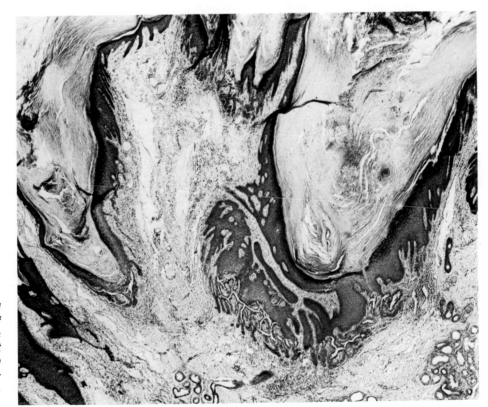

FIGURE 28–3.
Hypertrophic, verrucous, and pseudoepitheliomatous form of Darier's disease. Epidermis extends down to level of sweat coils. Similar pictures may be seen in isolated keratosis follicularis (warty dyskeratoma). H&E. X28.

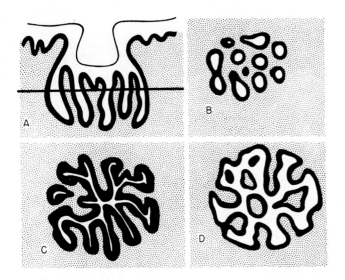

FIGURE 28–4.
*Diagram illustrating structural differences between a tubular adenoma (**B**), the cerebriform convolutions of hypertrophic Darier's disease (**C**), and a papilliferous cystadenoma (**D**), all of which may look deceptively similar in a vertical section (**A**). The heavy line in **A** designates the level at which a transverse section would reveal the three different configurations shown in **B**, **C**, and **D**. (From Pinkus. Arch Dermatol 82:681, 1960.)*

sections cut at different angles, and the hidradenomatous cyst (Fig. 38-5), which is filled with papilliform projections. Closer examination reveals the quite different character of the cells which line the clefts: a simple layer of basal cells in Darier's disease, a double layer of columnar and flat cells in syringadenoma. Dyskeratotic cells occur only in keratosis follicularis.

Inflammatory dermal infiltrate plays no significant role in Darier's disease, although it may become heavier in macerated or secondarily infected lesions. This is in contrast to the heavy infiltrate usually encountered in pemphigus vegetans and in syringadenoma papilliferum, both characterized by plasma cells, and in pemphigus vegetans by eosinophils.

Warty Dyskeratoma

In spite of the given name, the lesions of keratosis follicularis usually are restricted to the epidermis, but they can involve follicular epithelium and then may form deep saccular lesions. This feature is particularly prominent in the *isolated keratosis follicularis*[8] or *warty dyskeratoma*.[6,9] In other cases, the clinical picture may resemble comedones[10] or Kyrle's disease (Chap. 18).

BENIGN FAMILIAL CHRONIC PEMPHIGUS (HAILEY–HAILEY)

In contrast to the dry, open dyskeratotic cleft of Darier's disease, the *benign familial pemphigus* lesion (Fig. 28-5) shows extensive suprabasal splits, which are usually covered by coherent upper epidermal layers. These lakes (lacunae) commonly show evidence of having contained fluid in which isolated rounded prickle cells float.[11] The acantholytic cells have well-defined nuclei and sharply outlined cytoplasm, in contrast to the degenerating cells of pemphigus vulgaris or vegetans, and only occasionally show keratohyalin granules or a tendency to keratinize. They are acantholytic but generally not dyskeratotic. Basal layer budding often is pronounced, though never pseudoepitheliomatous. Hair follicles are spared by the process. In more acute or older lesions, the upper epidermal layers degenerate into a parakeratotic crust, and several such layers may be one on top of the other, somewhat resembling pemphigus foliaceus. Inflammatory infiltrate is variable but not significant.

A very astounding occurrence is the coexistence in the same patient, and even in the same lesion, of the acantholytic changes of benign familial pemphigus and of psoriasis, which has been reported at least three times.[12] We had occasion to study sections of the skin of one of the patients ourselves.[13] It is very difficult to explain how an epidermal cell that supposedly has the inherent tendency to psoriatic hyperproliferation can at the same time undergo the acantholytic change inherent in Hailey–Hailey's disease. The phenomenon is easier to explain if the primary disturbance of psoriasis is located in the dermis rather than in the epidermis (Chap. 8).

It may be recorded that small foci of Hailey–Hailey-like acantholysis are found occasionally in skin biopsied for entirely different purposes. Inquiry usually does not reveal any clinical symptoms of the disease. Such findings, therefore, may be disregarded as far as clinical significance is concerned.

Grover's Disease

Some years ago, however, a *transient acantholytic dermatosis*[14] was described in which papules and vesicobullous lesions, usually very pruritic, occur over a period of several months and subside spontaneously. The histologic picture (Fig. 28-6) shows similarity to Hailey-Hailey disease but may suggest

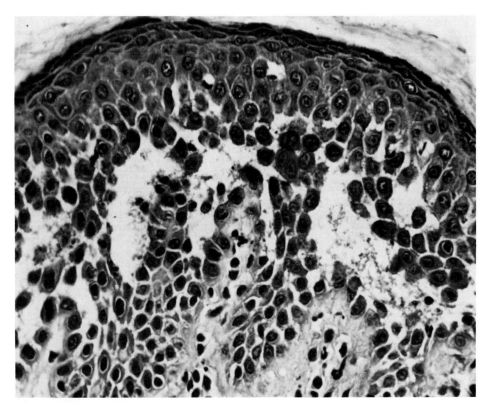

FIGURE 28–5.
Hailey–Hailey's disease. Acantholysis without dyskeratosis. H&E. X185. (From Sutton. Diseases of the Skin, 11th ed, 1956. Courtesy of Dr. R.L. Sutton, Jr. Contributed by H. Pinkus.)

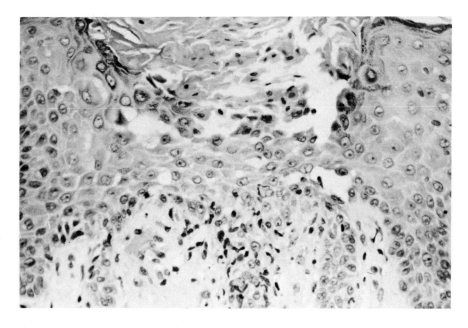

FIGURE 28–6.
Grover's disease. In this instance, the histologic picture is indistinguishable from Darier's disease, and clinical information must give the definitive diagnosis. H&E. X250.

true pemphigus vulgaris, Darier's disease, or a spongiotic dermatitis. There are always some acantholytic cells to suggest the correct diagnosis.

REFERENCES

1. Gottlieb SK, Lutzner MA: Darier's disease; an electron microscopic study. Arch Dermatol 107:225, 1973
2. Sato A, Anton-Lamprecht I, Schnyder UW: Ultrastructure of dyskeratosis in Morbus Darier. J Cutan Pathol 4:173, 1977
3. Pinkus F, Ledermann R: Beitrag zur Histologie und Pathogenese der Darierschen Krankheit. Arch Derm Syph (Berlin) 131:360, 1921
4. Goette DK: Zosteriform keratosis follicularis cleared with topically applied vitamin A acid. Arch Dermatol 107:113, 1973
5. Ackerman AB: Focal acantholytic dyskeratosis. Arch Dermatol 106:702, 1972
6. Tanay A, Mehregan AH: Warty dyskeratoma. Dermatologica 138:169, 1969
7. Beerman H: Hypertrophic Darier's disease and nevus syringocystadenomatosus papilliferus. Arch Dermatol 60:500, 1949
8. Graham JH, Helwig EB: Isolated dyskeratosis follicularis. Arch Dermatol 77:377, 1958
9. Szymanski FJ: Warty dyskeratoma. Arch Dermatol 75:567, 1957
10. Carneiro SJC, Dickson JE, Knox JM: Familial dyskeratotic comedones. Arch Dermatol 105:249, 1972
11. Pinkus H, Epstein S: Familial benign chronic pemphigus. Arch Dermatol 53:119, 1946
12. Heaphy MR, Winkelmann RK: Coexistence of benign familial pemphigus and psoriasis vulgaris. Arch Dermatol 112:1571, 1976
13. Fisher I, Orkin M, Bean S: Familial benign chronic pemphigus and psoriasis vulgaris in the same patient. Acta Derm Venereol (Stockh) 47:111, 1967
14. Chalet M, Grover R, Ackerman AB: Transient acantholytic dermatosis. A re-evaluation. Arch Dermatol 113:431, 1977

CHAPTER

29

Ichthyosiform Dermatoses

The ichthyosiform dermatoses are an example of how progress can be impeded by too rigid a classification and nomenclature and by a lack of coordination of clinical and histologic features. This situation had begun to be corrected by histobiologic and genetic analysis[1,2] at the time the first edition of the *Guide* was written. The prediction made at that time that many more variants would be uncovered has been fulfilled in the past 10 years, and Reed, in 1970, was able to list 13 different entities.[3] The field of ichthyosiform dermatoses[4] can be best understood by realizing that *ichthyosis* is one of those diagnostic terms that cover quite unrelated disorders and that it is a purely clinical designation for chronically hyperkeratotic skin.[5] Histologically, biologically, and genetically, it covers a variety of disorders of keratinization.[6] If one considers that specific disturbances of hair keratinization in mice are due to individual gene mutations and that the number of known mutations keeps increasing, it is not unreasonable to presume that there are many gene mutations in man which directly or indirectly affect epidermal keratinization in a manner that is clinically expressed as ichthyosis. It seems wise, therefore, to keep an open mind, to investigate every case and every family as a separate phenomenon, and to register histologic, histochemical, and other variations assiduously rather than to force them into preconceived diagnostic pigeonholes. That way, we may unravel pathogenetic mecha-

nisms, devise more than empirical therapy, and offer intelligent genetic counseling.

At the present time, the possibilities of producing an ichthyotic state listed in Table 29-1 are recognized.

If these qualities of the epidermis are related to involvement of follicular and eccrine ostia, abnormal features of hairs, presence or atrophy of sebaceous glands, and diffuse or localized involvement of the skin, a considerable number of combinations results, which might be increased if exact genetic factors were known in each case[7] and if the clinical development from infancy to adulthood were observed.[8,9] Table 29-2, based on Reed's 1970 tabulation, lists entities recognized at present.

ICHTHYOSIS

For practical diagnostic purposes, one should pay attention to thickness of the malpighian layer, the granular layer, and the horny layer, to presence or absence of nuclei in the latter, and to the number of mitoses. As a rule, *ichthyosis vulgaris*[10] has a rather thin stratum malpighi and a thick and compact horny layer without nuclei (Fig. 29-1). The granular layer is thin or interrupted in routine sections, but it is exaggeration to say that it is absent. Mitoses are scarce. Differentiation of *autosomal dominant* from *x-linked recessive* cases[11] remains

TABLE 29–1.
Histologic Pictures Found in Ichthyosiform Disorders

Orthokeratotic
  Granular layer thin or absent, horny layer compressed (superkeratinization) or thick
  Granular layer thick, epidermis acanthotic, horny layer stratified
  Granular cells ballooning, horny layer thick, verrucous (epidermolytic type)
Parakeratotic
  Granular layer absent, epidermis psoriasiform
  Granular layer present, nuclei preserved in horny layer

insecure in routine sections and may require histochemical, tissue cultural,[12] or ultrastructural methods.[4] So-called *lamellar ichthyosis* has a somewhat acanthotic epidermis (Fig. 29-2), with a slight or considerable increase of granular cells and a thick but loosely constructed horny layer. Turnover of keratinocytes may be sufficiently rapid that mitotic figures can be found on cursory examination. While the surface is orthokeratotic, pyknosis of nuclei in the granular layer may be delayed, and

some nuclei may persist in the stratum corneum. In some patients, the skin appears dark without containing melanin in the horny layer. Harlequin fetus usually is considered the most severe form of lamellar ichthyosis, but Buxman et al.[13] found distinct lipid abnormalities in the epidermis.

Cases presenting the clinical picture of *ichthyosis linearis circumflexa* have been associated with bamboo hairs (Fig. 46-8A) and other abnormalities.[14] The histologic picture (Fig. 29-3) varies in these cases depending on the relation of the specimen to the migrating active borders and the severity of the complicating eczematous dermatitis. More or less parakeratosis and inflammatory infiltrate are to be expected. In one personally observed case of *biphasic ichthyosiform dermatosis*,[9] an unusual clinical course was combined with unusual cytologic abnormalities (Fig. 29-4), consisting of a separation of the cytoplasm of prickle cells into edematous inner and tonofibril-rich outer zones, and thick orthokeratosis in spite of defective keratohyalin formation. Similar hereditary cases were analyzed by Anton-Lamprecht et al.[15] Such observations make

TABLE 29–2.
Major Forms and Some Rare Types of Ichthyosiform Dermatoses

	Inheritance	Presence at Birth	Histology
Ichthyosis vulgaris	Autosomal dominant	No	Compressed orthokeratosis, decreased granular layer, average epidermal thickness
Sex-linked ichthyosis	Sex-linked recessive	Yes	Stratified orthokeratosis, thick granular layer and rete malpighi, perivascular dermal infiltrate
Lamellar ichthyosis	Autosomal recessive	Yes (collodion baby)	Hyperkeratosis with focal parakeratosis, thickened granular and spinous layers, dermal infiltrate
Epidermolytic hyperkeratosis	Autosomal dominant	Yes	Marked thickening of all epidermal layers, vacuolar degeneration of granular cells
Harlequin fetus	Autosomal recessive	Yes	Extreme orthokeratotic hyperkeratosis, average granular layer, diffuse acanthosis, cholesterol and triglycerides high
Psoriasiform ichthyosis (congenital psoriasis?)	Psoriasis in family	Yes	Parakeratosis, loss of granular layer, acanthosis with thin suprapapillary plate, Munro abscesses?
Wile's ichthyosiform erythroderma[16]	Autosomal recessive?	Yes	General parakeratosis, absence of granular layer, acanthosis
Sjögren–Larsen syndrome	Autosomal recessive	Yes	Lamellated orthokeratosis, normal or diminished granular layer, acanthosis with papillomatosis
Netherton's syndrome (ichthyosis linearis circumflexa with bamboo hairs)	Autosomal recessive?	Soon after	Orthokeratosis and parakeratosis depending on stage of eruption, variable granular layer, acanthosis, changes may be obscured by coexisting eczematous dermatitis, trichorrhexis invaginata
Erythrokeratodermia variabilis	Autosomal dominant	Sometimes	Hyperkeratosis with focal parakeratosis, average granular layer, acanthosis and papillomatosis, all depending on stage of disease
Biphasic ichthyosiform dermatosis (ichthyosis hystrix Curth-Macklin)	Autosomal dominant	No	Orthokeratotic hyperkeratosis above an incomplete granular layer, acanthosis and papillomatosis with binucleate prickle cells and "intracellular edema"
Refsum's disease	Autosomal recessive	No	Moderate acanthosis, hypergranulosis, hyperkeratosis, lipid vacuoles in basal cells
Acquired ichthyosis	None	No	Similar to ichthyosis vulgaris

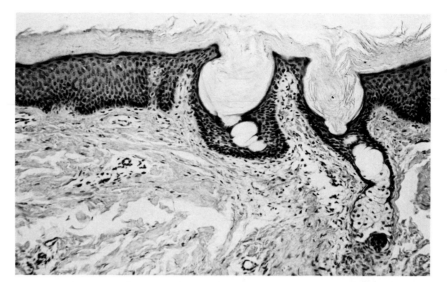

FIGURE 29–1.
Ichthyosis vulgaris. Compact othokeratotic layer above a thin or defective granular layer. Rete malpighi usually is thinner than in this case. Sweat ducts and hair follicles have keratotic plugs. Sebaceous glands are small. H&E. X135.

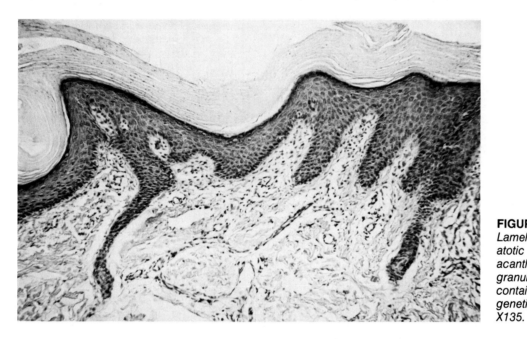

FIGURE 29–2.
Lamellar ichthyosis. Orthokeratotic horny layer rests on acanthotic epidermis with thick granular layer. Horny layer contains some melanin due to genetic pigmentation. H&E. X135.

FIGURE 29–3.
Ichthyosis linearis circumflexa. Intracellular edema and parakeratosis with slight crusting characterize the advancing border of the lesion. Practically no inflammatory infiltrate. H&E. X135. (From Nabai and Mehregan: J Cutan Pathol 6:144, 1979. Copyright © 1979 Munksgaard International Publishers, Copenhagen).

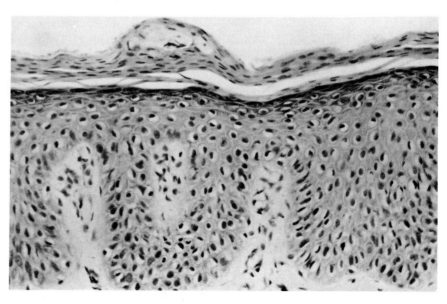

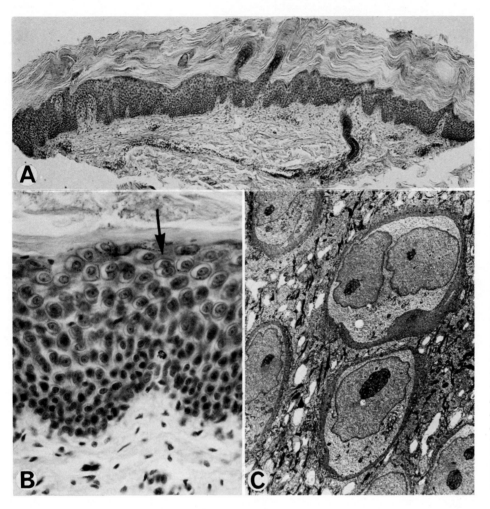

FIGURE 29–4.
*Biphasic ichthyosiform derma-
tosis (Pinkus-Nagao), probably
identical with ichthyosis hystrix
Curth-Macklin.* **A.** *Thick epidermis without keratohyalin
layer and very thick orthokeratotic horny layer into which individual long papillae project.
H&E. X45.* **B.** *At higher power,
epidermis shows several mitoses and exhibits peculiar
rings at some distance around
nuclei. Note one binucleated
cell (arrow). A few keratohyaline granules are visible. Cells
flatten out into stratum corneum. H&E. X370.* **C.** *Electron
micrograph shows the bi-
phasic structure of the cytoplasm. Mitochondria in inner
phase, tonofilaments in outer
realm separated by a shell.
One binucleated cell. X4,500.
(From Pinkus and Nagao. Arch
Klin Exp Dermatol 237:737,
1970.)*

one feel that more variants of the ichthyotic process await identification.

ICHTHYOSIFORM ERYTHRODERMAS

There are two principal forms of clinical disease fitting the descriptive diagnosis *ichthyosiform erythroderma.* Yet the attempted differentiation of
this picture into *bullous* and *nonbullous* forms dis-
regards the histobiologic facts. Histologically, there
is a clear distinction between those cases that have
a hyperplastic granular layer with ballooning cells
(Fig. 29-5) and those that have no granular layer and
are parakeratotic (Fig. 29-6).[16] It does not matter
whether or not the former ever show a clinical blister, since the structure of their stratum granulosum is the decisive defect (*epidermolytic hyperkeratosis*)[1] and renders them pomphogenic. The
parakeratotic cases have lately been termed *psoriasiform,* a comparison that seems not too well
founded, although congenital cases of psoriasis undoubtedly exist.[17] Rare cases of slowly migrating

plaques that exhibit both erythema and ichthyotic
hyperkeratosis have been described as *erythrokeratodermia variabilis*[18] and cocardioform genodermatosis.[19] They exhibit rather noncharacteristic changes
of acanthosis, hyperkeratosis, and some inflammatory infiltrate.

ICHTHYOSIS HYSTRIX
AND ICHTHYOSIFORM NEVI

Severe cases of the diffuse epidermolytic type of
ichthyosiform erythroderma may show patches and
streaks of heavy verrucous hyperkeratosis of the
porcupine-man type. There are other cases, in
which the epidermal malformation is entirely localized in segmental fashion and may be classified
as an epidermal nevus (Chap. 33). These are usually
called *ichthyosis hystrix* (Fig. 29-7). Families have
been described in which both the diffuse and segmental forms occurred. There are also occasional
cases in which a small localized epidermal nevus is
found to have the same histologic picture. These

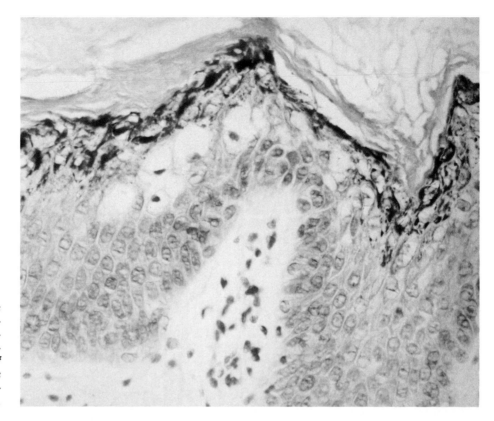

FIGURE 29–5.
Epidermolytic hyperkeratosis (so-called bullous type of ichthyosiform erythroderma). Ballooning pregranular and granular cells without signs of acantholysis predispose this epidermis to formation of bullae (see Fig. 29-7). H&E. X185.

observations and the concept of epidermolytic hyperkeratosis as a histobiologic entity, put forward in the first edition of the *Guide,* have been substantiated by several authors in recent years.[20,21] They have been extended to include cases of keratoderma palmare and plantare (Chap. 33)[22,23] and subclinical lesions.[24] Thus, somewhat similar to Darier's disease, a peculiar metabolic derangement of the epidermis can occur in a small island or in one or several dermatomes or can be more or less widespread or diffuse. Just as we base a diagnosis of ker-

atosis follicularis on the histologic substrate, all skin lesions exhibiting the characteristic granular cell ballooning belong to the group of epidermolytic hyperkeratosis[25] and should be differentiated from nonepidermolytic papillomatous affections, which also may present themselves as small verrucous nevi, segmental nevi unius lateris, or more widespread papillomatosis (Chap. 33). On the other hand, the obvious differences in prognosis and management of localized and diffuse cases warrant clinical diagnostic distinction.

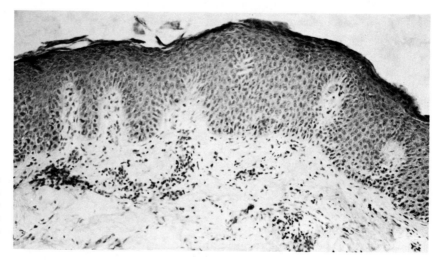

FIGURE 29–6.
Psoriasiform ichthyosis exhibits acanthosis and parakeratosis, but no evidence of squirting papillae. This biopsy was taken in adult life from the surviving member of the family whose cases were published by Wile.[16]

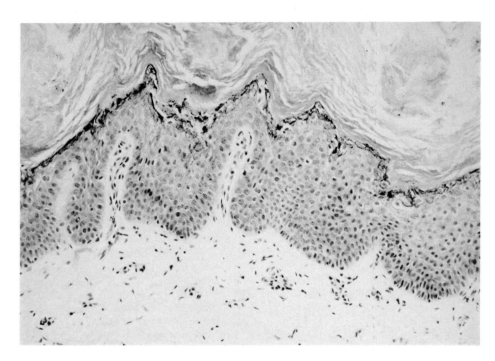

FIGURE 29–7.
Ichthyosis hystrix shows changes identical with epidermolytic hyperkeratosis (Fig. 29-5). H&E. X135.

Acquired Ichthyosis

Acquired ichthyosis is a term applied to ichthyotic states developing later in life, as a symptom of malignancy. Malnutrition in a wider sense has been implied as a cause, and dry ichthyotic skin is not infrequently seen on the lower legs in marasmic patients. The diagnosis should be reserved for severe generalized conditions.[26] The histologic picture resembles that of ichthyosis vulgaris.

HYPERKERATOSIS LENTICULARIS PERSTANS

It may seem incongruous to append an affection consisting of keratotic papules to the chapter on ichthyoses. There are, however, positive and negative reasons for the arrangement. The negative reason is the desire to separate *Flegel's disease* from Kyrle's disease (Chap. 19) to which it has been compared. The positive identification is the finding that the disorder is an example of hyperkeratosis occurring in the absence of membrane coating granules and, thus, constitutes a unique alteration of epidermal metabolism. It is a genetic disease of autosomal dominant type.[27]

Flegel's disease manifests itself as hyperkeratotic papules, mainly on the lower extremities. The histologic picture consists of bandlike inflammatory infiltrate in the papillary dermis and an epidermis that alternates between atrophy and acanthosis with peculiar tentlike elevations of the skin surface. Frenk and Tapernoux[28] found a complete absence of Odland bodies below the hyperkeratotic lesions, an observation confirmed by two other groups.[29,30]

REFERENCES

1. Frost P, Van Scott EJ: Ichthyosiform dermatoses. Classification based on anatomic and biometric observations. Arch Dermatol 94:113, 1966
2. Wells RS, Kerr CB: Genetic classification of ichthyosis. Arch Dermatol 92:1, 1965
3. Reed WB: Ichthyosiform dermatoses. Arch Dermatol 101:620, 1970
4. Marks R, Dykes PJ (eds): The Ichthyoses. New York, Spectrum, 1978
5. Schnyder UW: Inherited ichthyoses. Arch Dermatol 102:240, 1970
6. Goldsmith LA: Molecular mechanisms of genetic disorders of keratinization. Arch Dermatol 112:375, 1976
7. Harper PS: Genetic heterogeneity in the ichthyoses. In Marks R, Dykes PJ (eds): The Ichthyoses. New York, Spectrum, 1978, p 127
8. Lentz CL, Altman J: Lamellar ichthyosis. The natural clinical course of collodion baby. Arch Dermatol 97:3, 1968
9. Pinkus H, Nagao S: A case of biphasic ichthyosiform dermatosis: light and electron microscopic study. Arch Klin Exp Dermatol 237:737, 1970
10. Kuokkanen K: Ichthyosis vulgaris. A clinical and histopathologic study of patients and their close relatives in the autosomal dominant and sex-linked forms of the disease. Acta Derm Venereol (Stockh) 49 [Suppl 62]:1, 1969

11. Frakj JE, Kuokkanen K, Hopsu Harvu VK: Morphometric analysis of the dominant and sex-linked forms of ichthyosis vulgaris. Acta Derm Venereol 53:299, 1973
12. Shapiro LJ, Weiss R, Buxman MM, et al.: Enzymatic basis of typical x-linked ichthyosis. Lancet 2:756, 1978
13. Buxman MM, Goodkin PE, Fahrenbach WH, et al.: Harlequin ichthyosis with epidermal lipid abnormality. Arch Dermatol 115:189, 1979
14. Mevorah B, Frenk E: Ichthyosis linearis circumflexa Comel with trichorrhexis invaginata (Netherton's syndrome). A light microscopic study of the skin changes. Dermatologica 149:193, 1974
15. Anton-Lamprecht I, Curth HO, Schnyder UW: Zur Ultrastruktur hereditärer Verhornungsstörungen II. Ichthyosis hystrix Typ Curth-Macklin. Arch Dermatol Forsch 246:77, 1973
16. Wile UJ: Familial study of three unusual cases of congenital ichthyosiform erythroderma. Arch Dermatol 10:487, 1925
17. Henrickson L, Zachariae H: Pustular psoriasis and arthritis in congenital psoriasiform erythroderma. Dermatologica 144:12, 1972
18. Vandersteen PR, Muller SA: Erythrokeratodermia variabilis. Arch Dermatol 103:362, 1971
19. Castello CA, Jonquieres EDL: Cocardioform genodermatosis (Degos' disease). Dermatologica 13:37, 1971
20. Degos R, Civatte J, Belaïch S, et al.: Image histologique particulière de certains naevi verruqueux systématisés. Ann Dermatol Syphiligr 96:361, 1969
21. Shapiro L, Baraf CS: Isolated epidermolytic acanthoma: a solitary tumor showing granular degeneration. Arch Dermatol 101:220, 1970
22. Klaus S, Weinstein GD, Frost P: Localized epidermolytic hyperkeratosis: a form of keratoderma of the palms and soles. Arch Dermatol 101:272, 1970
23. Gomez-Orbaneja J, Sanchez Lozano de Sosa JL, Simon Huarte P: Hiperqueratosis palmo-plantar difusa y circumscrita (tipo Thost-Unna) con degeneracion reticular del cuerpo mucosa. Int J Dermatol 11:96, 1972
24. Mehregan AH: Epidermolytic hyperkeratosis. Incidental findings in the epidermis and in the intraepidermal eccrine sweat duct units. J Cutan Pathol 5:76, 1978
25. Ackerman AB: Histopathologic concept of epidermolytic hyperkeratosis. Arch Dermatol 102:253, 1970
26. Dykes PJ, Marks R: Acquired ichthyosis: multiple causes for an acquired generalized disturbance in desquamation. Br J Dermatol 97:327, 1977
27. Bean SF: The genetics of hyperkeratosis lenticularis perstans. Arch Dermatol 106:72, 1972
28. Frenk E, Tapernoux B: Hyperkeratosis lenticularis perstans (Flegel). A biological model for keratinization occuring in the absence of Odland-bodies? Dermatologica 153:253, 1976
29. Ikai K, Murai T, Oguchi M, et al.: An ultrastructural study of the epidermis in hyperkeratosis lenticularis perstans. Acta Derm Venereol (Stockh) 58:363, 1978
30. Squier LA, Eady RAJ, Hopps RM: The permeability of epidermis lacking normal membrane coating granules: an ultrastructural tracer study of Kyrle–Flegel disease. J Invest Dermatol 70:361, 1978

CHAPTER

30

Pigmentary Disorders

Pigmentary disorders not related to nevi or neoplasms manifest themselves clinically as either lightening or darkening of the skin. The histologic possibilities of producing these effects are manifold[1] and are listed in Table 30-1.

Quantity of melanin is difficult to judge in H&E sections, especially when they are deeply stained with eosin. Here, the O&G stain proves its worth because melanin granules, having a proteinaceous base, turn greenish black and appear much darker against the light blue background of the epidermal cells. In the dermis, the same reaction permits one to differentiate melanin from hemosiderin and other pigments that do not change color. For additional data on identification of various colored substances, see Chapters 3 and 27.

DECREASE AND INCREASE OF EPIDERMAL MELANIN

Changes in quantity of epidermal pigmentation can be judged only when normal tissue is available for comparison. The untanned skin of whites can resemble that of an albino or can contain considerable melanin in the basal layer, depending on complexion. Visible melanin granules usually are restricted to basal cells, except in suntan and other forms of hyperpigmentation. Again depending on complexion, the epidermis of blacks may resemble brunet white skin but usually contains variable amounts of dark melanin granules in higher strata, including the horny layer (Chap. 2). Oriental epidermis often contains a surprising amount of melanin granules, which, however, have a lighter hue in an unstained condition.

Depigmentation

If visible melanin is completely absent in epidermal cells, one must ascertain the condition of the junctional melanocytes. These may contain a few pigment granules even in very blond skin and in some conditions of hypopigmentation or may appear as clear cells of Masson, indistinguishable by light microscopy from similarly situated Langerhans cells.

Clear cells (nonkeratinocytes) are present in normal number in *total* and *partial albinism* but may be reduced in number in *vitiligo, secondary leukoderma,* and *nevus depigmentosus* (Chap. 32). Quantitative studies in vitiligo, using the electron microscope,[2] have shown that melanocytes are gradually replaced by indeterminate cells, containing neither melanosomes nor Langerhans granules, and that eventually Langerhans cells take the place of melanocytes at the junction.

In repigmenting vitiligo, it is commonly seen that pigment arises and spreads from hair follicles.

TABLE 30–1.
Histologic Substrates of Lightened or Darkened Skin

Clinical Lightening
  Absence of epidermal melanin (leukoderma, vitiligo, nevus depigmentosus, albinism)
  Reduction of epidermal melanin (hypopigmentation, Stufen-vitiligo, tinea versicolor achromians)
  Increased granular layer (lichen sclerosus et atrophicus, Wickham's striae)
  Increased dermal fibrosity (scars, lichen sclerosus et atrophicus, morphea)
  Diminished amount of blood (scars, nevus anemicus, Raynaud's phenomenon)
Clinical Darkening
  Increase of epidermal melanin (suntanning, chloasma, freckles, lentigines, nevus spilus, nevus Ota, nevus Becker, chronic inflammation)
  Increase of subepidermal melanin (postinflammatory pigmentation, incontinentia pigmenti, lichen planus, lupus erythematosus, Mongolian spot, nevus Ota, blue nevus)
  Increased horny layer (acanthosis nigricans, papillomas, tinea versicolor, ichthyosis)
  Blood in horny layer (thrombosed angiomas, warts, black heel)
  Increased amount of blood in dermis (various hemangiomas and angiectasias, superficial hemorrhage)
  Hemosiderin (hemosideroses)
  Other pigments in dermis (tattoos, ochronosis, apocrine cystadenoma)

This mechanism has been confirmed by histoenzymatic studies in patients under oral photochemotherapy.[3] Follicular melanocytes become active, migrate up the length of the follicle, and spread laterally in the epidermis in a manner comparable to the repigmentation of burn wounds (see below). In some biopsy specimens of vitiligo, an abnormally large and dendritic melanocyte is found at the very border. It is not known, however, whether this is an indication of repigmentation.

Another phenomenon seen occasionally in vitiligo is an erythematous infiltrated border.[4] Histologically, there is noncharacteristic inflammatory infiltrate with epidermal invasion by polymorphs and lymphocytes. The question whether this is an autoimmune mechanism, or whether some other inflammatory disease in the patient's skin leads to vitiliginous depigmentation has not been resolved. The electron microscope does not enable us to differentiate between vitiligo, piebaldism (partial albinism[5] and Waardenburg–Klein syndrome),[6] and leukoderma due to toxic or other causes. In the Vogt–Koyanagi syndrome which is certainly related to autoimmune processes, association of depigmenting melanocytes with lymphocytes has been reported.[7] *Albino melanocytes* contain nonfunctional melanosomes. In the Chediak–Higashi syndrome,[8,9] melanocytes have abnormal, incompletely melanized granules which may be very large. Leukocytes in blood smears also contain large granules. Some cases of vitiligo (Stufenvitiligo) have a broad zone of partial depigmentation between normal and totally blanched skin. This zone contains fairly active melanocytes. The leaf-shaped hypopigmented spots of the tuberous sclerosis syndrome have melanocytes exhibiting weak tyrosinase reaction and incompletely melanized melanosomes.[10]

So-called *incontinentia pigmenti achromians* (hypomelanosis of Ito)[11] is properly classified as a systematized hypochromic nevus[12] and may be associated with mental, ocular, and osseous manifestations. It differs from vitiligo in the presence of dyskeratotic epidermal cells and the persistence of some melanin formation.[13] For differential diagnosis from nevus depigmentosus, see Chapter 32.

A peculiar situation exists in epidermis that has regenerated after a *burn* or other denudation. The new epidermis usually carries a few melanocytes with it as it migrates over the wound surface. It is repopulated with melanocytes secondarily some weeks later[14] by migration from hair follicles and from the wound border and by local multiplication.

Epidermal pigment is reduced in all forms of *tinea versicolor*, but this effect becomes clinically visible only in the *achromians* type, or after treatment of the disease in a tanned skin. It seems to be due to inhibition of melanin production[15] but is overshadowed clinically by erythema and thickening of the horny layer. The depigmentation of Sutton's halo nevus and related phenomena will be discussed in Chapter 32.

Hyperpigmentation

Sharply localized increase of epidermal melanin is seen in freckles (ephelis), chloasma (melasma), nevus spilus, solitary pigment spots of the lips and volar surfaces, and the various forms of lentigo. All these lesions will be discussed in Chapter 32.

Generalized. General increase of epidermal melanization is responsible for the dark skin of *Addison's disease* and of *hemochromatosis*.[16] In the latter, hemosiderin appears in the integument much later than the clinical bronzing, which is due to epidermal hyperpigmentation with melanin, and one should advise internists to take liver biopsies rather than skin biopsies for early diagnosis. A very extraordinary case of gradually increasing universal epidermal hyperpigmentation (the carbon baby) was seen in a Mexican child.[17] Topically limited epidermal hyperpigmentation is encountered in *sun tanning*. In this condition, all layers of the epidermis contain visible granules during the active phase of melanin production.[18,19] If exposure is discontinued, the melanin content of the outer layers gradually diminishes, but basal cell pigment may persist for many months. The combined effect of oral methoxsalen and external long wave ultraviolet (PUVA) therapy seems to be a very complicated one,[20] the details and long-range results of which await further investigation.

Localized. *Erythromelanosis follicularis faciei et colli* is a fairly common condition, which is rediscovered every few years under a different name.[21,22] It owes its clinically poikilodermatous features to a combination of focal epidermal hyperpigmentation with large sebaceous glands and telangiectasia and is confined to sun-exposed areas of the face and neck. Other types of hyperpigmentation are restricted to the acra of the extremities and are also better sorted out on the basis of their clinical appearance than on the histologic substrate of epidermal melanization. *Reticulate acropigmentation of Kitamura*[23] and *acropigmentation of Dohi* (acromelanosis albo-punctata[24]) are examples.

Melanin Block. Many types of chronic inflammation induce some epidermal hyperpigmentation, while others produce hypopigmentation. These phenomena were mentioned in their respective chapters. A paradoxic situation exists in black skin in chronic eczematous and other forms of dermatitis. Clinical darkening in these cases is due to increased blood supply and increased pigmentation. However, under the low power of the microscope (Chaps. 2 and 5), the acanthotic and spongiotic epidermis actually appears lighter. Close examination reveals that the keratinocytes contain less or no melanin. On the other hand, melanocytes appear highly dendritic (Fig. 2-39B) and stuffed with pigment granules. This phenomenon of *melanin block* (Fig. 2-41), or disruption of the functional epidermal melanin unit, spreads melanin over a larger area and dilutes it as far as tissue sections are concerned. On the other hand, it produces a clinical darkening effect similar to the one a frog produces by spreading melanin in its dermal melanophores. For a review of pigment changes in diseased African skin see Sarrat and Nouhouayi.[25]

INCREASE OF SUBEPIDERMAL MELANIN

Subepidermal melanin may be found in macrophages or in dermal melanocytes, only rarely free in the tissue. Barring histochemical demonstration of acid phosphatase in macrophages or tyrosinase in melanocytes, the best available criterion for differentiation of these cell types is the size and distribution of the granules, which are of small, even size and diffusely distributed in the melanin-forming cell, with the nucleus plainly visible. They are of uneven size and clumped in the macrophage and often obscure the nucleus by their great quantity. In these respects, macrophages containing melanin resemble those containing hemosiderin. The Giemsa stain will differentiate the two pigments without recourse to special measures. Subepidermal pigmentation due to dermal melanocytes will be discussed in Chapter 32.

Subepidermal macrophage pigmentation is found in many chronic inflammatory diseases and may be associated either with epidermal hyperpigmentation or with epidermal pigment loss. The latter condition often exhibits focal damage to basal cells and melanocytes and is designated as *incontinentia pigmenti*. It is present in the disease of that name (see below) or as symptomatic incontinence in lichenoid tissue reactions, lupus erythematosus, lichen sclerosus et atrophicus, and poikilodermatous states. The leukomelanoderma of the chronically irritated skin in *vagabond's disease* also deserves mention here.[26]

Subepidermal melanophages are found without obvious basal layer derangement and often associated with some epidermal hyperpigmentation in *postinflammatory pigmentation* (Fig. 5-13). The pigment usually is retained for many months and may thus remain after all evidence of active disease, such as lichen planus or lupus erythematosus, has subsided. It is most prominently found in *fixed drug eruptions*. Its amount depends on the natural pigmentation of the skin and therefore is greatest in blacks, who exhibit the phenomenon of postinflammatory pigmentation following a variety of dermatoses which would not lead to appreciable deposition of pigment in macrophages in a light-complexioned skin. Postinflammatory pigmentation, therefore, is not diagnostic, although one may venture suggestions if there are associated remnants of a specific dermatosis or signs of acute flare-up of inflammation, as in a fixed drug eruption.

In cases in which neither clinical history nor histologic evidence suggests specific inflammatory disease, one may consider two rare dermatoses.

One is the so-called Naegeli type of incontinentia pigmenti *(reticular pigmented dermatosis)* in which, according to Whiting,[27] transitory fragility of the epidermal melanin unit leads to loading of macrophages along the venous network. The other one was described in Japan as *pigmentatio maculosa multiplex* and is characterized clinically by brownish gray or bluish gray macules measuring from a few millimeters to 1 cm in diameter. Histologically, there is macrophage pigmentation with or without epidermal hyperpigmentation, but no evidence of significant inflammation.[28]

The diffuse melanosis secondary to malignant melanoma is probably due to dissemination of melanin granules but was found in one case[29] to be caused by diffuse spread of melanoma cells in the dermis.

Incontinentia Pigmenti

More recent investigations of *Bloch–Sulzberger's disease* have shown that the characteristic streaky pigmentation is only the end stage of a chain of processes, which in the fully developed case start with blisters in the newborn period and often have an intermediate verrucous stage.[30] Incontinentia pigmenti, therefore, might as well have been discussed in Chapter 11 (Table 11-1), Chapter 29, or even Chapter 28. A worldwide analysis[31] revealed more than 600 reported cases.

Babies born with, or developing, vesicles or bullae soon after birth should be suspected to have incontinentia pigmenti, especially if they are female. The bulla, on histologic examination, shows accumulation of eosinophilic leukocytes (Fig. 30-1A) in

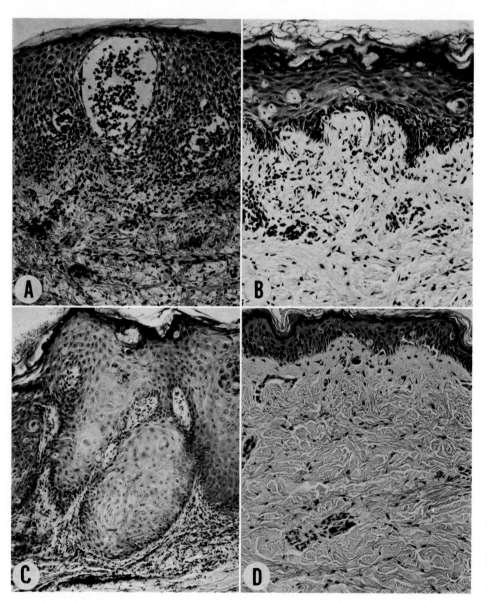

FIGURE 30–1.
Four stages of incontinentia pigmenti. **A.** *Intraepidermal vesicles filled with eosinophils in newborn period.* **B.** *Hyperkeratotic and dyskeratotic phase often preceding verrucous stage shown in* **C. D.** *End stage of macrophage pigmentation below a nonpigmented, but otherwise fairly normal, epidermis. All H&E. X135.*

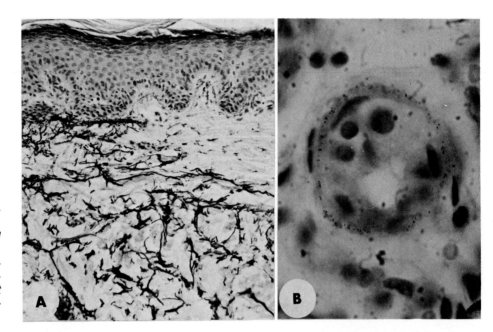

FIGURE 30–2.
Argyria. **A.** *Silver amalgam in-oculated into oral mucosa. Metal preferentially deposited on elastic fibers. H&E. X125.* **B.** *Argyria caused by ingestion. Silver granules preferentially deposited on basement membrane of eccrine secretory tubule. H&E. X540.*

the stratum spinosum. By the time the bullous stage subsides, the epidermis may become acanthotic and hyperkeratotic in a verrucous manner (Fig. 30-1C).

It usually contains large vacuolated cells (Fig. 30-1B), which electron microscopists have interpreted as degenerating melanocytes[32] or as macrophages.[33] The most characteristic feature is whorling of prickle cells with central keratinization (endokeratinization, Chap. 31), which simulates cross sections of intraepidermal sweat ducts in individual sections but may be shown in serial sections to be independent of acrosyringia. These first stages are variable in their clinical expression and usually subside by the time the baby is one year old. It is only then that pigmentation becomes clinically apparent. Histologically, it develops gradually and presents the contrast (Fig. 30-1D) between dermal melanophages and a practically nonpigmented epidermis. A histologic picture somewhat similar to that illustrated in Figure 30-1B may be seen in the unrelated *pseudoatrophoderma colli.*[34]

OTHER INTRADERMAL COLORED MATTER

Hemosiderin is a common cause of dermal pigmentation, as described in Chapter 27. It should not be confused with the artifactual formalin pigment sometimes observed in tissue sections (Chap. 3). Practically all other colored granular material is present in the skin, either due to *tattooing* (intentional or accidental) or to long-continued internal uptake of metals or certain modern drugs. Carbon

particles are used for blue tattoos and may get into the skin accidentally, mainly as a professional hazard of miners. They are recognized in sections because they are truly black. Other granules may appear black in transillumination, e.g., cinnabar and other pigments used in tattooing. Cinnabar crystals have a characteristic rounded shape, and examination with oil immersion usually brings out their red color. Sometimes examination in incident light may give a clue. White powders (such as the material contained in golf balls), which have been accidentally tattooed into the skin, appear black in transmitted light but chalky in incident light.

Metal pigmentation is most commonly due to silver *(argyria)*, which may be seen as tiny black granules (Fig. 30-2) deposited in dermal tissue cells and on the basement membrane of sweat coils, if it is present in profusion.[35] It is startlingly demonstrated, even in small amounts, by darkfield illumination (Chap. 3), but shares this property[36] with gold *(auriasis)* and mercury.[37] Amalgam is sometimes introduced into oral tissues by the slip of a dental drill (Chap. 45).

Peculiar discoloration of light-exposed skin has been observed after long-continued intake of certain tranquilizers, cardiac drugs, and other modern medicaments.[38-40] The nature of the responsible pigments is not fully elucidated, but they are not necessarily melanin. The specific pigment of *ochronosis*[41] occurs more commonly in cartilage, but masses of it may be found in the skin (Fig. 30-3) and stain specifically dark with methylene blue. An epidemic of cutaneous ochronosis associated with colloid milia was observed in South Africa

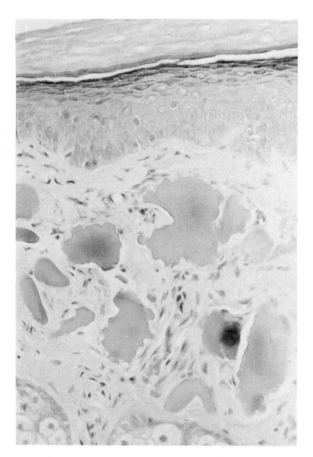

FIGURE 30–3.
Ochronosis. Irregular masses of brown material not related to cells in upper dermis of face. Unusually thick stratum granulosum and stratum corneum for this part of body. H&E. X250.

after prolonged use of strong hydroquinone bleaching creams.[42] The contents of epithelial cysts or apocrine cystadenomas (Chap. 37) may impart a dark blue hue to the overlying skin.

OTHER DERMAL CHANGES AFFECTING COLOR

Just as excessive blood makes the skin redder or darker, so does reduced content of blood make it look paler, as we can observe in cold weather when fingers and hands turn white. Permanently contracted vessels seem to be the only substrate in *nevus anemicus*,[43,44] while melanin, dermal structure, and structure of vessels appear normal in histologic section. Relative lack of vessels, together with increased density of collagen bundles, is the reason that *scars* remain lighter than surrounding skin long after the epidermis has regained its ability to pigment. The white color of lichen sclerosus et

atrophicus (Chap. 25) and of atrophie blanche (Chap. 15) also is in part due to these factors. It takes a sharp eye and an open mind to recognize such rather subtle changes in tissue sections. Distinctly yellow color may be imparted to the skin not only by lipids but also by elastic tissue, as in pseudoxanthoma elasticum and actinic elastosis (Chap. 26).

COLOR CHANGES DUE TO HORNY LAYER

On gross examination, thickened stratum corneum may look any hue from pale yellow (keratoderma palmare) to grayish black (ichthyosis). It may express the color of contained melanin but often owes its tinge to other, ill-defined substances. In *acanthosis nigricans* one is often surprised by the small amount of melanin contained in a clinically very dark epidermis. Similarly, other verrucous

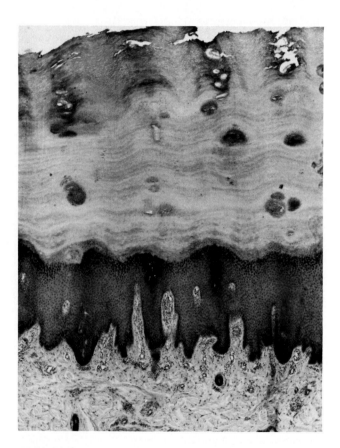

FIGURE 30–4.
Intrakeratinous hemorrhages of black heel (pseudochromidrosis). Dark areas in horny layer consist of inspissated erythrocytes, some of which are inside sweat ducts. Others result from capillary hemorrhage and enter the stratum corneum by transepidermal elimination. H&E. X45. (From Mehregan. Can Med Assoc J 95:584, 1966.)

papillomas, and particularly seborrheic verruca, may owe their dark color to keratin rather than melanin. The varied hues of *tinea versicolor* are due to a combination of erythema and thick horny layer, even in the presence of diminished melanization. That the peculiar orange-yellow color in *carotinemia* is most pronounced in volar skin indicates that it resides mainly in the horny layer. These and other possibilities must be kept in mind when the clinically evident color of the skin seems to have no substrate in histologic sections.

Intrakeratinous traumatic hemorrhage (Fig. 30-4) has been found to be the substrate of *black heel*, a condition encountered in young athletes.[45]

On the other hand, one has to remember that a thick stratum granulosum reflects and diffuses light. It can hide or change the color of underlying blood or melanin, giving it a bluish tinge. This was mentioned under lichen planus (Chap. 9). Keratohyalin may even give the surface a chalky white color, as in lichen sclerosus et atrophicus or leukoplakia of the mucous membranes.

REFERENCES

1. Mishima Y: Histopathology of functional pigmentary disorders. Cutis 21:225, 1978
2. Mishima Y, Kawasaki H, Pinkus H: Dendritic cell dynamics in progressive depigmentations: distinctive cytokinetics of dendritic cells revealed by electron microscopy. Arch Dermatol Forsch 243:67, 1972
3. Ortonne J-P, Macdonald DM, Micoud A, et al.: La repigmentation du vitiligo induite par la photochimiothérapie orale. Étude histoenzymologique (Split-Dopa) et ultrastructurale. Ann Dermatol Venereol 105:939, 1978
4. Ortonne J-P, Baran R, Civatte J: Vitiligo à bordure inflammatoire. A propos de 2 observations avec revue de la littérature (18 cas). Ann Dermatol Venereol 106:613, 1979
5. Bonerandi J-J, Baran R, Breton A, et al.: Piebaldisme. Étude anatomo-clinique et ultrastructurale de 3 cas. Ann Dermatol Venereol 105:67, 1978
6. Ortonne J-P, Perrot H, Beyvin A-J, et al.: Le syndrome de Waardenburg-Klein. Ann Dermatol Syphiligr 103:245, 1976
7. Bazex A, Balas D, Bazex J, et al.: Maladie de Vogt-Koyanagi-Harada. A propos de 2 observations. Ann Dermatol Venereol 104:849, 1977
8. Blume RS, Wolff SM: The Chediak-Higashi syndrome: studies in four patients and a review of the literature. Medicine 51:247, 1972
9. Deprez P, Laurent R, Griscelli C, et al.: La maladie de Chédiak-Higashi. A propos d'une nouvelle observation. Ann Dermatol Venereol 105:841, 1978
10. Denoeux J-P, Cesarini J-P, Carton F-X: Les mélanocytes dans l'épiloia; aspects ultrastructuraux (à propos de 7 cas). Ann Dermatol Venereol 104:845, 1977
11. Jelinek JE, Bart RS, Schiff GM: Hypomelanosis of Ito ("incontinentia pigmenti achromians"). Arch Dermatol 107:590, 1973
12. Maize JC, Headington JT, Lynch PJ: Systematized hypochromic nevus: incontinentia pigmenti achromians of Ito. Arch Dermatol 106:884, 1972
13. Grosshans E, Stoebner F, Bergoend H, et al.: Incontinentia achromians (Ito): étude clinique et histopathologique. Dermatologica 142:65, 1971
14. Staricco RG: Mechanism of migration of the melanocytes from the hair follicle into the epidermis following dermabrasion. J Invest Dermatol 36:99, 1961
15. Charles CR, Sire DJ, Johnson BL, et al.: Hypopigmentation in tinea versicolor; a histochemical and electron microscopic study. Int J Dermatol 12:48, 1973
16. Chevrant-Breton J, Simon M, Bourel M, et al.: Cutaneous manifestations of idiopathic hemochromatosis. Arch Dermatol 113:161, 1977
17. Ruiz-Maldonado R, Tamayo L, Fernando-Diaz J: Universal-acquired melanosis. The carbon baby. Arch Dermatol 114:775, 1978
18. Langner A, Kligman AM: Tanning without sunburn with aminobenzoic acid-type sunscreen. Arch Dermatol 106:338, 1972
19. Urbach F (ed.): The Biologic Effects of Ultraviolet Radiation (With Emphasis on the Skin). Oxford, New York, Pergamon, 1969
20. Braun-Falco O, Hofmann C, Plewig G: Photochemotherapy of psoriasis: clinical and histological findings. In Farber E, et al. (eds): Psoriasis. New York, Yorke Medical Books, 1977
21. Mishima Y, Rudner E: Erythromelanosis follicularis faciei et colli. Dermatologica 132:269, 1966
22. Colomb D, Racouchot J, Gho A, et al.: L'erythrosis interfollicularis colli de Leder. Ann Dermatol Venereol 104:238, 1977
23. Griffiths WAD: Reticulate acropigmentation of Kitamura. Br J Dermatol 95:437, 1976
24. Siemens HW: Acromelanosis albo-punctata. Dermatologica 128:86, 1964
25. Sarrat H, Nouhouayi Y: Les modifications du pigment melanique cutané rencontrées chez l'Africain au cours de diverses dermatoses. Int J Dermatol 10:44, 1971
26. Grosshans E, Stoebner F, Basset A: La leukomélanodermie des vagabonds; étude anatomopathologique et ultrastructurale. Ann Dermatol Syphiligr 99:141, 1972
27. Whiting DA: Naegeli's reticular pigmented dermatosis. Br J Dermatol 85 [Suppl 7]:71, 1972
28. Degos R, Civatte J, Belaïch S: La pigmentation maculeuse eruptive idiopathique. Ann Dermatol Venereol 105:177, 1978
29. Konrad K, Wolff K: Pathogenesis of diffuse melanosis secondary to malignant melanoma. Br J Dermatol 91:635, 1974
30. Epstein S, Vedder JS, Pinkus H: Bullous variety of incontinentia pigmenti (Bloch–Sulzberger). Arch Dermatol 65:557, 1952
31. Carney RS Jr: Incontinentia pigmenti. A world statistical analysis. Arch Dermatol 112:535, 1976
32. Wong CK, Guerrier CJ, MacMillan DC, et al.: An electron microscopical study of Bloch–Sulzberger syndrome (incontinentia pigmenti). Acta Derm Venereol (Stockh) 51:161, 1971
33. Schaumburg-Lever G, Lever WF: Electron micro-

scopy of incontinentia pigmenti. J Invest Dermatol 61:151, 1973

34. Kanan MW, Kendil E: Pseudoatrophoderma colli in a male. Br J Dermatol 81:65, 1969
35. Pariser RJ: Generalized argyria. Clinicopathologic features and histochemical studies. Arch Dermatol 114:373, 1976
36. Cox AJ, Marich KW: Gold in the dermis following gold therapy for rheumatoid arthritis. Arch Dermatol 108:655, 1973
37. Kennedy C, Molland EA, Henderson WJ, et al.: Mercury pigmentation from industrial exposure. An ultrastructural and analytical electron microscopic study. Br J Dermatol 96:367, 1976
38. Levantine A, Almeyda J: Drug induced changes in pigmentation. Br J Dermatol 89:105, 1973
39. Dyster-Aas K, Hansson H, Miörner G, et al.: Pigment deposits in eyes and light exposed skin during long-term methacycline therapy. Acta Derm Venereol (Stockh) 54:209, 1974
40. Lambert D, Noble J-P, Justrabo E, et al.: Pigmentation cutanée secondaire a l'administration d'amiodarone. Ann Dermatol Syphiligr 102:277, 1975
41. Attwood HD, Clifton S, Mitchell RE: A histological, histochemical and ultrastructural study of dermal ochronosis. Pathology 3:115, 1971
42. Findlay GH, Morrison JGL, Simson IW: Exogenous ochronosis and pigmented colloid milium from hydroquinone bleaching creams. Br J Dermatol 93:613, 1975
43. Greaves MW, Birkett D, Johnson C: Nevus anemicus: a unique catecholamine-dependent nevus. Arch Dermatol 102:172, 1970
44. Daniel RH, Hubler WR, Wolf JE, et al.: Nevus anemicus. Donor dominant defect. Arch Dermatol 113:53, 1977
45. Mehregan AH: Black heel: a report of two cases. Can Med Assoc J 95:584, 1966

CHAPTER
31

Virus Epidermoses

The causal association of virus with mammalian neoplasia, a subject which was taboo 25 years ago, is now rather generally admitted. However, those proliferative epidermal lesions for which an infectious etiology was established many years ago have characteristics sufficiently different from true neoplasms to treat them at this point. These are molluscum contagiosum and the infectious verrucae. Viral diseases causing predominantly inflammatory changes in the skin were treated in Chapter 12.

MOLLUSCUM CONTAGIOSUM

The agent of molluscum contagiosum belongs to the large intracytoplasmic viruses of the pox group. The umbilicated clinical papule is represented histologically in Figure 31-1 by an orderly, lobulated mass of stratified epithelium, which hangs down from the epidermis like a small septate tomato. Occasionally, the lesion may develop in the wall of an epidermoid cyst.[1] The keratinizing products of the thick wall of the molluscum are discharged into a central chamber which opens to the surface through a relatively narrow pore. It is characteristic that only a certain percentage of the epithelial elements show evidence of viral infection, leaving a majority of cells to keratinize fairly normally. The altered cells (Fig. 31-1B) become recognizable in the low layers of the stratum spinosum. They exhibit a small hazy mass in their cytoplasm, which increases in size in the higher layers, compressing the

nucleus and dislodging it to the periphery, where it is seen as a thin sickle in cross section. The cells assume large ovoid shape as they enter the keratohyaline layer and are transformed into basophilic ellipsoid bodies of hyaline appearance in the horny layer. These *molluscum bodies* can be seen in fresh unstained preparations of the material that can be squeezed from the pore of the *molluscum*. Special stains can demonstrate the *virus elementary bodies* in the intracytoplasmic mass. They are at the borderline of light microscopic visibility. Their cubelike shape has been demonstrated by electron microscopy.

Ordinarily, the molluscum is surrounded by a thin shell of finely woven connective tissue, and this permits the epithelial ball to be shelled out easily by firm lateral pressure. Occasionally, a lesion will become clinically inflamed. Histologically, there is then found a heavy mixed infiltrate that has granulomatous features and even may simulate lymphoma. It is our opinion, on the basis of experimental studies,[2] that this infiltrate is an immunologic reaction, and this view was supported by Kipping.[3] This inflamed type of lesion often is biopsied without the clinician's suspecting molluscum contagiosum.[4] Inasmuch as the epithelial part may have been largely destroyed by the time the specimen is obtained or may have been dislodged and lost during surgery, such lesions offer considerable diagnostic difficulties, and in some cases only the identification of a few molluscum bodies in the purulent surface crust solved the riddle for us.

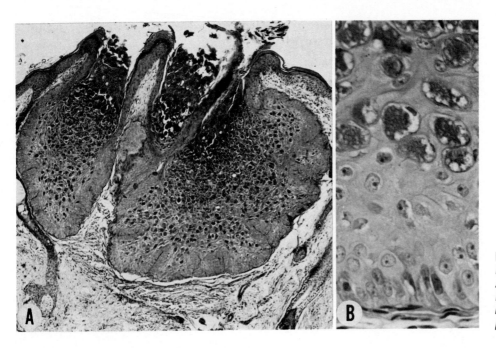

FIGURE 31-1.
Molluscum contagiosum. **A.**
Aggregate of three mollusca.
H&E. X60. **B.** *Formation of*
molluscum bodies in hyper-
plastic epithelium. H&E. X280.

VIRUS WARTS

Under the general heading of virus warts,[5] we discuss the variants of verruca plana juvenilis, verruca plana, verruca vulgaris, verruca filiformis, verruca digitata, verrucae of the plantar type, and condyloma acuminatum. Epidermodysplasia verruciformis, having been proved to be transferable and to contain viral particles, also will be included.

The virus or viruses of warts belonging to the papova group[6,7] are very small and intranuclear[8] and manifest themselves in routine sections only by the presence of stainable nuclei in the horny layer above a thick granular layer. While it has been shown by immunofluoroescence that the stainable material is viral DNA rather than human chromatin, it is their spheric shape (Fig. 31-2) that distinguishes these masses from ordinary flat parakeratotic nuclei in routine stains. Often, they are not present, and histologic diagnosis of the various types of virus warts must rely on other criteria.

One can put diagnosis on a more rational basis by remembering that all warts are verrucous papillomas and that cellular maturation is not impeded or grossly altered, in contrast to certain other papillomas (Chap. 33) and dysplastic precanceroses (Chap. 34). That a flat wart should be a papilloma may sound surprising. However, papilloma means circumscribed combined hyperplasia of epidermis and papillae, and one can usually find, even in a flat verruca (Fig. 31-3), one or two papillae that project so high that the suprapapillary plate is thin

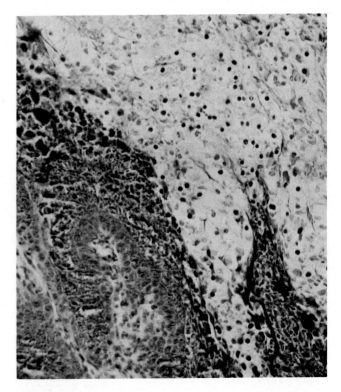

FIGURE 31-2.
Verruca vulgaris. Keratohyalin hyperplasia and spherical DNA inclusion bodies in horny layer simulating parakeratotic nuclei. H&E. X185.

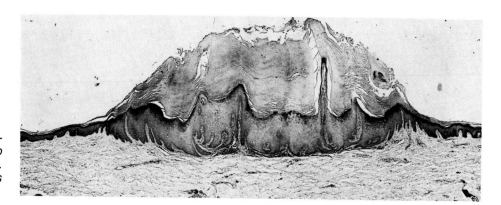

FIGURE 31–3.
Verruca vulgaris plana. Individual long papillae attest to papillomatous nature of lesion. Convergence of rete ridges is well shown. H&E. X35.

or elevated. In most viral warts, elongation of papillae is a prominent feature of diagnostic value. The term *verrucous papilloma* means that the papillomatous lesion is also hyperkeratotic and thus is actually synonymous with "verruca" (seborrheic verruca, Chap. 33).

Verruca Vulgaris

The prototype of all virus warts (Fig. 31-4) consists of thickened acanthotic epidermis, the mass of which greatly exceeds that of the thin, compressed, but elongated papillae. These cause the surface of the lesion to be elevated into cone-shaped projections covered with thin and often parakeratotic epithelium. While the granular layer is hyperplastic in the valleys, it becomes thinner on the slopes of the projections and is often absent at their tips, which appear covered with a stack of inverted hollow parakeratotic cones. The center contains scant connective tissue and a blood-filled capillary. The granular layer in the valleys is not only hyperplastic but contains unusually large and often angular blobs of keratohyalin, a very characteristic but not pathognomonic feature. In between, especially in young warts, there are large vacuolated cells with a central nucleus but few keratohyalin granules. Occasionally, a few of the above-mentioned spheric nuclei are seen in the thick, regularly lamellated, and otherwise orthokeratotic horny layer that fills the valleys. The living portion of the epidermis consists of large prickle cells in regular array, and the basal layer is well formed and shows a single row of cuboid or columnar cells. Inflammatory infiltrate is not a characteristic feature of common warts.

A very important feature is the centripetal direction of the tips of rete ridges (Fig. 31-3). This is due to the expansive growth of the upper layers, which have become voluminous and have displaced the surrounding normal structures, while the lowest point of the ridges and the corresponding bases of the papillae remain fixed near the site of origin of the lesion. This convergence of the ridges, which actually is a sign that the vascular papillae diverge like the stamens of a flower, is in contrast to the divergence of any invasive epithelial tumor and a valuable sign in differential diagnosis.

The foregoing detailed description of the common wart was given for two reasons. It is the basis for differential diagnosis from other types of verrucous and papillomatous lesions and from malignant tumors. It is also the basis for understanding the variable features of other virus warts. Those of oral mucosa will be mentioned in Chapter 45.

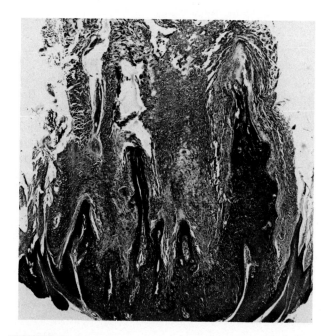

FIGURE 31–4.
Manifestly papillomatous verruca vulgaris combining features of digitate form with so much coherent hyperkeratosis that cutaneous horn (see Chap. 34) results. H&E. X14.

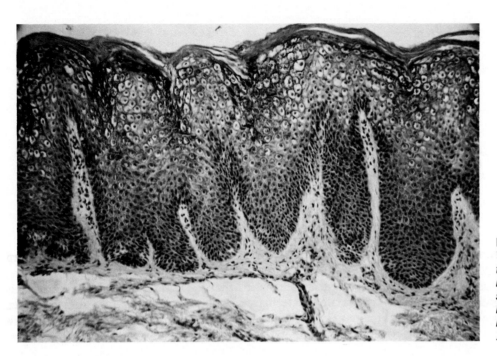

FIGURE 31–5.
Verruca plana. In this case, in-tracellular edema of the upper malpighian layers sets the stage for a basket-weave horny layer, but alteration has not reached stratum corneum. H&E. X135.

Verruca Plana

Reduction of the papillomatous features of the common wart makes the surface smoother and gives the aspect of *verruca vulgaris plana* (Fig. 31-3). Hypergranulosis, elongation of some papillae, and convergence of rete ridges are characteristic features. *Verruca plana juvenilis* (Fig. 31-5) may show compressed papillae in a platelike thickened epidermis. Vacuolated cells, hypergranulosis, and the basket-weave type of horny layer are the outstanding features. The latter is due to intracellular edema of prickle cells and is an exaggeration of an aspect of normal stratum corneum. In both cases, it is the walls of the keratinized cells that stain. The cells of the wart remain more bulky but look empty. It is not always easy to be sure of the border between normal and abnormal in this respect.

Plane warts occasionally undergo involution associated with clinical signs of inflammation. Histologically, the epidermis is infiltrated with inflammatory cells (Fig. 31-6), suggesting cell-mediated immunity.[9,10]

Verruca Filiformis and Verruca Digitata

Exaggeration of the papillomatous features and extremely elongated papillae are found preferentially on the face and neck and around elbows and knees. If only a single papilla is involved, a filamentous growth results, and only this should properly be

called *verruca filiformis*. If several papillae are forming long, fingerlike protrusions, we deal with *verruca digitata*. In both cases, the papillae may branch, and their terminal portions, including the engorged capillaries, often become dyhydrated in the thick horny layer, making the tips look black due to inspissated blood.

Verrucae of Plantar Type

Lesions with the histologic features of *verruca plantaris* (Fig. 31-7) may also be found on the volar surface of the hand, and even in the thickly keratinized dorsal portions of feet, hands, elbows, and knees. They represent an extreme degree of thickening of all epidermal layers above the stratum basale and grotesque exaggeration (Fig. 31-2) of the keratohyalin formation already described under verruca vulgaris. In addition, virus-laden nuclei are prominent in the horny layer, and thin papillae become extremely long and form columns of dehydrated blood in the upper strata. The resulting picture, with alternating columns of nucleated and nonnucleated horny layer, is highly characteristic but quite confusing to the uninitiated, especially if the sections were not cut vertically to the skin surface. A common error is to declare the large keratohyalin-filled cells as molluscum bodies. However, close examination shows that they contain a spheric nucleus near the center rather than a compressed sickle-shaped one at the periphery and that the stainable intracytoplasmic material consists of

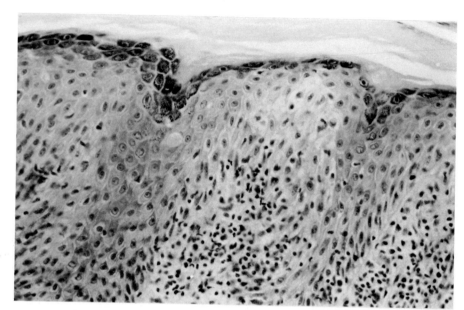

FIGURE 31–6.
Inflamed regressing verruca plana juvenilis. Keratinocytes of epidermis have small fading nuclei, and some vacuolated cells are left as the only characteristic of verruca. Cells of acrosyringium stain normally dark, have normal nuclei with nucleoli, and keratinize. H&E. X375.

irregular masses of keratohyalin rather than of homogeneous viral gloea. For this type of wart, the old term *myrmecia* has been revived.[11] The dehydrated blood in the long papillae is the basis for the diagnostic black dots which one sees shaving a plantar wart, and deeper shaving leads to fairly profuse bleeding from the exposed capillaries. The convergent rete ridges cause a plantar wart to have a smooth lower contour, and a sharp-spoon curette can shell out the entire lesion as a glistening ball, with minimal damage to connective tissue. Knowledge of histopathology thus aids in diagnosis and rational treatment. We do not advocate the blind use of the electric current but prefer clean sharp curettage as the most effective treatment of plantar warts.

Condyloma Acuminatum

The question whether warts in the moist skin of the genitoanal region owe their specific character to a different virus or just to the terrain in which they develop seems to be resolved in favor of a variant of HPV virus.[7,12] Actually, genital warts only rarely (Fig. 31-8) exhibit histologic evidence of the virus but are the purest example (Fig. 31-9A) of a cutaneous papilloma. The core consists of fairly loose collagenous tissue having a good blood supply and no or just a few thin elastic fibers. There is branching of papillae, and the epidermis is acanthotic with a variable amount of keratinization. There is no unusual hypergranulosis. The horny layer is orthokeratotic unless maceration causes

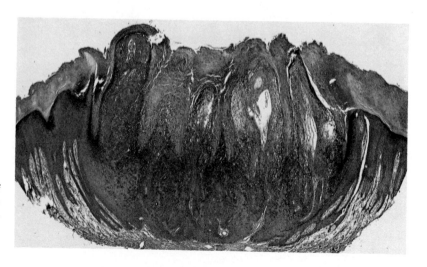

FIGURE 31–7.
Verruca vulgaris plantaris. Convergence of rete ridges makes possible removal of entire lesion with sharp curette without appreciable damage to underlying dermis. H&E. X14.

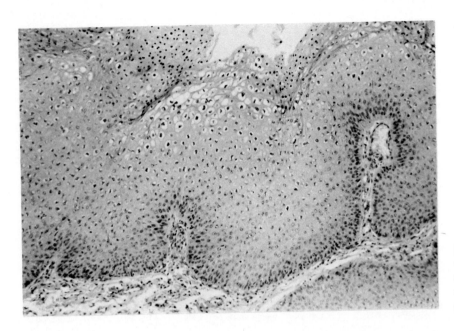

FIGURE 31–8.
Condyloma acuminatum showing vacu-olated cells and viral inclusion bodies resembling parakeratotic nuclei. H&E. X135.

parakeratosis. The large, well-developed prickle cells often were used by the old anatomists for the illustration of tonofibrils and intercellular bridges. The peculiar cytologic features caused by the therapeutic application of podophyllin are shown in Figure 31-9B.

Differential Diagnosis. It may be impossible to differentiate condyloma acuminatum histologically from a papillomatous epidermal nevus, especially when the lesion is situated in a relatively dry area,

such as the shaft of the penis. Lesions on the female genitalia are more often macerated and super-infected and exhibit inflammatory infiltrate and parakeratosis. On the other hand, it is usually easy to rule out malignancy if one pays attention to the presence of large stratified prickle cells above a single layer of basal cells. Mitoses often are seen in the basal layer, but rarely in great number. Nuclei are evenly sized and normochromatic, but occasional dyskeratotic *(individually keratinizing)* cells may be present. Difficulty arises in cases of *giant*

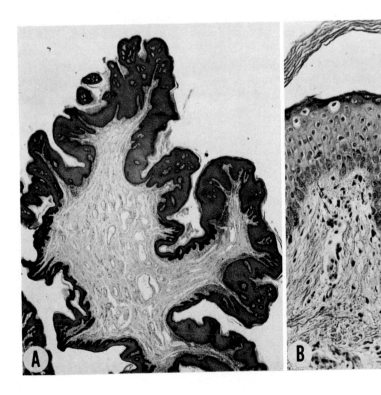

FIGURE 31–9.
Condyloma acuminatum. **A.** *Relatively dry lesion shows fibroepithelial, papillomatous character. H&E. X13.* **B.** *Shows effects of podophyllin treatment (podophyllin cells). H&E. X209.*

condylomata acuminata (Buschke–Loewenstein type), which develop in a preputial sac and break through the foreskin. Although these are as a rule clinically benign, malignant behavior and metastasis have been recorded, and histologic differentiation from *verrucous carcinoma* of mucous membranes[13] must be based on examination of ample material from the borders as well as the depth of the lesion (Chap. 45).

Some excitement was produced recently when a number of observers found histologic changes of Bowen's disease in lesions removed from penis and vulva of young people as condylomata acuminata. The question whether these changes mean Bowen's disease or are benign bowenoid dyskeratosis will be discussed in Chapter 45.

EPIDERMODYSPLASIA VERRUCIFORMIS

It had long been recognized that the microscopic picture of this disease is similar to that of verruca plana. Now, electron microscopy has demonstrated wart virus in the nuclei. Thus this condition, in which squamous cell cancer often supervenes,[14] (Fig. 31-10) appears to be a perfect homologue to the Shope rabbit papilloma, which also is the precursor of cancer. A review of the literature is found in the recent paper of Yabe et al.[15]

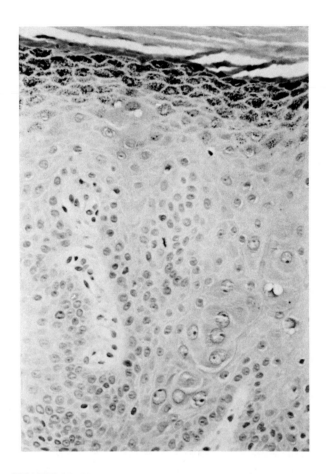

FIGURE 31–10.
Epidermodysplasia verruciformis exhibiting nests of large cells with large nuclei and prominent nucleoli suggesting transformation into malignant neoplastic cells. H&E. X400.

REFERENCES

1. Fellner MJ, Osowsky MJ: Molluscum contagiosum in an epidermal inclusion cyst. Int J Dermatol 18:160 1979
2. Pinkus H, Frisch D: Inflammatory reactions to molluscum contagiosum, possibly of immunologic nature. J Invest Dermatol 13:289, 1949
3. Kipping HF: Molluscum dermatitis. Arch Dermatol 103:106, 1971
4. Mehregan AH: Molluscum contagiosum. A clinicopathologic study. Arch Dermatol 84:123, 1961
5. Steigleder G-K: Histology of benign virus induced tumors of the skin. J Cutan Pathol 5:45, 1978
6. Thivolet J, Viac J: Immunologie des verrues humaines. Ann Dermatol 105:257, 1978
7. Orth G, Dompmartin D, Agache, P, et al.: Pluralité du virus des papillomes humains. Ann Dermatol 105:279, 1978
8. Almeida JD, Howatson, AF, Williams MG: Electron microscopic study of human warts; sites of virus production and nature of the inclusion bodies. J Invest Dermatol 38:337, 1962
9. Tagami H, Takigawa M, Ogino A, et al.: Spontaneous regression of plane warts after inflammation. Clinical and histologic studies in 25 cases. Arch Dermatol 113:1209, 1977
10. Berman A, Winkelmann RK: Flat warts undergoing involution. Histopathological findings. Arch Dermatol 113:1219, 1979
11. Lyell A, Miles JAR: The myrmecia; a study of inclusion bodies in warts. Br Med J 1:912, 1951
12. Coggin JR, zur Hausen H: Workshop on papilloma viruses and cancer. Cancer Res 39:545, 1979
13. Dawson, DF, Duckworth JK, Bernhardt H, et al.: Giant condyloma and verrucous carcinoma of the genital area. Arch Pathol 79:225, 1965
14. Orth G, Jablonska S, Jarzabek-Chorzelska M, et al.: Characteristics of the lesions and risk of malignant conversion associated with the type of human papilloma virus involved in epidermodysplasia verruciformis. Cancer Res 39:1074, 1979
15. Yabe Y, Yashi M, Yoshino N, et al.: Epidermodysplasia verruciformis: viral particles in early malignant lesions. J Invest Dermatol 71:225, 1978

VII

MALFORMATION AND NEOPLASIA

In the chapters dealing with inflammatory diseases in the widest sense, we are concerned with normal cells reacting to certain stimuli and either dying or returning to normal when the disease heals. Even though healing of the skin organ might take place with scar formation or atrophy, there is no permanent derangement of the tissue cells. When discussing certain epithelial diseases, such as Darier's or ichthyosis, we assume that the metabolism of all epidermal cells is genetically deranged but that the clinical and histologic expression of the derangement depends on internal or external regulatory factors and can be reversed or suppressed temporarily. Similarly, when the metabolism of mesodermal cells is deranged, as in angiokeratoma of Fabry or the mucopolysaccharidoses, we can expect to overcome the general but specific enzymatic deficiency by supplying the missing enzyme, withholding the substrate that can not be metabolized, or administering the lacking end product.

We discuss virus epidermoses as tumorlike but different from neoplasia because of the presence of an identifiable virus and because of known immunologic reactions that lead to spontaneous destruction or involution of the epidermal derangement. Possibility of progression from a viral papilloma to a true neoplasm underlines the distinction.

We now come to disorders which are *localized*, since only a local focus of cells is deranged, but which can be cured only by removal or destruction of the cells involved because the derangement is *permanent* and its expression more or less *independent* of regulatory influences. The cellular derangement may be present at birth, due either to inheritance or to prenatal events, or it may occur at any time in life due to internal or external factors (e.g., radiation). Once it has occurred, the change is permanent and is transmitted to the offspring of the deranged cell.

It is important, for diagnostic interpretation, to keep these concepts clearly in mind, even though there are borderline cases in which a decision is difficult. Exact definitions and distinct terminology take us further than a denial that limits can be drawn. Nobody denies the existence of male and female, even though intersexes occur. Having defined the field of this section as localized disturbances due to heritable derangement of specific tissue cells, we subdivide it into *malformation* and *neoplasia*. A malformation is stable, or relatively so. It consists of excess or deficiency of one or several of the normal constituents of the skin and usually is designated as a *nevus*. We shall, however, have to discuss the nevus concept in more detail later. A *neoplasm* consists of cells which not only are present in excess but also are retarded in their maturation and often deviate from normal cells in other morphologic or functional characteristics. One of the basic features of a neoplasm is that it is not stable but increases in size due either to excessive proliferation or delayed death of its constituent cells. A neoplasm may be benign or malignant, depending on the ability of its cells to destroy normal tissue and to metastasize. There are neoplasms which fit neither into the benign nor into the malignant classification, as we shall discuss later.

In *A Guide to Dermatohistopathology*, we shall not describe in detail every malformation or neoplasm that occurs in the skin. We shall rather give a conceptual frame into which the known nevi and tumors fit and into which unusual cases, and even as yet unclassified lesions, can be fitted, as we have done in previous publications when eccrine poroma, trichofolliculoma, and melanoacanthoma were recognized as entities worth identifying within the larger categories of benign sweat apparatus tumor (hidradenoma), benign follicular tumor, and benign epidermoid tumor.

NEVUS

The term *nevus* has been used and misused in so many ways that it has become almost meaningless. It deserves, however, to be preserved because, if properly defined, it describes one category of skin lesions for which no better name is available. The present confusion has its basis in history and stems from a time when the nature of the *nevus cell* was unknown and *nevus* was used for almost any inborn circumscribed mark on the skin. It came to mean what we call a "pigmented mole" just as well as a nevus sebaceus, epidermal nevus, or strawberry mark. We recommend a return to the classic concept outlined by Jadassohn[1] and Darier[2] and prefer to make their definition even more precise,[3] as follows: a nevus is a circumscribed stable malformation of the skin, not due to external causes and, therefore, thought to be of congenital origin. It consists of local excess of one or several of the normal mature constituents of the skin organ. Minus nevi are similarly defined as local deficiency due to underdevelopment of one or several constituents (aplasia cutis congenita, nevus depigmentosus, nevus anemicus). Jadassohn pointed out that a supernumerary digit is a malformation, but not a neoplasm (tumor) or a hyperplasia, and that, similarly, a localized excessive accumulation of sebaceous glands is not a neoplasm, nor is it described sufficiently as hyperplasia, but it deserves the name "nevus sebaceus," which implies congenital origin, stability, and maturity. The words *hamartoma* and *phakoma*[4] are not suitable substitutes because they are formed with the suffix *-oma*, indicating neoplasia, and they do not include the concept of mature tissue. We must, however, recognize that nevus as defined here includes tissue nevi and organoid nevi but excludes the *cellular nevus*

or *nevus cell nevus*, which is a benign tumor consisting of peculiar abnormal cells and undergoing evolution and involution. The definition also separates nevi from *nevoid tumors*, lesions that are thought to arise on a congenital basis but exhibit retarded maturation of cells, deviate in essential points from normal histologic structures, and show continued growth, even though this may be slow. For these nevoid tumors, the term *hamartoma* is well suited. We shall see later that these distinctions have practical as well as theoretical significance.

BENIGN VERSUS MALIGNANT TUMORS

Benign and *malignant* are old clinical terms which are not even restricted to the field of neoplasia. Malignant hypertension and Degos' malignant atrophic papulosis are examples. When a modern pathologist tries to define benign and malignant tumors, considerable difficulties are encountered.[5] The borderline is not sharp (Fig. VII-1), and malignant transformation may progress by steps (Fig. VII-2). Features such as rapid growth, cellular atypies, invasion, and metastasis usually are named as characteristic of malignant tumors. One needs only to think of keratoacanthoma, juvenile melanoma, and nodular fasciitis to find cutaneous lesions that have one or several of these attributes but are not biologically malignant. The only absolute proof of malig-

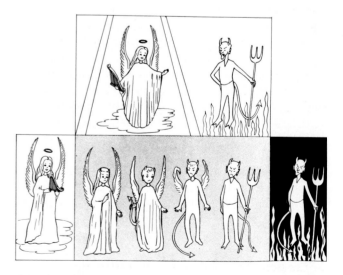

FIGURE VII–1.
The borderline between benign and malignant is not sharp; there is a broad, gray border zone. (Adapted from Fig. 183 in Hamperl. Lehrbuch der allgemeinen Pathologie und der pathologischen Anatomie, 28th ed. New York, Springer-Verlag, 1968.)

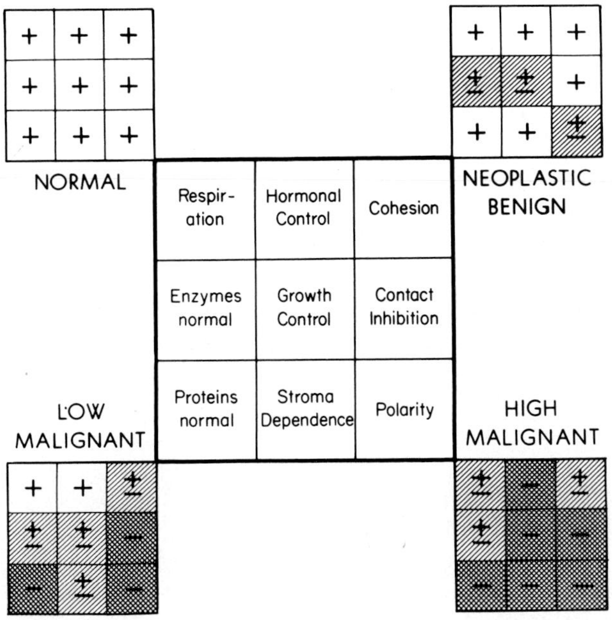

FIGURE VII–2.
Diagram showing step-by-step transformation of normal cells into cancer cells as loss or derangement of several cellular functions. Other functions might be added or substituted. (From Pinkus. In Kopf and Andrade (eds). Year Book of Dermatology, 1967. Courtesy of Year Book Medical Publishers.)

nancy in the sense of modern oncologic knowledge is metastasis because it proves the existence of a self-perpetuating and relatively autonomous cancer cell. Metastasis, however, is a clinical phenomenon and, as far as skin tumors are concerned, does not help the histopathologist in the evaluation of a given primary tumor.

It has become quite clear that as dermatopathologists we must include in our considerations not only quite benign tumors and definitely malignant tumors, but in-between categories of which there are three: precanceroses,[6] pseudocancers, and basaliomas. (These will be discussed in their respective chapters.) We must also keep in mind that our diagnosis includes prognostication and implied advice to the clinician on what to expect and how to handle a given tumor. We thus exceed the pathologist's basic task of doing morphologic interpretation, and we become partners in patient care. We must, therefore, know the therapeutic philosophy of the clinician in regard to a certain diagnosis. It is not wise to give a diagnosis of carcinoma in situ instead of actinic keratosis or of basal cell carcinoma instead of very superficial basal cell epithelioma to a practitioner to whom the word "carcinoma" is the trigger for extensive surgery or high-dosage X-ray therapy.

A general classification of epithelial nevi and neoplasms is given in Table VII-1. The table is based on degree of *maturation* (morphologic differentiation) of the constituent cells and on the direction in which they are *determined* (embryologic differentiation). Although histogenesis will be invoked in some instances (Chap. 38), origin from any specific normal structure is omitted from this classification because epithelial matrix cells in the skin are pluripotential (Fig. 2-13) and can undergo

TABLE VII–1.
Classification of Fibroepithelial Nevi and Neoplasms

Level of Maturation	Direction of Differentiation				
		Pilar Apparatus			
Normal	Epidermis	Sebaceous Gland	Hair Follicle	Apocrine Apparatus*	Eccrine Apparatus*
Malformation	Verrucous epidermal nevus	Nevus sebaceus	Hair nevus Hair follicle nevus	Apocrine nevus	Eccrine nevus
Adenomatous	Pale cell acanthoma Melanoacanthoma Seborrheic verruca, papillomatous Seborrheic verruca, solid Seborrheic verruca, reticulated	Sebaceous adenoma	Trichofolliculoma Trichoadenoma Tumor of follicular infundibulum Inverted follicular keratosis Trichilemmoma	Cystadenoma Papilliferous adenomas Syringoma	Eccrine poroma Tubular adenoma Nodular adenoma
Epitheliomatous		Sebaceous epithelioma	Pilomatricoma Trichoepithelioma	Cylindroma	Clear cell hidradenoma
Basaliomatous	Basal cell epithelioma				

*For more detailed classification of sweat gland tumors, see Table 39-1.

modulation (return to a quasi-embryonic state, Chap. 2) and later redifferentiate in other directions. While there is no good evidence that epidermis can generate new hairs or eccrine glands after birth, pluripotentiality is amply demonstrated whenever new epidermis is quickly formed by adnexal epithelia in planed facial skin, when new sebaceous glands are formed from follicular sheath epithelium in adult life, or when the eccrine duct including the acrosyringium is regenerated from the sweat coil during the healing of a deep wound. The germinative (basal) cells of normal cutaneous adnexa, therefore, are not fully differentiated in the embryologic sense of *determined toward maturation in a specific direction*. On the other hand, most tumor cells are differentiated in this sense. If they show any tendency to mature, this is fully determined in one specific direction: toward epidermis, sebaceous structure, follicular sheath, or eccrine duct, to name just a few examples. Some tumors can show multiple maturation within a fairly limited range, as will be discussed in their respective chapters.

The use of the word "differentiation" in the two very different meanings of determination (embryologists) and maturation (pathologists) has caused considerable confusion, because the undifferentiated (immature) cell of a malignant tumor is actually more highly differentiated (determined), being incapable of producing anything but more tumor cells of its own kind. While two rare neoplasms (teratocarcinoma of mice and neuroblastoma of infants) represent exceptions to this rule, it cannot be contended[7] that maturation of a squamous carcinoma cell into a keratinized flake means return to a more normal state. Certainly, a keratinizing cell that has left the mitotic pool is no longer malignant (Chap. 5), but only because it is committed to death, just as other cancer cells that die as mucinous blobs or just fade away. This example cannot be used to raise false hopes of our ability to revert malignant cells to viable normal ones. An exceptional situation seems to exist in the field of basaliomas[8] and will be discussed in Chapter 39. In the

following chapters we shall endeavor to make precise use of all the terms defined here.

The classification of epithelial lesions shown in Table VII-1 has been compared to Mendeléeff's Periodic Table of the Elements, and it actually has made it possible to predict the existence of certain tumors, which had not been identified at the time the table was first drawn up. The vertical arrangement, however, represents a spectrum rather than a set of pigeonholes. Not infrequently, tumors are encountered that do not exactly fit any of the slots. Classification, after all, is an ordering process of the human mind. The classification presented here has been the most satisfactory one in our work, but nature is apt to come up with exceptions that do not fit human rules, and it is not necessary to give new names to all minor variants.

Classifications of lesions of pigment-forming cells and of mesodermal cells will be given in their respective chapters.

REFERENCES

1. Jadassohn J: Bemerkungen zur Histologie der systematisierten Naevi und über "Talgdrüsen-Naevi." Arch Dermat Syph (Berlin) 33:355, 1895
2. Darier J, Civatte A, Tzanck A: Précis de Dermatologie. Paris, Masson et Cie, 1947
3. Pinkus H: Zur Begriffsbestimmung der Naevi, Organnaevi und naevoiden Tumoren. Hautarzt 16:184, 1965
4. Vinken PJ, Bruyn GW (eds): Phakomatoses. Handbook of Clinical Neurology, vol 14. New York: American Elsevier, 1973
5. Pinkus H: The borderline between cancer and noncancer. In Kopf AW, Andrade R (eds): Year Book of Dermatology, 1966–67. Chicago, Year Book, 1967, p 5
6. Newbold PCH: Precancer and the skin. Br J Dermatol 86:417, 1972
7. National Panel of Consultants on the Conquest of Cancer: Report, Pt 2. Washington, DC, US Government Printing Office, 1970, pp 73–74
8. Cooper M, Pinkus H: Intrauterine transplantation of rat basal cell carcinoma as a model for reconversion of malignant to benign growth. Cancer Res 37:2544, 1977

CHAPTER

32

Melanocytic and Nevocytic Tumors and Malformations

It is now generally conceded that the normal junctional melanocyte is a neuroectodermal derivative and that its stem cell, the melanoblast, arrives at the dermoepidermal junction during fetal life by migrating there from the neural crest through the dermis. Dermal melanocytes, which form so-called Mongolian spots, are thought to be of similar origin and to complete their migration within the reticular portion of the corium. The origin of nevus cells remains under discussion, although their neuroectodermal nature is accepted by most authors. We do not have to decide here whether all nevus cells are derived from adult junctional melanocytes, whether some or all of them are derived from Schwann cells of cutaneous nerves, or whether they are embryonically misdirected cells, although this last hypothesis (Fig. 32–1) explains many data most satisfactorily.[1] Our task is to identify benign nevus cells and to differentiate them from normal and pathologic melanocytes and from malignant melanoma cells. This task is interrelated with giving diagnostic criteria for the various forms of nevus cell nevi, benign melanocytic lesions, and malignant melanomas. The lesions discussed in this chapter are listed in Table 32–1. It is to be noted that some of these disorders were listed also in Chapter 30 as causing visible color changes of the skin.

HOW TO RECOGNIZE MELANOCYTES, NEVUS CELLS, AND MELANOPHAGES

Terminology in the field of pigment cells was confusing until it was reasonably clarified by common consent in 1958. According to that classification, the word *melanoblast* was restricted to fetal immature cells. All mature pigment-forming cells of mammals were *melanocytes*, while *melanophore* was restricted to the pigment cells of cold-blooded vertebrates, which show streaming of melanin granules in their dendrites. Histiocytes carrying phagocytized melanin were termed *melanophages* or *pigmented macrophages*. Cells of malignant melanomas became *melanoma cells*. Cells of benign cellular nevi remained *nevus cells*.

This classification satisfied the requirements of the pathologist and of many biologists, but it became less satisfactory when electron microscopy was developed to its present level. Therefore, at a later conference (1965) the terminology and definitions given in Table 32–2 were proposed.[2] While highly sophisticated and scientifically accurate, the new classification leaves the light microscopist in a quandary because most criteria can be ascertained only by electron microscopy. For our purposes, we will have to rely mostly on what we can see in paraffin sections stained with H&E or O&G.

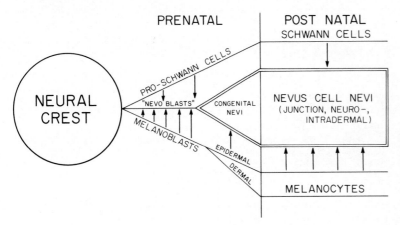

FIGURE 32–1.

Direct and indirect derivation of nevus cells from neural crest. The concept is illustrated that nevus cells, the benign neoplastic cells forming nevocytic nevi, may be derived early from neural crest cells as immature nevoblasts or later during fetal life from melanoblasts or pro-Schwann cells, or still later in postnatal life from melanocytes or Schwann cells.

If, in a particular case, fresh material is available, histochemical reactions for tyrosinase and cholinesterase are highly useful. Such occasions, however, will remain the exception, and there is little expectation that electron microscopy will become a routine tool for the pathologist.

Epidermal Melanocytes

The normal junctional or epidermal melanocyte was formerly known as *Masson's clear cell*. The

TABLE 32–1.
Malformations and Tumors Involving Pigment-Forming Cells

Epidermal Melanocytes
  Malformation (nevi)
    Ephelis
    Pigmented mascules of lip and volar skin
    Nevus spilus
    Nevus depigmentosus and partial albinism
  Neoplasia
    Lentigo simplex
    Lentigo senilis
    Melanoacanthoma
    Lentigo maligna
    Melanocytic malignant melanoma
Dermal Melanocytes
  Malformation
    Persistent Mongolian spot
    Nevi of Ota and Ito (oculomucocutaneous
      melanosis)
    Blue nevus
  Neoplasia
    Cellular blue nevus
    Malignant blue nevus
Nevus Cells
  Neoplasia
    Junction nevus
    Compound nevus
    Intradermal nevus, including neuronevus
    Balloon cell nevus
    Benign juvenile melanoma (Spitz nevus)
    Bathing-trunk type nevus
    Nevocytic malignant melanoma

term *clear cell* has been applied to a variety of cells. When it is employed, it should be qualified, as in this case by the author's name, but it is preferable to discontinue its use in the pigment cell field, because the name "Masson's clear cell" has also been applied in a wider sense to nevus cells, melanoma cells, and Langerhans cells. The normal melanocyte (Chap. 2) has a small, dark-staining, and often shrunken-looking nucleus, in which a nucleolus is not easily recognized. Its cytoplasm, when not occupied by melanin granules, stains pale and appears retracted from the surrounding keratinocytes, so that the cell seems to sit in a hole. Occasionally, thin dendritic processes are seen to insert themselves between prickle cells. These should not be mistaken for intercellular bridges. The cell (Fig. 2–39) usually is situated between the lower halves of neighboring basal cells, its lower border resting on the basement membrane, but it may sit a little higher, or it may bulge down and may actually seem to be attached to the lower epidermal surface like a spider. The melanocyte may contain a few or many evenly sized pigment granules, which, if numerous, outline the dendrites. These then can be followed for many microns along the basal membrane or upward between keratinocytes. The nucleus usually is not obscured by the melanin granules, although it may be tightly surrounded by them. Most normal melanocytes give a positive dopa reaction if the test is done on fresh or properly fixed tissue.

Intraepidermal and Junctional Nevus Cells

Nevus cells are a variant of melanocytes that are a specific human characteristic. Cellular nevi in animals are extremely rare, and animal malignant melanomas are mainly derived from dermal melanocytes, corresponding to the cells of blue nevi in humans. The nevus cell differs in important points

TABLE 32–2.
Terminology for Vertebrate Melanin-containing Cells, Their Precursors, Related Cells, and Specific Particles (1965)

Melanocyte*	A cell which synthesizes a melanin-containing organelle, the melanosome
Melanophore	A type of melanocyte that participates with other chromatophores in the rapid color changes of animals by intracellular displacement (aggregation and dispersion) of melanosomes
Melanoblast	A cell which serves at all stages of the life cycle as the precursor of the melanocyte (and melanophore)
Langerhans Cell†	A distinctive cell of the mammalian epidermis and dermis presumed to belong to the melanocyte series; revealed by gold impregnation and contains distinctive nonmelanized, disklike organelles
Melanosome‡	A discrete, melanin-containing organelle in which melanization is complete; shown to be more or less uniformly electron dense by electron microscopy; tyrosinase activity not usually demonstrable
Premelanosome	All distinctive particulate stages in the maturation of melanosomes; electron density variable; possesses an active tyrosinase system after the onset of melanin synthesis

*Included here are differentiated cells which synthesize nonmelanized or partly melanized premelanosomes as terminal products. It is suggested that in albinism the melanocytes containing nonmelanized premelanosomes be called "albino melanocytes."
†Definition outdated in 1980 (see Chap. 24).
‡Multiple melanosomes embedded in supporting matrices, for example, as in the macrophages and malpighian cells of mammals, may be designated "melanosome complexes."
From Fitzpatrick, Quevedo, Levene, et al.[2]

from the normal melanocyte as outlined in Table 32–3. The most important difference is its ethologic behavior. Normal melanocytes are dendritic, individualistic cells, each occupying its own territory as can be seen well in split skin preparations (Fig. 2–40). Nevus cells have a herd instinct, they crowd together in *theques.* This indicates specific differences in cell membrane constituents. It makes the nevus cell a benign tumor cell with diminished contact inhibition, a feature that becomes more outspoken in malignant melanoma cells. We differentiate sharply, therefore, between melanocytes and nevus cells and call the common junctional, compound, and intradermal moles *nevus cell nevi,* preserving the term *melanocytic nevi* for blue nevi and other lesions in which true territorial melanocytes exist.

Generally, the junctional nevus cell (see Fig. 32–18) is a little larger and looks more turgid than the melanocyte. In particular, it has a larger ovoid or round nucleus in which chromatin and nucleolus are plainly visible. It usually has a well-defined outline without dendrites, even if it contains a fair number of melanin granules. Most nevus cell theques consist of apposed rounded cells, but in some cases the cells are fusiform and stellate. This is particularly true in lesions related to the benign juvenile melanoma (see Fig. 32–26).

TABLE 32–3.
Benign Melanogenic Cells: The Melanocyte versus the Nevus Cell

	Melanocytes	Nevus Cells
Cell Shape	Epidermal: dendritic Dermal: fusiform, ameboid	Round-oval, fusiform, rarely dendritic
Nucleus	Dark-staining, shrunken	Vesicular with nucleolus
Enzymes	Dopa-oxidase-positive, cholinesterase-negative	Dopa- and/or cholinesterase-positive or negative
Ethology	Solitary, territorial even when crowded	Sociable, herd instinct, forming nests (theques)
Habitat	Epidermal: junction, basal layer, hair matrix Dermal: reticular dermis	All layers of epidermis and dermis

Intradermal Nevus Cells

Nevus cells, in contrast to melanocytes, occur in the dermis without contact with epithelial structures. They then are *intradermal nevus cells* in contrast to the *dermal melanocytes* that form blue nevi. Only the latter should be called dermal nevi or melanocytic nevi.

Nevus cells in the dermis are of three types, designated "A," "B," and "C" by Miescher and Albertini[3] and "epitheloid," "lymphocytoid," and "neuroid" by others. These are illustrated in Figures 32–19, 32–20, and 32–23. Other descriptive terms, such as "large," "small," and "fusiform," also have been used. The A type cells have nucleus and cytoplasm similar to junctional nevus cells, usually form nests in the papillary and subpapillary layer, and may or may not be pigmented. B type cells are smaller, with a small, dark-staining nucleus, and usually occupy the mid-dermis. They rarely contain melanin. C type cells are found still deeper, may form Meissner corpusclelike aggregates, and practically never contain pigment. Nevus cells, unless they contain melanin, are characterized mainly by their negative attributes: they do not contain other visible granulations or fibers and have no intercellular connections. They may lie singly in the dermis but, more commonly, form nests of a few to many cells. Nests may be surrounded by flattened elements (*thequocytes*[4]), producing the impression of nevus cells lying in an endothelium-lined space (see Fig. 32–19).[5] In some cases, larger masses may resemble basal cell epithelioma in H&E sections. O&G stain, however, usually reveals elastic fibrils (see Fig. 32–20) which surround smaller aggregates within the larger masses, and if need be, a reticulum stain will always show fine fibrils spun around small nests or even individual cells. When intradermal nevus cells contain melanin, it is present in evenly sized and fairly small granules. A peculiar phenomenon, not uncommonly found in old quiescent intradermal nevi, is the presence of large vacuoles in a few or many nuclei. These may be pale or diffusely brown. Electron microscopy has shown that they are not truly intranuclear, but are parts of cytoplasm surrounded by nuclear lobes.[6] Similar inclusions are also found in malignant melanoma cells,[7] and one should be aware of their occurrence in perfectly benign nevus cells.

Cellular characteristics of malignant melanoma and benign juvenile melanoma will be discussed under those headings later.

Pigmented Macrophages

Melanophages contain acid phosphatase activity and collect phagocytized melanin in lysosomal vacuoles, as electron microscopy has shown. In routine sections, the pigment forms clumps of uneven size. Often the cell has gorged itself to the point where the nucleus becomes obscured. In H&E sections, melanophages resemble macrophages containing similar clumps of hemosiderin. O&G stain easily distinguishes the two pigments.

Dermal Melanocytes

Dermal melanocytes derive from neuroectoderm but do not reach the epidermis. They stay permanently in the dermis. They are widely distributed in the skin of animals, but in man they are restricted to certain areas except under pathologic circumstances. They are commonly found in the back skin, especially the sacral area, of newborns of darker skinned races, where they form the so-called *Mongolian blue spot* (see below). Dermal melanocytes are individualistic cells having ameboid appearance. They are dopa positive and contain melanosomes.

DIAGNOSIS OF SPECIFIC LESIONS

Lesions Involving Epidermal Melanocytes

For further discussion of lesions involving epidermal melanocytes, see Chapter 30.

Ephelis. *Freckles* or *ephelides* may be considered a malformation because they consist of localized areas of functionally overactive melanocytes. It has been shown[8] that the junctional melanocytes are larger and somewhat more widely spaced in the freckle, and it has been suggested that, at least in red-haired, white-skinned people, these melanocytes are the only mature ones, those in the normal skin being functionally deficient. Histologic examination shows a structurally normal epidermis with a sharply defined area in which the basal cells contain more pigment. Junctional melanocytes are present in approximately normal number.

Pigmented Macules of Lip and Volar Skin. The *solitary pigment spot* of the lip[9] shows deep pigmentation of the basal keratinocytes (Fig. 32–2) and a fairly normal number of melanocytes. Some pigmented macrophages are present in the uppermost dermis. It is unexplained why the prickle cells remain quite free of pigment. *Pigmented macules* found commonly on the lightly pigmented palms and soles of black people usually show a picture[10] resembling that seen on the lips. However, other lesions show the melanosomes accepted by all keratinocytes and carried up into the horny layer, as is seen in lentigo simplex, and in still other areas, melanin is restricted to large dendritic melanocytes and does not enter keratinocytes (pigment block, Chap. 2). The three types of distribution are seen side by side in the same lesion (Fig. 32–3). These pigmented macules may clinically resemble macular secondary syphilis. They are not associated with

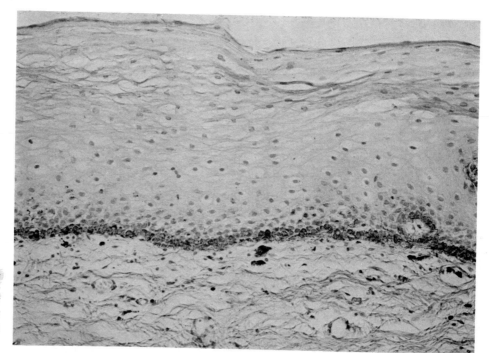

FIGURE 32–2.
Solitary labial pigment spot. Increased basal cell pigmentation due to increased activity of local melanocytes. A few pigmented macrophages in upper dermis. H&E. X185.

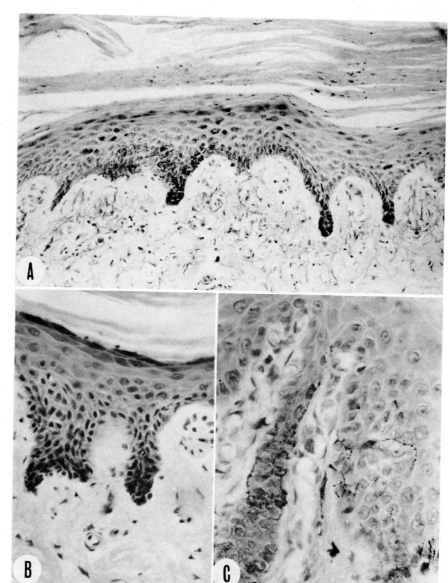

FIGURE 32–3.
*Volar melanotic macules. **A.** Pigment distribution similar to lentigo simplex in all epidermal layers including stratum corneum. O&G. **B.** Pigment concentrated in basal layer. Some rete ridges have a squared-off lower border that is very conspicuous in some lesions. H&E. **C.** Pigment block prevents melanin from being accepted by keratinocytes and remains in large dendritic melanocytes. H&E. Various magnifications. (From Chapel et al. Int J Dermatol 18:222, 1979.)*

inflammation. A peculiar, pigmented macule, not related to melanin, was described by Frenk and Delacrétaz.[11] The substrate of these spots is hydropic degeneration of prickle cells.

Nevus Spilus. Nevus spilus is a well-established term for macular hyperpigmented areas that are permanent and may be a few millimeters or several centimeters in diameter. Smaller macules often are grouped. That the hyperpigmentation is permanent and independent of insolation differentiates nevus spilus from freckles. Histologically, they are identical. Larger areas of hyperpigmentation, especially if they have light brown color, are also known as *café au lait spots*, a term used mainly for those associated with neurofibromatosis and the Albright syndrome. It has been shown by light and electron microscopy that the melanocytes in von Recklinghausen's disease contain giant melanosomes,[12] while those in Albright's syndrome do not.[13] These large round melanin granules, up to 5 μ in size, are also found in the macules of the *multiple lentigines* (leopard) syndrome[14,15] and in other situations. Thus, their diagnostic value is doubtful, since they also can be absent in neurofibromatosis.[16]

Cases of *cribriform and zosteriform hyperpigmentation* originating later in life and being progressive have recently been described.[17] They have increased basal layer pigmentation and no large melanin granules. They are of purely cosmetic impact.

Recent attempts to redefine nevus spilus as a lesion containing nevus cells[18] have caused some confusion and serve no useful purpose. Lesions containing papular nevus cell nevi on a light brown macular background are better kept apart as nevus on a nevus[19] or *speckled lentiginous nevus.*[20]

Nevus Depigmentosus and Partial Albinism. Histologic diagnosis of these conditions and the related *hypomelanosis of Ito*, all of which are minus nevi, is rather unsatisfactory in routine sections and should be investigated with dopa reaction or even electron microscopic melanocyte counts[21] in properly prepared specimens (Chap. 30). According to Jimbow et al.,[22] decreased synthesis and abnormal transfer of melanosomes are involved in *nevus depigmentosus.*

Lentigo Simplex. The histologic borderline between an ephelis and a lentigo simplex, which is the simplest form of melanocytic neoplasia, is not always sharp (Fig. 32–4). We use the term lentigo *simplex* in preference to lentigo *juvenilis* because it may persist unchanged into old age. In a typical lentigo simplex, melanin is present not only in the basal layer, but also in the upper layers of the epidermis, and some of these lesions present the most extreme degree of epidermal pigmentation, every cell including those of the horny layer being stuffed with brown granules. In addition, there is usually some acanthosis and accentuation of rete ridges, which may be bulbous. Deeply pigmented junctional melanocytes appear to be increased in number but are difficult to see, and there may be pigmented macrophages in the upper dermis. Inflammatory infiltrate in the papillary layer also is not uncommon and probably constitutes a reaction to melanin. Lentigines usually develop in the first years of life, and there is probably no human being who does not have at least one or several. Some in-

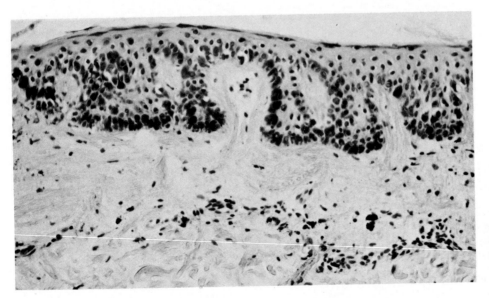

FIGURE 32–4.
Lentigo simplex. Rete ridges elongated and broadened at their tips. Increased amount of melanin in melanocytes, basal cells, and, to less degree, in prickle cells. Note dense collagen bundles in papillae, some melanized macrophages in subpapillary layer. H&E. X225.

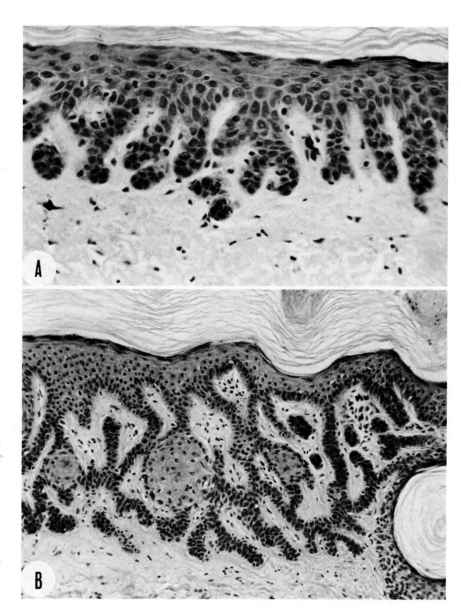

FIGURE 32–5.
Lentigo senilis. **A.** *Distorted budding rete ridges embedded in dense papillary stroma. No noticeable increase of melanocytes; pigment confined to tips of ridges. H&E. X225.* **B.** *More pronounced budding of narrow epidermal ridges approaches the picture of the reticulated type of seborrheic verruca (Fig. 33-10). Maturation of basal cells into prickle cells and horny cyst formation also points in that direction. H&E. X180.*

dividuals have many, and in some cases they are the cutaneous marker (dermadrome[23]) of the *multiple lentigines syndrome (leopard syndrome)*.[24,25] How lentigo simplex is related to junction nevus will be discussed under nevus incipiens.

Lentigo Senilis. In a wider sense, senile lentigines (senile freckles, liver spots) may be anything from flat seborrheic warts to Hutchinson's freckles. In a stricter histologic sense, lentigo senilis has a rather diagnostic picture (Fig. 32–5). It is characterized by club-shaped budding of the basal layer with hyperpigmentation. Junctional melanocytes may or may not be increased in number. The relation of this lesion to reticulated seborrheic verruca will be discussed in Chapter 33. Association with squamous cell carcinoma and melanocytic malignant melanoma probably is coincidental in actinically damaged skin. Lentigo senilis differs from lentigo simplex by the more irregular epidermal budding, which is not simple lengthening of rete ridges, by the tendency of pigmentation to be heaviest in the tips of the buds, and by the presence of dense, eosinophilic stroma between the buds.[26] Both types must be differentiated from so-called hard and soft epidermal nevi (Chap. 33).

Melanoacanthoma. Rare, but of considerable biologic interest, is a lesion, originally described by Bloch as nonnevoid melanoepithelioma, type I,[27] which represents combined benign neoplasia (Fig. 32–6) of epidermal keratinocytes and large dendritic melanocytes. It must be differentiated from the much more common type II of Bloch, which is sim-

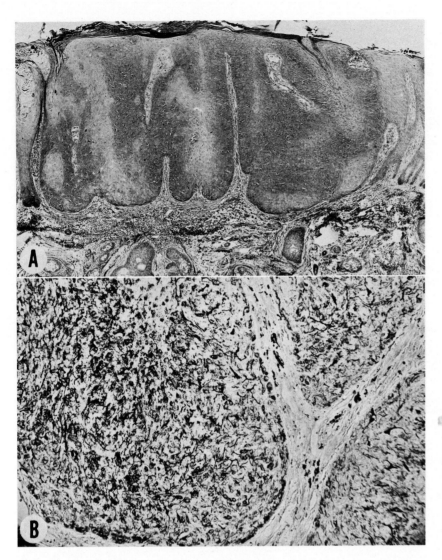

FIGURE 32–6.
Melanoacanthoma. **A.** *Massive papillomatous epidermis is composed of dark and light portions, the latter representing nonpigmented areas of prickle cells. O&G. X30.* **B.** *Most of melanin is contained in dendritic melanocytes, which are present in profusion between basaloid keratinocytes. Masson silver. X135. (From Mishima and Pinkus. Arch Dermatol 81:539, 1966.)*

ply a highly pigmented seborrheic verruca. In the latter, practically all of the melanin (Fig. 32–7) is in the keratinocytes, and relatively few small melanocytes are present at the junction. Occasional dendritic pigmented cells may be found in the substance of the tumor. Melanoacanthoma, on the other hand, shows the papillomatous epidermis pervaded with highly dendritic cells, which contain practically all of the pigment (Fig. 32–6B). We emphasize that this is an extremely rare tumor[28–30] but discuss it here as an example of benign neoplasia of melanocytes rather than of nevus cells.

Lentigo Maligna. Before the turn of the century, Hutchinson described as *infective melanotic freckle* a slowly spreading, macular pigmentation on the faces of elderly individuals, which was later referred to by Dubreuilh as *preblastomatous melanosis.* Unfortunately, in a subsequent paper Dubreuilh[31] widened and diluted his concept to include somewhat similar lesions occurring in younger people and on covered surfaces, lesions which we now separate as superficially spreading melanomas (see below). We decided to follow Clark's lead[32] and replaced the older terms with *lentigo maligna,* which emphasizes the entirely macular nature of the lesion. Hutchinson's picturesque but obsolete use of the word "infective" well expresses the peculiar clinical course of the disease, which progresses at a snail's pace and in stages from benign to malignant, a process that can be followed and analyzed microscopically.[33,34] Lentigo maligna is a distinct type of preinvasive melanoma, amounting to about 5 percent of all melanomas. The earliest stage (Fig. 32–8) is characterized by a somewhat larger number of more highly dendritic melanocytes at the junction. This may rarely be associated with basal layer budding.

We pointed out earlier that every normal melanocyte has a territory (epidermal melanin unit) and that larger melanocytes are spaced farther apart, e.g., in ephelids. Thus, a crowding together of

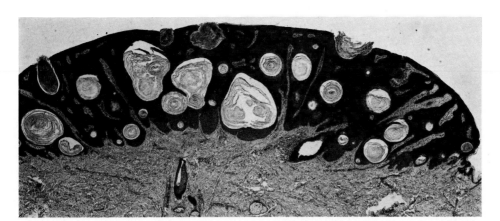

FIGURE 32–7.
Deeply pigmented seborrheic verruca. Practically every basaloid keratinocyte compos-
ing the lesion contains melanin. Melanocytes are few and small. Note papillomatous fea-
tures of lesion, which lacks any surface hyperkeratosis but contains characteristic horny
cysts. H&E. X8.

larger melanocytes may be taken as an early sign of loss of normal territorial behavior (contact inhibition) and, therefore, of neoplastic derangement of the cells. Yet, for a long time, the melanocytes remain dendritic individuals with small dark nuclei. They do not acquire the cytologic characteristics of nevus cells and do not form theques.[35] The epidermis thus has a peculiar, moth-eaten appearance in routine sections (Fig. 32–9).

Gradually, there occurs more pronounced focal crowding of cells (Fig. 32–9A), some of which may be carried into the higher epidermal strata (Fig. 32–9B) and shed with the horny layer. The number of such cells is relatively small, and the elements remain single and look shrunken and dying in contrast to the pagetoid picture we shall encounter in superficially spreading nevocytic melanoma. There is now present in the upper dermis a type of inflammatory infiltrate that we shall encounter in all precancerous epidermal lesions and shall discuss in more detail under keratosis senilis (Chap. 34). The upper dermis may contain pigmented macrophages (Fig. 32–8).

Malignant Melanocytoma. Still later, the melanotic cells become more atypical, show a tendency to migrate downward (Fig. 32–9A) within the basement membrane surrounding hair follicles, and be-

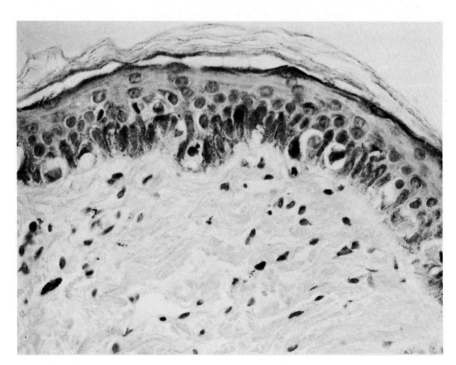

FIGURE 32–8.
Lentigo maligna (Hutchinson's me-
lanotic freckle), early stage. Epider-
mis thin without ridges. Increased
number of atypical melanocytes in
the basal layer. No tendency to nest
formation or migration into higher
layers. H&E. X600.

gin to form nests at the junction. These, however, are not nests of benign nevus cells but of dysplastic melanoma cells. We now have a melanocytic malignant melanoma in situ.

When cell nests are present also in the dermis, a full-blown *invasive melanocytic melanoma* (Fig. 32–36) has developed. It is well recognized by dermatologists that malignant melanomas arising in

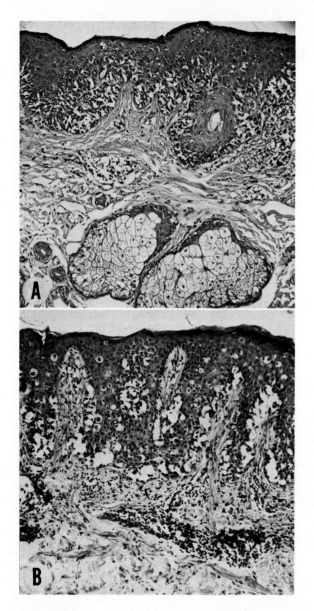

FIGURE 32–9.
Lentigo maligna. Some degree of epidermal hyperplasia. Crowding of atypical melanocytes in the basal layer produces moth-eaten appearance while only few dying cells are present in higher layers. Note atypical melanocytes in basal layer of hair follicle and sebaceous gland in **A.** *H&E. X90. Both features contrast with the picture of pagetoid melanoma shown in Figure 32-37, where nests of malignant nevus cells are present in the basal layer and viable tumor cells are disseminated through the prickle cell layers.*

lentigo maligna metastasize late and, therefore, often can be controlled by local excision. It has also been shown[36] that the radiosensitivity which distinguishes normal melanocytes from benign nevus cells is preserved to some degree in these malignant cells.

The biologic basis for these oncologic differences of lentigo maligna melanoma from nevocytic melanoma, as indicated in Figure 32–10, seems to reside in their origin from melanocytes rather than from nevus cells. Therefore, it is of the utmost importance to pay attention to the histologic and cytologic details described here, rather than to rely predominantly on the depth of invasion in a given lesion, and also to correlate microscopic data with the clinical factors of age of patient, site of lesion on exposed areas, and macular character of a slowly enlarging pigmented lesion. Although lentigo maligna usually occurs on the face, it may develop on the back of the hand and, in exceptional cases, on the tip of a finger[37] (Fig. 32–11). Rare instances of amelanotic lentigo maligna have been reported.[38]

Acral Lentiginous Melanoma. Lesions as described by Lupulescu et al.[37] (Fig. 32–11) have recently been given the name of *acral lentiginous melanoma*[39] for two reasons. They are not situated in normally light-damaged areas, and the progression to invasion and metastasis is accelerated. The term emphasizes the lentiginous macular character of the lesions but also really includes facial lesions in the designation "acral." It also is meant to include lesions on the genitals. If one remembers that 10 to 20 percent of malignant lentigos were reported from areas not exposed to sunlight, the appellation acral lentiginous melanoma is of questionable value but will probably prevail.

Lesions Related to Dermal Melanocytes

Mongolian Spot and Oculomucocutaneous Melanosis. Dermal melanocytes sometimes are called Mongolian cells because they form the substrate of the Mongolian spot of newborns. Actually, a blue sacral spot is not restricted to the Oriental gene pool.[40] It occurs, for instance, in 10 to 25 percent of babies of Southern European stock and in over 90 percent of American blacks. The presence of dermal melanocytes in the skin of the lower back is indeed a universal human attribute but is clinically inapparent in light-skinned children. In very dark-skinned children the spot may be overlooked, or it may not be recognized when it occupies most of the dorsal trunk, a not uncommon occurrence in blacks. The cells are large, ameboid-looking ele-

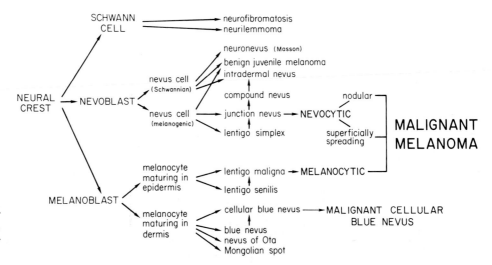

FIGURE 32–10.
Diagram of neural crest derivation of melanotic tumors. (Adapted from Mishima. Cancer 20:632, 1967.)

ments which are sparsely scattered in the reticular portion of the dermis and probably cease functioning shortly after birth, except in the relatively few cases of *persistent Mongolian spot*.[41] Because of their small number, they may be overlooked in H&E sections, and one has to search for them even in O&G sections. They also are the substrate of *nevus Ota* (nevus fuscoceruleus ophthalmomaxillaris, Fig. 32–12) and the similar *nevus Ito,* which is situated in the shoulder region. The cells of these lesions are unusually large and present in some-

what greater number in the upper corium. The peculiar powder-stain appearance of these macular melanocytic nevi is due to associated spotty epidermal pigmentation (freckling). Pigmentation of the ectodermal mucous membranes and the sclera of these patients is due to similar cells in the stroma.

Blue Nevus. Localized accumulation of dermal melanocytes forming a papule or small nodule is known as blue nevus of Jadassohn-Tièche.[42] While it usually is not present at birth, it persists through

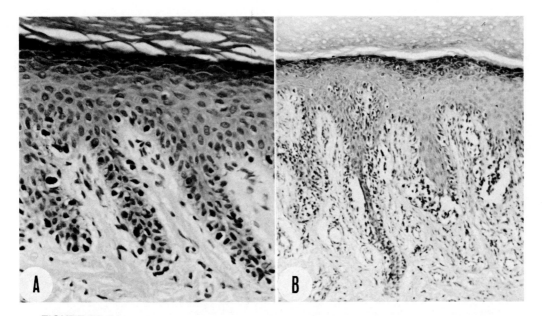

FIGURE 32–11.
Lentigo maligna of fingertip (so-called acral lentiginous melanoma) shows atypical melanocytic proliferation at the junction and extending downward around a sweat duct. Nests of atypical melanocytes project into the dermis. A few effete melanocytes are eliminated transepidermally. Very little reactive inflammatory infiltrate. H&E. X250. (From Lupulescu et al. Arch Dermatol 107:717, 1973. Copyright © 1973 American Medical Association.)

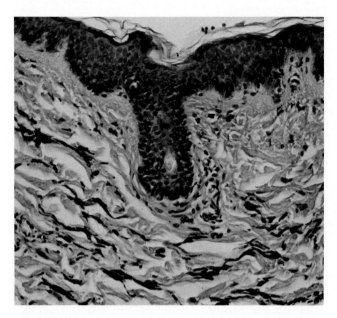

FIGURE 32–12.
Nevus Ota. Spotty hyperpigmentation of epidermis and huge dermal melanocytes in dermis. H&E. X180.

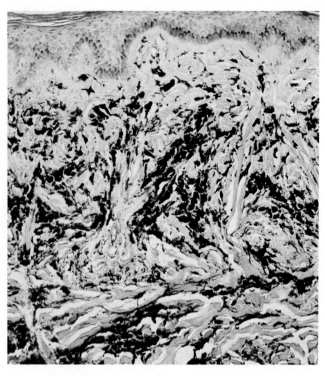

FIGURE 32–13.
Blue nevus. Strands of relatively little pigmented tumor cells are accentuated by massively melanized macrophages. H&E. X135.

life once it has formed and thus fulfills the criteria of a true nevus: stable, localized excess of a normal skin constituent. In rare cases, a large plaque studded with bluish black macules may be found.[43] The dermal melanocytes are present as a loose network and are mixed (Fig. 32–13) with a variable number of fibrocytes and melanophages, the latter often containing the bulk of the pigment. The fibrous portion of the dermis also is increased. If one bleaches the melanin in the sections with hydrogen peroxide, the lesion becomes almost indistinguish-

able from a histiocytoma or subepidermal nodular fibrosis (Chap. 41).

Cellular Blue Nevus and Malignant Blue Nevus. In contrast, the cellular blue nevus (Fig. 32–14) consists of densely packed and relatively large cells,

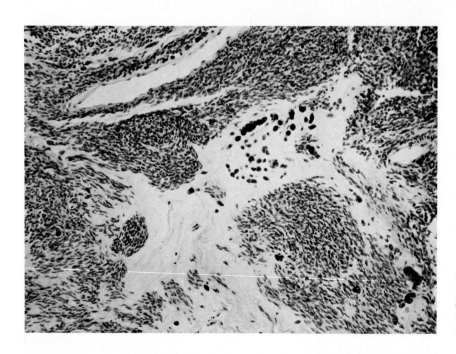

FIGURE 32–14.
Cellular blue nevus. Most of melanin is in macrophages, while nests of crowded tumor cells contain little pigment. H&E. X135.

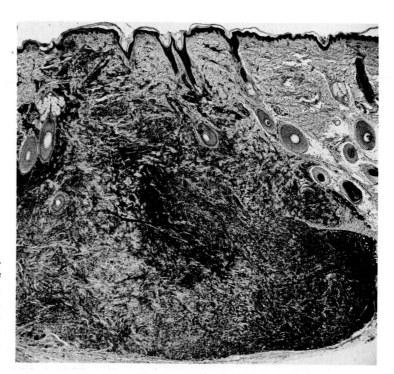

FIGURE 32–15.
Giant blue nevus. These lesions, which occur most commonly in the sacral area, on the back of hands and feet, and on the scalp, may reach a size of 2 cm or more and may extend deep into the subcutaneous tissue. Most of the melanin is contained in macrophages, which obscure the fusiform neoplastic, but usually benign, dermal melanocytes. H&E. X14.

which usually contain little pigment but are interspersed with many melanophages. The tumors may reach large size *(giant blue nevus)*[44] (Fig. 32–15). The tendency to grow and occasional instances of malignant transformation[45] speak for a neoplastic nature (Fig. 32–16). Histologic and cytologic characteristics have given rise to the suggestion that these lesions are *pigmented schwannomas.*[46] Electron microscopic studies[47] have shown that the tumor cells are melanogenic and are similar to dermal melanocytes. It is in the interpretation of data in these rare lesions that the diagram of Figure 32–10 proves its value. Evidently, neural crest derivatives occur in which enzyme systems and morphologic characteristics are mixed up and give tumor cells unusual features.

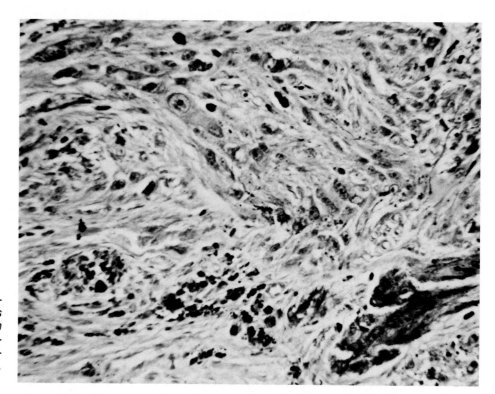

FIGURE 32–16.
Malignant blue nevus. Atypical, mainly fusiform tumor cells contain only few small melanin granules. Melanized macrophages attest to the melanogenic nature of the tumor. H&E. X225.

Lesions Containing Nevus Cells

The nevus cell, as described in the introduction to this chapter, is an abnormal cell, not a normal tissue constituent. Whether we consider it a derivative of normal melanocytes or of Schwann cells or of embryonically misdirected nevoblasts (Figs. 32–1, 32–10), lesions composed of nevus cells are neoplasms and not malformations (tissue nevi), as defined in the introduction to Section VII. On the other hand, nevus cells can occur in congenital lesions which otherwise satisfy the definition of a nevus, as will be discussed under bathing-trunk nevus. These paradoxes must be kept in mind. The *brown mole,* or *nevus cell nevus,* is a peculiar tumor. It develops some time after birth, grows, then may remain stable for many years or show renewed spurts of growth, and it often fibroses or atrophies (Fig. 32–28) late in life. It rarely undergoes malignant transformation.

Nevus Incipiens. Its first stage either is, or strongly resembles, a lentigo simplex (see above). While some lentigines persist indefinitely in their macular form, many become clinically palpable, and that coincides with the appearance of nests of nevus cells at the junction. A diagrammatic explanation is given in Figure 32–1. This nevus incipiens (Fig. 32–17), in which features of lentigo and junction nevus are combined, gradually transforms into the common *junction nevus,* or the latter may arise de novo. One may encounter tumors in which all stages from lentigo to intradermal nest formation are present simultaneously. Inflammatory infiltrate in the papillae and subpapillary layer is not uncommon in early junction nevi, seems to be related to the amount of melanin discharged into the dermis, and, like the presence of occasional mitosis, does not signify malignancy.

Junction Nevus and Compound Nevus. In a pure junction nevus (Fig. 32–18), theques or single nevus cells are intraepidermal, or their lower portion bulges downward, but there is no connective tissue between keratinocytes and nevus cells. It is difficult to ascertain the condition of the basement membrane in routine sections, but electron microscopy shows that it may be thin or absent around the lower pole of the nests. While there is no doubt that junctional nests are transformed into intradermal nests, Unna's classic concept of Abtropfung, meaning dropping down of nevus cells into the dermis, describes the process in the wrong terms. Actually, after the basement membrane has disappeared, reticulum and, later, collagen fibers and elastic fibers envelop the nests, pushing the epidermis away from them. This corresponds to the clinical phenomenon that a junction nevus becomes elevated when it transforms into a compound nevus (Fig. 32–19). The nevus cell nests do not migrate into preformed dermis but become surrounded by new connective tissue, which forms the stroma of the tumor. Nevi that extend deeper usually contain hairs, and one often sees nevus cell nests arising at the junction of follicular epithelium and fibrous root sheath. In rare cases, eccrine sweat ducts may serve as centers.[48] Every benign cellular nevus beyond the junction stage is a well-organized neuroectodermal-mesodermal tumor. With increasing distance from the epidermis, the nevus cells lose their melanin granules, and the dopa reaction becomes weaker. This does not mean that the cells become quiescent. It has been shown[49] that they maintain metabolic activity and that thymidine incorporation as an indication of mitotic activity persists at all levels of a mole.

Intradermal Nevus. We favor the designation intradermal over dermal nevus because the latter

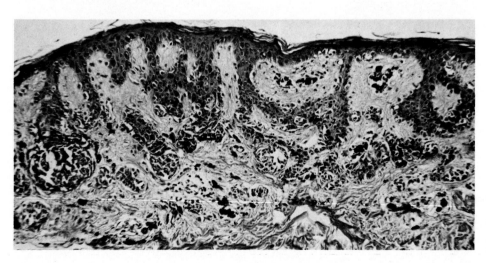

FIGURE 32–17.
Nevus incipiens. Theques of junctional nevus cells and individual large clear cells in a lesion which otherwise has characteristics of lentigo simplex (Fig. 32-4). H&E. X135.

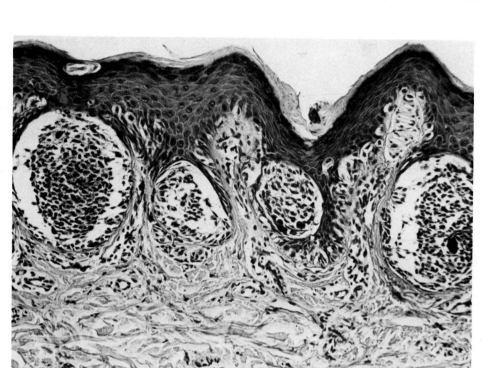

FIGURE 32–18.
Junction nevus of sole. Note Meissner's corpuscle, identifying hairless skin, in upper right corner. H&E. X185.

term may give rise to confusion with the blue nevus, which consists of dermal melanocytes. In most nevi, the new formation of theques at the epidermodermal junction subsides after some years, and all nests become intradermal (Fig. 32–20; see also Fig. 32–28). Most cellular nevi of postadolescent age are intradermal nevi, but new junction nevi may spring up in adult life and go through all the stages of their natural history without indication of malignancy. On the other hand, nevi in certain locations, especially on the hands and feet, may persist as junction or compound nevi (Fig.

32–18) throughout life. Finding a junction nevus on the sole of an elderly person does not imply malignancy unless there is cytologic evidence.

In many of the common brown moles of the face, new formation of junctional nests never ceases completely. Their prevalence in any pathologist's material depends on the number of sections of individual moles examined. It is likely that complete serial sections would reveal a few junctional nests in almost every mole. Thus, the presence of occasional nests and of single junctional nevus cells above an intradermal nevus does not indicate

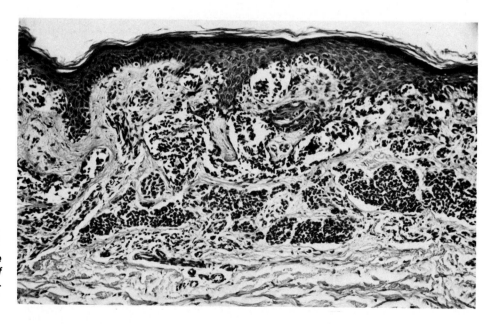

FIGURE 32–19.
Compound nevus. All of the nevus cells in this lesion are of the small (type B, lymphocytoid) variety. H&E. X135.

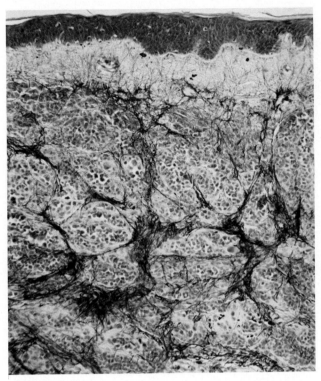

FIGURE 32–20.
Intradermal nevus with network of elastic fibers. Note difference in size between large superficial (type A) and smaller (type B) cells in the deep portions of the nevus. O&G. X135.

the line between the diagnosis of compound and intradermal nevus is not sharp, and terminology depends somewhat on personal preference. The diagnosis *predominantly intradermal nevus*, perhaps with the added notation "no unusual activity at the junction," seems to offer an acceptable compromise in many cases.

Many intradermal nevi (see above) show cells of different type and size. Those near the surface usually, but not always, possess a considerable amount of cytoplasm and an ovoid or round vesicular nucleus (type A). The uppermost row generally contains melanin granules, and these may be present in somewhat deeper nests. Melanization of nevus cells deep in the dermis arouses suspicion of malignant melanoma but may be related to the origin of nevus cells from hair roots. Cytologic analysis and evaluation of the entire lesion are necessary in every case. Old quiescent nevi not infrequently contain multinucleated giant cells (Fig. 32–34), which have no clinical significance. Nevus cells in the middle and deeper dermis often are small and may be almost indistinguishable from lymphocytes in H&E sections (type B). Their nature can be ascertained by finding them enmeshed in elastic fibers or reticulum fibers. Occasional association of intradermal nevus cell nests with dermal melanocytes, i.e., of a nevus cell nevus with a blue nevus, can be observed.

activity and certainly not malignancy. Nevus cell nevi having papillomatous configuration (Fig. 32–21), especially the type resembling a raspberry clinically, never loose their junctional element; they keep growing outward all the time. Therefore,

Eruptive Nevi. New nevi may appear in crops. They may seem to be quite spontaneous in some persons.[50] In other cases, an eruption of new nevi has been reported following an attack of toxic epidermal necrolysis or erythema multiforme.[51,52] While

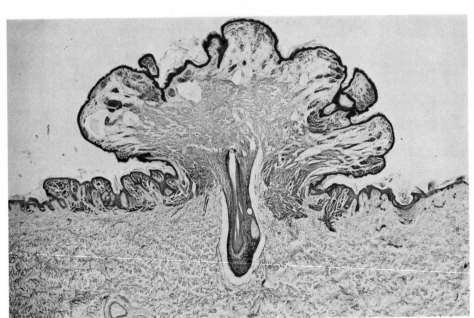

FIGURE 32–21.
Papillomatous nevus cell nevus with flat halo. Tumor is predominantly intradermal, but some nevus cell nests are present at the junction. Note involvement of perifollicular tissue. The superficial nests are surrounded by fat cells, producing the impression of lymph spaces. H&E. X30.

in these instances the new nevi follow the ordinary course and become stable, there is another type, occurring in families, which are precursors of malignant melanoma. They were described as the *B-K mole syndrome* by Clark[53] and have a somewhat uneven clinical configuration. Histologically (Fig. 32–22), they present atypical melanocytic hyperplasia at the junction and pagetoid invasion of the epidermis, together with inflammatory reaction in the dermis. The significance of crops of moles, especially if they occur in families, therefore, must be evaluated by careful observation.

Neuronevus. A special form of intradermal nevus, most commonly found about the head and neck, is *Masson's neuronevus.* The neuroid formations (Fig. 32–23) usually occupy the deep portion or the deep center of a lesion of long standing. The cells composing this part of a nevus are the type C cells of Miescher and Albertini and have been thought to be derived from neural Schwann cells rather than from melanocytes. Enzyme histochemistry[54] has shown that they contain the nonspecific cholinesterase characteristic of sensory corpuscles. Electron histochemistry has been able to find tyro-

sinase and cholinesterase activity in the same nevus cell,[55] thus suggesting unitarian origin rather than strict dichotomy of nevus histogenesis and supporting the concept that all nevus cells are deranged neuroectodermal elements distinct from melanocytes. Beginners are greatly helped in recognizing neuronevi in routine sections when they examine O&G sections. Here the neuroid structures, being of cellular nature, stain blue and are distinct from eosinophilic collagen. Mast cells, common in many nevi, and especially in this type, add to the distinctive appearance in O&G sections.

Balloon Cell Nevus. An always surprising and occasionally misleading histologic variant of nevus cell is the balloon cell (Blasenzelle). Balloon cells (Fig. 32–24) are up to 10 times larger than ordinary nevus cells and have a centrally or eccentrically placed vesicular nucleus and empty-appearing or foamy cytoplasm which stains faintly with PAS and Nile blue sulfate and perhaps contains phospholipids.[56] It may contain melanin granules. Balloon cells may be sparse or many, and some nevi consist entirely of these elements.[57] They are now acknowledged to be functional cells[58] capable of

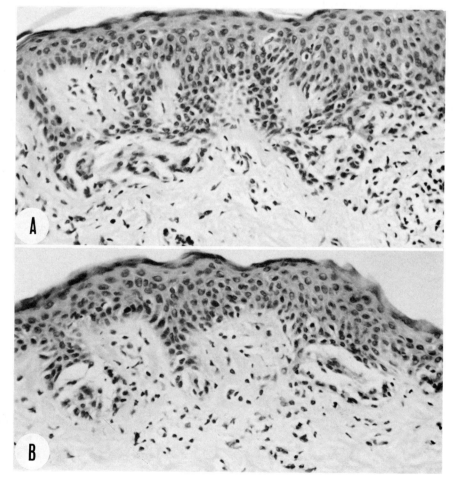

FIGURE 32–22.

B-K mole (Clark). Junction nevus with nests at tip of rete ridges uniting to form elongated theques parallel to skin surface. **A.** *Some nevus cells migrating upward in epidermis. H&E. X250.*

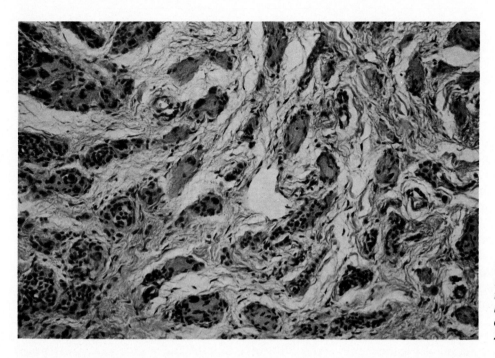

FIGURE 32–23.
Neuroid formations in an intradermal nevus. Type C cells usually exhibit nonspecific cholinesterase activity. H&E. X225.

mitosis. Malignant forms have been recorded[59,60] but, in general, presence of balloon cells does not alter either diagnosis or prognosis of a benign nevus.

Benign Juvenile Melanoma. The juvenile melanoma (Fig. 32–25) is an outstanding example of the

fact that the pathologist must constantly refine the diagnostic criteria in correlating them with clinical experience. When Spitz[61] first reviewed malignant melanomas in children because of their unusually favorable course, she could histologically identify a certain pattern common to those lesions that were clinically benign. At first, pathologists were hesi-

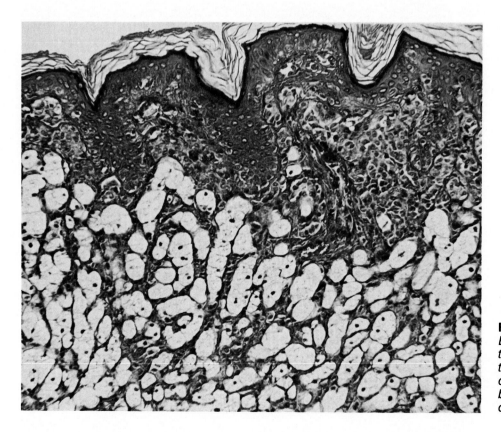

FIGURE 32–24.
Balloon cell nevus. Compare the type A nevus cells below the epidermis with the extraordinary size of the balloon cell bodies, while nuclei are reduced in size. H&E. X180.

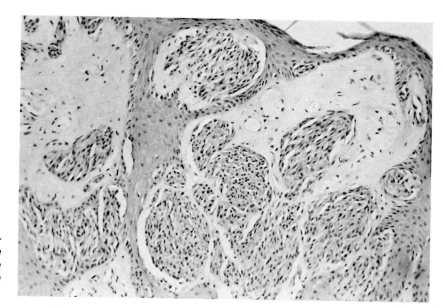

FIGURE 32–25.
Spitz nevus. The large nevus cells contain no melanin and are arranged in the epidermis, at the junction, and in the dermis. They have fusiform shape in this lesion. H&E. X125.

tant to trust histologic criteria when these were found in adults. Now, particularly based on the continued work of Allen,[62] one can again have confidence in one's ability to differentiate benign and malignant lesions under the microscope regardless of the age of the patient.[63,64] While Kopf and Andrade[65] recommend that the diagnosis benign juvenile melanoma be applied to such tumors at any age, others prefer the designations spindle cell or epithelioid cell nevus. The simplest designation is *Spitz nevus*.

One outstanding histologic feature of benign juvenile melanoma is the large size of its cells, but it shares this sign with most malignant melanomas.

Many lesions consist mainly of fusiform cells (Fig. 32–26), but others have rounded, ovoid, or irregularly bizarre elements (Fig. 32–27). Mitoses are not uncommon, and inflammatory infiltrate is often present. Many lesions contain little or no visible melanin, and not a few resemble malignant hemangioendotheliomas. Clinically, they are often considered granuloma pyogenicum. Differentiation from malignant tumors of nonmelanotic nature is usually assured when one finds at least some of the cells in junctional position. That means that they replace the basal layer of the epidermis or lie in niches within the lower contour of the epidermis. Relatively few benign juvenile melanomas are

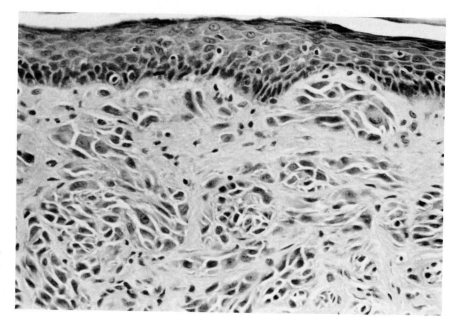

FIGURE 32–26.
Benign juvenile melanoma, intradermal. Plump large cells have predominantly spindle shape and are arranged in ill-defined nests. No melanin. H&E. X250.

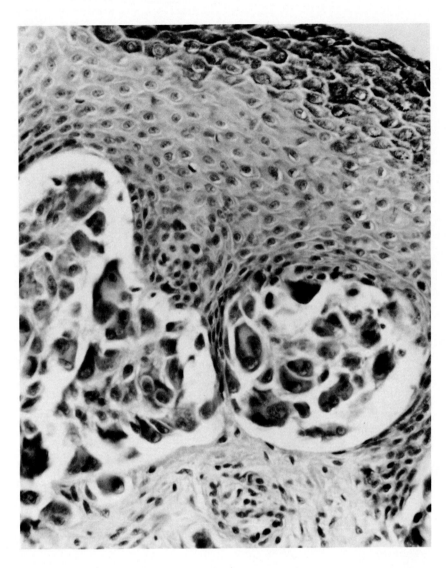

FIGURE 32–27.
Epithelioid cell nevus is another synonym for Spitz nevus. In this instance, very large and bizarre cells form nests in the epidermis and at the junction. H&E. X400. (From Kriner and Mehregan: J Cutan Pathol 5:90, 1978. Copyright © 1978 Munksgaard International Publishers; Copenhagen.)

completely intradermal (Fig. 32–26) at the time that they come to the pathologist's attention. The reason may be that these tumors grow rather rapidly and are excised during their period of growth. In the last analysis, diagnosis depends on recognition of a pattern, which requires experience with a good many lesions.

Regression of Nevus Cell Nevi and Sutton's Halo Nevus. An estimated 20 to 30 percent of nevi disappear through fibrosis or atrophy in old age. In others, the nevus cells seem to be crowded out by fat cells (Fig. 32–28), but this phenomenon is not atrophy but rather development of a lipomatous nevus in the mole. Some nevi, however, disappear in a most unusual manner and often early in life.[66] The nevus that is at the center of *leukoderma acquisitum centrifugum* (Fig. 32–29) is most commonly a compound nevus but may be predomi-

nantly intradermal. For unknown reasons (autoimmunity?),[67,68] a heavy inflammatory infiltrate develops, consisting mainly of small and larger round cells, histiocytes, and, occasionally, plasma cells. At the time the lesion is biopsied, nevus cells may be hard to recognize, pigment being present in macrophages. The surrounding epidermis is free of pigment, but nonpigmented melanocytes may be present. There are nevi that undergo the same process of destruction without development of a clinical white halo, and there is an occasional halo nevus without signs of inflammation.[69] It is important to be aware of these lesions in order to avoid mistaking them for malignant melanoma or for infectious granuloma or lymphoma.

Recurrence of Nevi after Removal. The desire of many patients to get rid of moles for purely cosmetic reasons has led to the practice of removing

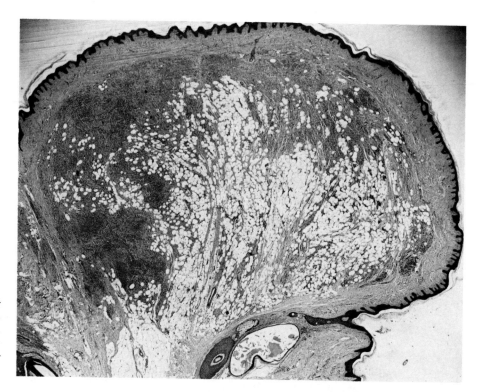

FIGURE 32–28.
Sessile intradermal nevus with fat tissue. Such pictures may be interpreted as combined nevocellular and lipomatous tumor, or as fat tissue replacing an old cellular nevus. H&E. X30.

only the protruding part either by shaving or by electrodesiccation. With both procedures, intradermal nests of nevus cells are left behind. Occasionally, some weeks or months after surgery, new pigment will become visible in the scar, causing concern to patient and physician alike. On excision of the lesion, a characteristic histologic picture (Fig. 32–30) is found.[70,71] Often, there are intradermal nests of nevus cells, separated from the epidermis by some scar tissue. The overlying epidermis contains individual and grouped nevus cells forming a new junction nevus. Sometimes, these cells are somewhat more irregular than spontaneous junction nevi, but in several fairly large series of

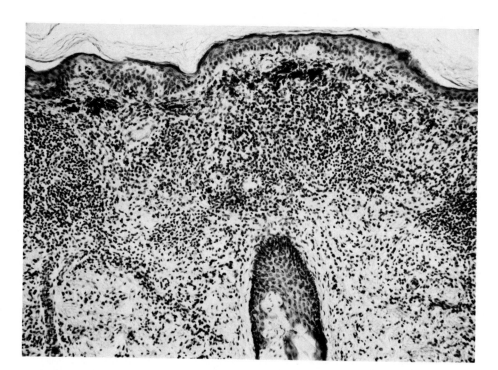

FIGURE 32–29.
Sutton's halo nevus. Practically all of nevus cells have been replaced by inflammatory, presumably reactive infiltrate. Such pictures may be encountered with or without clinical halo of leukoderma acquisitum centrifugum. H&E. X135.

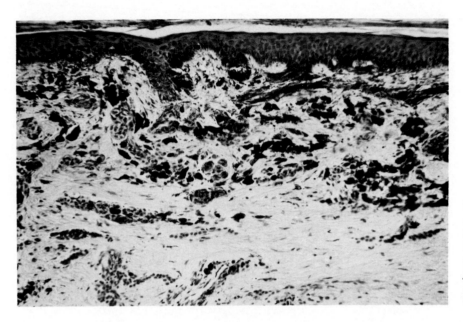

FIGURE 32–30.
Recurrence of nevus after cosmetic removal by shaving. Scar tissue at bottom of picture. The regenerated epidermis shows several typical junctional nests of pigmented nevus cells. Some melanophages below the epidermis. H&E. X250.

cases, no clinical or histologic evidence for development of malignancy was found in this situation. The new nevus probably arises from preexisting junctional cells either at the periphery of the incompletely removed lesion or in the epithelium of hair follicles within the mole. Such new lesions are diagnosed properly as *recurrent junction nevi*. The term "pseudomelanoma,"[72,73] which has been used in the past for hemosiderotic histiocytoma as well, is misleading and inappropriate.

Bathing-Trunk Nevus. There is one congenital malformation of the skin that contains nevus cells. Because of its preferred distribution it is often called bathing-trunk nevus. A German term is Tierfellnaevus, meaning a nevus simulating the pelt of an animal. This designation expresses the nevus nature, which consists in overdevelopment of perfectly normal strong hairs or entire pilar complexes. In these lesions, nevus cells develop during fetal life at stages at which the dermis is just maturing, and thus nevus cells are embedded in all layers of the corium without going through the sequence described earlier for the formation of postnatal moles. It is well known that in these individuals, melanotic lesions may also occur in the nervous system and that malignant melanoma may develop in any location involved.[74] The existence of this type of lesion lends support to the thesis that nevus cells are embryonically misdirected neuroectodermal elements (Fig. 32–1). Their presence in animal pelt nevi poses peculiar conceptual complications but does not invalidate the definition of nevus versus tumor. Giant pigmented nevi should be completely excised as early as feasible, but lesions measuring only a few centimeters in diameter are probably harmless.

Malignant Nevocytic Melanoma

For many years, the nevus cell was considered to be the only benign neoplastic form of melanogenic cells, and all malignant melanomas were thought to be *malignant nevocytomas*. Only the modern interpretation of Bloch's concept of "nonnevoid melanoma" and the demonstration that benign and precancerous melanocytomas, not related to nevus cells, do exist in the form of melanoacanthoma and lentigo maligna made possible a biologically based distinction between malignant nevocytoma (Figs. 32–31 and 32–32) and *malignant melanocytoma* (Fig. 32–36). We pointed out in the first edition of the *Guide* that this distinction has practical significance inasmuch as malignant melanocytomas, which are derived from lentigo maligna, metastasize late and have a much better prognosis[75] than do malignant nevocytomas, which have their origin in nevus cell nevi or pagetoid melanosis[76] unless they arise de novo.

Since that time, mainly through investigations in Australia and this country, many data have been added, and a refined concept and clinicopathologic classification have been developed[77,78] that permit the division of malignant nevocytomas into an immediately invasive nodular type and a superficially spreading (or pagetoid) type, in which a more or less prolonged, preinvasive (radial growth) phase precedes the metastasis-prone formation of invasive nodules (Figs. 32–33 and 32–37).

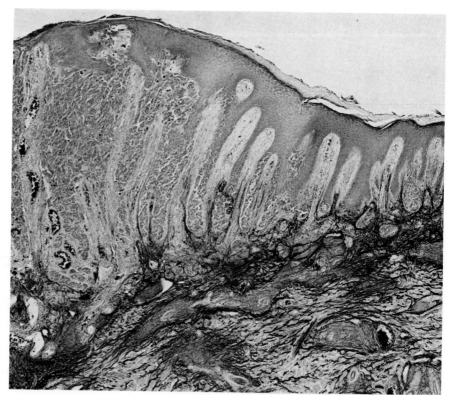

FIGURE 32–31.
Malignant melanoma developing above a benign intradermal nevus. Presence of elastic fibers in benign part (lower right) and absence in malignant portion (upper left) emphasize difference. O&G. X45.

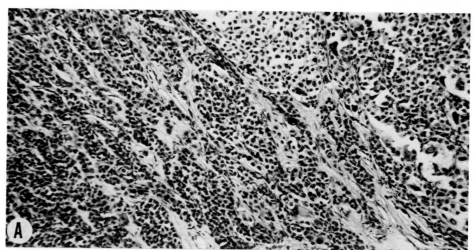

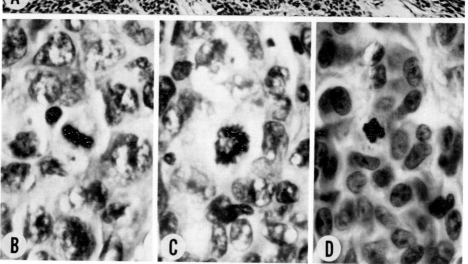

FIGURE 32–32.
*Malignant melanoma. **A.** At higher magnification, relatively large size of cells is evident, when compared with Figures 32-17 and 32-19. There is some indication of nest formation, cells form diffuse masses in other areas, and there is a minimum of stroma. In the fully developed malignant tumor, cytologic differentiation of melanocytic and nevocytic types becomes impossible. H&E. X124. **B, C,** and **D.** Characteristics of nuclei and mitotic figures. Aster in **C** has more than normal complement of chromosomes. H&E. X1012.*

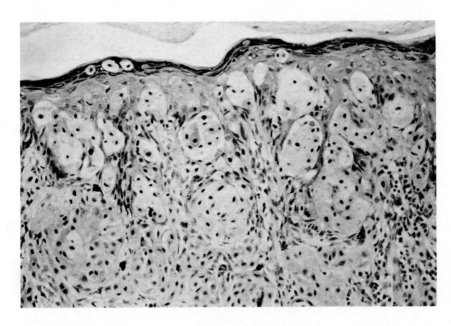

FIGURE 32–33.
Superficially spreading malignant melanoma producing pagetoid picture in its radial growth phase. Note that there is already vertical growth downward into the dermis. H&E. X250.

The histologic examination of a lesion suspected to be malignant melanoma, therefore, has three important goals. One is establishment of the diagnosis of a melanotic tumor, even though the lesion may be amelanotic, the second is the establishment of malignancy, and the third one is the decision whether the neoplasm is a *lentigo maligna melanoma*, a *superficially spreading melanoma*, or a *nodular malignant melanoma.*[79] Table 32–4 was adapted from a chart published by Mihm et al.[80]

The first goal is relatively easily attained, inasmuch as completely amelanotic melanomas are rare. If routine sections, especially those stained with O&G, do not reveal pigment, a stain with Masson's ammoniacal silver solution may show premelanin. Tyrosinase reaction is very helpful if

TABLE 32–4.
Differential Diagnosis of Malignant Melanomas

Diagnosis	Significant Histologic Features
Malignant Melanocytoma	
Lentigo maligna (Hutchinson's melanotic freckle)	Crowding of atypical (usually dendritic) pigmented melanocytes in the basal layer. Only minor degree of transepidermal elimination. Later formation of cell nests at the junction. Heavy lymphocytic and plasmacytic infiltrate with pigmented macrophages in upper dermis
Lentigo maligna melanoma	Similar. Nests formed by atypical melanocytes (dendritic or spindle shaped) at junction and in dermis. Often downgrowth of melanocytes in outer root sheath and eccrine ducts
Malignant Nevocytoma	
Superficially spreading malignant melanoma, noninvasive (pagetoid melanosis)	Large, more or less pigmented nevus cells (usually rounded) in basal layer with strong tendency to nest formation even in the periphery. Invasion of upper epidermal layers in pagetoid fashion and extensive transepidermal elimination. Moderately heavy lymphocytic and plasmacytic dermal infiltrate with pigmented macrophages
Superficially spreading malignant melanoma, invasive	Similar. Nests of malignant nevus cells also in dermis, extending to variable depth
Nodular malignant melanoma	Nests of malignant cells at junction and in dermis forming a more or less spherical tumor without appreciable peripheral spread in the epidermis. Variable amount of inflammatory infiltrate in dermis
Malignant Blue Nevus	Atypical fusiform cells, often with relatively little pigment, mixed with deeply pigmented macrophages in the dermis. No involvement of the epidermis. Variable amount of inflammatory infiltrate
Metastatic Malignant Melanoma	Malignant cell nests in dermis usually without involvement of the junction and often without much inflammatory infiltrate

Adapted from Mihm et al.[80]

fresh tissue is available, although an occasional melanoma may even lack this critical enzyme. The disposition of tumor nests in junctional arrangement is an important clue, but metastatic malignant melanoma usually does not approach the epidermis.

Criteria for Malignancy. There are several criteria for malignancy of a melanotic tumor, some more significant than others. The presence of mitoses (Figs. 32–32B,C,D) is of primary importance, although some mitotic figures may be found in benign juvenile melanomas and an occasional one even in benign nevi. The absence of mitosis does not rule out malignancy. The next important feature is inflammatory reaction composed of lymphocytes and possibly plasma cells. It is practically always present but may be absent in rapidly growing tumors and, on the other hand, may also be found in benign juvenile melanoma, nevus incipiens, and Sutton's halo nevus. This reactive infiltrate must not be confused with the acute or granulomatous infiltrate (Fig. 21–14) that may be caused in a benign intradermal nevus by infection of a hair root or breakdown of a follicular cyst.[81] Cell size has considerable significance. Cells of malignant melanomas (Figs. 32–32 and 32–35) usually are much larger than even the large A type cells of benign nevi, a feature also true for benign juvenile melanoma. One should not be confused by large multinucleated nevus giant cells (Fig. 32–34) occurring in benign lesions. The distribution and amount of pigment usually are more variable in malignant melanoma, some nests containing much, others little or none. Particularly characteristic is a dustlike pigmentation (Fig. 32–35) of large-celled junctional nests. One should not be deceived by the presence of pigmented macrophages, which occur in benign as well as in malignant lesions.

It is almost dogmatic, although bathing-trunk nevus and malignant blue nevus are exceptions, that all types of malignant melanoma start at the dermoepidermal junction. It is not essential for diagnostic purposes to decide whether the cell that was converted to malignancy had been a melanocyte or a junctional nevus cell. It is, however, essential to ascertain whether the cells have a strong tendency to form nests or whether they retain individuality even where crowded. From the junction, cells may be carried into the higher epidermal layers and be excreted to the surface.

It has been said that suspicious melanocytic hyperplasia can be discounted if the intradermal part of a nevus is obviously benign. However, if we accept the thesis that malignant melanoma starts at the junction and often starts in a preexisting nevus, we must find, every once in a while, a tumor in which smaller or larger remnants of the benign intradermal nevus are still present, although a malignant strain of cells, once started, will soon overgrow and eliminate its benign prototype neighbors. The clinical outcome is apt to be favorable in cases in which remnants of the benign nevus persist because the cancer was in an early stage and had not

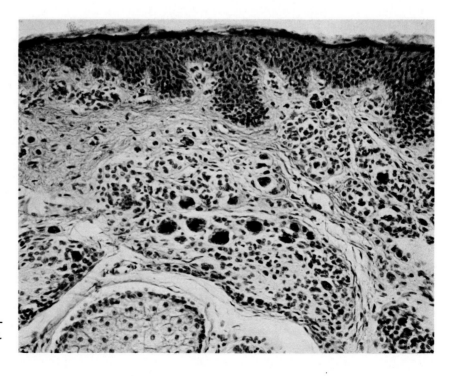

FIGURE 32–34.
Variability of nevus cells in benign intradermal nevus. Nevus giant cells. H&E. X180.

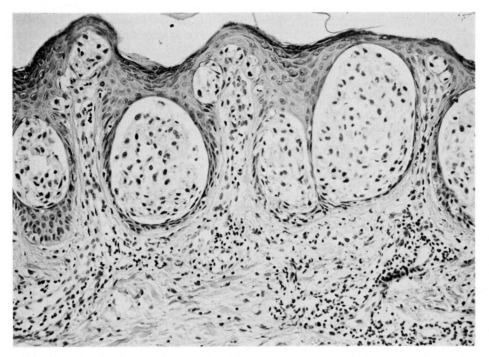

FIGURE 32–35.
Intraepidermal nests of large malignant nevus cells in a superficially spreading malignant melanoma, level 1. Cells contain tiny dustlike pigment granules, not visible at this magnification. H&E. X225. (From Pinkus and Mehregan. In Schnyder UW (ed). Haut und Anhangsgebilde, 1973. Courtesy of Springer-Verlag.)

yet invaded deeply or metastasized. Therefore, clinical proof of malignancy will be lacking. It seems, however, to be abrogating the last claim of the pathologist to make a microscopic diagnosis of malignancy if we define benign lesions as those that do not kill the patient owing to timely surgical interference.

Another factor helpful in some cases is the constitution of the dermal stroma. It was mentioned earlier that nests of benign nevus cells are often surrounded by collagen bundles and, even in their absence, by fine elastic fibers (Fig. 32–20) and reticulum fibers, making an orderly and distinct pattern.[82] This is not so in malignant melanoma (Fig. 32–31), which outgrows and destroys stroma.[83] Elastic fiber and reticulum stains can assist in differential diagnosis between benign and malignant intradermal tumors.

The third goal, differentiation of melanocytic and the two types of nevocytic malignant mela-

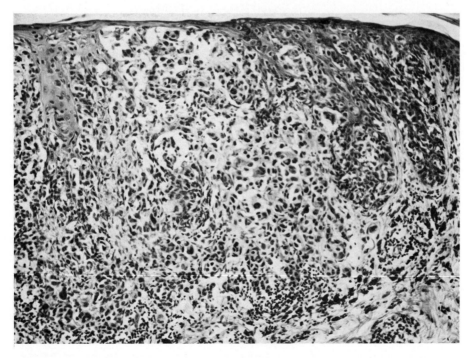

FIGURE 32–36.
Malignant melanoma developing in lentigo maligna (Hutchinson's melanotic freckle). Persistence of individualized atypical melanocytes in edge of lesion permits diagnosis. H&E. X135.

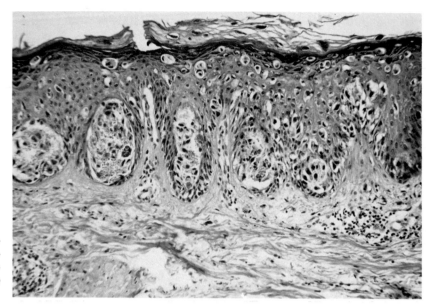

FIGURE 32–37.
Pagetoid premalignant melanosis.[76] If tumor is amelanotic, and no suitable material is available for enzyme studies, absence of mucin may be used as a clue to identification (see Fig. 40-6). H&E. X185.

noma, cannot be achieved by examination of the invading tumor. Only if we have favorable sections, large enough to show the epidermal rim around the tumor,[84] can we hope to find evidence of any preexistent lesion and of the mode and degree of lateral advance of the melanoma. Crowding of atypical melanocytes, as in Figures 32–8, 32–9, and 32–36, establishes a diagnosis of malignant melanocytoma, while pictures, such as those illustrated in Figures 32–35 and 32–37, represent superficially spreading nevocytoma. If there is no lateral exten-

sion for more than a couple of rete ridges, the diagnosis of nodular malignant melanoma (Fig. 32–38) is established, even if one is dealing with an early tumor that has not yet invaded deeply.

There are three terms we avoid. "Junction activity" really means no more than that increased numbers of either melanocytes or benign nevus cells or malignant melanoma cells are present at the dermoepidermal junction. The observation that there is melanocytic hyperplasia should put the pathologist on guard, and the benign or malignant na-

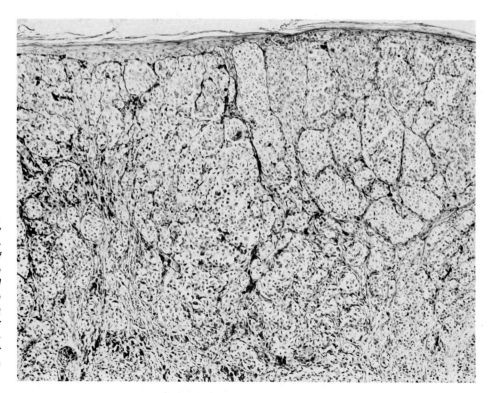

FIGURE 32–38.
Nodular malignant melanoma. This general view of a bulky and relatively amelanotic tumor illustrates the variability of the tumor cells, which are gathered into unevenly sized nests by scanty stroma. While there is a thin layer of stroma between epidermis and tumor in the left half of the picture, tumor cells replace the lower half of the epidermis in the right half. H&E. X60.

ture of the lesion must be determined. One should not transmit the expression "junction activity" as such to the clinician, for whom it has an ominous meaning. The second term, "active junction nevus," has no place in our nomenclature because it has been used mistakenly in the past to include lentigo maligna. We diagnose either a *growing benign junction nevus* or *superficially spreading malignant melanoma* in its early phase. If all nests of the latter lesion are definitely above the basement membrane, it may in fact be preferable to make a diagnosis of *precancerous pagetoid melanosis*. The third undesirable term is "superficial melanoma" because it describes only the momentary status of the lesion without saying anything about its history and biologic behavior. A young nodular melanoma may be restricted to the superficial layer of the dermis but may be expected to invade more deeply within a few weeks. A superficially spreading melanoma, on the other hand, may remain superficial for many months or even some years, and lentigo maligna for many years. One should, therefore, give the specific diagnostic term and add to it the descriptive facts: whether the tumor cells are restricted to the junctional zone, the pars papillaris, the upper half of the dermis, or extend into the deep dermis and subcutis.

We repeat a statement concerning the intraepidermal spread of malignant melanoma cells. The melanocytes of lentigo maligna prefer to stay in the basal and immediate suprabasal layers. Relatively few single pigmented cells, most of them in an obviously degenerating state, are carried upward into the horny layer (Fig. 32–9). The cells of superficially spreading melanoma, on the other hand, have a strong tendency for intraepidermal spread, singly or in small groups of well-preserved large elements. This phenomenon caused McGovern to coin the name *pagetoid melanoma* (Fig. 32–33, 32–37), and the resemblance to Paget's disease (Fig. 40–6A) can indeed be striking, especially if the cells contain little or no melanin. In the latter case, and if the lesion is in the intraepidermal phase, one may have to resort to histochemical procedures. A positive Fontana-Masson silver stain or a positive dopa or tyrosinase reaction identifies the melanotic lesion, while the presence of glycogen or acid mucopolysaccharides is strong evidence for Paget's disease (Chap. 40).

Prognostic Interpretation Concerning Metastasis. The gravest responsibility of the pathologist in the field of malignant melanoma is the prognostication of metastatic spread. We owe a debt to Clark and his collaborators,[32] who showed that not every malignant melanoma carries the expectation of metastasis. In statistical terms, the depth of penetration is important, and Clark's grading of invasion into levels 2, 3, 4, and 5 has become very helpful in predicting which tumors have a high chance of having

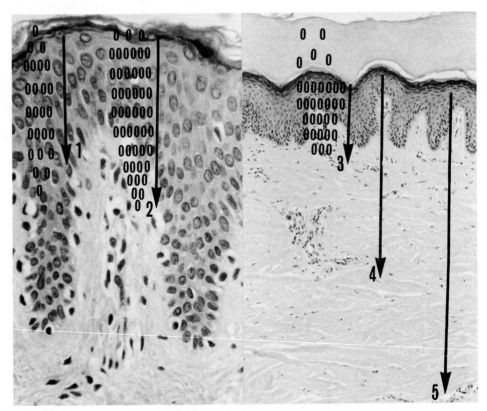

FIGURE 32–39.
The levels of dermal invasion according to Clark are indicated: level 1, intraepidermal; level 2, invasion of papillae; level 3, involvement of superficial vascular plexus; level 4, invasion of reticular dermis; level 5, involvement of subcutaneous tissue.

already seeded themselves in the lymph stream (Fig. 32–39). His level 1 means precancerous melanosis in the epidermis; level 2, invasion of the papillary layer; level 3, involvement of the superficial vascular plexus; level 4, invasion of the reticular dermis; and level 5, involvement of the subcutaneous tissue. The breaking point, according to Clark, is between level 2 and level 3, indicating the advisability of prophylactic lymph node dissection for any level 3 lesion. The difficulty is the accuracy of individual judgment of level 2 and level 3 penetration.

A newer rule has been advanced by Breslow,[85] who advocates actual measurement of maximal tumor thickness under the microscope. Tumors less than 0.75 mm in thickness are not apt to have metastasized; tumors more than 1.5 mm thick most likely have. This method is more easy to follow and seems to fit the clinical data better.[86]

The foregoing discussion was lengthy and detailed because the diagnosis of malignant melanoma constitutes a frequent problem for any pathologist. The responsibility of ruling it in or out is greater than in any other field of cutaneous pathology, owing to the propensity for rapid metastasis of the nodular types of malignant nevocytoma, and the resulting importance of prompt adequate therapy. In spite of, or perhaps because of, all the diagnostic refinements, there will be irreconcilable differences of opinion in individual cases.

REFERENCES

1. Mishima Y: Macromolecular changes in pigmentary disorders. III. Cellular nevi: subcellular and cytochemical characteristics with reference to their origin. Arch Dermatol 91:536, 1965
2. Fitzpatrick TB, Quevedo WC, Levene AL, et al.: Terminology of vertebrate melanin-containing cells: 1965. Science 152:88, 1966
3. Miescher G, Albertini A: Histologie de 100 cas de naevi pigmentaires d'après les méthodes de Masson. Bull Soc Fr Dermatol Syphiligr 42:1265, 1935
4. Kriner J, Crivelli MR: Determinación de elementes structurales en 10 casos de nevo dermal. Arch Argent Dermatol 20:13, 1970
5. Sagebiel RW: Histologic artefacts of benign pigmented nevi. Arch Dermatol 106:691, 1972
6. Mishima Y: Unpublished data
7. Tarnowski WM: Nuclear pseudoinclusions in melanoma cells. Br J Dermatol 81:709, 1969
8. Breathnach AS: Melanocyte distribution in forearm epidermis of freckled human subjects. J Invest Dermatol 29:253, 1957
9. Shapiro L, Zegarelli DJ: The solitary labial lentigo: a clinicopathologic study of twenty cases. Oral Surg 31:87, 1971
10. Chapel TA, Taylor RM, Pinkus H: Volar melanotic macules. Int J Dermatol 18:222, 1979
11. Frenk E, Delacrétaz J: Hydropic degeneration of epidermal keratinocytes. An alteration leading to patchy hyperpigmentation. Dermatologica 148:135, 1974
12. Jimbow K, Szabo G, Fitzpatrick TB: Ultrastructure of giant pigment granules (macromelanosomes) in the cutaneous pigmented macules of neurofibromatosis. J Invest Dermatol 61:300, 1973
13. Frenk E: Étude ultrastructurale des tâches pigmentaires du syndrome d'Albright. Dermatologica 143:12, 1971
14. Bhawan J, Purtilo DT, Riordan JA, et al.: Giant and "granular melanosomes" in leopard syndrome: an ultrastructural study. J Cutan Pathol 3:207, 1976
15. Weiss LW, Zelickson AS: Giant melanosomes in multiple lentigines syndrome. Arch Dermatol 113:491, 1977
16. Silvers DN, Greenwood RS, Helwig EB: Café au lait spots without giant pigment granules; occurrence in suspected neurofibromatosis. Arch Dermatol 110:87, 1974
17. Rower JM, Carr RD, Lowney ED: Progressive cribriform and zosteriform hyperpigmentation. Arch Dermatol 114:98, 1978
18. Cohen HJ, Minkin W, Frank SB: Nevus spilus. Arch Dermatol 102:433, 1970
19. Piñol Aguadé J, Peyri Rey J: Nevus sobre nevus. Med Cutan 7:85, 1973
20. Stewart DM, Altman J, Mehregan AH: Speckled lentiginous nevus. Arch Dermatol 114:895, 1978
21. Grupper C, Pruniéras M, Hincky M, et al.: Albinisme partial familiale (piebaldisme): Étude ultrastructurale. Ann Dermatol Syphiligr 97:267, 1970
22. Jimbow K, Fitzpatrick TB, Szabo G, et al.: Congenital circumscribed hypomelanosis: a characterization based on electron microscopic study of tuberous sclerosis, nevus depigmentosus, and piebaldism. J Invest Dermatol 64:50, 1975
23. Wiener K: Skin Manifestations of Internal Disorders (Dermadromes). St. Louis, Mosby, 1947
24. Selmanowitz VJ: Lentiginosis profusa syndrome II. Histological findings, modified Crow's sign, and possible relationship. Acta Derm Venereol (Stockh) 51:387, 1971
25. Norlund JJ, Lerner AB, Braverman IM, et al.: The multiple lentigines syndrome. Arch Dermatol 107:259, 1973
26. Mehregan AH: Lentigo senilis and its evolutions. J Invest Dermatol 65:429, 1975
27. Bloch B: Über benigne, nicht naevoide Melanoepitheliome der Haut nebst Bemerkungen über das Wesen und die Genese der Dendritenzellen. Arch Dermatol Syphiligr 153:20, 1927
28. Mishima Y, Pinkus H: Benign mixed tumor of melanocytes and malpighian cells. Melanoacanthoma; its relationship to Bloch's benign non-nevoid melanoepithelioma. Arch Dermatol 81:539, 1960
29. Delacrétaz J: Melano-acanthoma. Dermatologica 151:236, 1975
30. Schlappner OLA, Rowden G, Philips TN, et al.: Melanoacanthoma. Ultrastructural and immunological studies. J Cutan Pathol 5:127, 1978
31. Dubreuilh MW: De la mélanose circonscrite précancereuse. Ann Dermatol Syphiligr 3:129, 1912
32. Clark WH Jr, From L, Bernardino EA, et al.: The histogenesis and biologic behavior of primary human malignant melanoma of the skin. Cancer Res 29:705, 1969

33. Mishima Y: Melanosis circumscripta praecancerosa (Dubreuilh): a non-nevoid premelanoma distinct from junction nevus. J Invest Dermatol 34:361, 1960
34. Anton-Lamprecht I, Schnyder U, Tilgen W: Das Stade éphélide der melanotischen Präcancerose; eine vergleichende klinisch-histopathologisch-elektronenmikroskopische Studie. Arch Dermatol Forsch 240:61, 1971
35. Paul E, Illig L: Fluorescence-microscopic investigations of pigment cells of lentigo maligna (melanosis circumscripta praeblastomatosa Dubreuilh) and lentigo maligna melanoma. Arch Dermatol Res 256:179, 1976
36. Petratos MA, Kopf AW, Bart RS, et al.: Treatment of melanotic freckle with x-rays. Arch Dermatol 106:189, 1972
37. Lupulescu AP, Pinkus H, Birmingham DJ, et al.: Lentigo maligna of the finger tip; clinical, histologic, and ultrastructural studies of two cases. Arch Dermatol 107:717, 1973
38. Burket JM: Amelanotic lentigo maligna. Arch Dermatol 115:496, 1979
39. Coleman WP, Loria PR, Reed RJ, Krementz EF: Acral lentiginous melanoma. Arch Dermatol 116:773, 1980
40. Pinkus H: Die makroskopische Anatomie der Haut. In Jadassohn J: Handbuch der Haut-und Geschlechtskrankheiten. Ergänzungswerk, vol 1, pt 2. Berlin, Springer-Verlag, 1965, p 44
41. Hidano A: Persistent Mongolian spot in the adult. Arch Dermatol 103:680, 1971
42. Dorsey CS, Montgomery H: Blue nevus and its distinction from Mongolian spot and the nevus of Ota. J Invest Dermatol 22:225, 1954
43. Pittman JL, Fisher BK: Plaque-type blue nevus. Arch Dermatol 112:1127, 1976
44. Epstein E, Pinkus H: Giant blue nevus: cellular blue nevus as a clinical concept. Cutis 5:309, 1969
45. Hernandez FJ: Malignant blue nevus. Arch Dermatol 107:741, 1973
46. Santa Cruz DJ, Yates AJ: Pigmented storiform neurofibroma. J Cutan Pathol 4:9, 1977
47. Mishima Y: Cellular blue nevus: melanogenic activity and malignant transformation. Arch Dermatol 101:104, 1970
48. Mishima Y: Eccrine-centered nevus. Arch Dermatol 107:59, 1973
49. Bentley-Phillips CB, Marks R: Cell division and metabolic activity of nevus cells. The relationships between anatomy and behaviour in moles. Br J Dermatol 94:559, 1976
50. Eady RAJ, Gilkes JJH, Wilson-Jones E: Eruptive nevi: report of two cases, with enzyme histochemical, light and electron microscopical findings. Br J Dermatol 97:267, 1977
51. Kopf AW, Grupper C, Baer RL, et al.: Eruptive nevocytic nevi after severe bullous disease. Arch Dermatol 113:1080, 1977
52. Goerz G, Tsambaos D: Eruptive nevocytic nevi after Lyell's syndrome. Arch Dermatol 114:1400, 1978
53. Clark WH Jr, Reimer RR, Greene M, et al.: Origin of familial malignant melanomas from heritable melanocytic lesions. "the B-K mole syndrome." Arch Dermatol 114:732, 1978
54. Winkelmann RK: Cholinesterase nevus: cholinesterases in pigmented tumors of the skin. Arch Dermatol 82:17, 1960
55. Mishima Y: Cellular and subcellular activities in the ontogeny of nevocytic and melanocytic melanomas. In Montagna W, Hu F (eds): The Pigmentary System. Advances in Biology of Skin, vol 8. Oxford, New York, Pergamon, 1967, p 545
56. Schrader WA, Helwig EB: Balloon cell nevi. Am J Pathol 48:60, 1966
57. Goette DK, Doty RD: Balloon cell nevus. Summary of the clinical and histologic characteristics. Arch Dermatol 114:109, 1978
58. Hashimoto K, Bale G: An electron microscopic study of balloon cell nevus. Cancer 30:530, 1972
59. Ranchod M: Metastatic melanoma with balloon cell changes. Cancer 30:1000, 1972
60. Hüla M: Clear cell melanoblastoma. Dermatologica 146:86, 1973
61. Spitz S: Melanomas of childhood. Am J Pathol 24:591, 1948
62. Allen AC: Juvenile melanomas of children and adults and melanocarcinomas of children. Arch Dermatol 82:325, 1960
63. Weedon D. Little JH: Spindle and epithelioid cell nevi in children and adults. A review of 211 cases of the Spitz nevus. Cancer 40:217, 1977
64. Paniago-Pereira C, Maize JC, Ackerman AB: Nevus of large spindle and/or epithelioid cells (Spitz's nevus). Arch Dermatol 114:1811, 1978
65. Kopf AW, Andrade R: Benign juvenile melanoma. In Year Book of Dermatology, 1965–1966. Chicago, Year Book, 1966, p 7
66. Kopf AW, Morrill SD, Silberberg I: Broad spectrum of leukoderma acquisitum centrifugum. Arch Dermatol 92:14, 1965
67. Copeman PWM, Lewis MG, Phillips TM, et al.: Immunological associations of the halo naevus with cutaneous malignant melanoma. Br J Dermatol 88:127, 1973
68. Roenigk HH Jr, Deodhar SD, Krebs JA, et al.: Microcytotoxicity and serum blocking factors in malignant melanoma and halo nevus. Arch Dermatol 111:720, 1975
69. Gauthier Y, Surlěve-Bazeille J-E, Texier L: Halo nevi without dermal infiltrate. Arch Dermatol 114:1718, 1978
70. Schoenfeld RJ, Pinkus H: The recurrence of nevi after incomplete removal. Arch Dermatol 78:30, 1958
71. Walton RG, Cox AJ: Electrodesiccation of pigmented nevi. Arch Dermatol 87:342, 1963
72. Kornberg R, Ackerman AB: Pseudomelanoma: recurrent melanocytic nevus following partial surgical removal. Arch Dermatol 111:1588, 1975
73. Reed WB: Pseudomelanoma. Arch Dermatol 112:1611, 1976
74. Lorentzen M, Pers M, Bretteville-Jensen G: Incidence of malignant transformation in giant pigmented nevi. Scand J Plast Reconstr Surg 11:163, 1977
75. Mishima Y: Melanocytic and nevocytic melanomas; cellular and subcellular differentiation. Cancer 20:632, 1967b
76. Mishima Y, Matsunaka M: Pagetoid premalignant melanosis and melanoma: differentiation from Hutchinson's melanotic freckle. J Invest Dermatol 65:434, 1975
77. McGovern VJ, Lane Brown MM: The Nature of Melanoma. Springfield, Ill, Thomas, 1969

78. Kopf AW, Bart R, Rodríguez-Sains R, et al.: Malignant Melanoma. New York, Masson, 1979
79. McGovern VJ, Mihm MC, Bailey C, et al.: The classification of malignant melanoma and its histologic reporting. Cancer 32:1446, 1973
80. Mihm MC Jr, Clark WH Jr, From L: The clinical diagnosis, classification and histogenic concepts of the early stages of cutaneous malignant melanomas. N Engl J Med 284:1078, 1971
81. Duperrat B: Suppurations folliculaires torpides sous les naevi mélaniques. Ann Dermatol Syphiligr 81:251, 1954
82. Mehregan AH, Staricco RG: Elastic fibers in pigmented nevi. J Invest Dermatol 38:271, 1962
83. Scott IP, Venter IJ, Lups JGH: Malignant change in nevi: a supplementary histological feature. Br J Dermatol 85 [Suppl 7]:50, 1971
84. Cochran AJ: Studies of the melanocytes of the epidermis adjacent to tumors. J Invest Dermatol 57:38, 1971
85. Breslow A: Tumor thickness, level of invasion and node dissection in stage I cutaneous melanoma. Ann Surg 182:572, 1975
86. Breslow A: Prognostic factors in the treatment of cutaneous melanoma. J Cutan Pathol 6:208, 1979

CHAPTER
33

Epidermal Nevi and Benign Epidermoid Tumors

Circumscribed areas of skin exhibiting hyperplasia or hypoplasia of the epidermis, without appreciable alteration of the normal structure or maturation process and without external cause, may be called *epidermal nevi* regardless of their becoming manifest before or after birth. If circumscribed hyperplasia is associated with retarded but relatively normal maturation of cells and with some alteration of structure, the lesion is then a *benign epidermoid tumor* (Table 33–1). Considerable disruption of normal epidermal organization, dysplasia of cells, and atypical keratinization are the marks of *malignant epidermoid tumors*, which may be precancerous, carcinoma in situ, or invasive carcinoma. The term *epidermoid* is used because such tumors may take their origin not only from epidermal but also from adnexal keratinocytes. Site of origin is not important, and direction of maturation of the tumor cells in an epidermoid manner is the diagnostic feature. Malignant epidermoid tumors will be discussed in Chapter 34, where we shall say more about the clonal origin of neoplasms. Here we deal with epidermal nevi and benign epidermoid tumors, both of which manifest their relatively high level of organization through associated characteristic dermal changes. In fact, most benign epidermoid tumors are fibroepithelial in character. Just as inflammatory epidermal hyperplasia is practically always associated with increase of papillary tissue and just as viral warts have a papillomatous pattern, so do most epidermal nevi and benign epidermoid tumors exhibit papillary hyperplasia. They are papillomas as defined in Chapter 31. The increasing awareness of ectodermal-mesodermal interaction in skin disorders and especially in neoplasia has led to the publication of two books,[1,2] which are worth consulting. We shall refer to these phenomena repeatedly in the chapters to follow.

EPIDERMAL NEVI

Verrucous Epidermal Nevus. *Verrucous epidermal nevi* (Fig. 33–1) are flesh colored or brown lesions with a smooth or hyperkeratotic surface. They may be present at birth or appear during childhood or adolescence. The lesion is either localized or is arranged in linear fashion (linear verrucous epidermal nevus). Extensive involvement of one extremity or one side of the trunk is known as *nevus unius lateris*. Histologically, these lesions show hyperplasia of the epidermis and papillary connective tissue in varying degrees, which is responsible for the hyperkeratotic warty appearance or soft pedunculated lesions. A special form is the *hard nevus of Unna* (Fig. 33–1A) in which all dermal papillae in the area are evenly elongated and produce a serrated configuration of the epidermis which itself is moderately acanthotic and hyperkeratotic.

Verrucous epidermal nevi are differentiated from

TABLE 33–1.
Epidermal Nevi and Tumors by Level of Maturation

Malformation	Linear verrucous epidermal nevus
	Ichthyosis hystrix
	Pigmented hairy epidermal nevus (Becker)
	Inflammatory linear verrucous epidermal nevus
Adenomatous	Seborrheic verruca
	Melanoacanthoma
	Clear (pale) cell acanthoma
Epitheliomatous	Palmar pits of nevoid basal cell epithelioma syndrome

the organoid nevi by lack of adnexal participation in the nevoid lesion and by the absence of secondary development of nevoid tumors.

Ichthyosis Hystrix. This histologically distinctive lesion may be considered as a variant of verrucous epidermal nevus or a form fruste of epidermolytic hyperkeratosis (Chap. 29). Clinically, brown, verrucous, hyperkeratotic lesions appear in linear bands or may involve one segment of the body.

Histologically (Fig. 29–7), the verrucous hyperplastic epidermis shows marked hypergranulosis and vacuolization of the epidermal cells with basket-weave type hyperkeratosis.[3,4]

Inflammatory Linear Verrucous Epidermal Nevus. ILVEN is characterized by the appearance of scaling, erythematous, and dermatitic lesions in linear fashion.[5,6] The lesion is persistent and is refractory to treatment. Histologically, the acanthotic epidermis shows well-defined areas of hypergranulosis and hyperkeratosis alternating with foci of loss of granular layer and parakeratosis[7] (Fig. 33–2). Telangiectasia and mild lymphocytic infiltrate may be present in the underlying dermis.

Pigmented Hairy Epidermal Nevus. *Nevus of Becker* becomes manifest usually during adolescence over one side of the upper back and shoulder.[8,9] In the early stage, velvety macular areas of hyperpigmentation appear in this location and later show hypertrichosis. Smaller, macular, hyperpigmented lesions with or without hypertrichosis may

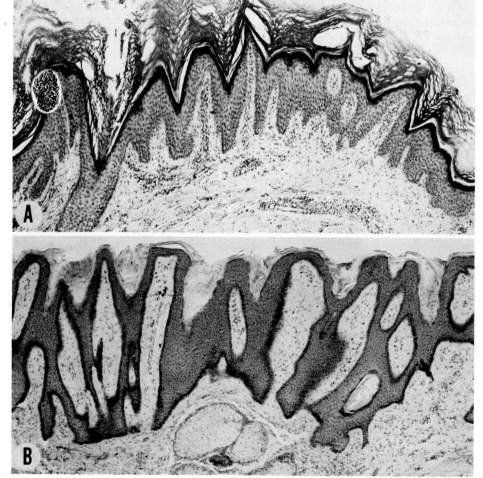

FIGURE 33–1.
Epidermal nevus. Both lesions are papillomatous. **A.** *Hard epidermal nevus with hyperkeratosis and relatively minor connective tissue component.* **B.** *Soft epidermal nevus which is also pigmented. There is little keratin, and papillae are large. H&E. X70.*

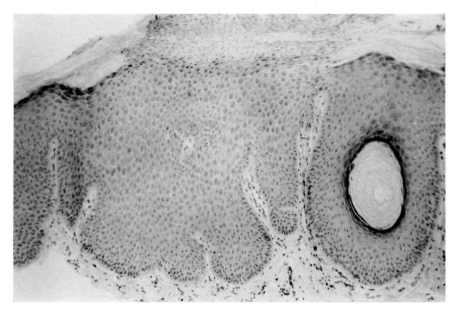

FIGURE 33–2.
Inflammatory linear verrucous epidermal nevus. Sharply limited blocks of pale-staining parakeratotic epidermis alternate with dark-staining, normally keratinizing blocks, only some of which are associated with follicular openings (right). H&E. X135.

also occur in other parts of the body. Histologic sections (Fig. 33–3) show mild epidermal thickening and uniform epidermal hyperpigmentation. Hyperpigmentation results from an overload of melanin in the keratinocytes.[10] There is an increase in the number or size of the hair follicles in the area. There also may be an increase in the number of smooth muscles.[11]

Epidermal Nevus Syndrome. This syndrome is characterized by an association of linear verrucous epidermal nevus with skeletal abnormalities and central nervous system manifestations.[12] The majority of cases show histologic changes of hyperkeratotic linear verrucous epidermal nevus, but, cases with features of ichthyosis hystrix and inflammatory linear verrucous epidermal nevus also have been reported.[13,14]

Nevoid Hyperkeratosis of Nipples and Areolae. Velvety hyperkeratotic and hyperpigmented lesions occur bilaterally over the nipples and areolae of

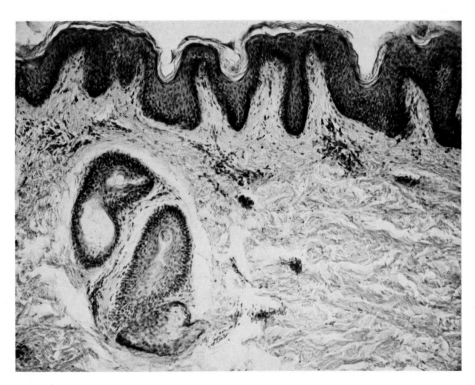

FIGURE 33–3.
Pigmented hairy epidermal nevus of Becker. Papillomatous, hyperpigmented epidermis associated with hyperplastic pilar complexes. H&E. X135.

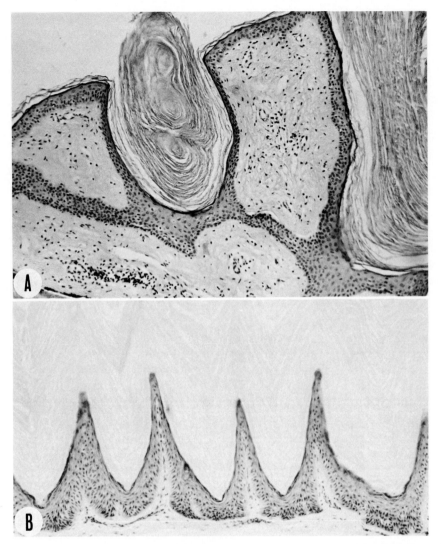

FIGURE 33–4.
A. *Nevoid hyperkeratosis of nipple. Papillomatosis and lamellated hyperkeratosis in association with rather thin epidermis. H&E. X135. (From Mehregan and Rahbari: Arch Dermatol 113:1691, 1977. Copyright © 1977 American Medical Association.)* **B.** *Acrokeratosis verruciformis of Hopf. Church spire appearance of long papillae covered by unremarkable heavily kerantinized epidermis. H&E. X125.*

young women.[15] Histologically (Fig. 33–4A), there is a marked papillomatous configuration of the epidermis and hyperkeratosis with minimal epidermal acanthosis.

Acrokeratosis Verruciformis of Hopf. Acrokeratosis verruciformis of Hopf appears to be a manifestation of Darier's disease in some cases, but it is questionable if one should consider it a form fruste of that disease when it occurs without other manifestations. Histologically (Fig. 33–4B), there is marked papillomatosis of the epidermis, with acanthosis and hyperkeratosis resembling church spires.[16]

Acanthosis Nigricans. Velvety hyperkeratotic and hyperpigmented plaques that occur in axillae and in other flexural areas show histologic changes (Fig. 33–5) very similar to those with a verrucous epidermal nevus. Papillomatous hyperplasia of the epidermis and hyperpigmentation occur with min-

imal epidermal thickening. There are no histologic differences between the benign and malignant varieties.[17,18]

Reticulated and Confluent Papillomatosis (Gougerot and Carteaud). The papillomatosis of Gougerot and Carteaud often is found heavily colonized by *Pityrosporum orbiculare*, and there is an indication that the papillomatosis is a peculiar tissue reaction to this organism.[19] Histologically, there is mild hyperkeratosis, epidermal acanthosis, and hyperpigmentation.[20]

Multiple Minute Digitate Hyperkeratoses. Minute digitate hyperkeratotic lesions that occur over the chest wall and shoulder show areas of hyperkeratosis with elongation of the epidermal rete ridges and hypergranulosis (Fig. 33–6). Minimal lymphocytic infiltrate is present in the underlying dermis.[21,22]

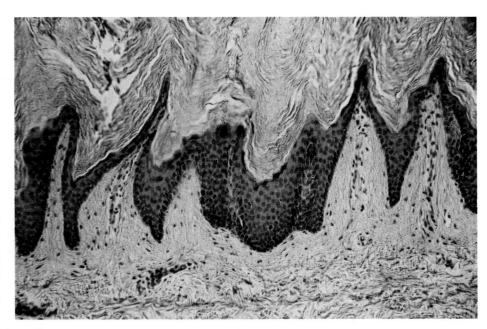

FIGURE 33–5.
Acanthosis nigricans. The epidermis is neither significantly acanthotic nor hyperpigmented. The clinical picture is due mainly to elongation and increased bulk of papillae and to hyperkeratosis. The dark color has its seat in the horny layer. H&E. X135.

Stucco Keratosis. Small grayish white keratotic lesions occur over the distal portions of the lower extremities.[23] Histologically, there is papillomatous hyperplasia of the epidermis with hyperkeratosis in church spire fashion.

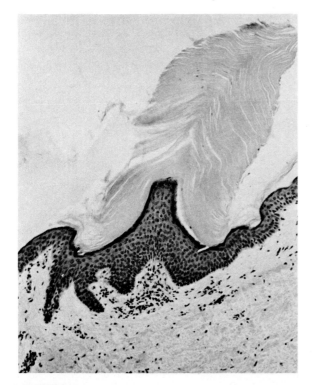

FIGURE 33–6.
Minute digitate hyperkeratosis. One papilla contains some inflammatory cells. The overlying epidermis has a thick granular layer and is covered by a minute cutaneous horn. H&E. X125.

SEBORRHEIC VERRUCA

Seborrheic verruca is the prototype of a benign epidermoid neoplasm corresponding in its structural organization and degree of maturity to an adenoma in the spectrum of glandular tumors[24] (Table 33–1). Structure is mildly distorted, and maturation is retarded but proceeds along normal channels. The tumors, therefore, show an increased proportion of basaloid cells, while typical light-staining prickle cells often are restricted to a few layers below the stratum granulosum. All three major patterns of seborrheic verruca—the solid, the papillomatous, and the reticulated types—basically are combined hyperplasia of epidermis and papillary dermis. The latter is minimal in the solid type (Figs. 32–7 and 33–7), which also shows little or no hyperkeratosis. Ectodermal and mesodermal components are fairly well balanced in the common papillomatous types (Fig. 33–8), characterized by an onionlike lamellation of horny material in recesses and intralesional cysts (Fig. 33–9). The latter are due to *endokeratinization.* They originate in deep portions of the thick epithelium and are gradually pushed upward and outward as they enlarge until they merge with the surface keratin. The hypothesis of invagination of the horny layer is ill conceived, inasmuch as all movement in the epidermis is outward, and examination of suitable lesions in serial sections leaves no doubt about the intraepidermal origin and truly cystic nature of many of these horny pearls. Other cornified cysts and cystlike structures are due to retention of keratin in hair follicles and sweat ducts traversing the verruca. Sweat ducts can be recog-

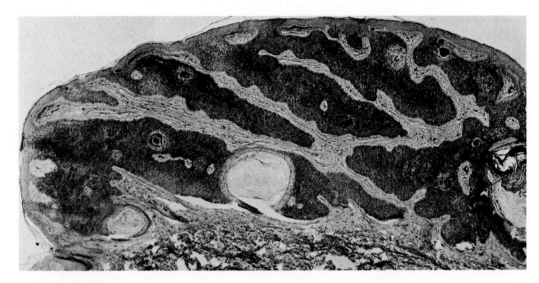

FIGURE 33–7.
Seborrheic verruca, solid type. This sessile, protruding lesion consists of masses of deeply pigmented basaloid cells changing rather abruptly into a relatively thin stratified layer of larger prickle cells. There is no surface hyperkeratosis and only few keratinizing foci in the substance of the tumor. O&G. X30.

nized in O&G sections by the eosinophilic staining of their keratin.

The *reticulated* type of seborrheic verruca is fairly rare and has structural relations to *lentigo senilis*.[25] The typical histologic picture of lentigo senilis (Fig. 32–5) shows peculiar club-shaped downward projections of the epidermis which seem to be true buds of the basal layer and usually are deeply pigmented, especially at the bulbous tips (Chap. 32). They do not penetrate the papillary layer but often are embedded in dense, eosinophilic connective tissue. From this simple pattern, one can find transitions to the complicated lacy appearance of the reticulated type of seborrheic verruca (Fig. 33–10).

Seborrheic verrucae have a normal complement of inconspicuous melanocytes and often contain moderate amounts of melanin in their keratino-

cytes. Some are deeply pigmented (Figs. 32–7 and 33–7). The amount of melanin has no clinical significance, and it seems unnecessary to use special names (Bloch's nonnevoid melanoepithelioma, type II, pigmented papilloma of skin) for these lesions, which the clinician sometimes mistakes for melanomas. The only form deserving recognition as a special biologic phenomenon is melanoacanthoma (Chap. 32).

Activated Seborrheic Verruca

Seborrheic verrucae have clinical and histologic aspects of sluggishness. They grow very slowly, and the accumulation of large amounts of stagnating keratin and often of pigment supports the impression of slow turnover. Under certain conditions,

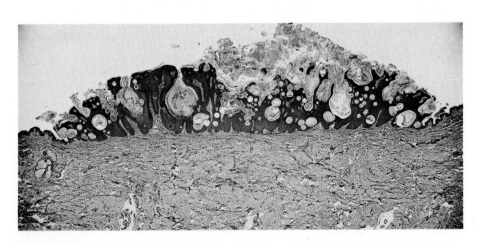

FIGURE 33–8.
Common type of seborrheic verruca in which many horny cysts move upward to become incorporated in surface hyperkeratosis. Note superficial stuck-on nature of papillomatous lesion. H&E. X14.

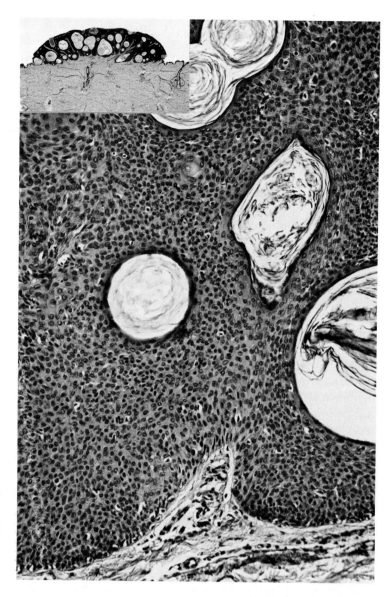

FIGURE 33–9.
Seborrheic verruca showing development of horny cysts deep in the body of the lesion (endokeratinization) and moving upward to join the surface stratum corneum. In between is another cyst that is a dilated hair follicle containing a few tiny hairs. The isolated cells in the substance of the verruca are probably Langerhans cells. H&E. X225.

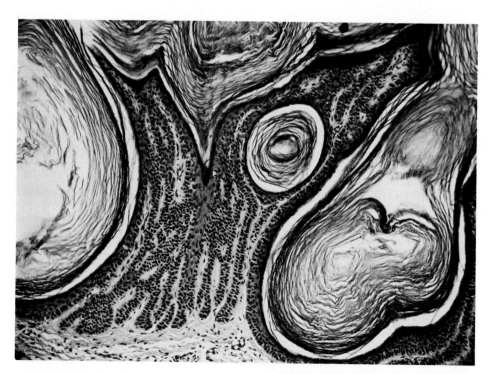

FIGURE 33–10.
Seborrheic verruca, reticulated type. Note similarity to pattern of lentigo senilis in Figure 32–5. H&E. X135.

however, the lesions may increase rather suddenly in size and change their histologic character. Some elderly people suffering from widespread eczematous dermatitis may develop many small papular lesions, which become manifest when the dermatitis subsides—and then subside gradually themselves. Histologically, they are papillomatous acanthomas[26] in the sense that they have layers of prickle cells above a single basal layer. Biologically, they are tiny seborrheic verrucae, temporarily stimulated into proliferation and precipitous maturation along with the surrounding acanthotic and exfoliating epidermis.

If one irritates a seborrheic verruca, for instance by the application of croton oil, conversion of basal cells into prickle cells also is accelerated, and the proportion of the latter increases.[27] This experience supports the view that the keratinocytes of this benign tumor are not materially deranged in their metabolism but are retarded in their maturation, which is one of the essential criteria of neoplasia. Occasionally, one encounters lesions which present the characteristic structure of the benign epidermoid neoplasm in one part, while another part presents a most unusual architecture (Fig. 33–11) consisting of numerous tiny or larger spheres of prickle cells in concentric arrangement, the larger ones undergoing central keratinization. The spheres, or *squamous eddies*,[28] are embedded (Fig. 33–11) in a mass of basaloid cells. This picture, to which the name *basosquamous acanthoma* was given by Lund[29] when it was found as the sole substrate of lesions, suggests that a seborrheic verruca has been activated by some inflammatory stimulus, perhaps by infection, and that basaloid cells have been explosively converted into maturing prickle cells in numerous foci. One has to be acquainted with this picture of the activated seborrheic verruca, which otherwise may be misdiagnosed as squamous cell carcinoma.

Intraepidermal Nests

While intralesional nests of prickle cells (squamous eddies) are found in activated seborrheic verrucae and inverted follicular keratosis, other types of seborrheic verruca are characterized by sharply defined nests of basaloid cells.[30] These lesions usually are flat clinically and occur most commonly on the lower extremities. While the histologic picture (Fig. 33–12) closely resembles certain types of intraepidermal epithelioma (Chap. 39), it is identified by finding a transition zone to the surrounding epidermoid tumor somewhere along the periphery of the nest. The nests are not true islands of cells but are *basaloid eddies*.

Seborrheic verrucae are benign tumors and are not precancerous. All cases in which development of basal cell epithelioma was reported are either instances of coincidental development of two common tumors of senile skin in close proximity or are due to histologic misinterpretation. The same holds true for the development of squamous cell carcinoma in seborrheic verruca. Bowenoid dysplastic cellular changes, however, can occur in se-

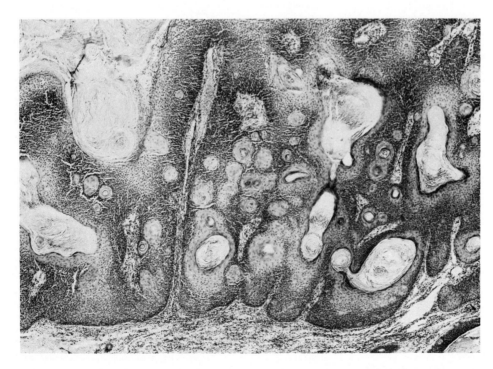

FIGURE 33–11.
Activated seborrheic verruca with numerous keratinizing centers. This is the pattern of Lund's basosquamous acanthoma and is encountered also in Helwig's inverted follicular keratosis. H&E. X45.

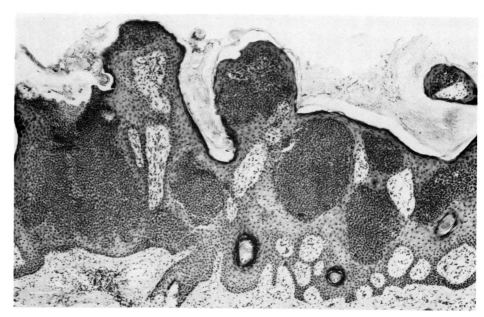

FIGURE 33–12.
Seborrheic verruca with basaloid nests resembling intraepidermal epithelioma of Jadassohn type. H&E. X45.

borrheic verruca in rare instances and in longstanding lesions.[31,32] Sudden appearance and rapid increase in size and number of seborrheic verrucae associated with internal malignancy is known as the sign of Leser-Trélat.[33]

PALE CELL ACANTHOMA (DEGOS)

A striking appearance, both clinically and histologically, is presented[34–37] by the rare tumor described as *acanthome à cellules claires* by Degos. The tumor, often localized on the leg, resembles an exuberant granuloma clinically and consists of a greatly thickened epidermis composed of unusually large keratinocytes, which stain pale in routine sections (Fig. 33–13) because they contain much glycogen.[38] The altered epithelium has cell-sharp margins against normal surrounding epidermis and adnexal units traversing the tumor—a hallmark of all epidermal neoplasms. Long papillae with blood-filled capillaries characterize Degos' acanthoma as a papilloma and, together with incomplete keratinization, account for the clinical aspect.

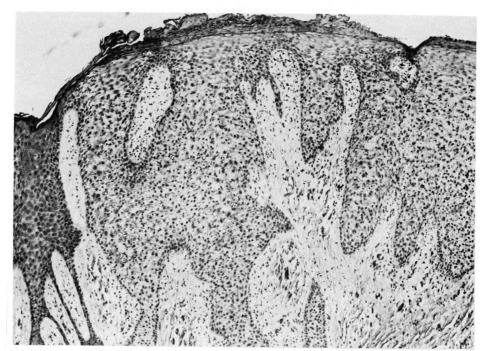

FIGURE 33–13.
Pale cell acanthoma. Sharp delineation between the dark-staining epidermis at left and the light-staining tumor cells. Both types of epithelium are similarly acanthotic. Nuclei of tumor cells are not enlarged. H&E. X75.

PALMAR PITS

Another instance of localized retarded maturation of epidermis, but with a quite different and peculiar connotation, is palmar pits, which are a marker of the nevoid basalioma syndrome.[39,40] They exhibit an increase of basaloid cells and diminished coherence of keratinocytes (Fig. 33–14), which leads to premature shedding of horny cells and a localized defect in the keratin layer. Disturbances of the papillary dermis indicate that they are, in fact, tiny fibroepithelial neoplasms.[41] In several cases, they progressed to basalioma formation.[42] Clinically similar pits occur in Darier's disease, have been described in association with internal malignancy, and are occasionally seen without any known disease association. These pits, however, resemble keratoderma punctatum (see below) on microscopic examination.

POROKERATOSIS

Porokeratosis of Mibelli is a misnomer based on the failure to view the skin in three dimensions. The sweat pore is a dot, and the cornoid lamella which encircles the lesion of porokeratosis is a ring which slowly moves eccentrically, crossing the fixed ostia of sweat ducts and hair follicles as it travels. In cutting biopsy sections, we try to orient

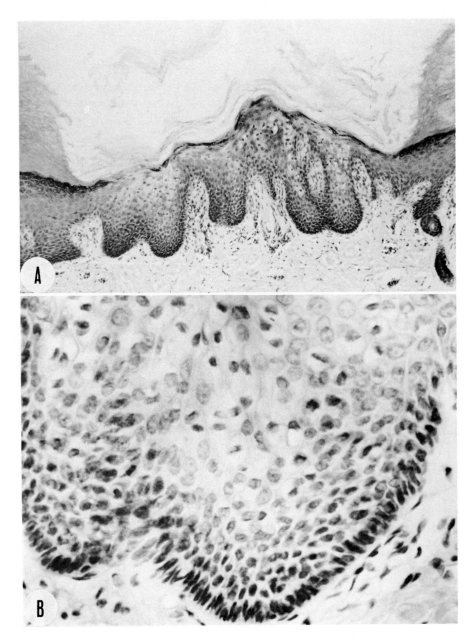

FIGURE 33–14.
*Palmar pit in nevoid basalioma syndrome. **A.** Sharply limited area of epidermis with decreased keratinization. Increased cellularity of papillary dermis. H&E. X125. **B.** Palisading basal layer beneath disordered prickle cells resembles somewhat a basal cell epithelioma. H&E. X400.*

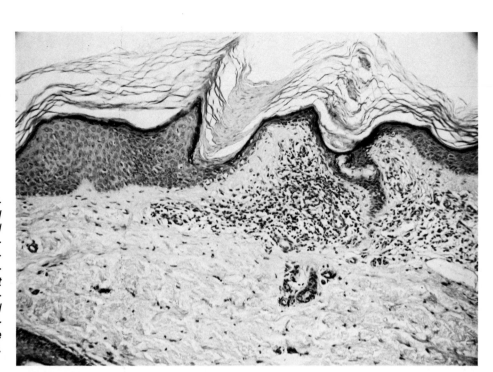

FIGURE 33–15.
Porokeratosis of Mibelli. Border of lesion is characterized by break in granular layer and oblique parakeratotic plug representing cross section of cornoid lamella. Note that this lesion has no relation to sweat duct, epidermis does not return to normal inside ring, and sweat duct in this area is dilated and hyperkeratotic. Note also inflammatory infiltrate. H&E. X135.

the tissue so that the lamella is shown in cross section. It then appears as a funnel-shaped depression in the epidermis (Fig. 33–15) usually not associated with a sweat pore. The granular layer is missing in the depth of the depression, and a column of parakeratotic cells rises obliquely from it. It must be emphasized once more that the column is but a cross section of the ring-shaped cornoid lamella. The nature of the lesion is puzzling if we concentrate attention on the ring. Closer examination, however, shows that the entire disk of epidermis inside the ring is abnormal, often hypoplastic, sometimes verrucous.[43] While keratinization usually is normal, parakeratotic plugs resembling the cornoid lamella may be found in follicular and eccrine ostia within the lesion. We pointed out in the first edition that one might consider porokeratosis as a benign heritable derangement of the metabolism of some epidermal cells. These form a slowly enlarging disk, in which only the active rim expresses the disturbance in the form of parakeratosis. A similar hypothesis has been independently voiced and documented by Reed and Leone,[44] and we, therefore, feel safe in listing Mibelli's disease as a benign epidermal neoplasm. Clinically in the classic form, single or multiple circular lesions show an elevated, hyperkeratotic, and ridged border.[45] Other morphologic forms include the superficial disseminated type[46] and the linear nevoid[47] and punctate varieties.[48] Facial foci and lesions of lips or buccal mucosa may be present.[49,50] Solitary lesions involving the plantar surface of the foot are

known as porokeratosis plantaris discreta.[51] Lesions of porokeratosis can become complicated by Bowen's disease,[52] squamous cell carcinoma,[53,54] or basal cell epithelioma.[55]

LARGE CELL ACANTHOMA

Not exceedingly rare, but rarely diagnosed, is another benign epidermal neoplasm which produces slightly scaling discolored spots and barely infiltrated plaques in the sun-exposed skin of elderly persons, with a decided preference for the female sex. Biopsies are usually submitted to rule out actinic keratosis, or the lesions are removed for cosmetic reasons.[56] The histologic picture at first suggests normal skin or a flat papilloma until one becomes aware of the unusually large size not only of the cytoplasm but of the nuclei of keratinocytes as well. There may be slight anisocytosis but never enough to confuse the lesion with Bowen's dermatosis. The granular and keratin layers are thickened, and the epidermis often is hyperpigmented. Mild inflammatory infiltrate may be present in the upper dermis. Closer examination reveals that the nuclei are larger, but not paler staining, than the nuclei of normal epidermis and adnexa and that mitoses, when present, also are bulkier but do not seem to contain a larger number of chromosomes. Photocytometry[57] confirmed that the nuclei are hyperploid. The lesions, which were described as *large cell acanthoma* (Fig. 33–16), appear to be entirely benign.[58]

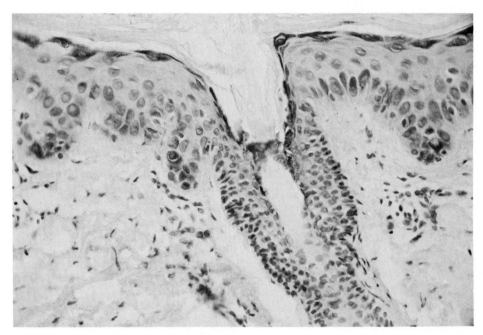

FIGURE 33–16.
Large cell acanthoma. Sharp contrast between the normal sized cells of a hair follicle and abnormally large cells forming an epidermislike surface epithelium with normal keratinization. Nuclei and cytoplasm are large, and the nuclei are sufficiently variable to arouse suspicion of Bowen's dermatosis. However, there are no dyskeratotic cells, and mitoses, if present, are restricted to the basal layer. H&E. X225.

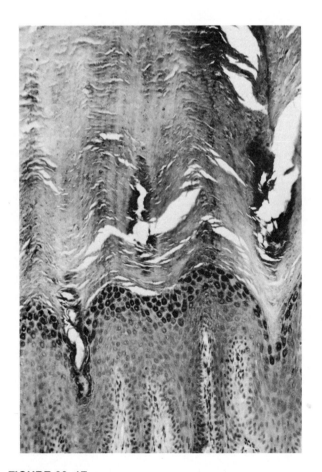

FIGURE 33–17.
Keratoderma palmare. Diffuse acanthosis, hypergranulosis, and hyperkeratosis. Sweat ducts normal (compare to Fig. 2–36). H&E. X125.

KERATODERMA PALMARE ET PLANTARE

The various heritable forms of diffuse keratoderma of palms and soles represent peculiar intermediates between generalized nevoid disturbances of the integument, which we discussed in Chapter 29, and the localized malformations, with which we deal in this chapter. This ambivalence is accentuated by rare cases in which diffuse volar keratoderma has the histologic features of epidermolytic hyperkeratosis (Chap. 29). Keratodermas of palms and soles, whether occurring in families or as isolated cases, show pure epidermal hypergranulosis and hyperkeratosis (Fig. 33–17). Clinical manifestation may be localized or diffuse or may show linear configuration *(striate keratoderma)*. Reed and Porter[59] listed 25 different types of volar keratoderma, and at least three more have been added since.[60–62] *Keratoderma punctatum palmare et plantare* refers to discrete lenticular lesions histologically characterized by a small cup-shaped area of epidermal depression containing dense orthokeratotic material (Fig. 33–18A). At the base of the lesion, the epidermis shows mild thickening and hypergranulosis.

CALLOSITIES AND CLAVUS

Callosities are localized areas of hyperkeratosis in response to chronic irritation and can occur in any location. Clavus refers to lesions appearing most commonly over the weight-bearing areas of the sole. They are histologically characterized by a cen-

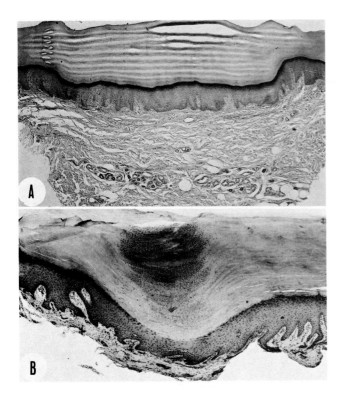

FIGURE FIGURE 33–18.
A. *Keratoderma palmare punctatum. Sharp-edged depression of epidermis. Striated appearance of the keratotic plug is shattering artifact caused by its brittleness. Epidermis has normal structure; dermis is slightly compressed. H&E. X45.* **B.** *Clavus. Relatively small lesion shows cup-shaped depression and thinning of epidermis, loss of granular layer, and parakeratosis of center of horny plug, all of which characterize the clavus. H&E. X45.*

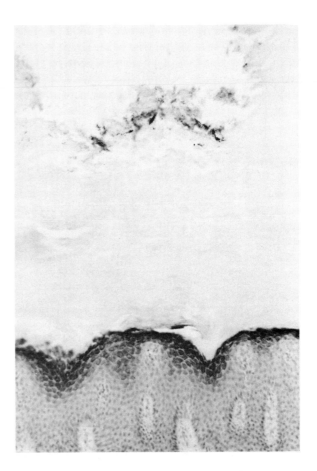

FIGURE 33–19.
Pitted keratolysis. Keratin layer partly destroyed by Corynebacterium growing in the upper layers of entirely normal stratum corneum. H&E. X125.

tral parakeratotic horny plug situated within a funnel-shaped area of epidermal depression (Fig. 33–18B). The epidermis may become very thin under the center of the lesion.

PITTED KERATOLYSIS

Superficial dissolution of the plantar keratin layer by species of *Corynebacterium*[63] produces shallow circular or circinate erosions (Chap. 13). Filamentous and coccoid microorganisms are present within the keratin layer in eroded areas (Fig. 33–19).

RETICULATED PIGMENTED ANOMALY OF THE FLEXURES

Dowling–Degos disease[64] shows diffuse reticulated and dark brown macular pigmentation of face, trunk, and extremities more pronounced over the flexural areas. Histologically (Fig. 33–20), there are

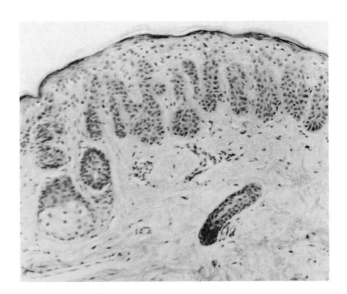

FIGURE 33–20.
Reticulated pigmented anomaly of the flexures. Picture resembles lentigo senilis or reticulated seborrheic verruca. H&E. X250.

areas of hyperpigmentation and downward budding of basaloid cells in connection with the lower surface of the epidermis, resembling a lentigo senilis or reticulated form of seborrheic verruca.[65] Similar budding of basaloid cells occurs in connection with the infundibular portion of the hair follicles.

REFERENCES

1. Fleischmajer R, Billingham RE (eds): Epithelial-Mesenchymal Interactions. Baltimore, Williams & Wilkins, 1968
2. Tarin D (ed): Tissue Interactions in Carcinogenesis. New York, Academic Press, 1972
3. Zeligman I, Pomeranz J: Variations of congenital ichthyosiform erythroderma. Report of cases of ichthyosis hystrix and nevus unius lateris. Arch Dermatol 91:120, 1965
4. Adam JE, Richards R: Ichthyosis hystrix: epidermolytic hyperkeratosis; discordant in monozygotic twins. Arch Dermatol 107:278, 1973
5. Altman J, Mehregan AH: Inflammatory linear verrucose epidermal nevus. Arch Dermatol 104:385, 1971
6. Kaidbey KH, Kurban AK: Dermatitic epidermal nevus. Arch Dermatol 104:166, 1971
7. Dupré A, Christol B: Inflammatory linear verrucous epidermal nevus: a pathologic study. Arch Dermatol 113:767, 1977
8. Becker SW: Concurrent melanosis and hypertrichosis in distribution of nevus unius lateris. Arch Dermatol 60:155, 1949
9. Copeman PWM, Wilson-Jones E: Pigmented hairy epidermal nevus (Becker). Arch Dermatol 92:249, 1965
10. Boiron G, Surlève-Bazeille JE, Maleville J: Ultrastructure of Becker's melanosis. J Cutan Pathol 5:299, 1978
11. Haneke E: The dermal component in melanosis naeviformis Becker. J Cutan Pathol 6:53, 1979
12. Solomon LM, Fretzin DF, Dewald RL: The epidermal nevus syndrome. Arch Dermatol 97:272, 1968
13. Golitz LE, Weston WL: Inflammatory linear verrucous epidermal nevus. Association with epidermal nevus syndrome. Arch Dermatol 115:1208, 1979
14. Haustein UF, Süss E: Inflammatorischer linearer verruköser epidermaler naevus (ILVEN). Dermatol Monatsschr 164:120, 1978
15. Mehregan AH, Rahbari H: Nevoid hyperkeratosis of nipples and areolae. Arch Dermatol 113:1691, 1977
16. Schneller WA: Acrokeratosis verruciformis of Hopf. Arch Dermatol 106:81, 1972
17. Curth HO: Significance of acanthosis nigricans. Arch Dermatol 66:80, 1952
18. Garrott TC: Malignant acanthosis nigricans associated with osteogenic sarcoma. Arch Dermatol 106:384, 1972
19. Roberts SOB, Lachapelle JM: Confluent and reticulate papillomatosis (Gougerot-Carteaud) and *Pityrosporum orbiculare.* Br J Dermatol 81:841, 1969
20. Baden HP: Familial cutaneous papillomatosis. Arch Dermatol 92:394, 1965
21. Goldstein N: Multiple minute digitate hyperkeratoses. Arch Dermatol 96:692, 1967
22. Yoon SW, Gibbs RB: Multiple minute digitate hyperkeratoses. Arch Dermatol 111:1176, 1975
23. Willoughby C, Soter NA: Stucco keratosis. Arch Dermatol 105:859, 1972
24. Mehregan AH, Rahbari H: Benign epithelial tumors of the skin. Part 1: Epidermal tumors. Cutis 19:43, 1977
25. Mehregan AH: Lentigo senilis and its evolutions. J Invest Dermatol 65:429, 1975
26. Barriere H, Litoux P, Bureau B, et al.: Acanthomes post-eczema. Bull Soc Fr Dermatol Syphiligr 79:555, 1972
27. Mevorah B, Mishima Y: Cellular response of seborrheic keratosis following croton oil irritation and surgical trauma. Dermatologica 131:452, 1965
28. Helwig EB: Inverted follicular keratosis. In Seminar on the Skin: Neoplasms and Dermatoses. American Society of Clinical Pathologists, International Congress of Clinical Pathology, Washington, Sept 1954. Chicago, American Society of Clinical Pathology, 1955
29. Lund HZ: Atlas of Tumor Pathology: Tumors of the Skin. Sec. 1. Fascicle 2. Washington, Armed Forces Institute of Pathology, 1957
30. Mehregan AH, Pinkus H: Intraepidermal epithelioma. A critical study. Cancer 17:609, 1964
31. Bloch PH: Transformation of seborrheic keratosis into Bowen's disease. J Cutan Pathol 5:361, 1978
32. Rahbari H: Bowenoid transformation of seborrheic verrucae (keratoses). Br J Dermatol 101:459, 1979
33. Dantzig PI: Sign of Leser-Trélat. Arch Dermatol 108:700, 1973
34. Degos R, Civatte J: Clear cell acanthoma; experience of eight years. Br J Dermatol 83:248, 1970
35. Brownstein MH, Fernando S, Shapiro L: Clear cell acanthoma; clinico-pathologic analysis of 37 new cases. Am J Clin Pathol 59:306, 1973
36. Landry M, Winkelmann RK: Multiple clear cell acanthoma and ichthyosis. Arch Dermatol 105:371, 1972
37. Witkowski JA, Parish LC: Clear cell acanthoma. Int J Dermatol 18:162, 1979
38. Desmons F, Breuillard F, Thomas P, et al.: Multiple clear cell acanthoma (Degos): histochemical and ultrastructural study of two cases. Int J Dermatol 16:203, 1977
39. Howell JB, Mehregan AH: Story of the pits. Arch Dermatol 102:583, 1970
40. Hashimoto K, Howell JB, Yamanishi Y, et al.: Electron microscopic studies of palmar and plantar pits of nevoid basal cell epithelioma. J Invest Dermatol 59:380, 1972
41. Covo JA: The pits in the nevoid basal cell carcinoma syndrome. Arch Dermatol 103:568, 1971
42. Holubar K, Matras H, Swalik AV: Multiple palmar basal cell epitheliomas in basal cell nevus syndrome. Arch Dermatol 101:679, 1970
43. Pinkus H: In discussion of Saunders TS: Porokeratosis. A disease of epidermal eccrine sweat duct unit. Arch Dermatol 84:142, 1961
44. Reed RJ, Leone P: Porokeratosis; a mutant clonal keratosis of the epidermis. I. Histogenesis. Arch Dermatol 101:340, 1970
45. Mikhail GR, Wertheimer FW: Clinical variants of porokeratosis (Mibelli). Arch Dermatol 98:124, 1968
46. Chernosky ME: Disseminated superficial actinic po-

rokeratosis (DSAP). Int J Dermatol 12:152, 1973

47. Rahbari H, Cordero AA, Mehregan AH: Linear porokeratosis. A distinctive clinical variant of porokeratosis of Mibelli. Arch Dermatol 109:526, 1974

48. Rahbari H, Cordero AA, Mehregan AH: Punctate porokeratosis. A clinical variant of porokeratosis of Mibelli. J Cutan Pathol 4:338, 1977

49. Dupré A, Christol B: Porokeratosis of the lips. Arch Dermatol 114:1841, 1978

50. Nabai H, Mehregan AH: Porokeratosis of Mibelli. A report of two unusual cases. Dermatologica 159:325, 1979

51. Montgomery RM: Porokeratosis plantaris discreta. Cutis 20:711, 1977

52. Coskey RJ, Mehregan AH: Bowen disease associated with porokeratosis of Mibelli. Arch Dermatol 111:1480, 1975

53. Ehlers G, Rothe A: Porokeratosis Mibelli mit multiplen Präcancerosen und Plattenepithelcarcinomen. Hautarzt 2:68, 1971

54. Cort DF, Abdel-Aziz AM: Epithelioma arising in porokeratosis of Mibelli. Br J Plast Surg 25:318, 1972

55. Sarkany I: Porokeratosis Mibelli with basal cell epithelioma. Proc R Soc Med 66:435, 1973

56. Rahbari H, Pinkus H: Large cell acanthoma. One of the actinic keratoses. Arch Dermatol 114:49, 1978

57. Fand SB, Pinkus H: Polyploidy in benign epidermal neoplasia. J Cell Biol 47:2, pt 2, 1970, p 52a

58. Pinkus H: Epidermal mosaic in benign and precancerous neoplasia (with special reference to large-cell acanthoma). Acta Dermatol (Kyoto), 45:75, 1971

59. Reed WB, Porter PS: Keratosis. Arch Dermatol 104:99, 1971

60. Brown FC: Punctate keratoderma. Arch Dermatol 104:682, 1971

61. Onwukwe F, Mihm MC, Toda K: Hereditary papulotranslucent acrokeratoderma; a new variant of familial punctate keratoderma? Arch Dermatol 108:108, 1973

62. Herman PS: Punctate keratoderma. Arch Dermatol 109:910, 1974

63. Tilgen W: Pitted keratolysis (keratolysis plantare sulcatum). J Cutan Pathol 6:18, 1979

64. Wilson-Jones E, Grice K: Reticulated pigmented anomaly of the flexures. Arch Dermatol 114:1150, 1978

65. Howell JB, Freeman RG: Reticular pigmented anomaly of the flexures. Arch Dermatol 114:400, 1978

CHAPTER

34

Epidermal Precancer, Squamous Cell Carcinoma, and Pseudocarcinoma

In this chapter we discuss purely epithelial neoplasia in contrast to the organoid fibroepithelial lesions[1] dealt with in the previous chapter. Whether and to what extent the mesoderm is involved in the causation of human cutaneous precanceroses and carcinomas[2] is a question irrelevant to diagnostic interpretation of characteristic histologic changes. We can diagnose a dysplastic precancerous stretch of epidermis regardless of the presence of actinic elastosis and other dermal changes, and their presence or absence should not influence our judgment. The significant features are cytologic alteration of keratinocytes in a manner leading to an abnormal end product. This change involves a limited number of cells which are distinctly different from their normal neighbors, on which they abut with a sharp border. From this no-mixing, no-transition feature we deduct that the neoplastic cells are a clone or stock, heritably deranged and not just temporarily altered through external influences emanating from the body in general (e.g., hormones) or from supporting connective tissue.

A clone of irreversibly altered neoplastic cells may replace a stretch of epidermis, yet remain in the boundaries of a basement membrane. Alternately, it may form distinct nests within a framework of persistent epidermis, or it may grow invasively down into the dermis. In the latter case, the basement membrane, which is evidence of epithe-

lial-mesenchymal interrelations, usually is lost, and all trace of fibroepithelial coordination has disappeared. In any of the three situations, the mesoderm does not participate in forming the tumor. At most it exhibits an inflammatory reaction and other secondary changes found commonly in cancer of any organ.

PRECANCEROUS KERATOSES

Keratosis is a clinical term and has been applied rather loosely to many lesions exhibiting increased and usually adherent keratin formation thought not to be due to an inflammatory process. Histopathologic study cannot really accept "keratosis" as a diagnostic term, and it was pointed out that seborrheic keratosis is a papilloma and better designated a seborrheic verruca (disregarding that seborrheic is also inappropriate). One might say that all neoplasms of keratinocytes are *acanthomas*, and this term has been applied to some recently delineated lesions (pale cell acanthoma, large cells acanthoma, Chap. 33). The name keratosis, however, is ingrained, and we shall continue using it for actinic and other *precancerous keratoses*. Objections have frequently been raised against the use of "precancerous" in histologic diagnosis because it includes prophecy. It is, however, one of the principal tasks

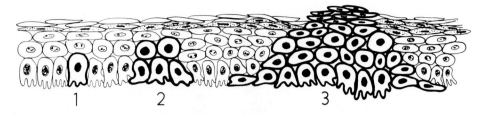

FIGURE 34–1.
*Diagram illustrates three stages of development of a solar keratosis as prototype of epidermal malignant transformation. **1**. Heritable perversion of a single basal germinal cell which by multiplication **(2)** produces more abnormal basal cells and keratinizing cells. **3**. When abnormal products reach surface, clinical keratosis results. Meanwhile abnormal germinal cells undermine normal epidermis, thus producing a slanting cell-sharp border. (From Pinkus. In Kopf and Andrade (eds). Year Book of Dermatology, 1967. Courtesy of Year Book Medical Publishers.)*

of the pathologist to imply prognosis in his diagnostic interpretation. While the concept of *precancerosis* is based essentially on statistical data which show the more or less frequent association of a certain type of lesion with cancer developing in it, we can apply Pusey's pertinent remark that he had known many a premedical student who never became a physician (quoted by Rattner[3]). Similarly, we can diagnose a precancerous lesion by certain histologic and cytologic criteria without waiting for it to progress to invasive carcinoma, and this can be done electron microscopically much earlier[4] than by light microscopy. On the other hand, if we accept the thesis that the cells composing the keratosis are irreversibly altered[5] and have acquired some of the properties characteristic of malignant neoplasia (Fig. 34–1), we can apply the term *carcinoma in situ*. Which term we prefer to use depends on personal choice and extraneous circumstances (see introduction to this section).

The two principal lesions in this group are actinic keratoses and the precancerous dermatosis of Bowen. Certain variants, like erythroplasia of Queyrat and lichenoid actinic keratosis, will also be discussed, as well as cutaneous horns. Xeroderma pigmentosum will be mentioned. The outstanding differential feature between a typical actinic keratosis (keratosis senilis) and a typical Bowen lesion is that the former consists of fairly even squamous cells ending in parakeratosis without a granular layer, while the latter consists of uneven cells exhibiting dyskeratosis, but may have a granular layer and orthokeratosis. We shall see that transitions exist.

Keratosis Senilis (Freudenthal)

Although the diagnosis *keratosis senilis* has been supplanted in clinical usage by *actinic keratosis*, it remains a useful histologic diagnostic term if we define it by the features originally delineated by Freudenthal and reemphasized and biologically interpreted by Pinkus.[6] The diagram (Fig. 34–2) illustrates that keratosis senilis consists of deranged epidermal keratinocytes which are demarcated sharply from hyperplastic but otherwise normal adnexal

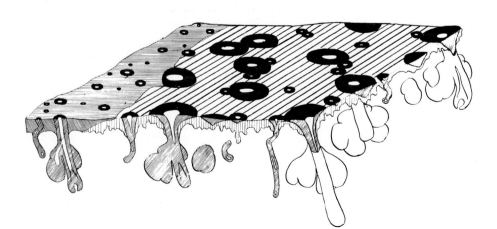

FIGURE 34–2.
Diagram illustrating three-dimensional architecture of actinic keratosis. Cut borders of epidermal plate show what is seen in two-dimensional vertical sections. Dysplastic epidermis borders on and creeps under normal epidermis and adnexal epithelium. The latter forms hyperplastic umbrellas which may merge on surface, thus submerging dysplastic epithelium. (From Pinkus. Am J Clin Pathol 29:193, 1958.)

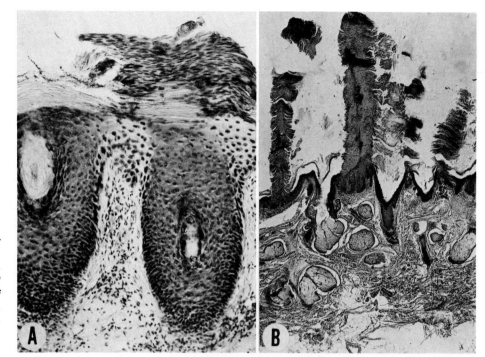

FIGURE 34–3.
Keratosis senilis type of solar keratosis. Illustrated are sharp borders of dysplastic epidermis and hyperplastic adnexal epithelium with production of alternating stretches or columns of parakeratotic and orthokeratotic horny material. **A.** *H&E. X135.* **B.** *H&E. X35.*

keratinocytes and from the normal surrounding epidermis. In a histologic section (corresponding to the cut edges of the three-dimensional diagram), we see (Figs. 34–3 and 34–4) lighter staining, more eosinophilic epidermal prickle cells arising from an often irregular basal layer and ending as nucleated (parakeratotic) flakes without the formation of a granular layer. In between, there are follicular and eccrine ostia lined with multiple layers of darker-staining cells which form a hyperplastic granular

layer and orthokeratotic horny material. It is characteristic that the border between the two types of epithelium is sharp and that it usually does not run vertically but forms a slant or slanting curve (Fig. 34–4). Most often, the adnexal keratinocytes cover more surface, while epidermal keratinocytes cover more dermal junction and often extend like a collar downward around adnexal ostia (Fig. 34–5). In some spots (Fig. 34–5B), however, adnexal epithelium barely reaches the surface, a sign that the balance

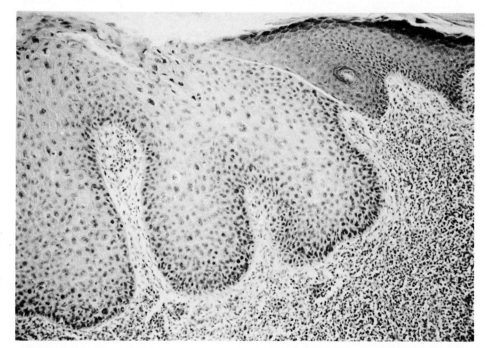

FIGURE 34–4.
Keratosis senilis (Freudenthal), lateral edge. Sharp slanting border of bowenoid epithelium and normal epidermis, including a sweat duct. Lack of cohesion between the two types of epithelium. Strong reactive inflammatory infiltrate in dermis. H&E. X135.

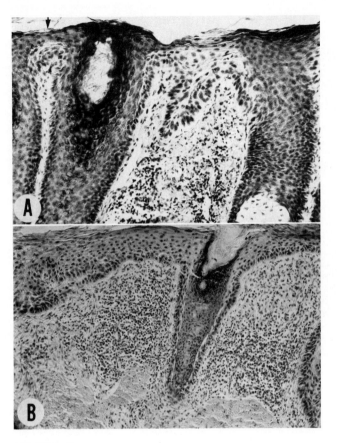

FIGURE 34–5.
Keratosis senilis. **A.** *Atypical budding of dysplastic epidermis between hair follicles. Dysplastic epithelium also creeps down around the follicles, which form umbrellas on the surface. Adnexal epithelium has joined at left side of picture (arrow), cutting dysplastic epithelium off from access to the surface. H&E. X135.* **B.** *Dysplastic epidermis has crept far down on outside of sweat duct and begins to overpower it. While ductal keratinocytes still spread on surface to left and form keratohyalin layer, they do not reach surface on right. Note reactive inflammatory infiltrate in* **A** *and* **B.** *H&E. X70.*

in the struggle between the competing keratinocytes is being tipped. Occasionally, adnexal epithelium is completely submerged by dysplastic epidermis (Fig. 34–6). In other areas, the umbrellalike spreading of adnexal keratinocytes from adjacent ostia may merge on the surface (Figs. 34–3A and 34–5A) and submerge the dysplastic epidermal cells. Such pictures falsely suggest that only the lower part of the epidermis is deranged, the upper being normal. Examination of the diagram and biologic interpretation of the events explain the situation. There is over- and undersliding of normal and dysplastic keratinocytes of different provenience, not maturation of atypical basal strata into normal upper strata. The basal layer of the keratosis may be straight or may show mild or pronounced atypical budding.

These matters are discussed in detail because biologic insight into the mechanics of keratosis senilis helps the student to grasp the concepts of cutaneous carcinogenesis and also assists in the diagnosis of unusual lesions and in the interpretation of small fragments of tissue obtained from curettings of this type of lesion.

If we retrace theoretically the development of keratosis senilis to its beginning, we arrive at the one deranged stem cell of the carcinoma in situ, as illustrated in Figure 34–1. A clinical lesion is not apparent until the third stage has been reached, and histologic diagnosis is possible only slightly earlier. The diagram illustrates that actinically damaged skin can carry many more foci of deranged epidermis than are clinically visible, a fact nicely demonstrated by the effects of local application of 5-fluorouracil, which seeks out the parakeratotic, vulnerable areas, and supported by findings that the epidermis surrounding a keratosis is not normal.[7]

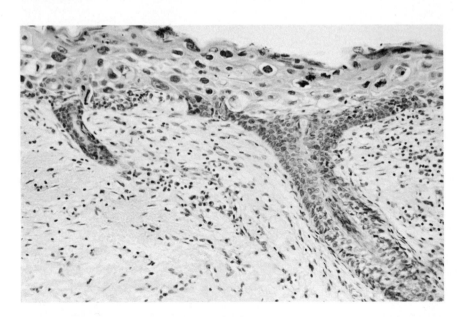

FIGURE 34–6.
Unusual picture of keratosis senilis in which a solid layer of dysplastic epidermis covers the surface, while a sweat duct and a hair follicle spread below it. H&E. X125.

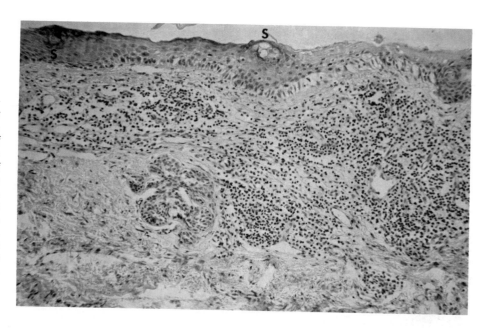

FIGURE 34–7.
Atrophic keratosis senilis. Dysplastic basal cells form quickly degenerating upper layers without keratohyalin in right half of picture and extend below normally keratinizing epidermis of adnexal provenience almost to left border of picture. Two intraepidermal centers (s) are cross sections of sweat duct lumina. Branching epithelial island in dermis is a tangential section of bulge proliferation of a hair follicle (Chap. 2). Note heavy inflammatory reaction. H&E. X135.

Any actinic keratosis, whether keratosis senilis or other type, is of course associated with actinic changes in the dermis, especially with elastotic alteration. In addition, there is an infiltrate of round cells which may be mild or heavy and which often includes plasma cells and, occasionally, eosinophils.[8] This type of infiltrate is associated with practically all malignant neoplastic skin lesions, whether they are invasive or not, and is of considerable diagnostic significance even though it may be absent in rare cases. It should alert the pathologist to look for the diagnostic epidermal changes, as in the atrophic form of actinic keratosis (Fig. 34–7). Our early hypothesis that it is a tissue immune reaction to the neoplastic cells which the organism recognizes as nonself long before they become invasive has become much more acceptable in the last 10 years. A similar interpretation has been advanced to explain the polymorphous infiltrate of mycosis fungoides.[9]

Variants of Keratosis Senilis. One of the more common variants of classic keratosis senilis is the *Darierlike form* (Fig. 34–8), in which a section will show a single layer of dysplastic cells at the dermoepidermal junction separated by a cleft from fairly normal upper layers of epidermis. Acantholytic degenerating or dyskeratotic cells may float in the fluid-filled cleft.[10] This picture is explained as an extreme case of the biologic process. The deranged and highly dysplastic epidermal epithelium has been completely submerged by a new epidermis originating from the adnexa. If the dysplastic cells become more vigorous and invasive, they then form the *acantholytic type of squamous cell carcinoma* (Fig. 34–18).

Another common variant is produced by the epidermal cells becoming more dyskeratotic in a bowenoid manner. The histologic picture then resembles that of Bowen's dermatosis, and it is difficult to decide in some cases whether one is dealing

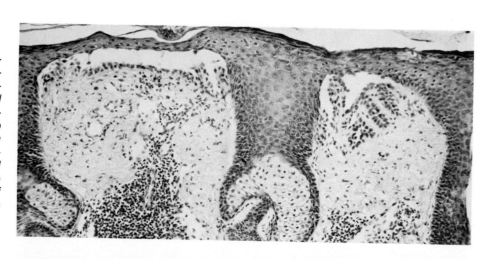

FIGURE 34–8.
Highly dysplastic actinic keratosis. Nothing is left of original epidermis except a layer of basaloid cells which sends atypical buds downward and sheds occasional acantholytic cells into cleft which separates it from new epidermis formed by confluence of modulated adnexal keratinocytes. Darier-like picture thus produced is extreme of process seen at far left in Figure 34–5A and indicated by arrow. H&E. X135.

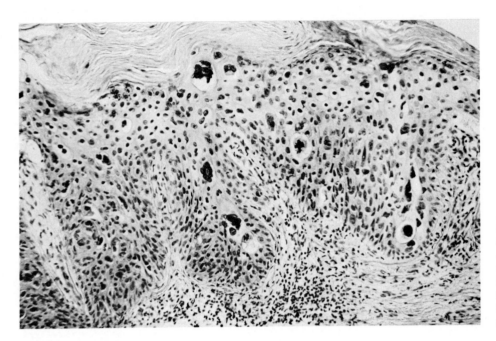

FIGURE 34–9.
Bowenoid keratosis senilis. Extreme dysplasia of epidermis is indistinguishable from pictures seen in Bowen's dermatosis (Fig 34–11). Presence of actinic elastosis and information that the lesion is situated in actinic skin influence the judgment. H&E. X135.

with true Bowen's disease in a sun-exposed area or with a *bowenoid actinic keratosis* (Fig. 34–9). The significance of differentiation is clinical because an actinic keratosis is more apt to become invasive. In cases of the bowenoid type, but also in some lesions of less dysplastic character, the epidermis may become quite hyperplastic, and, at low power, the picture may resemble a cutaneous papilloma. Attention to cytologic detail will lead to the correct diagnosis of a *hyperplastic variant* of keratosis senilis.

A fourth variant may be called *atrophic keratosis senilis*. These lesions look red and atrophic clinically, have an adherent scale, and are painful on blunt pressure. They resemble discoid lupus erythematosus in all these respects and usually are biopsied for differential diagnosis. Histologically (Fig. 34–7), the epidermis is atrophic, and the upper corium contains heavy round cell infiltrate associated with some telangiectasia. The zone of actinic elastosis is more or less destroyed. At first glance, the infiltrate may appear to be the most significant feature, and the resemblance to lupus erythematosus may be striking, but closer inspection reveals the distinguishing features. The epidermis has no granular layer and is parakeratotic. It also may show some cellular atypicality and always is sharply delineated against the hyperplastic and hyperkeratotic adnexal ostia. In discoid lupus, ostial and epidermal epithelia are equally atrophic and orthokeratotic. The dermal infiltrate usually contains plasma cells in the keratosis.

A fifth variant is the *spreading pigmented actinic keratosis*[11] (Fig. 34–10). Usually, melanocytes

do not survive long in the deranged epithelium. If they do, the question of lentigo maligna may arise but is usually ruled out by the dysplastic changes of the keratinocytes. Pigmented lesions often spread beyond the usual dimensions of a keratosis senilis.

Other Actinic Keratoses

That exposure to ultraviolet rays causes the formation of pyknotic cells in the epidermis has been known for many years[12] (Chap. 3). The recent introduction of combined psoralen and long-wave ultraviolet ray exposure (PUVA) in the treatment of psoriasis and other disorders has caused new interest in the effect of UV on the epidermis. Focal dysplasia was found in about one half of the cases[13] and persisted for one year after the start of the therapy.

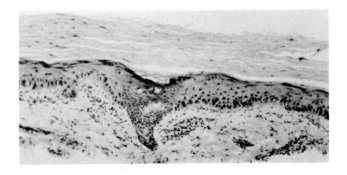

FIGURE 34–10.
Pigmented keratosis senilis. Melanocytes persist and form melanin in a keratosis of the back of the hand. Melanin is being carried into the horny layer. H&E. X125.

Whether such cells may survive after the discontinuance of treatment remains to be seen, but clinical experience of larger numbers of squamous cell carcinomas in treated skin leads to that conclusion.

Other abnormalities occur in the epidermis due to light and produce not only inflammatory lesions (Chap. 14) but recognizable neoplastic processes either on the basis of preexistent flaws, such as in actinic lichenoid keratosis, or perhaps on the basis of genetic predisposition, as in actinic porokeratosis and xeroderma pigmentosum.

The *lichenoid actinic keratosis (lichen planus-like keratosis, isolated lichen planus)* (Chap. 9) was identified only recently. It exhibits considerable histologic similarity (Fig. 9–12) to lichen planus, and diagnosis is based largely on clinicohistologic correlation. It may develop from lentigo senilis (Chap. 30). *Disseminated actinic porokeratosis* (Chap. 33) and *large cell acanthoma* (Chap. 33) are other lesions found in actinically damaged skin. All three were discussed in other chapters because they are not definitely precancerous and have other histologic differential associations. Their existence, however, emphasizes our contention that actinic keratosis is a group designation and not synonymous with *keratosis senilis of Freudenthal.*

Bowen's Precancerous Dermatosis and Erythroplasia of Queyrat

The *precancerous dermatosis* described by Bowen in 1912[14] is the first recognized example of carcinoma in situ, and although it is not often mentioned in pathologic or gynecologic literature, it has all the structural and cytologic aberrations observed much later in the cervix uteri. Clinically, it forms flat scaly or elevated crusted plaques, and some lesions may be exuberantly papillomatous—features expressed in the microscopic picture of individual lesions. The cytologic alterations (Fig. 34–11) are the outstanding examples of dyskerato-

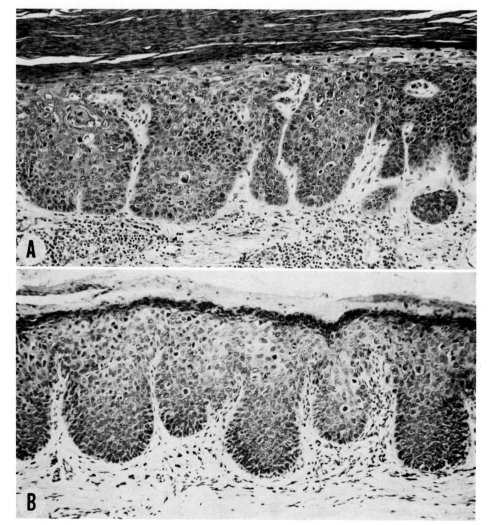

FIGURE 34–11.
*Bowen's precancerous dermatosis. Acanthosis and dyskeratosis are shown in both figures. **A.** Parakeratosis and considerable inflammatory infiltrate. **B.** Horny layer is mainly orthokeratotic and includes some dyskeratotic cells. Inflammatory infiltrate is unusually mild. H&E. X135.*

sis but should not be called anaplastic (Chap. 5). Because Bowen's disease has little tendency to progress toward invasive carcinoma, there is not much point distinguishing dysplastic stages from carcinoma in situ. The general features consist of a loss of stratification (unrest, windblown appearance), great variability of nuclear size and depth of staining *(poikilokaryosis)*, occurrence of mitoses in all layers of the living epidermis, and presence of atypical cells, some with multiple nuclei, others representing clumped mitoses. The surface may be parakeratotic or orthokeratotic. There is usually some degree of acanthosis, and the rete ridges are uneven and plump. Papillae may be inconspicuous or elongated. No characteristic dermal changes have been described in connection with Bowen's disease, except the aforementioned inflammatory infiltrate.

Similar changes are found in keratoses due to sunlight, X-rays or other ionizing radiation, and arsenic. These lesions are called *bowenoid*. The questions of arsenical causation of conventional Bowen's dermatosis and of its association with internal cancer are not pertinent to our discussion. It is debatable whether Bowen's name should be attached to localizations other than the open skin surface. There is, however, no doubt that exactly similar changes of carcinoma in situ occur on mucous membranes, such as cornea, conjunctiva, and urethra (Chap. 45), and in the nail bed and nail matrix.[15,16]

The therapeutic conclusions to be drawn from this discussion are that complete removal of the involved epidermis is essential but that no deep excision of dermis or amputation of a limb is necessary.

The balance between dysplastic epidermis and adnexal epithelium often is disturbed in Bowen's disease to the disadvantage of the adnexa. Instead of forming hyperkeratotic umbrellas (Fig. 34–12), the follicular epithelium often just reaches the skin surface (Fig. 34–12C). In many cases, dyskeratotic epidermis invades ostial territory (Fig. 34–12D) and may replace follicular epithelium all the way down to the sebaceous duct without disturbing the basement membrane. The symbiosis between keratinocytes and melanocytes is disturbed in Bowen's dermatosis, and melanocytes disappear gradually, just as they do in actinic keratoses. Plaques of the anogenital region, however, are often deeply pigmented[17-19] and may be multiple.

Epithelial cells of Bowen's disease characteristically have a nucleus that is large in relation to cytoplasm (Fig. 34–13A). The number of individually keratinizing cells often is relatively small. If it is large, the picture may simulate Paget's disease

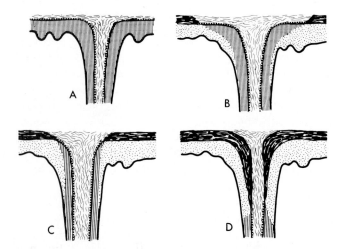

FIGURE 34–12.
Diagram illustrating shifting balance between adnexal and dysplastic epidermal keratinocytes in Bowen's disease and other precancerous conditions. **A.** *In normal skin, epidermal and infundibular keratinocytes are indistinguishable and form orthokeratotic keratin through intermediate stage of a granular layer indicated by dots.* **B.** *Umbrellalike spread of orthokeratotic adnexal epithelium while parakeratotic epidermis forms a collar around the follicle. (Compare with Figs. 34–2 to 34–5)* **C.** *Beginning repression of adnexal epithelium which just reaches skin surface corresponding to situation in Figure 34–5B on right.* **D.** *Follicular territory taken over by dysplastic epidermis. Adnexal epithelium is present deeper down. Basement membrane (heavy black line) remains intact. Careful examination of tissue sections shows this situation not infrequently in Bowen's disease. (From Pinkus. In McKenna (ed). Modern Trends in Dermatology, 1966. Courtesy of Butterworth & Co., Ltd.)*

(Chap. 40) but can be differentiated from it by finding the entire epidermis dysplastic, while the remaining keratinocytes of Paget's dermatosis are quite normal (Fig. 40–6). If the number of plainly dysplastic cells (clumping cells, giant cells) is small in a particular case and the epidermis consists mainly of relatively small, dark-staining cells, we have the *basal* type (or, rather, *basaloid* type) of Bowen's dermatosis. This is commonly found on the semimucous membranes and merges into the full-blown histologic picture of the épithélioma nu (Fig. 34–14) of *Queyrat's erythroplasia*. The latter is usually accompanied by very heavy dermal infiltrates of lymphocytes and plasma cells, and this factor, as well as the clinical feature of velvety redness, is shared by *Zoon's plasma cell balanitis*, which, however, has a thin epithelium and shows none of the cytologic features of Queyrat's or Bowen's affections. Plasma cell balanitis (Chap. 45) is not related to neoplasia.

The relationship of condyloma acuminatum and Bowen's disease will be discussed in Chapter 45.

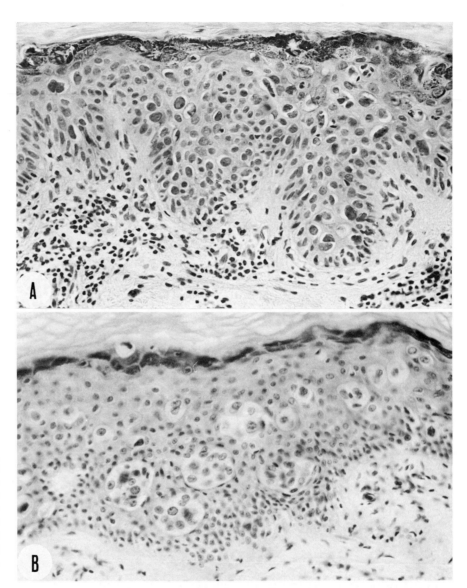

FIGURE 34–13.
Bowen's disease. **A.** *Cell details, especially the relatively large size of many nuclei in relation to cytoplasm. H&E. X250.* **B.** *Borst phenomenon (Fig. 39–13) lateral to replacement of entire epidermis by dysplastic cells. Such pictures are found occasionally and indicate the mobility of the malignant cells. H&E. X250.*

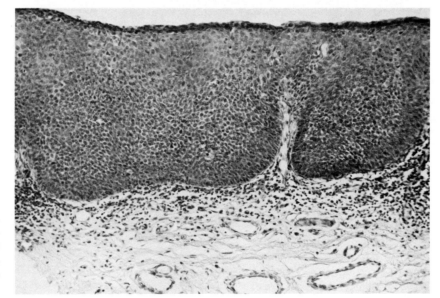

FIGURE 34–14.
Erythroplasia of Queyrat. Thick epidermis consists almost entirely of nonkeratinizing basaloid cells (épithéliome nu) with only slight indication of dysplasia. Relatively mild inflammatory infiltrate. H&E. X135.

CUTANEOUS HORN

Cutaneous horn is a clinical diagnosis. The pathologist[20,21] is compelled to diagnose the underlying condition, which might be an epidermal nevus, ichthyosis hystrix, verruca vulgaris, actinic keratosis (Fig. 34–3B), other precancerous keratosis, or invasive squamous cell carcinoma (Fig. 34–15). In other cases, such diverse lesions as seborrheic verruca, basal cell epithelioma,[22] molluscum contagiosum, or trichilemmal or epidermoid cysts may produce cutaneous horns. Cutaneous horn is not an acceptable histologic diagnosis.

XERODERMA PIGMENTOSUM

One precancerous condition is in a class by itself. It has been shown,[23] although there are excep-

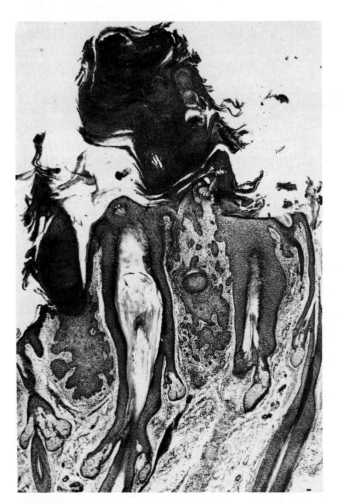

FIGURE 34–15.
Early squamous cell carcinoma arising in keratosis senilis. Atypical interfollicular budding (Figs. 34–3B and 34–5A) has been replaced by frank invasion of dermis down to level of sebaceous glands. Massive parakeratotic material forms a small cutaneous horn. H&E. X35.

tions, that all the cells of patients afflicted with xeroderma pigmentosum are unable to repair ultraviolet-induced DNA damage properly. A proportion of the defective cells acquire the properties of neoplastic cells early in life and progress from precancer to manifest cancer. Squamous cell carcinomas, basal cell epitheliomas, malignant melanomas, and cutaneous sarcomas may arise. These lesions do not differ histologically from other tumors of their respective types, and no special discussion is needed. Xeroderma pigmentosum, however, is of tremendous biologic and pathogenetic interest because it proves the direct damaging influence of ultraviolet rays on the genetic material of those cells which later become neoplastic. Similar mechanisms[25] may act much more slowly in normal skin.

PROGRESSION FROM PRECANCEROSIS TO CANCER

If we accept the concept that any epidermal precancerous lesion is, in fact, carcinoma in situ, we can rephrase the heading and discuss histomechanisms by which an in situ lesion becomes invasive. Attention has been focused on the basement membrane by old authors and new.[26] Redefinition of the basement membrane (Chaps. 2 and 5) as that thin layer between mesoderm and epithelium that can be demonstrated by the PAS method has led to a fairly general agreement that the basement membrane disappears wherever squamous epithelium becomes invasive. This fact should not be interpreted to mean that the neoplastic epithelium has acquired the power to break through the confining barrier or that a hole in the barrier permits the cells to slip through. Basement membrane formation is an expression of ectodermal-mesodermal interaction.[27] Its disappearance indicates cessation of this intertissue coordination and, therefore, is a secondary, although highly valuable, diagnostic feature.[28]

Actinic and other keratoses, including Bowen's disease, can become invasive by three different routes. The most direct and obvious one is increased budding of the neoplastic epithelium into the dermis between the adnexa (Fig. 34–15). A second route is the creeping of epithelium (Figs. 34–5 and 34–12) on the outer surface of hair follicles and sweat ducts within the basement membrane. The third one is repression of adnexal epithelium (Fig. 34–12) and occupation of follicular territory (Fig. 34–16), as discussed for Bowen's disease. In all cases, the basement membrane eventually disappears, and the epithelium becomes truly invasive and destructive. It is important to realize that recurrences of keratoses after relatively superficial

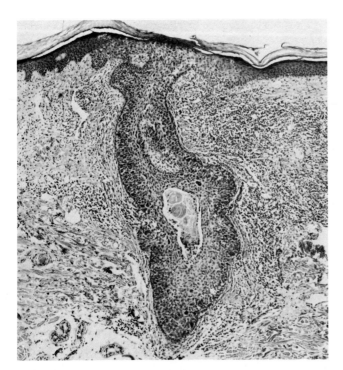

FIGURE 34–16.
Extensive invasion of a hair follicle by dysplastic epidermis of Bowen's disease. Patient had been treated locally with 5-fluorouracil, and lesion appeared clinically cured. Drug did not destroy cells hidden in follicle, and surviving dyskeratotic epithelium is now secondarily spreading on surface. Clinical history is essential to explain paradoxical picture. H&E. X60.

excision or destruction may have their origin in epithelia that have reached mid-dermis by the last two routes without actually having invaded the corium. It is wise to point this out to the clinician in appropriate cases.

SQUAMOUS CELL CARCINOMA

The diagnosis of squamous cell carcinoma is generally accepted and understood in the United States. British usage prefers "epithelioma," which American dermatologists, following Lever's example, restrict to the group of organoid adnexal tumors including basal cell epithelioma (Chaps. 35 to 39). Other synonymous terms are *epidermoid carcinoma, prickle cell cancer, spinous cell carcinoma,* or *spinalioma,* the latter being common usage in German. Darier's designation *épithélioma pavimenteux typique* has been replaced by *carcinoma* (or *épithélioma) spinocellulaire* in French.

While cutaneous squamous cell carcinoma (Fig. 34–17) most commonly arises in the epidermis, it may arise in adnexal epithelium and in keratinous cysts, most of which are of adnexal origin. Derivation, therefore, is not important for diagnosis. All true carcinomas of the skin are squamous cell carcinomas, with the exception of rare adenocarcinomas of a sebaceous and sudoriparous nature. Basal cell carcinomas (discussed in Chap.

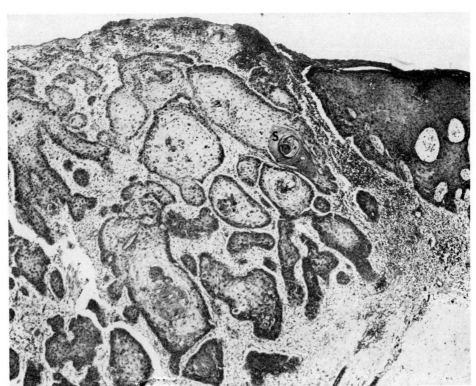

FIGURE 34–17.
Invasive squamous cell carcinoma, keratinizing. Tumor would be Broders' grade II. Hyperplastic obstructed sweat duct (s) is enveloped by malignant epithelium. H&E. X70.

39) belong to a different class of tumors. They are members of the tribe of organoid adnexoid tumors and, therefore, are now designated as *basal cell epitheliomas* by many American dermatologists. The tumor cell of squamous cell carcinoma is a heritably deranged keratinocyte (Fig. VII–2) which has escaped from the regulatory influences of the organism to the extent that it grows invasively and destructively into the mesoderm and may demonstrate its relative autonomy by metastasis, although this event occurs relatively late and is encountered but rarely in modern practice. The squamous cancer cell preserves its ability for maturation in the form of keratinization to a greater or lesser degree and may lose it completely. *Histologic grading* of squamous cell carcinoma was put on this basis by Broders,[29] who devised four classes: tumors in which more than 75 percent of cells are maturing (differentiating) are grade I; 75 to 50 percent differentiating cells put the tumor into grade II; 50 to 25 percent into grade III; and fewer than 25 percent into grade IV. Although this system has many practical and theoretic flaws, it remains a simple means of descriptively expressing degree of maturation. Many pathologists prefer to say well-differentiated, poorly differentiated, and undifferentiated. We discussed in the opening pages of this section the greater biologic accuracy resulting from the substitution of *mature* for *differentiated* in this respect. One might then use such terms as highly mature, fairly mature, or immature in one's description.

The derangement of the epidermoid cancer cell changes its morphology so that no normal basal cells are present. Even the outermost cells of a cancer nest are relatively large and pale-staining elements in most instances and exhibit little tendency to palisading. They are closely applied to the surrounding connective tissue, and the retraction spaces which we shall encounter in basal cell epithelioma are absent. Yet PAS stain reveals the absence of a basement membrane in most instances. Nuclei have large nucleoli. Mitotic figures, sometimes atypical, may be found in all layers of a nodule. Toward the center of larger nests, the cells may undergo fairly normal keratinization with formation of keratohyalin, but, more commonly, they form parakeratotic material. Thus, irregular horn pearls are produced that must be separated from the squamous eddies and horny pearls seen in activated seborrheic verruca (Chap. 33). Individual cell keratinization may occur. If it predominates, the lesion assumes a bowenoid character.

Acantholytic Squamous Cell Carcinoma

Pronounced acantholytic tendency may lead to the formation of irregular cavities lined with atypical cells and filled with dyskeratotic or plainly degenerating elements. Such cancers often are derived from Darier-like keratosis senilis and have been called "adenoacanthomas,"[30] a term that should be abandoned. Acantholytic squamous cell carcinoma

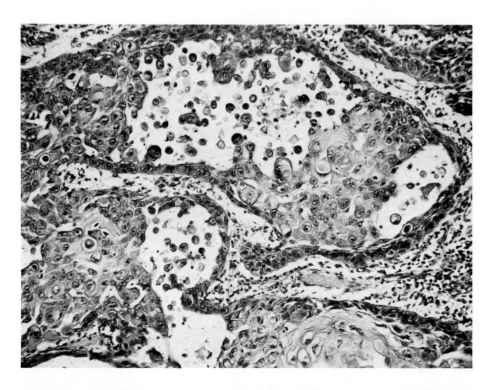

FIGURE 34–18.
Acantholytic squamous cell carcinoma. Often arises in Darier-like Keratosis senilis (Fig. 34–8). H&E. X135.

(Fig. 34–18) appears to be the most straightforward and unmistakable designation, but *adenoid* or *pseudoglandular carcinoma*[31] and *carcinoma segregans*[32] also have been used.

Immature Tumors

Even squamous cell carcinomas that have lost all ability to keratinize (Fig. 34–19) do not resemble basal cell epitheliomas, one of the best arguments against Darier's old classification (Chap. 39). They usually consist of large, pale-staining cells in compact array. However, if one encounters a completely immature tumor, the differential diagnosis between squamous cell carcinoma, adenocarcinoma, and amelanotic melanoma must be weighed carefully. In some cases, it may be impossible without resorting to special histochemical methods. Silver and dopa reactions can be used to identify amelanotic melanomas. Stains for acid mucopolysaccharides, lipids, and certain enzyme activities may be positive in adenocarcinomas, while glycogen may be found in adenocarcinomas and some squamous cell carcinomas but practically never in malignant melanomas.

Small Cell Squamous Carcinomas

There are a few actinic keratoses of keratosis senilis type in which the dysplastic cells are small and basaloid and may give rise to small-celled carcinomas simulating basal cell epithelioma in their early

stages. However, the absence of retraction spaces and PAS-positive basement membrane identifies these lesions as squamous cell cancers.

Spindle Cell Squamous Carcinomas

Spindle cell squamous carcinomas were first described as recurrent tumors after X-ray treatment.[33] More recently, their close histologic resemblance to atypical fibroxanthomas[34] has forced electron microscopic study to demonstrate tonofilaments and desmosomes in and between the cells. The tumors consist of large, often atypical cells with multinucleated elements, and there may not be any visible relation to the epidermis. Light microscopic examination may not always be sufficient, and even formalin-fixed material may be suitable for electron microscopic examination.[35]

Verrucous Carcinoma of Skin

Under the picturesque name of *epithelioma cuniculatum*,[36] deeply invasive and destructive forms of squamous carcinoma were described, which penetrate the foot from the volar surface and resemble a rabbit warren on cross section. These tumors (Fig. 34–20) have recently been compared to the *verrucous carcinoma* of the oral mucosa (Chap. 45) and the destructive lesions of giant condyloma acuminatum.[37,38] These three varieties of carcinoma do not show much cellular atypicality or tendency to squamous pearl formation. Their frontal edge ad-

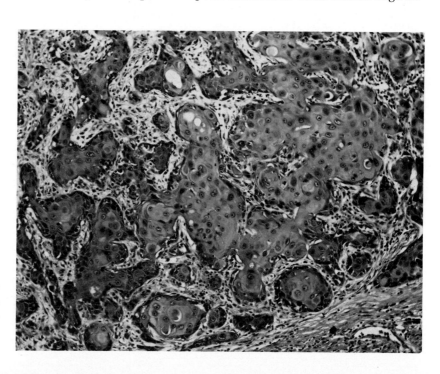

FIGURE 34–19.
Squamous cell carcinoma exhibiting only a few individually keratinizing cells. Note absence of retraction spaces in all photographs of squamous cell carcinoma. H&E. X135.

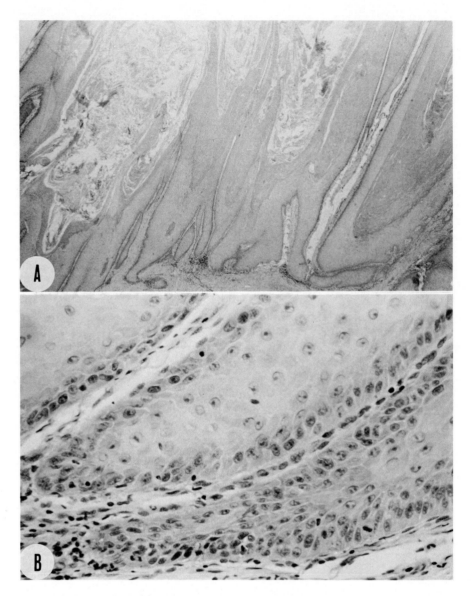

FIGURE 34–20.
Verrucous carcinoma of skin. **A** *demonstrates the deceptively benign aspect at low power. H&E. X10.* **B** *shows absence of a well-formed basal layer and slight atypicality of cells. Mitoses and large nucleoli. H&E. X250.*

vances in a pushing manner, destroying tissue without obvious invasion by individual sprouts. Sufficiently large and deep biopsies are needed for diagnosis.

Squamous cell carcinoma of the ectodermal mucous membranes and its precursor lesions have special features and require special differential considerations. They will be discussed in Chapter 45.

PSEUDOCARCINOMA

Under this heading we have to discuss two separate phenomena: one usually referred to as *pseudoepitheliomatous proliferation* associated with various inflammatory processes, the other known as *keratoacanthoma* or self-healing squamous cell carcinoma.

Pseudoepitheliomatous Proliferation

In ordinary acanthosis and in papillomatosis, the rete ridges and papillae increase in length and bulk and lift the suprapapillary epidermis above the level of the surrounding skin. Although often described in the literature, there is no downgrowth of rete ridges in any of these conditions.[39] The true baseline of the papillae–epidermis unit remains undisturbed, as can be shown simply by staining for elastic fibers (Chap. 2). However, in some inflammatory diseases, usually in the group of granulomatous inflammation, rarely in severe lichen simplex chronicus and hypertrophic lichen planus, the nonneoplastic epidermis indeed grows down into the pars reticularis (Figs. 7–13, 9–9, 21–2, 21–4, 21–13, and 28–3), although one cannot always be sure how much of the stratified epithelium found deep in the skin may take its origin from hair roots and eccrine glands. The general configuration of the invasive formations may be indistinguishable from true carcinoma, but pronounced cellular atypy is absent, and nuclei usually are normochromatic and relatively small in relation to cytoplasm. Nucleoli may be as large as in carcinoma, and a basement membrane between epithelium and mesoderm commonly is absent. Central keratinization may occur. It often contains an admixture of inflammatory cells in which infective microorganisms may be found (Figs. 21–2 and 21–4) (Chap. 21). In most cases, the underlying inflammatory process is sufficiently evident to permit diagnosis, but awareness and careful examination may be needed to avoid mistakes. We shall see that at least one mesodermal tumor, granular cell myoblastoma, also provokes pseudoepitheliomatous epidermal proliferation.

In contrast to neoplastic epithelium, the epidermis returns to normal when the primary condition heals. While this knowledge does not help in the examination of specific specimens, it is one of the best arguments against any concept that development of carcinoma depends only on the opportunity for normal cells to break through the basement membrane.

Papillomatosis Cutis Carcinoides

A special case is Gottron's *papillomatosis cutis carcinoides*.[40] These broad plaques located on the lower extremities have a clinical resemblance to so-called pyoderma vegetans (Chap. 27, lymphedema) but are (in spite of a mistaken quotation[38]) in no way related to verrucous carcinoma of the sole of the foot. Histologically, they show great acanthosis and papillomatosis, often extending downward into the dermis, but the cells are relatively normal prickle cells and keratinize normally in association with a vascular connective tissue stroma.

Keratoacanthoma

The concept of *self-healing squamous cell carcinoma* is relatively new and, just like the concept of benign juvenile melanoma, was developed on a catamnestic clinical basis. Pathologists then forced to refine their histologic criteria and, in many cases, to change their diagnoses on specimens previously diagnosed as cancer.

We describe a keratoacanthoma (Fig. 34–21) as a heavily keratinized squamous cell lesion which is definitely destructive and invasive but stops growing spontaneously and subsides, leaving a scar. It spreads laterally below the epidermis, leading to a picture of buttress formation on cross section with a horn-filled, very irregular crater in the center. Histologic criteria include the presence of mitoses only in the outermost layer, growth not deeper than the sweat coils, relatively normal nuclear-cytoplasmic ratio, absence of dyskeratosis, and mainly orthokeratotic maturation of central cells. However, none of these rules is without exception, and invasion of blood vessels and neural sheaths in the subcutaneous tissue may occur. The characteristic buttress formation by the surrounding epidermis may also be seen in some slow-growing, well-

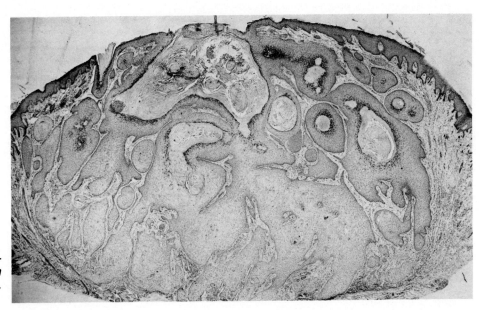

FIGURE 34–21.
Keratoacanthoma. Note pale-staining nuclei and cytoplasm of invasive epithelium. H&E. X14.

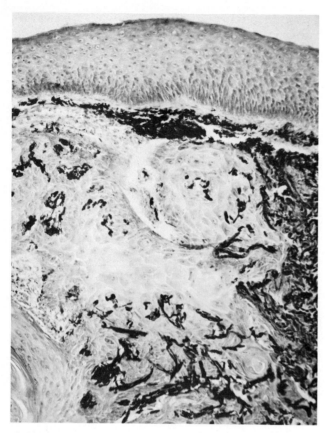

FIGURE 34–22.
Keratoacanthoma invading elastotic dermis and containing undigested remnants of elastic fibers. O&G. X135.

differentiated carcinomas without a tendency to spontaneous involution. Tangential sectioning and convolution of the advancing margin may cause difficulties in exactly locating mitoses. A rarely mentioned but striking and helpful feature in O&G sections (Fig. 34–22) is survival of elastic fiber remnants in the epithelial masses. Collagen fibers may also be demonstrated by specific stains.[41] Although histologic diagnosis usually is possible on an adequate biopsy specimen,[42] which must include the edge and the lower pole of the tumor, there remain cases in which the final decision has to be based on clinicopathologic correlation: a rapidly growing tumor exhibiting histologic features of a well-differentiated squamous cell carcinoma is a keratoacanthoma, while a very slowly growing lesion with similar histology but no self-healing tendency during a year or more is a carcinoma.

Cytologic criteria are important. Most keratoacanthomas do not exhibit cytologic abnormalities, and a highly dysplastic epithelium is not compatible with the diagnosis even if the pattern of the entire tumor is classic. This differentiation is, of course, impossible to prove because total excision

of the lesion will lead to cure whether it was a keratoacanthoma or an early squamous cell carcinoma. It is, however, of value to advise the clinician not to neglect a dysplastic tumor because it has the configuration of keratoacanthoma. This advice becomes more important in view of the fact that in their recent review, such experienced authors as Rook and Whimster[43] feel that keratoacanthoma today is the most common single precursor of squamous cell carcinoma in the exposed skin of the elderly.

Multiple[44] and generalized forms[45] occur occasionally and pose problems in diagnosis and management because lesions may be small and histologically noncharacteristic or may involve difficult areas of the body, such as eyelids and penis. Diagnosis also is more difficult when the nail bed is involved.[46]

Self-Healing Squamous Cell Carcinoma. The self-healing squamous epitheliomas of Ferguson-Smith[47] are probably a condition different from keratoacanthoma. They are familial in many cases, especially in Scotland. Their histologic appearance suggests a squamous cell carcinoma, and after a number of lesions heal spontaneously, the last one kills the patient in spite of therapeutic attempts.[48]

REFERENCES

1. Pinkus H: Epithelial and fibroepithelial tumors. Arch Dermatol 91:24, 1965
2. Pinkus H: Malignant transformation of epithelium. In McKenna RMB (ed): Modern Trends in Dermatology, vol 3. London, Butterworth, 1966, p 275
3. Rattner H: William Allen Pusey at close range. Arch Dermatol 35:25, 1937
4. Everett MA, Nordquist J, Olson RL: Ultrastructure of human epidermis following chronic sun exposure. Br J Dermatol 84:248, 1971
5. Pinkus H: The borderline between cancer and noncancer. In Year Book of Dermatology, 1966–67. Chicago, Year Book, 1967, pp 5–34
6. Pinkus H: Keratosis senilis. Am J Clin Pathol 29:193, 1958
7. Pearse AD, Marks R: Actinic keratoses and the epidermis on which they arise. Br J Dermatol 96:45, 1977
8. Pinkus H, Jallad MS, Mehregan AH: The inflammatory infiltrate of precancerous skin lesions. J Invest Dermatol 41:247, 1963
9. Clendenning WE, Brecher G, Van Scott EJ: Mycosis fungoides. Arch Dermatol 85:785, 1964
10. Carapeto FJ, García-Perez A: Acantholytic keratosis. Dermatologica 148:233, 1974
11. James MP, Wells GC, Whimster IW: Spreading pigmented actinic keratoses. Br J Dermatol 98:373, 1978
12. Olson RL, Gaylor J, Everett MA: Ultraviolet-induced

individual cell keratinization. J Cutan Pathol 1:120, 1974

13. Cox AJ, Abel EA: Epidermal dystrophy. Occurrence after psoriasis therapy with psoralen and long-wave ultraviolet light. Arch Dermatol 115:567, 1979

14. Degos R, Civatte J, Belaïch S, et al.: Maladie de Bowen cutanée ou muceuse. A propos de 243 cas. Ann Dermatol Syphiligr 103:5, 1976

15. Coskey RJ, Mehregan AH, Fosnaugh R: Bowen's disease of the nail bed. Arch Dermatol 106:79, 1972

16. Dieteman DF: Bowen's disease of the nail bed. Arch Dermatol 108:577, 1973

17. Lloyd KM: Multicentric pigmented Bowen's disease of the groin. Arch Dermatol 101:48, 1970

18. Burket JM: Dark plaques in nether regions. JAMA 230:439, 1974

19. Emerson RW: Multicentric pigmented Bowen's disease of the perineum. Proc R Soc Med 68:345, 1975

20. Mehregan AH: Cutaneous horn. A clinicopathologic study. Dermatol Digest 4:45, 1965

21. Bart RS, Andrade R, Kopf AW: Cutaneous horn; a clinical and histopathologic study. Acta Derm Venereol (Stockh) 48:507, 1968

22. Sandbank M: Basal cell carcinoma at the base of cutaneous horn. Arch Dermatol 104:97, 1971

23. Reed WB, Landing B, Sugarman G, et al.: Xeroderma pigmentosum: clinical and laboratory investigation of its basic defect. JAMA 207:2073, 1969

24. Cleaver JE: Xeroderma pigmentosum: genetic and environmental influences in skin carcinogenesis. Int J Dermatol 17:435, 1978

25. Jung EG: Das pigmentierts Xerodermoid, ein Defekt der Rekombinations-Erholung von U-V Schaden. Arch Dermatol Forsch 241:33, 1971

26. Cawley EP, Hsu YT, Weary PE: The basement membrane in relation to carcinoma of the skin. Arch Dermatol 94:712, 1966

27. Gay S, Kresina TF, Gay R, et al.: Immunohistochemical demonstration of basement membrane collagen in normal human skin and in psoriasis. J Cutan Pathol 6:91, 1979

28. Tarin D (ed): Tissue Interactions in Carcinogenesis. New York, Academic Press, 1972

29. Broders AC: Practical points on the microscopic grading of carcinoma. NY State J Med 32:667, 1932

30. Carapeto FJ, García-Perez A: Adenoacanthoma: a review of twenty cases, compared with the literature. Dermatologica 145:269, 1972

31. Lever WF, Schaumberg-Lever G: Histopathology of the Skin, 5th ed. Philadelphia, Lippincott, 1975, p 481

32. Jablonska S, Chorzelski T: Dyskeratoma and epithelioma (carcinoma) dyskeratoticum segregans. Dermatologica 123:24, 1961

33. Martin HE, Stewart FW: Spindle cell epidermoid carcinoma. Am J Cancer 24:273, 1935

34. Feldman PS, Barr RJ: Ultrastructure of spindle cell squamous carcinoma. J Cutan Pathol 3:17, 1976

35. Hudson AW, Winkelman RK: Atypical fibroxanthomas of the skin: A reappraisal of 19 cases in which the original diagnosis was spindle-cell squamous carcinoma. Cancer 29:413, 1972

36. Aird I, Daintree Johnson H, Lennox B, et al.: Epithelioma cuniculatum. A variety of squamous carcinoma peculiar to the foot. Br J Surg 42:45, 1954

37. Headington JT: Verrucous carcinoma. Cutis 21:207, 1978

38. Seehafer JR, Muller SA, Dicken CH, et al.: Bilateral verrucous carcinoma of the feet. Arch Dermatol 115:1222, 1979

39. Pinkus H: The direction of growth of human epidermis. Br J Dermatol 83:556, 1970

40. Nikolowski W: Papillomatosis cutis carcinoides. In Braun-Falco O, Petzold D (eds): Fortschritte der praktischen Dermatologie und Venerologie, vol 7. Berlin, Springer-Verlag, 1973, p 36

41. Bakker PS, Tjon A Joe SS: Inclusion of elastic and collagen fibers in keratoacanthoma. NedTijdschr Geneeskd 112:1358, 1968; 113:371, 1969

42. Baer RL, Kopf AW: Keratoacanthoma. In Year Book of Dermatology 1962–1963. Chicago, Year Book, 1963, p 7

43. Rook A, Whimster I: Keratoacanthoma—a thirty year retrospect. Br J Dermatol 100:41, 1979

44. Reid BJ, Cheesbrough MJ: Multiple keratoacanthoma. A unique case and review of the current classification. Acta Derm Venereol (Stockh) 58:169, 1978

45. Winkelmann RK, Brown J: Generalized eruptive keratoacanthoma and report of cases. Arch Dermatol 97:615, 1968

46. Mehregan AH, Fabian L: Keratoacanthoma of nail bed; a report of two cases. Int J Dermatol 12:149, 1973

47. Rook A, Moffat JC: Multiple self-healing epithelioma of Ferguson-Smith type. Report of a case of unilateral distribution. Arch Dermatol 74:525, 1956

48. Pinkus H: Personal observation in Glasgow, Scotland, 1973

Nevus Sebaceus and Sebaceous Tumors

The spectrum of adnexoid neoplasia discussed in the introduction to Section VII (Table VII–1) is most clearly seen in tumors related to sebaceous glands. We use the cautious expression "related" because the possibility exists that tumors of sebaceous structure may arise in the epidermis or in nonsebaceous adnexal matrix, although most sebaceous tumors probably have their origin in sebaceous glands.

ORGANOID NEVUS (NEVUS SEBACEUS OF JADASSOHN)

It is not uncommon to find two or more of the adnexa participating in nevus formation, and these lesions often also involve the epidermis and the supporting connective tissue. Such nevi are best diagnosed as organoid nevi (Fig. 35–1), since they involve the entire skin organ. To focus diagnosis on only that structure which happens to be most prominent in the individual lesion leads to confusion, while realization of the true, complicated nature of such organoid nevi (Fig. 35–2) creates a unified concept and leads to proper prognostic and therapeutic conclusions. Organoid nevi are most commonly located on the scalp but may be found on face, neck, trunk, or extremities in descending frequency. They have a definite life history[1] in three stages, usually becoming manifest at birth or in childhood as hairless areas (hair minus nevus),

often with associated papillomatous epidermal hyperplasia. Pilosebaceous complexes[2] frequently are underdeveloped (Fig. 35–3) until puberty, when sebaceous glands may manifest tremendous hyperplasia, and apocrine glands appear in a minority of cases. In this second stage, the lesion usually is diagnosed as *nevus sebaceus of Jadassohn*, whereby attention is unduly focused on only one of the components. The second, mature phase of the organoid nevus is followed in 10 to 20 percent of cases by a third phase. A variety of benign tumors of epidermis and adnexa (Fig. 35-4) may develop secondarily (by progression) in the malformed epithelium. The incidence of basal cell epithelioma has been reported as high as 10 percent in some published series, although one has to realize that many organoid nevi never come to the attention of a pathologist if they remain quiescent.[3] An even more serious, but fortunately rare, association is that of other malformations and mental defects.[4]

To diagnose an organoid nevus as an aplastic birth defect or nevus verrucosus in childhood and overlook its potential to develop as nevus sebaceus later, does a disservice to the patient because it prevents correct prophylactic treatment, which ideally consists of complete excision deep enough to remove apocrine coils. Furthermore, failure to be cognizant of the broad concept of organoid nevus results in confusion of a field that can be understood clearly by synthesis of biologic and pathologic facts.

Generally, a nevus contains only elements that

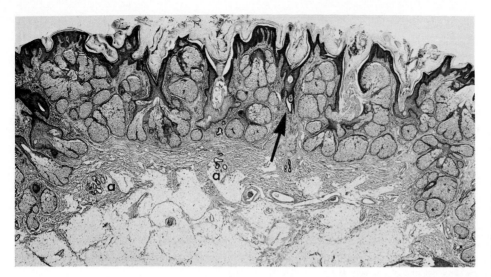

FIGURE 35–1.
Organoid nevus of scalp in adult life. While in this case preponderance of large sebaceous glands seems to justify diagnosis of nevus sebaceus, one should not overlook papillomatous hyperplasia of epidermis, underdevelopment of hair roots, and presence of apocrine glands (a). Arrow points to dilated apocrine duct. H&E. X30.

are at least potentially present in the affected area. For instance, apocrine glands (Fig. 38–1) are not ectopic on scalp and face, although most people probably have only a few in these areas. Similarly, free sebaceous glands are so common in the labial and buccal mucosa that they constitute a normal component. Very rare, indeed, are cases in which hairs are found in normally glabrous areas. Two such instances were recorded in association with nevus cell nevi of the sole,[5] and two families with circumscribed patches of vellus hair on the palms were observed recently.[6,7]

SENILE SEBACEOUS HYPERPLASIA

These are small yellowish nodular lesions occurring on the faces of middle-aged or older individuals. They consist of excessively large and crowded lobes of sebaceous glands[8] (Fig. 35–5). There is some accentuation of the basal layer, which exhibits a low labeling index when injected with tritiated thymidine. The process of maturation proceeds in the normal fashion. Labeled cells are retained in acini much longer, and the sebocytes are smaller.[9]

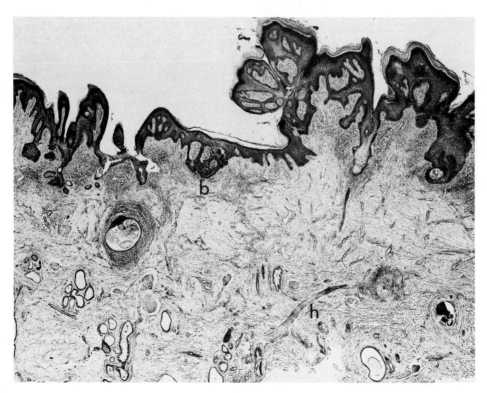

FIGURE 35–2.
Organoid nevus of scalp in adult life. In this case, not only hair roots but also sebaceous glands are underdeveloped. Epidermis is papillomatous, apocrine glands are present, and mesodermal portion of skin is obviously abnormal. h, hair muscle; b, atypical basaloid proliferation which may be a malformed hair root or a tiny basal cell epithelioma. H&E. X28. (From Mehregan and Pinkus. Arch Dermatol 91:574, 1965.)

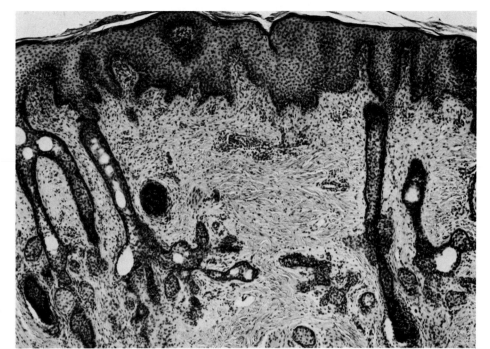

FIGURE 35–3.
Infantile form of organoid nevus of scalp (Wolters' nevus epitheliomatosus capitis). Acanthotic, somewhat papillomatous epidermis, malformed and underdeveloped pilosebaceous complexes, abnormal connective tissue. H&E. X75. (From Mehregan and Pinkus. Arch Dermatol 91:574, 1965.)

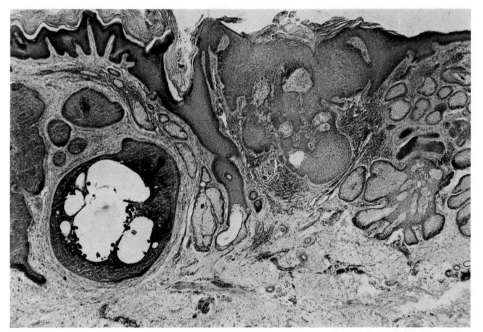

FIGURE 35–4.
Third phase in life history of organoid nevus of scalp. In this case, pigmented basal cell epithelioma (left) and solid hidradenoma of clear cell type (center) have developed in nevus sebaceus which persists in right third of picture. H&E. X21. (From Mehregan and Pinkus. Arch Dermatol 91:574, 1965.)

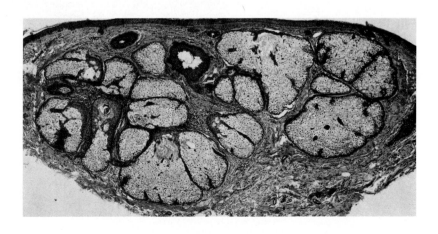

FIGURE 35–5.
Senile sebaceous hyperplasia. H&E. X30.

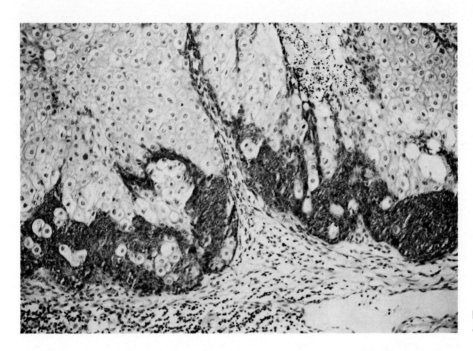

FIGURE 35–6.
Sebaceous adenoma. H&E. X135.

SEBACEOUS ADENOMA

True sebaceous adenomas are rare. These lesions show aggregation of sebaceous lobules with multiple layers of basaloid cells and relatively small sebocytes (Fig. 35–6). The lobular structure, however, is well preserved. Multiple sebaceous adenomas may occur in association with internal malignancy.[10,11]

SEBACEOUS EPITHELIOMA

In sebaceous epithelioma (Fig. 35–7), the architecture of the gland is more or less completely obliterated, and the tumors consist mainly of basaloid cells displaying focal ability for sebaceous maturation. Below this type of tumor on the ladder of maturity are tumors that we may call *basal cell epitheliomas* with *sebaceous differentiation* because

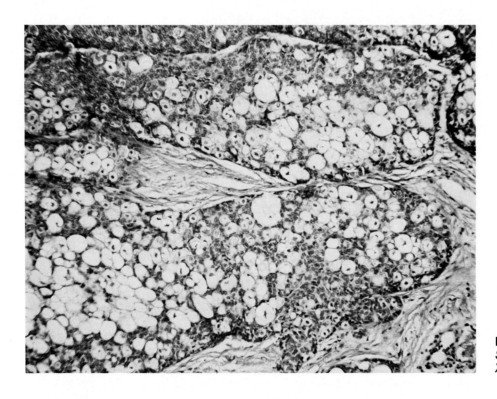

FIGURE 35–7.
Sebaceous epithelioma. H&E. X135.

only small groups or single cells show this tendency. The last step down the ladder takes us into the large pool of completely immature *basal cell epitheliomas* (basaliomas) (Table VII-1).

REFERENCES

1. Mehregan AH, Pinkus H: Life history of organoid nevi. Special reference to nevus sebaceus of Jadassohn. Arch Dermatol 91:574, 1965
2. Steigleder GK, Cortes Cortes A: Verhalten der Talgdrüsen im Talgdrüsennaevus während des Kindesalters. Arch Klin Exp Dermatol 239:323, 1971
3. Wilson-Jones E, Heyl T: Naevus sebaceus: A report of 140 cases with special regard to the development of secondary malignant tumors. Br J Dermatol 82:99, 1970
4. Bianchine JW: Nevus sebaceus of Jadassohn. Am J Dis Child 120:223, 1970
5. Mehregan AH, Coskey RJ: Pigmented nevi of sole. Report of two cases with histologic evidence of hair follicle formation. Arch Dermatol 106:886, 1972
6. Schnitzler ML: Dysembryoplasie pilaire circonscrite des paumes: Un cas familial. Bull Soc Fr Dermatol Syphiligr 80:323, 1973
7. Jackson CE, Callies OC, Krull EA, Mehregan AH: Hereditary hairy cutaneous malformation of palms and soles. Arch Dermatol 111:1146, 1975
8. Mehregan AH, Rahbari H: Benign epithelial tumors of the skin II. Benign sebaceous tumors. Cutis 19:317, 1977
9. Luderschmidt C, Plewig G: Circumscribed sebaceous gland hyperplasia: Autoradiographic and histoplanimetric studies. J Invest Dermatol 70:207, 1978
10. Leonard DD, Deaton WR Jr: Multiple sebaceous gland tumors and visceral carcinomas. Arch Dermatol 110:917, 1974
11. Tschang TP, Poulos E, Ho CK, Kuo TT: Multiple sebaceous adenomas and internal malignant disease: a case report with chromosomal analysis. Hum Pathol 7:589, 1976

CHAPTER

36

Hair Nevi and Hair Follicle Tumors

HAIR NEVI

Hair and hair follicle are involved in several nevi. Localized growth of unusually strong hairs is a hair nevus, while crowding of many tiny mature follicles (Fig. 36–1) constitutes a hair follicle nevus. Circumscribed patches of scalp hair of divergent color or texture may be classified as nevi. The most common form is the *white forelock (poliosis)*, which may occur alone or as part of piebaldism (Chap. 30), but patches of red hair in a brown scalp or other abnormalities may be observed *(dichromism)*. The *woolly-hair nevus* of Wise[1–3] in a straight-haired scalp has found its counterpart in the *straight-hair nevus* in a negroid scalp.[4,5] The excessive development of hairs in common pigmented moles and in bathing-trunk (animal-pelt) nevi can properly be classified as hair nevus *(nevus pilosus)*.

Nevus Comedonicus

In this nevoid lesion, a number of cystic dilated hair follicles containing pigmented horny plugs (Fig. 36–2) occur in a localized area or in a linear arrangement.[6,7] Sebaceous lobules may be observed in connection with the wall of the cystic follicles in early lesions.[8] Acneiform inflammation may complicate these lesions. Secondary tumors or malignant changes do not occur. Nevus comedonicus may occur in association with skeletal abnormalities and central nervous system manifestations.[9]

HAIR FOLLICLE TUMORS

A number of hair follicle tumors were listed in Table VII-1 in descending order of maturation. In recent years, the variety of such tumors has greatly increased due to more thorough observations of a multiplying number of investigators of dermal pathology. This tendency is welcome, although conservative pathologists offer the question: "Would it not be just as well to call all these lesions *benign adnexal tumors*?" It seems advisable to organize and subdivide the field for several reasons. The question of benign versus malignant can be answered with more confidence if one is familiar with all varieties of tumors. Several variants have unexpected associations with generalized systemic disease, while this association is uncommon in others. Finally, we must take into consideration the tendency of the mind of the inquisitive pathologist, who is not satisfied until a definite diagnostic term can be affixed to particular tumor. We shall, on the next pages, describe a fairly long list of tumors, longer than can be accommodated in Table 36–1, and it will become obvious that hair follicular epithelium can deviate from normal not only in the vertical order of maturity but also in several horizontal directions of organization. How much of this intellectual differentiation between various tumors is of practical significance to the clinician is a question that every pathologist has to answer in considering the circumstances of the individual case.

423

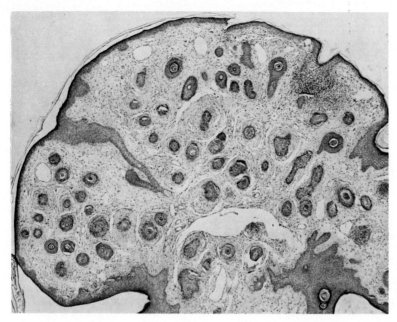

FIGURE 36–1.
Hair follicle nevus. Numerous tiny but mature hair follicles with thick fibrous root sheath in a pedunculated papillomatous papule. H&E. X60.

Trichofolliculoma

The most organized nevoid tumor related to the entire hair follicle has been appropriately called trichofolliculoma. It consists of one or several keratinized sinuses (Fig. 36–3) into which dozens of abortive hair roots enter from all sides. Some of these produce nothing but a rudimentary matrix,

others form inner root sheath, and some produce tiny colorless filaments (trichoids) which may appear on the skin surface as cottony or silky strands.[10] That many hair roots open into a common sinus and that they may have secondary branches constitutes adenomatous deviation from normal organization. The lower degree of maturation fits this pattern, distinguishing trichofolliculoma as an adenomatous neoplasm from mature hair follicle nevus.[11,12] Trichofolliculoma is a well-

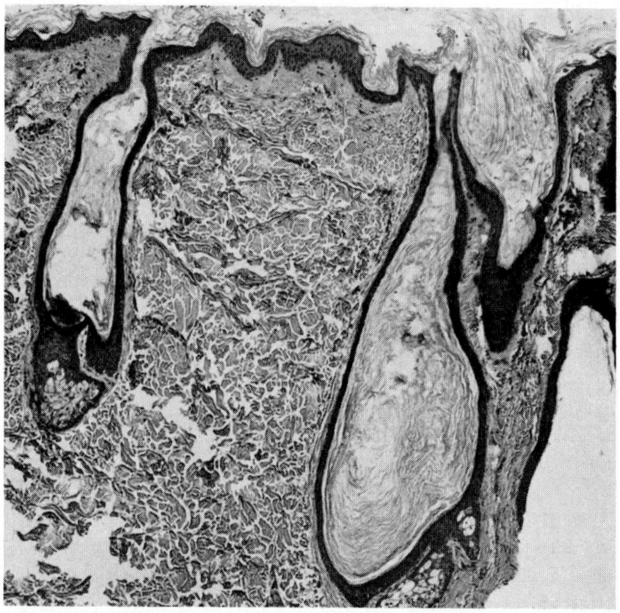

FIGURE 36–2.
Nevus comedonicus. Saccular dilatation of the lengthened pilosebaceous duct. Sebaceous glands situated at an unusually deep level in the dermis. Hair roots atrophic. H&E. X75.

TABLE 36–1.
Follicular Nevi, Tumors, and Cysts

	Pilosebaceous Complex	Follicular Sheath
Hair Matrix	Hair nevus	
	Hair follicle nevus	Dilated pore
	Trichofolliculoma	Epidermoid cyst
	(Steatocystoma multiplex)	Trichilemmal cyst
		Pilar sheath acanthoma
		Trichoadenoma
	Trichoepithelioma	Inverted follicular keratosis
	Desmoplastic trichoepithelioma	Tumor of follicular infundibulum
Piloma-tricoma	Premalignant fibro-epithelial tumor	Trichilemoma
	Trichoepithelioma-like basal cell epithelioma	Proliferating trichilemmal cyst
	Basal cell epithelioma	Cylindroma

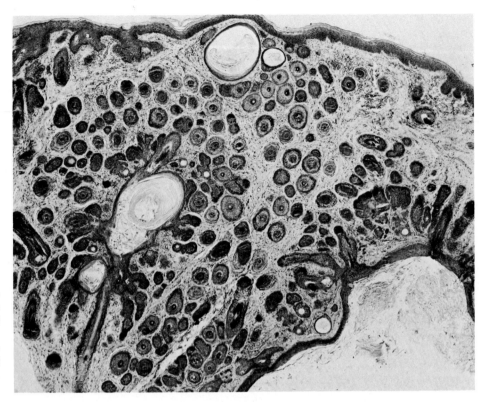

FIGURE 36–3.
Trichofolliculoma. Branching hair follicles achieve varying degrees of maturation, and some form tiny hairs. H&E. X45. (From Pinkus and Mehregan. In Schnyder (ed). Haut und Anhangsgebilde, 1973. Courtesy of Springer-Verlag.)

defined fibroepithelial growth. A case described as trichofolliculocarcinoma with irregular epithelial proliferation and perineural invasion does not seem to belong in this category.[13]

Trichoadenoma

Solitary intracutaneous nodule of trichoadenoma occurs over the face or on the trunk.[14] This is a moderately well-differentiated tumor (Fig. 36–4) consisting of solid masses of cells and small horny cysts with stratified epithelium of outer root sheath character, which keratinizes in the epidermoid manner with keratohyalin and flaky or dense keratin.[15] No hair roots are formed. It therefore is a tumor of the adenomatous level of organization and exhibits differentiation toward the pilosebaceous canal.

Dilated Pore

Dilated pore of Winer[16] may be considered as a simple type of follicular sheath neoplasm (Fig. 36–5). Thick proliferating folds of outer root sheath epithelium line a central cystic space that contains a horny plug and clinically resembles a large blackhead.[17]

Pilar Sheath Acanthoma

Related to dilated pore, this lesion appears most commonly over the upper lip area (Fig. 36–6). Massive proliferation of follicular sheath epithelium occurs, extending from the wall of a central cystic

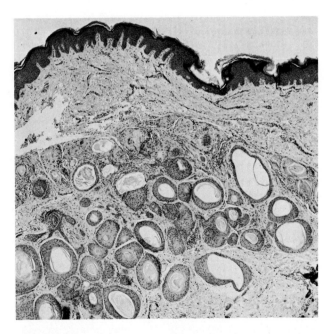

FIGURE 36–4.
Nikolowski's trichoadenoma. H&E. X70.

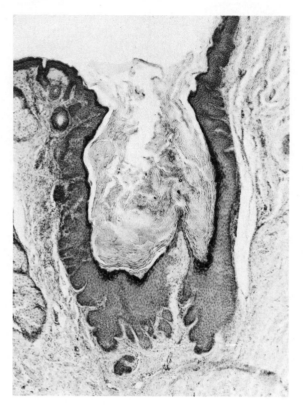

FIGURE 36–5.
Winer's dilated pore. H&E. X45.

cavity into the surrounding dermis in all directions. Keratinization is with formation of keratohyalin granules. Occasional abortive hair follicles may be present.[18]

Tumor of Follicular Infundibulum

A less mature follicular neoplasm suggesting a relationship to the infundibulum is the tumor of follicular infundibulum,[19] in which masses of rather light staining cells (Fig. 36–7) form a shelf or fenestrated plate below the epidermis, which they penetrate wherever there is a follicular opening. This tumor resembles, in some respects, the growth pattern of the very superficial type of basal cell epithelioma but seems to be even more benign in its clinical behavior and consists of cells resembling those of follicular infundibulum.[20]

Inverted Follicular Keratosis

Also known as *follicular poroma,*[21] it appears as keratotic nodular lesions over the face and occasionally elsewhere.[22] Hyperplastic follicular epithelium (Fig. 36–8) extends from the surface into the dermis surrounded by fibrovascular stroma. Maturation is retarded so that the percentage of small

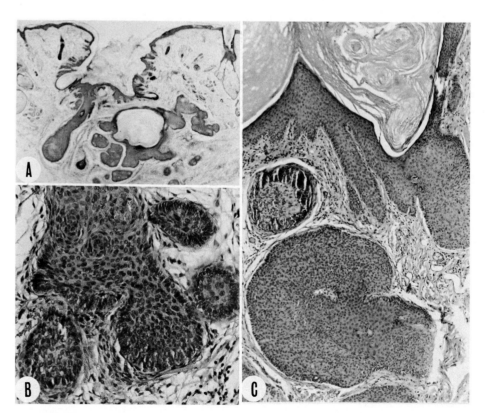

FIGURE 36–6.
*Pilar sheath acanthoma. Similar to dilated pore in the formation of a horny plug, it branches out in its deeper portions with massive solid proliferations of follicular sheath epithelium and contains rudimentary hair roots. H&E. **A.** X5. **B.** X400. **C.** X125. (From Mehregan and Brownstein. Arch Dermatol 114:1495, 1978. Copyright © 1978 by the American Medical Association.)*

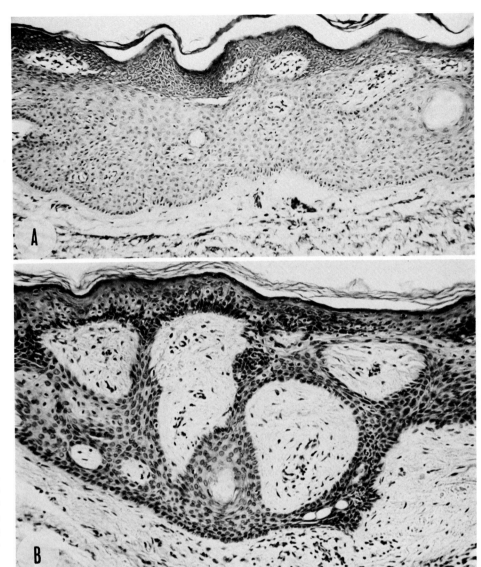

FIGURE 36–7.
*Tumor of follicular infundibulum. Benign neoplastic epithelium forms a plate below the epidermis, with which it is in multiple contact. The tumor stains lighter than the epidermis, is not pigmented, and is embedded in moderately mature stroma. **A.** Van Gieson. X70. **B.** H&E. X180.*

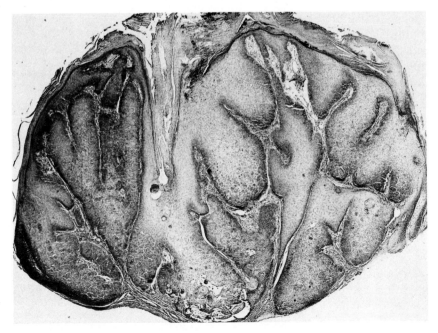

FIGURE 36–8.
Follicular poroma (inverted follicular keratosis) contains recognizable remnant of involved hair follicle in center and is characterized by smooth outline of the proliferating epithelium that contains numerous squamous eddies (see Fig. 36–9). Compare with Figure 34–21 (keratoacanthoma) consisting of large, light-staining prickle cells. H&E. X23. (From Mehregan. Arch Dermatol 89:229, 1964.)

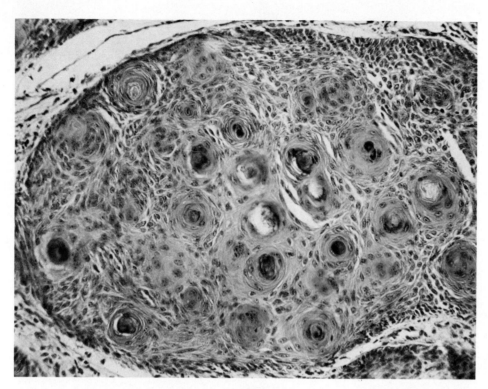

FIGURE 36–9.
Squamous eddies in inverted follicular keratosis (follicular poroma). H&E. X185. (From Mehregan. Arch Dermatol 89:229, 1964.)

basaloid cells is increased at the periphery of the tumor lobules. In the center, numerous foci of keratinization occur forming squamous eddies[23] (Fig. 36–9). Early lesions may show a connection with an underlying hair follicle or sebaceous gland.

Trichilemoma

Massive proliferation of follicular sheath epithelium (Fig. 36–10) is seen in connection with the lower surface of the epidermis.[24,25] The tumor epithelium (Fig. 36–11) is made up of light-staining cells with abundant glycogen granules. At the periphery, the tumore cells palisade and rest on a thick basement membrane, thus resembling the outer root sheath of the hair follicle.[26] Recent studies have suggested that multiple facial trichilemomas are an important cutaneous marker of Cowden's disease.[27–30]

Pilomatricoma

The single tumor definitely related to hair matrix is *Malherbe's calcifying epithelioma*, which therefore may be properly called pilomatricoma.[31,32] The living portions of this tumor (Fig. 36–12) strongly resemble the nonstratified mass of small, dark-staining cells of the pilar matrix. In one early tumor of this type in our collection, the upper part of a hair follicle persisted in almost normal fashion,

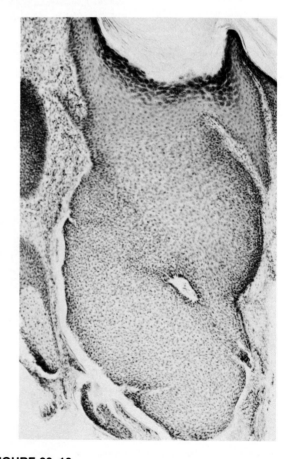

FIGURE 36–10.
Trichilemoma. Solid plug of follicular sheath epithelium extends into the dermis. The cells are fairly small but light-staining because they contain glycogen. There is no resemblance to verruca vulgaris. H&E. X125.

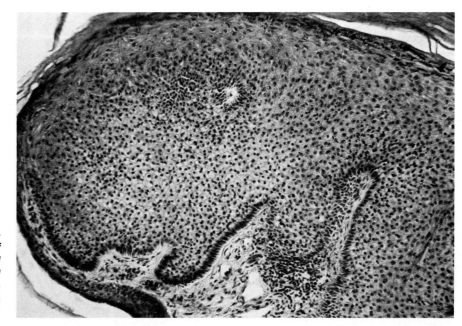

FIGURE 36–11.
Trichilemoma. Small portion of lesion to show clear cell character of epithelium and palisading basal layer which rests on a well-defined basement membrane. Tumor cells keratinize in epidermoid fashion on surface. H&E. X135.

while the deep portion was occupied by a pilomatricoma. The peculiar transformation of these germinative cells into shadow cells resembling epidermal prickle cells and their strong tendency to calcify are evidence of profound disruption of normal cellular metabolism.[33] A foreign-body-type granuloma is often present around the keratinized areas within the fibrous stroma of the lesion. Anetodermic changes due to loss of collagen and elastic fibers may be clinically observed.[34] Unusually large

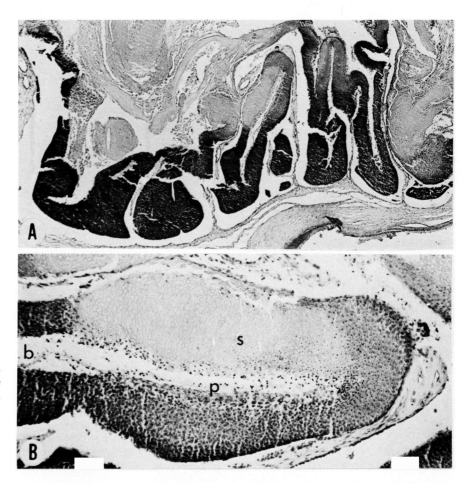

FIGURE 36–12.
Pilomatricoma. Calcification was not present in this case. A. Masses of small dark-staining cells contrast with ligher-staining squamous cells and shadow cells. H&E. X60. B. Details of three cellular components: basaloid (b), prickle (p), and shadow (s) cells. H&E. X135.

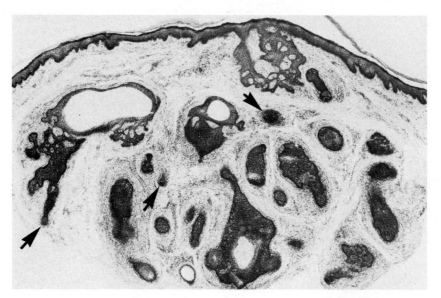

FIGURE 36–13.
Trichoepithelioma. Rudimentary hair papilla-matrix configurations indicated by arrows. The name trichoblastoma *was proposed for tumors of this type by Headington (1976). H&E. X45.*

lesions with deep dermal involvement occur.[35] Superficial perforation may lead to elimination of the tumor epithelium and calcified material.[36] Another development is the association of pilomatricomas with myotonic dystrophy.[37]

TRICHOEPITHELIOMA

In the systematic spectrum of adnexoid tumors there is a level of maturity at which much of the tumor may have the characteristics of quite immature basalioma, while small foci or larger parts show maturation in the direction of sebaceous gland, hair root, or other recognizable adnexal features.[38] Tumors with features of maturation resembling various parts of the hair follicle are common and vary from basal cell epitheliomas with peculiar antlerlike type of growth (Fig. 36–13), or with occasional rudimentary hairbulblike structures, to typical trichoepitheliomas.

Trichoepithelioma may be solitary or multiple (*epithelioma adenoides cysticum*). The multiple variety may be familial, transmitted by an autosomal dominant trait.[39]

Histologically, in addition to solid epithelial nests, which often show antlerlike branching, there often are tiny keratinizing cysts resembling milia and rudimentary hair papillae (Fig. 36–14). Formation of an organized hair is extremely rare. The nests usually show peripheral palisading, and the central cells may be lighter staining and larger, like those of premalignant fibroepithelial tumors (Chap. 39). The stroma also shows a relatively high degree of maturity and may form sulfated mucopolysaccharides and elastic fibers. Alkaline phosphatase activity has been found in rudimentary hair pap-

illae, while this enzyme seems to be absent from morphologically similar areas in true basal cell epitheliomas.[40]

In routine diagnosis, it is not always simple to classify one or the other tumor as either trichoepithelioma or basal cell epithelioma. The absence or

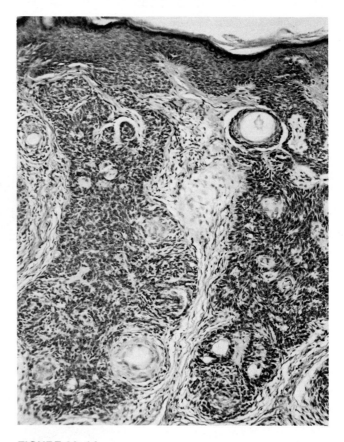

FIGURE 36–14.
Trichoepithelioma. Cellular details of epithelial and meso-dermal portions. Multiple connections with epidermis are secondary. H&E. X135.

presence of inflammatory infiltrate, characteristic of basalioma, is a helpful clue. For practical purposes, one should keep in mind that the individual tumor of cases of multiple epithelioma adenoides cysticum tends to remain small, while solitary trichoepitheliomas of similar histologic appearance grow progressively larger and should be treated like basaliomas.

Desmoplastic Trichoepithelioma

This is usually a solitary, firm nodule with a central depressed area appearing over the facial skin in all ages.[41,42] Histologically (Fig. 36–15), there is marked resemblance to a morphealike type of basal cell epithelioma consisting of small nests and thin strands of basaloid cells embedded in dense fibrotic stroma. They show, however, foci of keratin cyst formation, areas of calcification, and foreign-body granuloma.[41] Lesions with this histologic pattern have been reported in association with nevocytic proliferation as a combined malformation.[43,44]

Atrophodermia Vermicularis and Other Follicular Hamartomas

Long known as a clinical curiosity, atrophodermia vermicularis, which produces a worm-eaten appearance of the skin of the cheeks, has been shown to be due to malformation of all portions of the skin (Fig. 36–16) and may be considered another form of

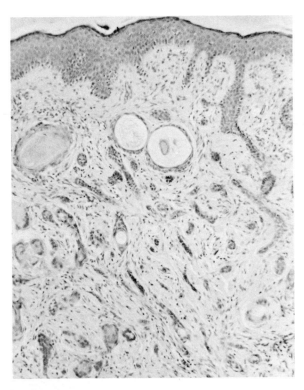

FIGURE 36–15.
Desmoplastic trichoepithelioma. Compare with Figure 39–12. H&E. X125.

peculiarly localized organoid nevus. Small sebaceous glands, incompletely formed hair follicles, and abnormal connective tissue characterize the histologic findings in this condition.[45] Haber's syndrome is a rare familial condition characterized by

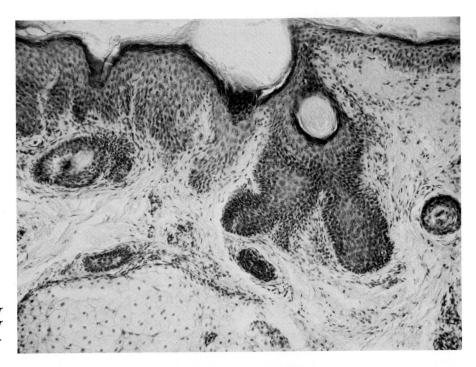

FIGURE 36–16.
Atrophodermia vermiculata. Minor malformation of epidermis, pilar apparatus, and dermis. H&E. X180.

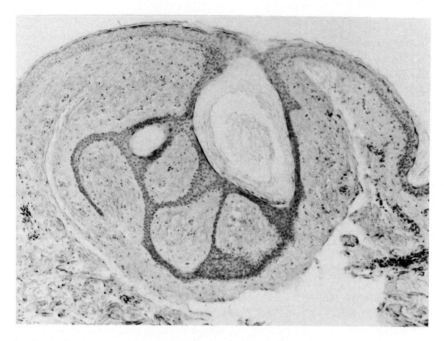

FIGURE 36–17.
Fibrofolliculoma (Birt-Hogg-Dubé). The upper part of the follicle is surrounded by a well-defined fibrous sheath tumor supporting a netlike proliferation of the upper outer root sheath. Follicle plugged with keratin. The sebaceous gland (not shown in this section) is displaced downward. H&E. X125. (From Weintraub and Pinkus, J Cutan Pathol 4:289, 1977. Copyright © 1977 by Munksgaard-International Publishers, Copenhagen.)

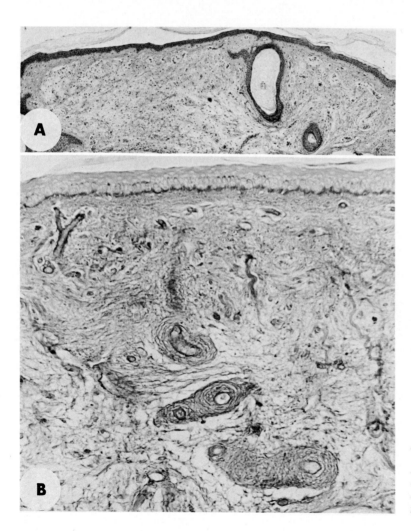

FIGURE 36–18.
*Trichodiscoma. **A.** Picture includes the greater portion of a flat sessile papule. Oblique sections of two hair follicles, which open near the rim of the tumor. H&E. X30. **B.** Blood vessels enveloped in PAS-positive lamellae are embedded in ground-substance-rich connective tissue. Alcian blue-PAS. X180.*

rosacealike facial dermatosis, keratotic plaques, and pitted scars. Follicular atrophy and budding of basaloid cells in connection with comedolike follicles are seen in the facial lesions.[46,47] There are other conditions in which clinical atrophy, hypotrichosis, or alopecia totalis was found to be due to histologic malformation or benign neoplasia of the pilar apparatus.[48,51]

TUMORS OF PERIFOLLICULAR CONNECTIVE TISSUE

The connective tissue component of the pilar apparatus gives rise to three different forms of neoplasms (Chap. 41), including perifollicular fibroma, fibrofolliculoma, and trichodiscoma.[52]

Perifollicular Fibroma. Single or multiple firm papulonodular lesions of perifollicular fibroma appear most commonly over the face and head and neck regions (Fig. 41–4). Histologically, there is concentric proliferation of fibrous connective tissue surrounding small vellus-type follicles.[53–55]

Fibrofolliculoma. These are usually multiple, firm papules 2 to 4 mm in diameter, some of which show a central hair. Histologically, in the center of each lesion is a cystic follicle containing keratinous material. The infundibular epithelium shows outward epithelial projections surrounded by proliferation of connective tissue fibers[56,57] (Fig. 36–17).

Trichodiscoma. The hair disk (haarscheibe) is a slowly adapting touch receptor in mammalian skin occurring in close vicinity to the hair follicles (Chap. 2). It consists of a well-vascularized dermal connective tissue and thick myelinated nerves in contact with Merkel cells in the basal layer of epidermis. Neoplasia of the dermal pad of this organ is manifest as numerous, small, 1 to 3 mm papular lesions. Histologically (Fig. 36–18), the dome-shaped parafollicular lesion is made up of richly vascular connective tissue with abundant alcian-blue-reactive material.[58]

REFERENCES

1. Domonkos A: Wooly hair nevus. Arch Dermatol 85:568, 1962
2. Hutchinson PE: Woolly hair. Trans St Johns Hosp Dermatol Soc 60:160, 1974
3. Lantis SDH, Pepper MC: Woolly hair nevus. Two case reports and a discussion of unruly hair forms. Arch Dermatol 114:233, 1978
4. Gibbs RC, Berger RA: The straight hair nevus. Int J Dermatol 9:47, 1970
5. Downham TF, Chapel TA, Lupulescu AP: Straight hair nevus syndrome: a case report with scanning electron microscopic findings of hair morphology. Int J Dermatol 15:438, 1976
6. Leppard B, Marks R: Comedone nevus: a report of nine cases. Trans St Johns Hosp Dermatol Soc 59:45, 1973
7. Abdel-Aal H, Abdel-Aziz AHM: Nevus comedonicus; report of three cases localized on glans penis. Acta Derm Venereol (Stockh) 55:78, 1975
8. Nabai H, Mehregan AH: Nevus comedonicus. A review of the literature and report of twelve cases. Acta Derm Venereol (Stockh) 53:71, 1973
9. Engber PB: The nevus comedonicus syndrome. A case report with emphasis on associated internal manifestations. Int J Dermatol 17:745, 1978
10. Pinkus H, Sutton RL Jr: Trichofolliculoma. Arch Dermatol 91:46, 1965
11. Kligman A, Pinkus H: Histogenesis of nevoid tumors of skin. Arch Dermatol 81:922, 1960
12. Lee S, Nasemann T: Das Trichofollikulom. Hautarzt 22:165, 1971
13. Stern JB, Stout DA: Trichofolliculoma showing perineural invasion. Trichofolliculocarcinoma? Arch Dermatol 115:1003, 1979
14. Rahbari H, Mehregan AH, Pinkus H: Trichoadenoma of Nikolowski. J Cutan Pathol 4:90, 1977
15. Nikolowski W: "Tricho-adenom" (organoides Follikel-Hamartom). Arch Klin Exp Dermatol 207:34, 1958
16. Winer LH: The dilated pore, a trichoepithelioma. J Invest Dermatol 23:181, 1954
17. Mehregan AH, Rahbari H: Benign epithelial tumors of the skin. Part III. Benign hair follicle tumors. Cutis 19:595, 1977
18. Mehregan AH, Brownstein MH: Pilar sheath acanthoma. Arch Dermatol 114:1495, 1978
19. Mehregan AH, Butler JD: Tumor of follicular infundibulum. Arch Dermatol 83:924, 1961
20. Mehregan AH: Tumor of follicular infundibulum. Dermatologica 142:177, 1971
21. Duperrat B, Mascaro JM: Une tumeur bénigne développée aux depens de l'acrotrichium ou partie intraépidermique du follicule pilaire: porome folliculaire (acanthome folliculaire intraépidermique; acrotrichoma). Dermatologica 126:291, 1963
22. Mehregan AH: Inverted follicular keratosis. Arch Dermatol 89:229, 1964
23. Helwig EB: Inverted follicular keratosis. In Seminar on the Skin: Neoplasms and Dermatoses. American Society of Clinical Pathology, International Congress of Clinical Pathology, Washington, DC, Sept 1954. Chicago, American Society of Clinical Pathology, 1955
24. Ackerman AB, Wade TR: Tricholemma. Amer J Dermatopathol 2:207, 1980
25. Headington JT: Tricholemmoma. To be or not to be? Amer J Dermatopathol 2:225, 1980.
26. Brownstein MH, Shapiro L: Trichilemmoma: analy-

sis of forty new cases. Arch Dermatol 107:866, 1973

27. Brownstein MH, Mehregan AH, Bikowski JB: Trichilemmomas in Cowden's disease. JAMA 238:26, 1977

28. Brownstein MH, Wolf M, Bikowski JB: Cowden's disease: a cutaneous marker of breast cancer. Cancer 41:2393, 1978

29. Nuss DD, Aeling JL, Clemons DE, Weber WN: Multiple hamartoma syndrome (Cowden's disease). Arch Dermatol 114:743, 1978

30. Brownstein MH, Mehregan AH, Bikowski JB, et al.: The dermatopathology of Cowden's syndrome. Br J Dermatol 100:667, 1979

31. Forbis R Jr, Helwig EB: Pilomatrixoma (calcifying epithelioma). Arch Dermatol 83:606, 1961

32. Wong WK, Somburanasin R, Wood MG: Eruptive multicentric pilomatricoma (calcifying epithelioma). Arch Dermatol 106:76, 1972

33. Wiedersberg H: Die Metamorphose des Epithelioma calcificans Malherbe. Virchows Arch [Pathol Anat] 349:236, 1970

34. Moulin G, Bouchet B, DosSantos G: Les modifications anétodermiques du tégument au-dessus des tumeurs de Malherbe. Ann Derm Venereol 105:43, 1978

35. Sasaki CT, Yue A, Enriques R: Giant calcifying epithelioma. Arch Otolaryngol 102:753, 1976

36. TarPorten HJ, Sharbaugh AH: Extruding pilomatricoma. Report of a case. Cutis 22:47, 1978

37. Chiaramonti A, Gilgor RS: Pilomatricomas associated with myotonic dystrophy. Arch Dermatol 114:1363, 1978

38. Lasser A, Carter DM: Multiple basal cell epitheliomas with sebaceous differentiation. Arch Dermatol 107:91, 1973

39. Gaul LE: Heredity of multiple benign cystic epithelioma "the Indiana family." Arch Dermatol 68:517, 1953

40. Kopf AW: The distribution of alkaline phosphatase in normal and pathologic human skin. Arch Dermatol 75:1, 1957

41. Brownstein MH, Shapiro L: Desmoplastic trichoepithelioma. Cancer 40:2979, 1977

42. MacDonald DM, Wilson-Jones E, Marks R: Sclerosing epithelial hamartoma. Clin Exp Dermatol 2:153, 1977

43. Schellander F, Marks R, Wilson-Jones E: Basal cell hamartoma and cellular nevus: an unusual combined malformation. Br J Dermatol 9:413, 1974

44. Rahbari H, Mehregan AH: Trichoepithelioma and pigmented nevus. A combined malformation. J Cutan Pathol 2:413, 1974

45. Rozum TL, Mehregan AH, Johnson SAM: Folliculitis ulerythematosa reticulata. Arch Dermatol 106:388, 1972

46. Sanderson KV, Wilson HTH: Haber's syndrome: Familial rosacea-like eruption with intraepidermal epithelioma. Br J Dermatol 77:1, 1965

47. Seiji M, Otaki N: Haber's syndrome. Familial rosacea-like dermatosis with keratotic plaques and pitted scars. Arch Dermatol 103:452, 1971

48. Brown AC, Crounse RG, Winkelmann RK: Generalized hair follicle hamartoma. Arch Dermatol 99:478, 1969

49. Pierard J, Dhondt F, Geerts ML, et al.: Atrophodermie folliculaire; proliferations basocellulaires et hypotrichose. Arch Belg Dermatol 27:55, 1971

50. Johnson WC, Hookerman BJ: Basal cell hamartoma with follicular differentiation. Arch Dermatol 105:105, 1972

51. Mehregan AH, Hardin I: Generalized follicular hamartoma. Arch Dermatol 107:435, 1973

52. Headington JT: Tumors of the hair follicle. Am J Pathol 85:480, 1976

53. Zackheim HS, Pinkus H: Perifollicular fibromas. Arch Dermatol 82:913, 1960

54. Cramer HJ: Multiple perifollikuläre Fibrome. Hautarzt 19:228, 1968

55. Freeman RG, Chernosky ME: Perifollicular fibroma. Arch Dermatol 100:66, 1969

56. Weintraub R, Pinkus H: Multiple fibrofolliculomas (Birt-Hogg-Dubé) associated with a large connective tissue nevus. J Cutan Pathol 4:289, 1977

57. Rahbari H, Mehregan AH: Benign follicular neoplasias. J Dermatol Surg Oncol 5:295, 1979

58. Pinkus H, Coskey R, Burgess GH: Trichodiscoma. Benign tumor related to haarscheibe (hair disk). J Invest Dermatol 63:212, 1974

CHAPTER

37

Cysts Related to the Adnexa

Cysts are properly considered simple benign neoplasms, even though they increase in size more through accumulation of keratinous or fluid contents than through proliferation of the cells in their walls and may be morphologically indistinguishable from retention cysts in some cases. One may introduce a classification (Fig. 37–1) based, as we have done in most of this section, on histologic resemblance rather than on origin. There are two principal types of cutaneous cysts, each with two subdivisions. One type has glandular epithelium in its wall; the other has keratinizing lining. A few cysts are combinations of the two types.

GLANDULAR CYSTS

Hidrocystomas

Cysts having two concentric layers of nonkeratinizing epithelium (Fig. 37–2) can be assumed to be related to sweat glands.[1] When the wall is very thin, one may have to examine it closely at high power in order to recognize the double row of flat nuclei. Tangential sectioning, on the other hand, may produce the false impression of multilayered stratification. Classification as eccrine or apocrine may be arbitrary or impossible in some cases. The presence of columnar, or at least bulging, luminal cells speaks for apocrine maturation, which is

made certain if intracellular lipid or pigmented granules can be demonstrated.[2]

Steatocystoma Multiplex

Sebaceous cysts, in spite of the widespread use of the name, are exceedingly rare.[3] The only type of cyst that definitely has sebaceous cells and lobules in its wall is steatocystoma multiplex (Fig. 37–3).[4] This is characterized by the appearance of numerous small intracutaneous cystic lesions usually over the trunk and occasionally elsewhere.[5] Even in these lesions, large portions of the cyst lining consist of thin, stratified, and partly keratinizing epithelium, perhaps related to the sebaceous duct. However, since these cysts often contain hairs and must, therefore, have hair roots in their makeup, they are actually pilosebaceous cysts, and perhaps simple dermoids.[6]

KERATINOUS CYSTS

All keratinous cysts are lined by stratified epithelium, which may be thin or thick. They keratinize either with formation of keratohyalin, forming a relatively loosely lamellated horny material resembling that of epidermis, or without keratohyalin, in which case the contents are dense and may look

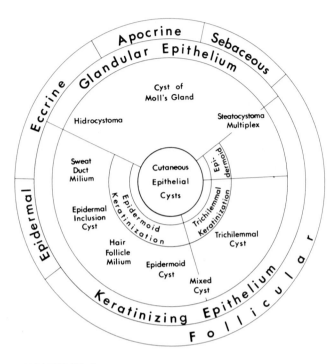

FIGURE 37–1.
Diagram showing diagnostic names of cutaneous epithelial cysts in relation to type of maturation of their epithelium. There is overlap between glandular and keratinizing maturation in eccrine and pilosebaceous cysts. In keratinizing group, epidermoid and trichilemmal types of maturation occur.

amorphous in H&E sections but can be shown to resemble trichilemmal keratin by a variety of other staining procedures.

Epidermoid Cysts

Because the epidermal type of keratinization is encountered in several extraepidermal tissues in the skin (acrosyringium, follicular infundibulum, sebaceous duct) and outside the skin (esophagus, cervix uteri), and can be induced in many other epithelia (squamous metaplasia), it appears wise not to speculate about the origin of cysts containing this type of maturation and to call them epidermoid cysts rather than epidermal cysts. Actually cysts of this type may originate in occluded hair follicles, in outer root sheath epithelium (facial *milia*), in obstructed eccrine ducts (retention *milia* in blistering dermatoses), and perhaps in buried epidermis (*epidermal inclusion cysts*), although this appears questionable.[7] The only basis for diagnosing an epidermoid cyst (Fig. 37–4) is the presence of stratified epithelium with a well-developed and (at least almost) continuous layer of flattened cells containing keratohyalin granules and transforming into soft epidermal-type horny material. Epidermoid cysts may contain considerable melanin in heavily pigmented individuals. Progressive darkening of cysts without increase of general skin color has been reported as a sign of hemochromatosis.[8]

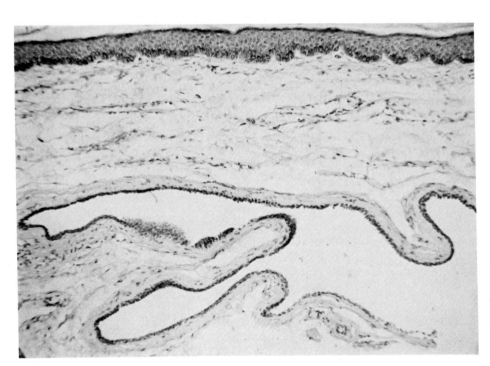

FIGURE 37–2.
Eccrine hidrocystoma. Collapse of the ruptured cyst gives the false impression of papilliferous projections of the wall, which is lined by two rows of flat or cuboid cells. H&E. X135.

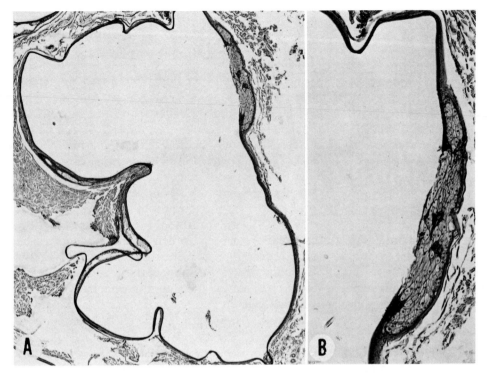

FIGURE 37–3.
*Steatocystoma multiplex. The contents of the cyst consisting of a soft mixture of keratinous flakes and sebum have disappeared during preparation of the paraffin sections. **A.** H&E. X27. **B.** Detail of part of wall in which sebaceous cells border lumen. Rest of cyst wall consists of stratified epithelium. H&E. X73.*

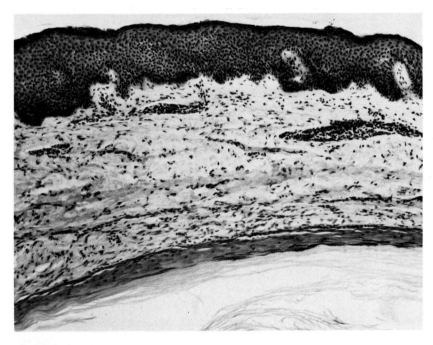

FIGURE 37–4.
Part of wall of an epidermoid cyst in comparison with epidermis. Cyst consists of flat basal and squamous cells with thin granular layer and flaky epidermoid keratin. H&E. × 135.

Eruptive Vellus Hair Cysts

Hyperpigmented papular eruption over the chest wall or extremities of children is the clinical manifestation of eruptive vellus hair cysts.[9,10] Cystic dilated vellus hair follicles are present in mid-dermis containing keratinous material and thin hair shafts. Breakdown of the cyst wall gives rise to foreign-body granuloma. Some lesions regress spontaneously (Fig. 37–5).

Trichilemmal Cysts

The other type of keratinous cyst has been recognized as having its prototype in the outer root sheath (trichilemma) at the level of the follicular isthmus and in the sac surrounding the lower end of the catagen and telogen hair (Fig. 2–30) which produces the hair club.[11,12] Thus, trichilemmal cyst is the new term to replace the misnomer "sebaceous cyst." Trichilemmal cysts (Fig. 37–6) are common, most frequently encountered on the scalp, and have a tough stratified lining resting on a well-developed, but usually not thick, basement membrane which permits one to shell them out without breaking the wall. Histologically, in young cysts, the epithelium consists of large, rather pale-staining cells which do not flatten but become more bulky toward the inside. The large vesicular nucleus fades, and the cell joins the dense central mass of keratin. Keratohyalin usually is absent but may occur in occasional cells. There is a characteristic interlocking of nucleated and keratinized cells similar to that seen in the formation of the club hair. Cell boundaries of complicated pattern can be demonstrated by PAS stain. In older cysts, the epithelium may be flattened and the boundary between wall and contents more smooth. The dense keratin often breaks down into granular masses and may calcify. If the wall ruptures, foreign-body granulation tissue may replace it partly or completely. Cutaneous horn that is made up of dense keratotic material with the base showing trichilemmal keratinization may represent a trichilemmal cyst that has opened to the surface and should be differentiated from a horn developing over a trichilemoma.[13]

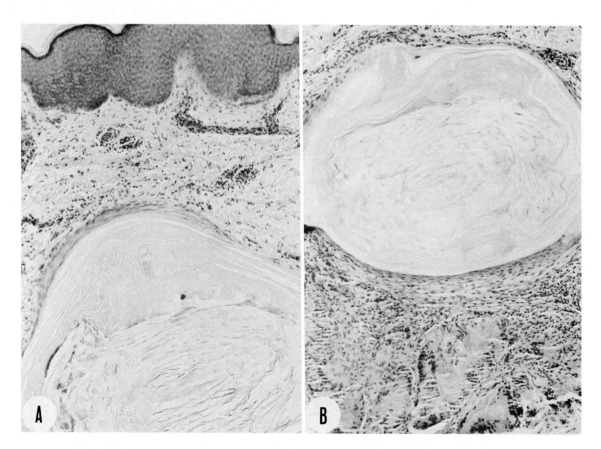

FIGURE 37–5.
Eruptive vellus hair cyst is a follicular retention cyst. **A.** *Cross sections of coiled-up vellus hair in cyst.* **B.** *Foreign-body granuloma below cyst. H&E. X125.*

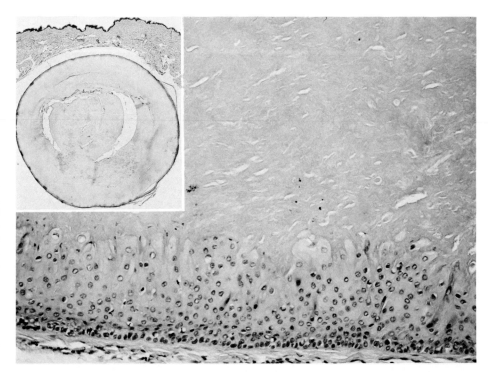

FIGURE 37–6.
Trichilemmal cyst. Inset shows the entire cyst in typical location in the deep dermis and below. The main picture shows part of the thick wall consisting of stratified epithelium. The cells get larger toward the lumen and fade individually into the dense keratinized mass without formation of keratohyalin. A few remnants of nuclei survive. Compare with Figure 2–30, cross section of catagen hair club. H&E. X5, X250.

Proliferating Trichilemmal Cyst (Pilar Tumor)

While we have listed this tumor in the classification of the follicular neoplasms (Table 36–1), we have elected to discuss it in this chapter. We have observed histologic indication that inflammation due to rupture of the wall of a trichilemmal cyst sets into motion a new proliferative cycle leading to the formation of a lobulated lesion.

Proliferating trichilemmal cysts are usually large intracutaneous multilobulated nodules or exophytic lesions, which have been described under various names.[14–17] Large infiltrative lesions may lead to areas of alopecia. Histologically (Fig. 37–7), massive proliferation of follicular sheath epithelium occupies a major portion of the dermis and extends into the subcutaneous fat tissue.[18] There are many central areas of trichilemmal keratinization and keratin cyst formation. Some areas may consist of

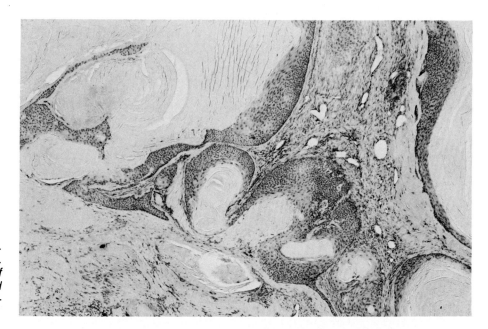

FIGURE 37–7.
Proliferating trichilemmal cyst. Part of large tumor is shown. Secondary cysts form in wall of larger ones, break down, and disappear with foreign-body reaction. H&E. X54.

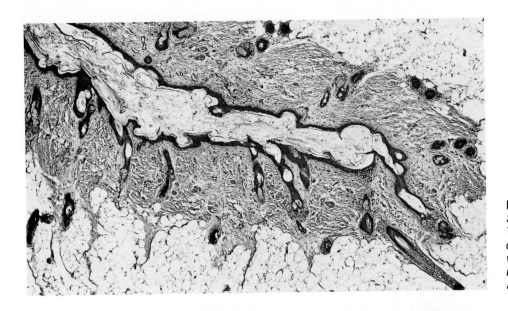

FIGURE 37–8.
Small dermoid cyst of ovary. The lining of the cyst consists of epidermislike epithelium from which cutaneous adnexa grow into the surrounding dermis and fat tissue. H&E. X5.

proliferating, glycogen-laden clear cells resembling the outer root sheath epithelium.[19] Abnormally large cells with hyperchromatic nuclei may give the impression of dysplasia. PAS-positive basement membrane is preserved in many areas. Fibrovascular proliferation and foci of foreign-body granuloma are present.

Other Types

True *dermoid cysts* (Fig. 37–8) usually localized in the subcutis[20] are rarely encountered in dermatologic practice. We mentioned that steatocystoma multiplex may be of this type. Whether the forma-

tion of a well-developed papillary body with epithelial ridges and vascular papillae constitutes evidence of dermoid remains questionable. Small hair follicles, sebaceous lobules, and, occasionally, sweat ducts may be present in the cyst wall.

Solitary and multilobulated cystic lesions in the lower extremities of women in their second or third decades of life occur in deep dermis or subcutaneous fat tissue lined by a simple columnar ciliated epithelium and have been described as cutaneous ciliated cyst.[21,22] An embryonal developmental defect of the male genitalia is median raphe cysts near the glans penis. The cystic spaces are lined by pseudostratified columnar epithelium of one to four cells in thickness.[23] Sinuses containing intes-

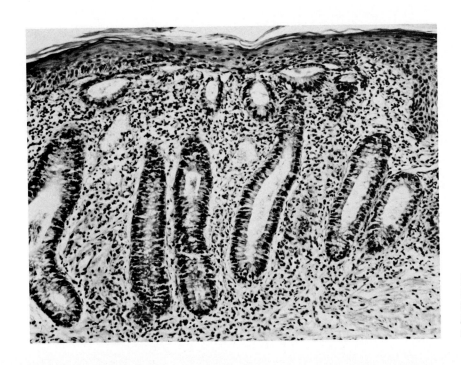

FIGURE 37–9.
Omphaloenteric polyp. Glandlike structures lined with intestinal crypt epithelium beneath epidermoid surface in an umbilical polyp. H&E. X150.

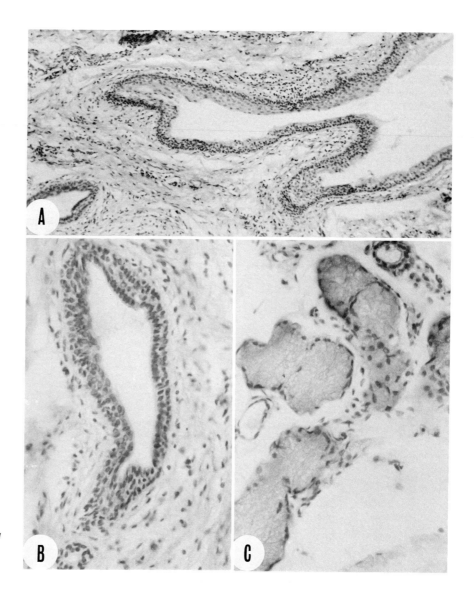

FIGURE 37–10.
Bronchogenic cyst. Pseudostratified epithelium and mucous cells. H&E.
A. *X125.* **B.** *and* **C.** *X250.*

tinal mucosa (Fig. 37–9) occur in the umbilicus as remnants of the omphaloenteric canal. Over the manubrium, one encounters occasional bronchogenic cysts (Fig. 37–10), which are lined with pseudostratified, ciliated epithelium containing goblet cells.[24] Smooth muscle, seromucous glands, and, rarely, lymphoid nodules and cartilage may be present. Branchial cleft cyst shows a lining of stratified squamous epithelium and often lymphoid structures. The occurrence of endometriosis in the skin should also be mentioned.[25]

REFERENCES

1. Smith JD, Chernosky ME: Hidrocystomas. Arch Dermatol 108:676, 1973
2. Mehregan AH: Apocrine cystadenoma. Arch Dermatol 90:274, 1964
3. Kligman AM: The myth of the sebaceous cyst. Arch Dermatol 89:253, 1964
4. Abdel-Aziz AM, El Khashab MM: Steatocystoma multiplex: histologic studies and histogenesis. J Egypt Med Assoc 55:292, 1972
5. Egbert BM, Price NM, Segal RJ: Steatocystoma multiplex. Report of a florid case and a review. Arch Dermatol 115:334, 1979
6. Kligman AM, Kirschbaum J: Steatocystoma multiplex: a dermoid tumor. J Invest Dermatol 42:383, 1964
7. Pinkus H: Epidermoid cysts or epidermal inclusion cysts? Arch Dermatol 111:130, 1975
8. Leyden JJ, Lockshin NA, Kriebel S: The black keratinous cyst: a sign of hemochromatosis. Arch Dermatol 106:379, 1972
9. Esterly NB, Fretzin DF, Pinkus H: Eruptive vellus hair cysts. Arch Dermatol 113:500, 1977
10. Bovenmyer DA: Eruptive vellus hair cysts. Arch Dermatol 115:338, 1979
11. Holmes EJ: Tumors of the lower hair sheath: common histogenesis of certain so-called "sebaceous cysts," acanthomas and "sebaceous carcinomas." Cancer 21:234, 1968
12. Pinkus H: "Sebaceous cysts" are trichilemmal cysts. Arch Dermatol 99:554, 1969
13. Brownstein MH: Trichilemmal horn: Cutaneous

horn showing trichilemmal keratinization. Arch Dermatol 114:1831, 1978

14. Wilson-Jones E: Proliferating epidermoid cysts. Arch Dermatol 94:11, 1966
15. Dabska M: Giant hair matrix tumor. Cancer 28:701, 1971
16. Yoshikawa K, Nakanishi A: A proliferating trichilemmal cyst on the back. J Dermatol (Tokyo) 5:279, 1978
17. Stranc MF, Bennet MH, Mehmed EP: Pilar tumour of the scalp developing in hereditary sebaceous cysts. Br J Plast Surg 24:82, 1971
18. Rahbari H, Mehregan AH: Benign follicular neoplasia. J Dermatol Surg Oncol 5:295, 1979
19. Mehregan AH, Hardin I: Generalized follicular hamartoma. Arch Dermatol 107:435, 1973
20. Brownstein MH, Helwig EB: Subcutaneous dermoid cysts. Arch Dermatol 107:237, 1973
21. Farmer ER, Helwig EB: Cutaneous ciliated cysts. Arch Dermatol 114:70, 1978
22. Clark JV: Cutaneous ciliated cysts. Arch Dermatol 114:1246, 1978
23. Asarch RG, Golitz LE, Sausker WF, Kraye SM: Median raphe cysts of the penis. Arch Dermatol 115:1084, 1979
24. Fraga S, Helwig EB, Rosen SH: Bronchogenic cysts in skin and subcutaneous tissue. Am J Clin Pathol 56:230, 1971
25. Premalatha S, Augustine SM, Thambia AS: Umbilical endometrioma. Clin Exp Dermatol 3:35, 1978

CHAPTER

38

Sweat Apparatus Tumors

With tumors related to sweat glands, our ability to diagnose and classify is taxed by several complications. Many of these tumors were recognized and named before a distinction between eccrine and apocrine glands had been established. Various authors used different principles of classification or did not bother with classification at all when they chose their names. The morphology encountered in sweat apparatus tumors is bewildering in its variability, and, finally, the criteria considered significant for classification are not fully agreed on.

In trying to organize the field on a biologic basis according to modern standards, we are using the term *sweat apparatus* for all parts of the gland: secretory, ductal, and poral. This is necessary because the old classification of tumors of the duct (syringadenomas) and of the coil (spiradenomas) does not take into consideration that a good portion of the eccrine coil also consists of duct and does not make allowance for the specific properties of the intraepithelial duct. Next, it is undeniable for anyone acquainted with principles of terminology that *hidradenoma* means sweat adenoma and, therefore, stands for benign sweat apparatus tumor in a general sense. Hidradenoma cannot be used for any particular tumor without adding a qualifying adjective, be it in the classic Latin form or in modern French or English, e.g., hidradenoma papilliferum, hidradénome éruptif, nodular hidradenoma. Other names that have been generally accepted, e.g., syringoma, eccrine spiradenoma, and eccrine poroma, may well be continued in use if their meaning is

clearly understood as designating certain types of hidradenoma and not being outside the limits of that general term. We discourage, however, the growing tendency to describe and name every new hidradenoma because of minor variation and will attempt a classification on sound general principles.

We therefore use the same two principles we outlined for sebaceous tumors: degree of maturation and morphologic resemblance to normal parts of the sweat apparatus, after first sorting out eccrine from apocrine tumors, inasmuch as these two types of glands are distinct in embryologic origin, anatomic structure, and secretory function (Table 38–1).

However, such an attempt meets obstacles in the unusually great variability of morphologic expression in sweat apparatus tumors and in the lack of agreement on valid criteria for the definition of eccrine or apocrine nature. Thus, while distribution of syringomas and cylindromas in areas of potential apocrine distribution (Fig. 38–1) and their absence in areas where apocrine glands are practically never found seemed to be fair evidence for their relation to apocrine glands, recent histochemical and electron microscopic studies favor an eccrine nature. More about this will be said later.

SWEAT GLAND NEVI

Hyperplasia of mature eccrine or apocrine glands in a localized area constitute a sweat gland nevus. *Ec-*

TABLE 38–1.
Classification of Sweat Apparatus Nevi and Tumors

Level of Maturation	Eccrine	Debated	Apocrine
Malformation	Eccrine nevus		Apocrine nevus

Adenomatous	Hidrocystoma
	Syringocystadenoma
	  papilliferum
	Papillary eccrine
	  adenoma
	Eccrine poroma
	Dermal duct tumor
	Nodular hidradenoma
	Eccrine spiradenoma
			Apocrine cystadenoma
			Syringocystadenoma
			  papilliferum
			Tubular apocrine
			  adenoma
			Hidradenoma
			  papilliferum of
			  vulva

Epitheliomatous	Hidroacanthoma
	  simplex
	Mixed tumor of skin
	Clear cell
	  hidradenoma
		Syringoma
		Cylindroma	

Carcinomatous	Eccrine
	  adenocarcinoma
			Apocrine
			  adenocarcinoma
			Extramammary Paget's
			  disease

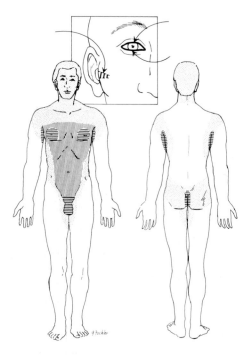

FIGURE 38–1.
Diagram of apocrine gland distribution. Heavily shaded areas—genitoanal, axillary, perimammary, periocular, auditory canal—regularly have well-developed apocrine glands. Lightly shaded area is axillary-pubic triangle in which accessory mammae are most often found. Stippled areas are those in which most people are apt to have some apocrine glands. Rest of skin surface never or rarely develops them. (From Pinkus. In Jadassohn. Handbuch der Haut-und Geschlechtskrankheiten, Ergänzungswerk 1, 2, 1965. Courtesy of Springer-Verlag.)

crine nevus[1] is rare and can be manifest as an area of hyperhidrosis. (Fig. 38–2). A very rare lesion is pure *apocrine nevus*.[2] Apocrine hyperplasia occurs within an organoid nevus, and lesions of this type have been reported as apocrine nevus.[3]

Supernumerary Nipple. Supernumerary nipple (polythelia) usually appears along the embryonic milk lines which run from the anterior axillary fold to the inner thighs. It may be single or multiple and can occasionally occur in other locations. The lesion usually is a light brown nodule often associated with hairs. Histologically (Fig. 38–3), it shows a corrugated pattern of epidermis over a central pilosebaceous structure. In the dermis are a number of smooth muscles and sometimes mammary glands.

APOCRINE TUMORS

Apocrine Cystadenoma

The cystic nodular lesion of apocrine cystadenoma appears most commonly over the face and occasionally elsewhere.[4–8] The growth may be skin color or deeply pigmented, resembling a blue nevus or a pigmented basal cell epithelioma. Histologically (Fig. 38–4), multiple cystic spaces containing secretory material are present in the dermis. Deep cystic spaces are lined with apocrine-type secretory epithelium of high columnar cells with basilar nuclei

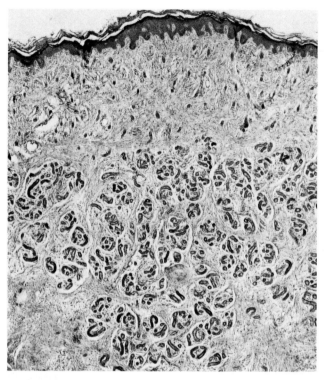

FIGURE 38–2.
Eccrine nevus (nevus sudoriparus). Increased number and size of structurally normal eccrine apparatuses. Epidermis slightly papillomatous. H&E. X60.

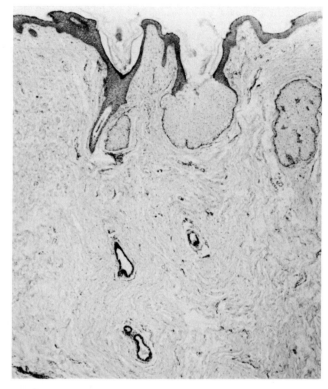

FIGURE 38–3.
Supernumerary nipple. Hair follicles, free sebaceous glands, and milk ducts in the dermis which contains multiple strands of smooth muscle. H&E. X25.

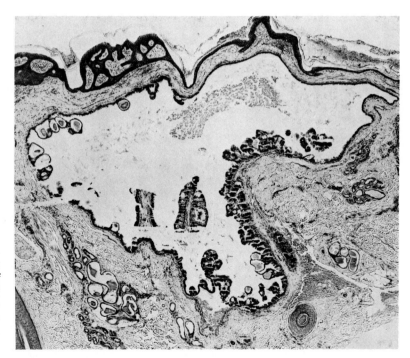

FIGURE 38–4.
Apocrine cystadenoma developed in organoid nevus. Apocrine and eccrine coils are present near tumor, which consists mainly of two-layered epithelium lining a large cyst and papilliferous projections into lumen. Papillomatous epidermal lesion is part of the preexistent nevus. H&E. X30. (From Mehregan. Arch Dermatol 90:274, 1964.)

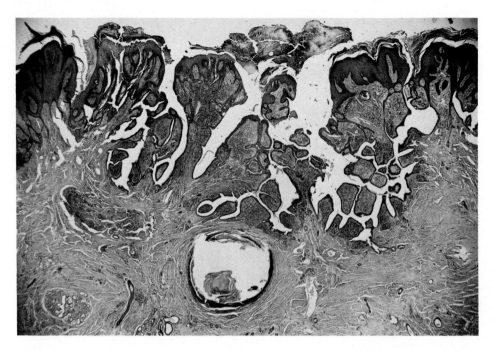

FIGURE 38–5.
Syringocystadenoma papilliferum developed in organoid nevus. Apocrine duct (arrow) opens into a sinus in lower right corner. Multiple papilliferous sinuses open to surface. Normal and atypical apocrine glands are present below tumor and are part of preexistent nevus. Keratinized cyst in lower center may be follicular retention cyst. H&E. X30.

resting over an outer layer of elongated myoepithelial cells.[9] Small papillomatous projections of secretory epithelium extend into the central cavity. Superficial cysts are lined by a thin layer of ductal epithelium. Lipochrome granules present in the cytoplasm of high columnar cells and in the secretory material inside the cysts are most likely responsible for the deep pigmentation of some lesions.[10]

Syringadenoma Papilliferum

Syringadenoma papilliferum occurs most commonly on the scalp over a preexisting organoid nevus but may also appear by itself and elsewhere.[11,12] Papilliferous and tubular structures (Fig. 38–5) extend from the surface into the dermis surrounded by fibrovascular stroma that contains an unusually

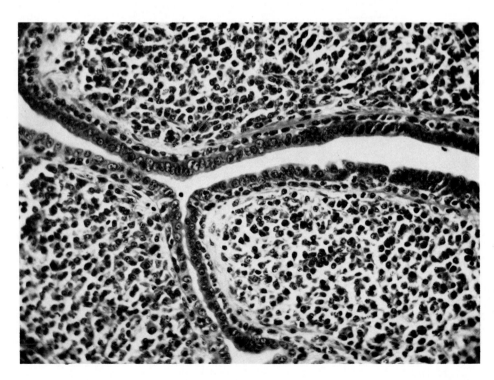

FIGURE 38–6.
Cellular details of papilliferous syringocystadenoma. Lumen-lining columnar or cuboidal cells rest on outer layer of flat epithelial cells. Stroma contains many plasma cells. H&E. X280.

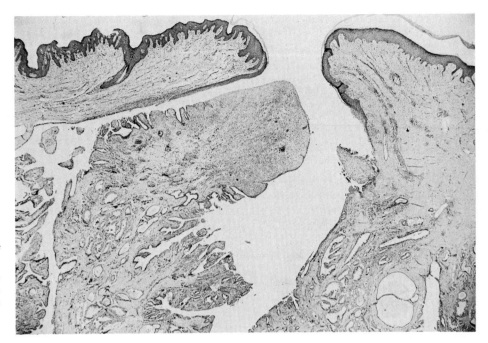

FIGURE 38–7.
Hidradenoma papilliferum of vulva. Large sinus filled with, and surrounded by, adenomatous tissue. Epithelial cells appear light because they have eosinophilic cytoplasm. H&E. X30.

large number of plasma cells.[13,14] The epithelial lining usually consists of high columnar luminal cells resting on a row of flat or cuboidal cells (Fig. 38–6).

Hidradenoma of Vulva (Hidradenoma Papilliferum)

This freely movable nodular lesion of vulva may show superficial erosion and moisture, suggesting active secretion.[15,16] Microscopically (Fig. 38–7), numerous papilliferous projections lined by high col-

umnar apocrine-type secretory epithelium extend from the wall of the cyst into the central cavity.[17]

Tubular Apocrine Adenoma

A well-defined, solitary, intracutaneous, nodular growth is histologically distinctive by the presence of cystic dilated tubular structures surrounded by fibrovascular stroma.[18] In the lining of the tubular structures is an inner layer of columnar cells resting over an outer layer of flattened or cuboidal cells and a basement membrane (Fig. 38–8). The enzyme

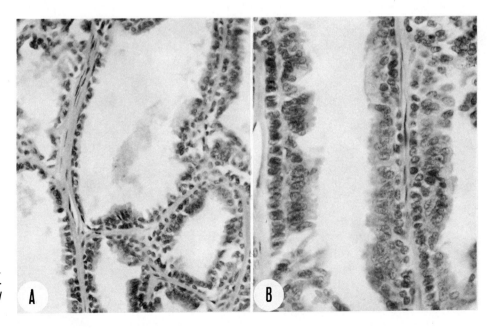

FIGURE 38–8.
*Tubular apocrine adenoma. Two rows of cells line basement membrane. H&E. **A** and **B.** X250.*

pattern and electron microscopic findings suggest apocrine differentiation.[19]

Erosive Adenomatosis of the Nipple

This lesion, also called *florid papillomatosis of the nipple ducts*, shows nodular enlargement of the nipple with superficial erosions and blood-stained or serous discharge.[20,21] The growth is well defined and shows numerous branching ducts and glandular structures extending from the surface deep into the dermis (Fig. 38–9). The papillary structures are lined by an inner layer of columnar cells and an outer layer of flattened or cuboidal cells resting on the basement membrane.[22]

Cutaneous Cylindroma

As the epitheliomatous representative of apocrine tumors, we discuss here with deliberation the cutaneous cylindroma. This tumor (Fig. 38–10) is not related to malignant cylindromatous tumors of other organs. Its name is old and derived from the hyalin sheaths which remained after maceration, one of the favorite methods of nineteenth century pathologists. After Spiegler's view that these "turban tumors" are endotheliomas had been replaced by recognition of their epithelial nature, discussions were centered for many years on their relation to either hair follicle or apocrine gland. Some years ago, their eccrine derivation was championed on the basis of histochemical evidence.[23]

It is our opinion that histochemical evidence

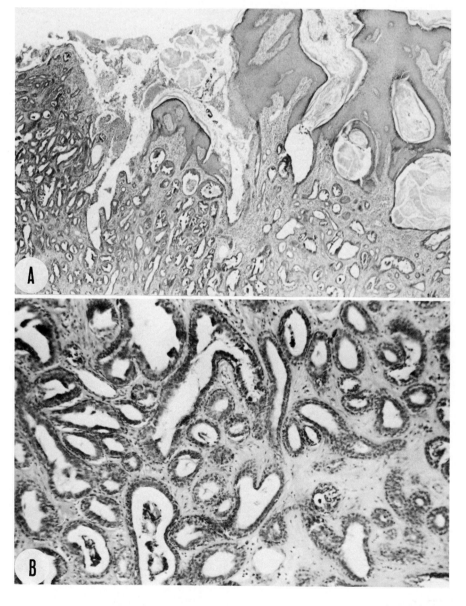

FIGURE 38–9.
Erosive adenomatosis of nipple. Similar to Figure 38–5, but no plasma cell infiltrate. H&E. **A.** *X45.* **B.** *X125.*

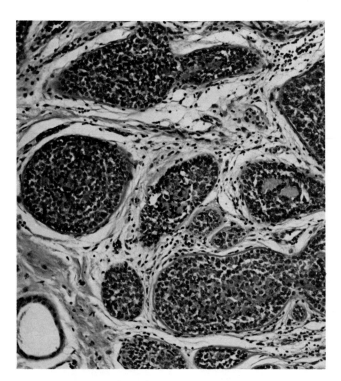

FIGURE 38–10.
Cutaneous cylindroma. In this case, intralobular hyaline clumps are more prominent than hyaline sheaths. Dilated duct in lower left corner is not part of the tumor. H&E. X135.

(enzyme signature) is not as stringent in the field of cutaneous neoplasia as it is claimed to be, and that is particularly true in deciding between the eccrine and apocrine nature of a tumor. The most basic feature of neoplastic growth is heritable disturbance of cellular metabolism (Fig. VII–2), and all metabolism involves enzymes. Presence or absence of gland-specific enzymes cannot be made the sole criterion of the direction of maturation in a tumor. We only have to think of the not uncommon production of ectopic hormones by lung and other carcinomas, a process that obviously involves enzyme aberrations. It appears quite possible that in those tumors, in which cellular morphology and other physiologic phenomena are so altered that our older histopathologic procedures gave equivocal results, enzyme histochemistry may meet a similar fate. Moreover, the absence of enzyme activity in a certain normal tissue usually is not absolute. For instance, apocrine secretory epithelium may show spotty reactivity for phosphorylase. In addition, the relatively few enzyme studies of apocrine duct have shown all the so-called eccrine enzymes to be present.[24]

Although we favor classifying skin tumors mainly by the direction of their differentiation (introduction to Sec. VII), it seems more rational in this in-

stance to base conclusions on a combination of all available embryologic, anatomic, and biologic evidence, and all these point toward the relation of cylindroma to the pilar apparatus. Cylindromas are most common on the scalp where pilary complexes are most numerous, and where occasional apocrine glands are known to occur (Fig. 38–1). They are absent in the eccrine territory of palms and soles but have been described in the external ear canal, one of the few regions where eccrine glands are lacking and hair follicles and apocrine (ceruminous) glands are present. Actually, the main features of cylindroma speak for its relation to both hair follicle and apocrine gland, the occasional lumina for the latter, while the hyaline sheaths resemble the vitreous membrane of the hair root. Formation of hyalin droplets within the tumor substance has its prototype in similar droplets occasionally found in bulge proliferations. The not infrequent association of trichoepitheliomas of the face and cylindromas of the scalp point to predisposition to pilary complex hamartomas in these patients, and there are cases on record where both components were combined in the same sumor.[25] Cutaneous cylindromas may well be an example of a pilar apparatus tumor of a fairly low level of maturity.

Cutaneous cylindroma may be a solitary lesion or multiple nodular or exophytic growths involving the scalp and forehead in turban areas (turban tumors[26]). Histologically, solid masses of small basaloid cells are closely applied to one another like pieces of a jigsaw puzzle[27] (Fig. 38–11). The tumor

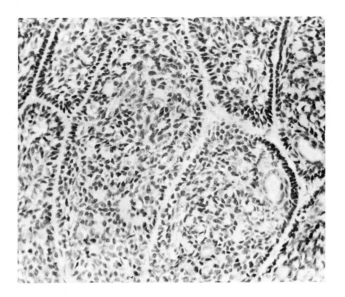

FIGURE 38–11.
Cutaneous cylindroma. Small basaloid cells and occasional ductlike lumina (at right). Light areas between cells contain hyaline material. The scant stroma between tumor lobes does not exhibit hyalinization. H&E. X125.

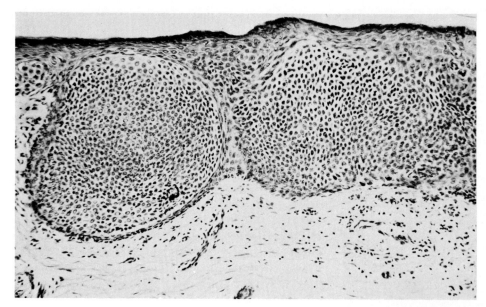

FIGURE 38–12.
Hidroacanthoma simplex. Intraepidermal nests of poroma-like cells (Fig. 38–13) are sharply delineated around their entire periphery and are in cytoplasmic (desmosomal) contact with surrounding epidermal keratinocytes in many places. H&E. X180.

lobules are surrounded by a layer of hyaline sheath and show globes of hyalin among the basaloid cells. There are occasional sweat glandular lumen formations.[28] Multiple cylindromas can occur with multiple trichoepitheliomas as a dominantly inherited trait.[29,30] Malignant degeneration of cylindroma can occur, leading to invasion of subcutaneous tissues or distant metastasis.[31–33]

ECCRINE TUMORS

Hidroacanthoma Simplex

This is a superficial eccrine neoplasm clinically resembling a flat type of seborrheic verruca or a plaque of Bowen's disease.[34] Histologically (Fig. 38–12), there are well-defined islands of small and uniform basaloid cells in the confines of an acanthotic epidermis.[35] The tumor cells contain glycogen granules and are well defined from the surrounding epidermal keratinocytes.

Eccrine Poroma and Dermal Duct Tumor

Eccrine poroma has become the accepted name for benign tumors (Fig. 38–13) which manifest ductal as well as keratinizing epidermoid maturation similar to the epithelium of the sweat pore (acrosyringium, eccrine epidermal sweat duct unit).[36] While they are most common on the nonhairy parts of the foot, they have been found in most regions of the body surface, hairy or nonhairy.[37] They are almost always single, but cases of eccrine poromatosis[38–40] have been described in which hundreds of tiny le-

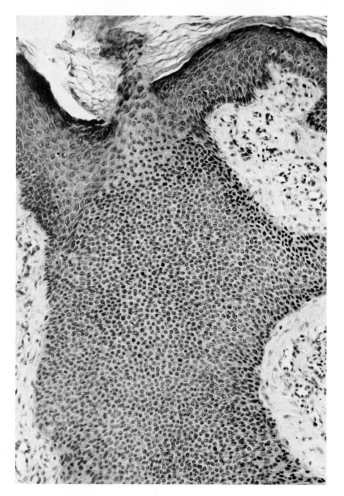

FIGURE 38–13.
Eccrine poroma. Part of a tumor shows even, small epithelial cells without a palisading outer layer. Sharp dividing line between tumor and normal epidermis which it penetrates. Near the skin surface, tumor cells become larger, prickle cell-like and show incomplete keratinization. In other areas, keratohyalin may be formed. H&E. X135.

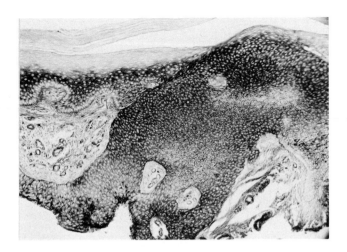

FIGURE 38–14.
Eccrine poroma stained for glycogen shows sharp division between epidermis (no glycogen in basal layer, considerable glycogen in lower prickle cells) and tumor (glycogen in every cell, including peripheral cells). Where tumor reaches the skin surface, it begins to keratinize, and the cells lose their glycogen. PAS-light green. X90. (From Pinkus, Rogin, and Goldman. Arch Dermatol 74:511, 1956. Copyright © 1956 by the American Medical Association.)

sions were present. Typically, they are superficial, often protruding or sessile, but occasionally they may project down into the dermis or form the superficial portion of a nodular hidradenoma.

The degree of organization of eccrine poroma usually is on the epitheliomatous rather than the adenomatous or acanthomatous level. The tumor consists mainly of peculiar small and even epithelial cells with only occasional slitlike or cystic lumina. PAS stain shows abundant glycogen granules in the tumor cells and a sharp line of demarcation between the tumor epithelium and the surrounding epidermis (Fig. 38–14). Tumors of similar structure situated entirely in the dermis (Fig. 38–15) have been described as dermal duct tumor.[41,42] Histochemical and electron microscopic findings suggest differentiation toward the dermal portion of the eccrine sweat duct unit.[43] Occasionally, these tumors may show melanin pigmentation.[44]

Papillary Eccrine Adenoma

Papillary eccrine adenoma is a counterpart of the tubular apocrine adenoma occurring as a solitary nodular lesion over the extremities. Histologically (Fig. 38–16), it is characterized by the presence of cystic dilated and branching ductal structures with areas of papillary projections into the central lumen.[45,46] Ductal structures are lined by an outer layer of flattened or cuboidal cells. The inner cells

may be flattened, cuboidal, or columnar. The central cystic lumen contains an amorphous eosinophilic secretory material.

Syringoma

Another tumor, which formerly was favored to be apocrine and now is considered to be eccrine by many, is the syringoma.[47] Again enzyme histochemistry tipped the balance, and, again, we feel that anatomic and biologic arguments should be given weight. Syringomas occur as multiple, small, skin-colored papules predominantly in orbital skin, an area in which well-developed Moll's glands and rudimentary apocrine glands occur. If the tumors are widespread, they prefer the apocrine triangle between axillae and pubes, including the vulva.[48–50] While they may spread laterally to the flanks, their occurrence on the back of the trunk and the distal extremities is rare. An anatomic relation of syringomatous epithelium to hair follicles has been documented at least as often as connection to the epidermis.[51] Syringomas (Fig. 38–17) are tumors of such variable organization of their epithelial portion, which is capable of producing horny material, foamy cells, and fairly good ductal pictures, that enzymatic derangement is well within

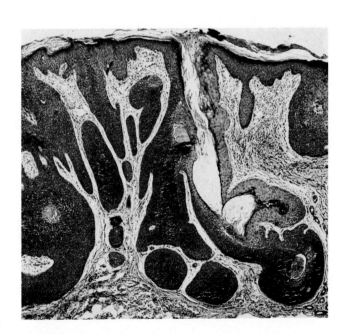

FIGURE 38–15.
Nodular hidradenoma combining features of eccrine poroma and Winkelmann's dermal duct tumor. Note edematous and vascular stroma. Tumor masses are in multiple broad contact with epidermis and a deformed hyperplastic eccrine duct. This cannot be interpreted as denoting origin of neoplasm from either. H&E. X30.

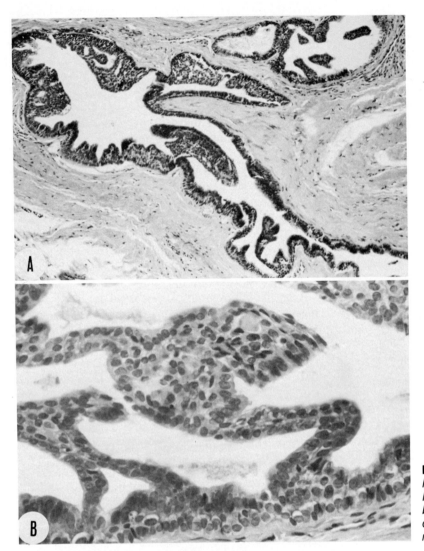

FIGURE 38–16.
Papillary eccrine adenoma. Compare with Figure 38–8. Two or more rows of cells line basement membrane but do not show apocrine configuration. The cells lining the lumen are cuboidal. H&E. **A.** *X125.* **B.** *X250.*

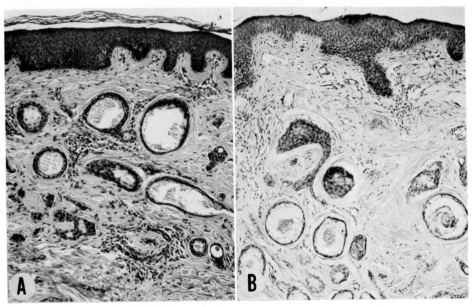

FIGURE 38–17.
Syringoma. Cysts in continuity with solid cords produce tadpole configurations. Most cysts have two-layered walls. The inner cells often have vacuolated cytoplasm resembling sebaceous cells in paraffin sections. In other cases, keratinizing cysts may be present. Deranged structure of the copious stroma is evident. Lymphocytic infiltrate present in **A** *has no significance.* **A** *and* **B.** *H&E. X90.*

the limits of possibility and even probability. Electron microscopic evidence is not applicable until it will have been shown that the apocrine duct is distinctly different from the eccrine duct. Whatever the nature of syringomas will eventually be determined to be, it is well to remember that they are also an outstanding example of the fibroepithelial nature of adnexal tumors. In many papules, specific stromal connective tissue constitutes by far the greater part of the tissue volume. Peculiarly clumped elastic fibers are common in the stromal portion.

Eccrine Spiradenoma

Eccrine spiradenoma provides a good example of a well-defined entity, some variants of which preserve enough tubular structure to impress as adenomas, while most of them have so low an organization that they are on the level of epitheliomas. In some tumors, the stroma is so prominent and vascular that they may be mistaken for hemangiomas or glomangiomas.[52] The term *spiradenoma*, based on Unna's old classification, does not specify ductal or secretory maturation, and the wisdom of this restraint has been shown by electron microscopic investigation.[53] That eccrine spiradenoma usually is situated deep in the skin or in the hypoderm may be taken as additional evidence for its relation to the sweat coil.

The growth is made up of two types of cells. One larger, light-staining cell, closely packed and often surrounding a central lumen, and the other, smaller cell with compact nuclei arranged at the periphery (Fig. 38–18). Malignant transformation of eccrine spiradenoma is a rare occurrence.[54]

Nodular Hidradenoma

Nodular hidradenoma seems to be the most noncommittal and the preferable term for a large group of tumors that have been given different names, *clear cell hidradenoma, solid cystic hidradenoma, eccrine acrospiroma,* according to structure and cellular differentiation and have the basic feature of

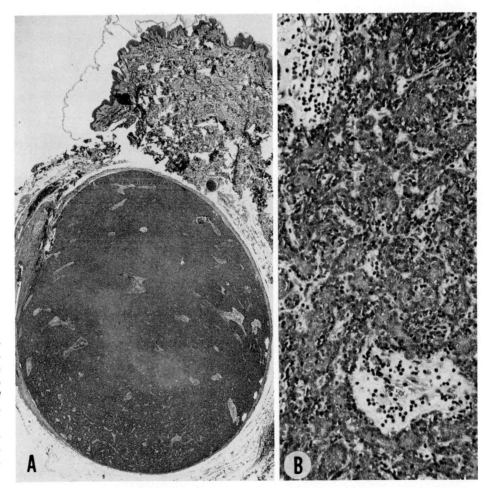

FIGURE 38–18.
*Eccrine spiradenoma. **A.** Typical picture of a well-demarcated tumor in deep dermis and subcutaneous tissue. Note vascular stroma in interior and a few ductlike lumina in periphery of epithelial nodule. H&E. X14. **B.** Two types of epithelial cells form interconnected cords closely interwoven with stroma. H&E. X225.*

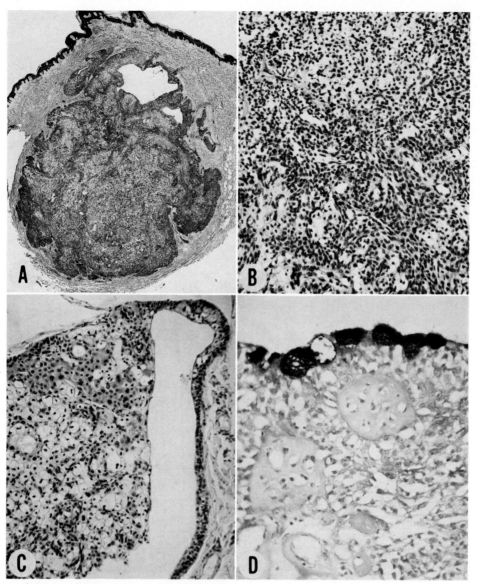

FIGURE 38–19.
Nodular hidradenoma, clear cell type. **A.** *Solid tumor which was connected to epidermis in other parts of block consists of lighter- and darker-staining areas, contains several duct-like lumina, and a few larger cystic spaces (solid-cystic hidradenoma). H&E. X8.* **B** *and* **C.** *Cellular patterns indicating that large clear cells are modifications of smaller cells with more solid cytoplasm. Tumor cells border lumen without arranging themselves into a definite lining; note appearance of goblet cells in right upper corner. H&E. X90.* **D.** *Goblet cells containing PAS-positive material which was found to stain with aldehyde fuchsin and alcian blue, an indication that it is sialomucin. Diastase-digested PAS. Hematoxylin. ×185.*

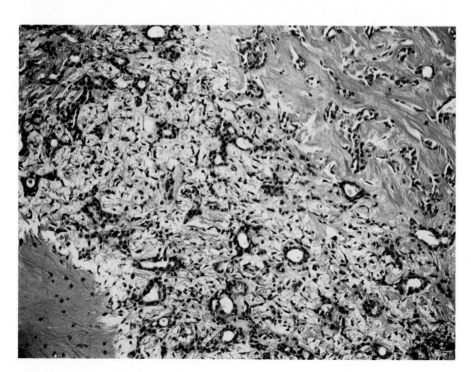

FIGURE 38–20.
Chondroid syringoma (mixed tumor of skin). In this type of tumor, tubular epithelial structures seem to dissolve into individual cells, which eventually are embedded in amorphous metachromatic matrix resembling cartilage, a process also seen in mixed tumors of salivary glands. H&E. X135.

their cells being arranged in solid masses with only occasional organization into lumen-lining order.[55] Lumina may be slitlike or cystic.[56] The tumor cells may have solid (epidermoid) cytoplasm or may be larger clear cells (Fig. 38–19). This last modification may be found in small areas of a tumor or may be widespread (clear cell hidradenoma).[57] Stroma may be scant or copious but does not usually exhibit the maturation encountered in tubular hidradenomas. Therefore, this group of tumors is on a lower (epitheliomatous) level of organization. They often occupy the entire width of the dermis and may be connected to the surface, with the superficial parts resembling eccrine poroma. Electron microscopy has shown that ductal as well as secretory features may be found in the cell.[58] While practically all clear cell hidradenomas are benign, a few malignant tumors have been found in which clear cells predominate.[59]

Chrondroid Syringoma (Mixed Tumor of the Skin)

This cutaneous neoplasm has many structural resemblances to the mixed tumor of salivary glands.[60] The clinical manifestation is a solitary intradermal or subcutaneous firm nodule.

Histologically (Fig. 38–20), the growth is made up of closely packed ductal structures and individual epithelial cells embedded in a distinctively myxomatous stroma which often shows chondroid areas.[61]

REFERENCES

1. Pippione M, Depaoli MA, Sartois S: Nevus eccrine. Dermatologica 152:40, 1976
2. Rabens SF, Naness JI, Gottlieb BF: Apocrine gland organic hamartoma (apocrine nevus). Arch Dermatol 112:520, 1976
3. Civatte J, Tsoïtis G, Préaux J: Le naevus apocrine. Étude de deux cas. Ann Dermatol Syphiligr 101:251, 1974
4. Ahmed A, Jones AW: Apocrine cystadenoma: A report of two cases occurring on the prepuce. Br J Dermatol 81:899, 1969
5. TerPoorten HJ: Apocrine hidrocystoma of the right scapula. Arch Dermatol 113:1730, 1977
6. Powell RF, Palmer CH, Smith EB: Apocrine cystadenoma of the penile shaft. Arch Dermatol 113:1250, 1977
7. Armijo M, De Unamuno P, Herrera E: Cystadénome apocrine. A propos de 3 observations dont une de siège balanique. Ann Dermatol Venereol 105:411, 1978
8. Kruse TV, Khan MA, Hassan MO: Multiple apocrine cystadenomas. Br J Dermatol 100:675, 1979
9. Hassan MO, Khan MA, Kruse TV: Apocrine cystadenoma: an ultrastructural study. Arch Dermatol 115:194, 1979
10. Mehregan AH: Apocrine cystadenoma. Arch Dermatol 90:274, 1964
11. Helwig EB, Hackney VC: Syringadenoma papilliferum lesions with and without naevus sebaceous and basal cell carcinoma. Arch Dermatol Syph 71:361, 1955
12. Rostan SE, Waller JD: Syringocystadenoma papilliferum in an unusual location. Report of a case. Arch Dermatol 112:835, 1976
13. Pinkus H: Life history of naevus syringadenomatosus papilliferus. Arch Dermatol Syph 69:305, 1954
14. Nizuma K: Syringocystadenoma papilliferum. Light and electron microscopic studies. Acta Derm Venereol (Stockh) 56:327, 1976
15. Meeker JH, Neubecker RD, Helwig EB: Hidradenoma papilliferum. Am J Clin Pathol 37:182, 1962
16. Woodworth H Jr, Dockerty MB, Wilson RB, et al.: Papillary hidradenoma of the vulva: A clinicopathologic study of sixty-nine cases. Am J Obstet Gynecol 110:501, 1971
17. Mehregan AH, Rahbari H: Benign epithelial tumors of the skin. IV. Benign apocrine gland tumors. Cutis 21:53, 1978
18. Civatte J, Belaïch S, Lauret P: Adénome tubulaire apocrine (quatre cas). Ann Dermatol Venereol 106:665, 1979
19. Umbert P, Winkelmann RK: Tubular apocrine adenoma. J Cutan Pathol 3:75, 1976
20. Jones DB: Florid papillomatosis of the nipple ducts. Cancer 8:315, 1955
21. Perzin KH, Lattes R: Papillary adenoma of the nipple (Florid papillomatosis, adenoma, adenomatosis). Cancer 29:996, 1972
22. Smith NP, Wilson-Jones E: Erosive adenomatosis of the nipple. Clin Exp Dermatol 2:79, 1977
23. Crain RC, Helwig EB: Dermal cylindroma (dermal eccrine cylindroma). Am J Clin Pathol 35:504, 1961
24. Svob M: Histochemistry of sweat glands. Radovi Akademije Nauka BiH, XLIV 16:71, 1972
25. Pinkus H: Pathobiology of the pilary complex. Jpn J Dermatol [B] 77:304, 1967
26. Reingold IM, Keasbey LE, Graham JH: Multicentric dermal type cylindromas of the parotid glands in a patient with florid turban tumor. Cancer 40:1702, 1977
27. Mehregan AH, Rahbari H: Benign epithelial tumors of the skin. V. Benign eccrine gland tumors. Cutis 23:573, 1979
28. Reynes M, Puissant A, Delanoe J, et al.: Ultrastructural study of cylindroma (Poncet–Spiegler tumor). J Cutan Pathol 3:95, 1976
29. Rasmussen JE: A syndrome of trichoepitheliomas, milia and cylindromas. Arch Dermatol 111:610, 1975
30. Gottschalk HL, Graham JH, Aston EE IV: Dermal eccrine cylindroma, epithelioma adenoides cysticum of Brooke and eccrine spiradenoma. Arch Dermatol 110:473, 1974
31. Lyon JB, Rouillard LM: Malignant degeneration of turban tumor of the scalp. Trans St Johns Hosp Dermatol Soc 46:74, 1961
32. Korting GW: Maligne entarteter Spiegler tumor. Dermatol Monatsschr 156:141, 1970
33. Tsambaos D, Greither A, Orfanos CE: Multiple malignant Spiegler tumors with brachydactyly and racket-

nails. Light and electron microscopic study. J Cutan Pathol 6:31, 1979

34. Mehregan AH, Levson DN: Hidroacanthoma simplex: a report of two cases. Arch Dermatol 100:303, 1969

35. Smith JLS, Coburn JG: Hidroacanthoma simplex: assessment of selected group of intraepidermal basal cell epitheliomata and of their malignant homologues. Br J Dermatol 68:400, 1956

36. Pinkus H, Rogin JR, Goldman P: Eccrine poroma: tumors exhibiting features of epidermal sweat duct unit. Arch Dermatol 74:511, 1956

37. Pinkus H: The discovery of eccrine poroma. Dermatology 2 (2):26, 1979

38. Goldner R: Eccrine poromatosis. Arch Dermatol 101:606, 1970

39. Ogino A: Linear eccrine poroma. Arch Dermatol 112:841, 1976

40. Wilkinson RD, Schopflocher P, Rozenfeld M: Hidrotic ectodermal dysplasia with diffuse eccrine poromatosis. Arch Dermatol 113:472, 1977

41. Winkelmann RK, McLeod WA: The dermal duct tumor. Arch Dermatol 94:50, 1966

42. Apisarnthanarax P, Mullins JF: Dermal duct tumor. Arch Dermatol 111:1171, 1975

43. Hu C-H, Marques AS, Winkelmann RK: Dermal duct tumor. A histochemical and electron microscopic study. Arch Dermatol 114:1659, 1978

44. Wilson-Jones E: Pigmented nodular hidradenoma. Arch Dermatol 104:117, 1971

45. Rulon DB, Helwig EB: Papillary eccrine adenoma. Arch Dermatol 113:596, 1977

46. Elpern DJ, Farmer ER: Papillary eccrine adenoma. Arch Dermatol 114:1241, 1978

47. Winkelmann RK, Gottlieb BE: Syringoma: an enzymatic study. Cancer 16:665, 1963

48. Brown SM, Freeman RG: Syringoma limited to the vulva. Arch Dermatol 104:331, 1971

49. Carneiro SJC, Gardner HL, Knox JM: Syringomas: Three cases with vulvar involvement. Obstet Gynecol 39:93, 1972

50. Thomas J, Majumdar B, Gorelkin L: Syringoma localized to the vulva. Arch Dermatol 115:95, 1979

51. Daiker B: Das Lidsyringom; Studien über seinen geweblichen Aufbau und seine Histogenese. Dermatologica 128:417, 1964

52. Kersting DW, Helwig EB: Eccrine spiradenoma. Arch Dermatol 73:199, 1956

53. Hashimoto K, Gross BG, Nelson RG, et al.: Eccrine spiradenoma. Histochemical and electronmicroscopic studies. J Invest Dermatol 46:347, 1966

54. Evans HL, Su WPD, Smith JL, Winkelmann RK: Carcinoma arising in eccrine spiradenoma. Cancer 43:1881, 1979

55. Johnson BL Jr, Helwig EB: Eccrine acrospiroma: a clinicopathologic study. Cancer 23:641, 1969

56. Winkelmann RK, Wolff K: Solid-cystic hidradenoma of the skin. Clinical and histopathologic study. Arch Dermatol 97:651, 1968

57. Brownstein MH, Shapiro L: The sweat gland adenomas. Int J Dermatol 14:397, 1975

58. Hashimoto K, DiBella RJ, Lever WF: Clear cell hidradenoma: histological, histochemical, and electron microscopic studies. Arch Dermatol 96:18, 1967

59. Headington JT, Niederhuber JE, Beals TF: Malignant clear cell acrospiroma. Cancer 41:641, 1978

60. Hirsch P, Helwig EB: Chondroid syringoma: mixed tumor of skin, salivary gland type. Arch Dermatol 84:835, 1971

61. Hernandez FJ: Mixed tumors of the skin of the salivary gland type. A light and electron microscopic study. J Invest Dermatol 66:49, 1976

39

Basal Cell Epithelioma

It was indicated in Table VII–1 that basal cell epithelioma is the least mature member of the large tribe of organoid adnexal tumors. It is found at the bottom of the tabulation below all the columns of the different adnexal maturations and comprises all tumors that do not have morphologic differentiating characters of one type or other. The fact that some basal cell epitheliomas have a few rudimentary foci of differentiation, such as small keratinizing foci or a few lipocytes, and that their peripheral cells often have palisading arrangement indicates the relationship. We emphasize that we talk about diagnostic criteria and systematics of classification.[1] We do not mean to say that a sebaceous adenoma or a benign hair follicle tumor often progresses to basal cell epithelioma. This may occur rarely, as discussed under sebaceous epithelioma and trichoepithelioma (Chaps. 35 and 36).

The most important point of this discussion is the sharp dividing line it makes between the two most common types of skin carcinoma. We have outlined the progression of epidermal precancerosis to invasive squamous cell carcinoma in Chapter 34, and we spoke about cancerization of individual squamous cells. A squamous cell carcinoma (or adnexal carcinomas, to be discussed in the next chapter) is a "carcinoma" to the general pathologist and is capable of individual cell metastasis.

The basal cell cancer, to which we, therefore, apply the term *basal cell epithelioma*[2] (or *basalioma*), is, on the contrary, a fibroepithelial tumor that consists, as do all benign adnexal tumors, of epithelial parenchyma interdependent with mesodermal stroma. This interdependence makes epithelial cell metastasis a very rare event and leads to various morphologic features important in diagnosis. Our whole presentation of basal cell epithelioma will be based on this concept.

We must train our eyes and our minds to consider the outer, peripheral border of a basal cell epithelioma not to coincide with the periphery of the epithelial part but with the periphery of its stroma. This concept is demonstrated in Figure 39–1, where the normal epidermal and adnexal basal cell is shown closely united with its stromal counterpart. Benign epidermoid and adnexal tumor cells, including basalioma cells, preserve this interdependence, while carcinomas of epidermis and of adnexa have lost it and devour stroma (the action of a tumor angiogenesis factor is present in both types of tumor and does not affect this discussion).

There is no doubt that basaliomas are destructive, locally malignant tumors. This is expressed in an almost obligatory association of the hallmark of malignancy in the skin: a focal lymphocytic infiltrate often containing plasma cells. The important point to remember is the interdependence of epithelial and stromal components that is practically never mentioned in descriptions in articles and textbooks.

We describe basal cell epitheliomas (Fig. 39–2) as tumors consisting of nests, cords, or masses of

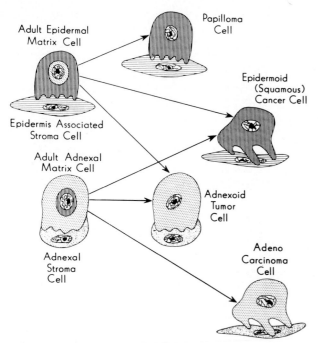

FIGURE 39–1.
Diagram illustrating contrast between fibroepithelial (benign and basaliomatous) neoplasia and destructive carcinomatous neoplasia. Either type can originate in epidermal or adnexal matrix cells but, once established, is differentiated and inexorably committed to formation of its specific type of tumor cell. Normal matrix cells, on the other hand, are pluripotential. (Compare with Fig. 2–13.)

small, dark-staining epithelial cells and of an envelope of specific mesodermal stroma. Interaction between the two components often is expressed in polar arrangement of the peripheral epithelial cells (palisading), the existence of a PAS-positive basement membrane, and elaboration of specific mesodermal products, most commonly collagenous and mucinous in character, occasionally elastic fibers. An inflammatory infiltrate consisting of small round cells and sometimes plasma cells is an al-

most obligatory feature, denoting local malignancy and separating basal cell epitheliomas from trichoepitheliomas and other benign adnexoid tumors. The advancing edge of basaliomatous structures may fuse with, and eventually destroy, epidermis, hair follicles, and glands. Pictures of this type (Figs. 39–3, 39–6, and 39–9) have been interpreted only too often as showing points of origin of the epithelioma. Application of the rules of biologic growth makes one realize that the point of origin of most tumors, just as that of a bacterial or fungal colony, is near their center and certainly not in their advancing edge. It is, moreover, inconsequential to try to demonstrate the point of origin of any adnexoid tumor as long as we are convinced that they may arise anywhere in the pluripotential epithelial system of the skin. Diagnosis, as a rule, is based on resemblance to, rather than origin from, any specific structure.

Epithelial Portion

While resembling epidermal or pilar basal cells, the epithelial cells (see Figs. 39–3, 39–7, and 39–8) are at most *basaloid*, a fact confirmed by electron microscopic studies.[3–6] The peripheral cells often form a continuous layer of columnar cells resting in palisade arrangement on a basement membrane, but this feature may be absent, especially if the tumor cells occur in small nests or cords. More centrally situated cells may show no particular arrangement or may be more or less fusiform. They often have a larger amount of somewhat lighter-staining cytoplasm.

Routine stains usually show no intercellular connections, and the supposed absence of prickles was originally thought to be the differentiating feature between prickle and basal cell cancer. For a discussion of the confused subject of prickles, see

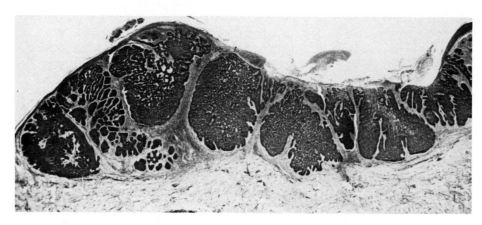

FIGURE 39–2.
Basal cell epithelioma. Tumor is centrally ulcerated. Its peripheral extension below normal epidermis produces pearly border seen by clinician. Epithelial portion is embedded in mesodermal stroma distinct from underlying dermis. Note different pattern (adenoid, solid, branching) in several epithelial nodules. Connections with epidermis are secondary. Tumor probably originated near ulcerated center. H&E. X9.

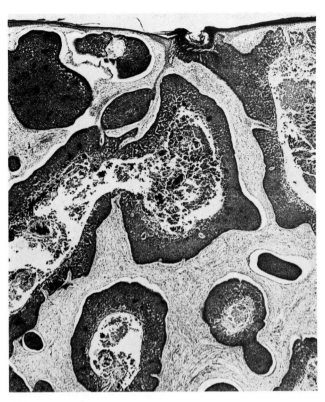

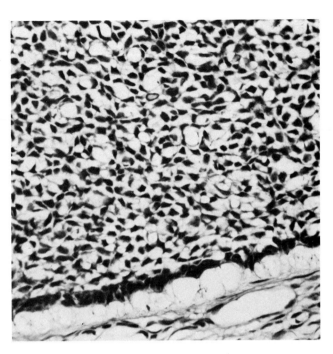

FIGURE 39–4.
Adamantinoid pattern in basal cell epithelioma. H&E. X370.

FIGURE 39–3.
Pseudocystic basal cell epithelioma. Cells degenerate (apoptosis) and disappear in central cavities. Note retraction spaces between epithelial nests and organoid stroma. Tumor approaches and invades epidermis. H&E. X30.

Chapters 2 and 5. It is a fact that the cells of basal cell epithelioma usually do not have a well-developed system of tonofibrils. The absence of tonofibrils may account for their relatively small size, for the softness of their cell bodies, which are apt to shrink during histologic processing, and for the inability to keratinize. On the other hand, intercellular bridges (desmosomes) are present, and in some tumors in which the intercellular spaces contain mucin, a peculiar picture of stellate interconnected cells results (Fig. 39–4), which may lead the novice to a diagnosis of prickle cell carcinoma. Similar pictures are not infrequently found in *ameloblastomas* (synonym: *adamantinoma*, an adnexoid epithelioma related to the tooth organ), and basal cell epitheliomas of this type are called *adamantinoid.*[7]

Keratinization with keratohyalin is very rare in basal cell epithelioma. Its occasional occurrence can be related to epidermoid keratinization in the sebaceous duct and the follicular infundibulum. Cornification in the so-called *keratotic basal cell epitheliomas* (Fig. 39–5A) usually is parakeratotic

and often incomplete. In most other cases, tumor cells probably just break down and disappear (apoptosis[8,9]). If breakdown becomes a prominent feature, cystic (or rather pseudocystic) tumors (Fig. 39–3) result, and the cavities may reach clinically perceptible size. Still other tumors (Fig. 39–5B) may show cells arranged somewhat regularly around numerous small mucin-filled spaces. The words *adenoid* or *pseudoadenomatous* are strictly descriptive when applied to such tumors and do not imply truly glandular nature. Yet another variant is the *plexiform epithelioma* (Fig. 39–6), in which two-rowed cords and sheets seem to bend around and connect with each other, embedded in rarefied stroma. In this type, there are no definable epithelial nests, but the entire tumor usually is well circumscribed by a stromal envelope.

Occasionally, all or some of the tumor nests contain multinucleated cells[10] or show so much variability of cell size and shape that a bowenoid picture results (Fig. 39–7). Such lesions support the conclusion that cytologic characteristics are less important in differentiating basal cell epithelioma from squamous cell carcinoma than evidence or absence of epithelial–mesodermal coordination.

Yet another variant contains melanin produced by symbiotically present melanocytes. The melanin granules may be present mainly in macrophages in the stroma[11] or in large dendritic cells[12]

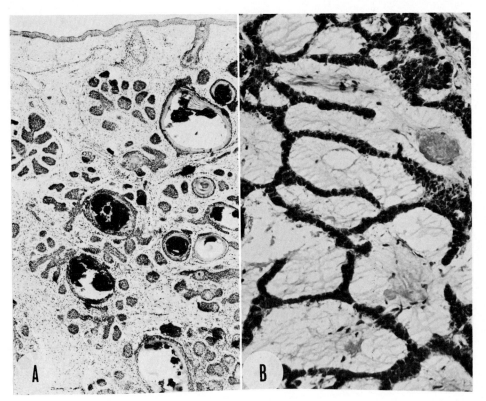

FIGURE 39–5.
Histologic patterns of basal cell epithelioma. **A.** *Keratotic basal cell epithelioma of trichoepitheliomatous pattern. Calcification (dark) of keratinized cysts. Organization into fibroepithelial lobules is well shown in this relatively benign tumor, but diffuse tissue-destroying growth of entire tumor and presence of scattered round cell infiltrate speak for a diagnosis of basal cell epithelioma. H&E. X75.* **B.** *Adenoid appearance is due to accumulation of mucin between epithelial cells and in stroma. H&E. X180.*

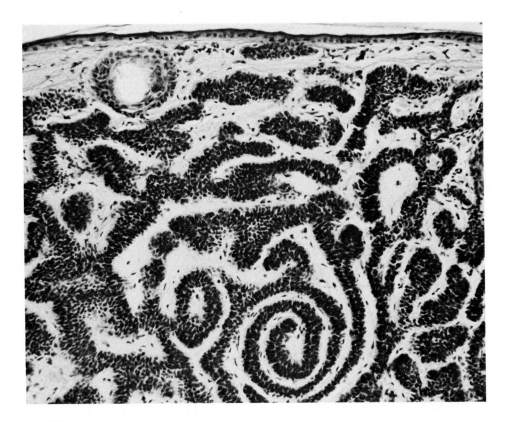

FIGURE 39–6.
Histologic patterns of basal cell epithelioma. Lacy or plexiform pattern results when myxomatous stroma envelops and separates thin cords and septal sheets of epithelium. H&E. X180.

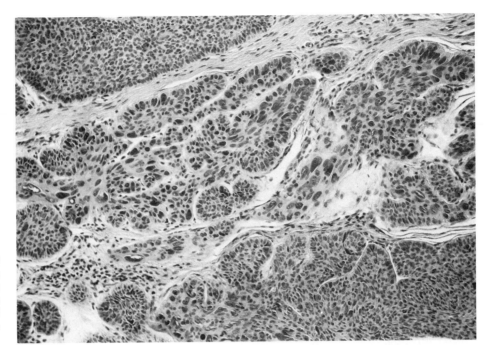

FIGURE 39–7.
Basal cell epithelioma with bowenoid pattern. Note more conventional appearance in upper left corner. Pattern has no clinical significance and does not denote basosquamous carcinoma. H&E. X135.

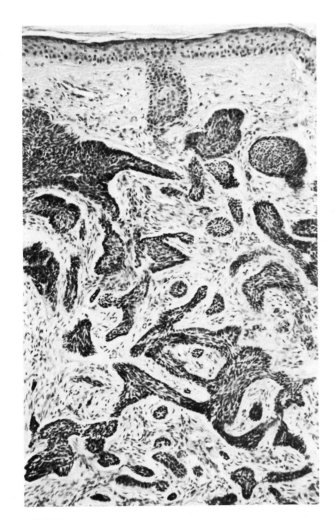

FIGURE 39–8.
Sclerosing basal cell epithelioma. H&E. X135.

without entering the tumor cells themselves. In some instances, however, the basaloid cells retain the capacity to accept pigment from the dendritic cells, and the tumor is truly a *pigmented basal cell epithelioma.*[13]

All these variants seem to have no great clinical significance, and neither does the relative incidence of mitotic figures.[14] Most tumors show few mitoses, but occasional ones may show many, perhaps in balance with accelerated cell death.[8] There is, however, one other morphologic variant which has clinical import.[15] This comprises tumors in which thin and compressed-looking epithelial cords are embedded in much fibrous stroma. This *sclerosing* form (Fig. 39–8) merges morphologically into the true *morphealike* type (see below) but grows much faster. Both are hard to eradicate. The difficulty probably lies more in the inability of the clinician to judge the extent of the lesion than in any unusual growth potential of the tumor. The pathologist who observes one of these lesions should forewarn the clinician. Excision or destruction must take in larger territory. X-ray treatment is not very effective, perhaps owing to the mass of sclerotic stroma.

Mesodermal Portion

Much too little attention has been paid to the stroma of basal cell epitheliomas. Just as stroma is a characteristic feature of benign adnexoid tumors and may constitute the major part of their volume, so is it in basal cell epithelioma.[16,17] The stroma often is somewhat less mature, more cellular, and less fibrous. A PAS-positive basement membrane usually surrounds the epithelial portions. Mucinous ground substance, mainly hyaluronic acid, is increased, and mucin formation may reach considerable proportions around the epithelial nests. H&E sections then show empty halos, so-called retraction spaces (Figs. 39–3 and 39–8). While some retraction takes place during fixation and dehydration, owing to the softness of the tissues, one can usually show that most of this space is occupied by metachromatic and alcian blue-positive substance. Its presence is evidence of specific synthesis, especially when sulfated mucopolysaccharides are formed, and should not be dismissed as mucinous degeneration. The tumor–stroma interface also should not be compared to the epidermal–dermal junction[18] of normal skin (Chap. 2). The concept of specific constructive metabolic processes in the stroma is supported by the fact that new elastic fibers (Fig. 3–12) in typical perifollicular arrangement are found in a small percentage of lesions.[19-21] In some tumors, they form a dense coat resembling the hyaline sheaths of cylindromas in H&E sections. Cartilage may rarely develop, but amyloid is a not uncommon deposit in the stroma of basal cell epithelioma[22] where it is produced in fibroblasts.[23]

The most important point to be aware of is that the tumor does not end at the periphery of the epithelial nests and that these are embedded in newly formed connective tissue which is part of the tumor,[24] at the same time containing and influencing the epithelial growth. Attentive examination will show that the entire preexisting dermis has disappeared in the area and has been replaced by fibroepithelial neoplasia. Recognizing this phenomenon helps considerably in the differentiation of basal cell epithelioma from squamous cell carcinoma in doubtful cases (Chap. 34, small cell squamous carcinoma).

While emphasis is placed here on epithelial-stromal relations because of their practical diagnostic and therapeutic significance—a point we shall return to in the following pages—the interactions between ectodermal and mesodermal portions are also of theoretical importance. They indicate stroma dependence of the neoplastic epithelium in a more specific manner than the well-accepted need of a growing cancer for vascular supporting tissue. Specific stroma dependence provides a hypothetical explanation for the almost universal absence of metastasis of basaliomas. There were less than 80 published cases of metastasizing basal cell cancer

in 1970,[25] a few cases per year have been added since.[26-28] Considering that some of these cases presumably were implantations of aspirated tumor fragments in the lung from highly invasive facial lesions,[29] it is, in fact, astounding that true single-cell metastasis is observed so rarely. Therapy for basalioma is confidently based on the expectation that local treatment will eradicate the neoplasm. It is to be hoped that future cases of *metastasizing basal cell carcinomas* will be investigated by modern techniques in order to prove that they truly are basaliomas and not basaloid squamous cell carcinomas or adenocarcinomas.[30]

Terminology

Krompecher's term, "basal cell carcinoma," has been attacked often and from many quarters. Yet it seems indestructible. The designation is bad because the tumor does not consist of epidermal basal cells, nor is it generally derived from epidermal basal cells, and it is not a carcinoma in the true sense (see above). The critics, however, have not been able to agree on a generally acceptable term. American dermatologists more and more prefer to say *basal cell epithelioma*, indicating a less malignant process. This does not conform with British usage, which calls squamous cell cancer of the lip an epithelioma. Belisario[31] introduced "rodent carcinoma," derived from the old *rodent ulcer* of Jacob. We might say "rodent epithelioma" in this country, but so far Belisario has not found many followers. A simple solution has been offered in the word *basalioma* which is used generally in Germany and is understood in other European countries. The word is short and circumvents the difficulty of classifying these tumors as either benign or fully malignant. As a matter of fact, it indicates that they are in a class by themselves, and we use basalioma in this sense in this book.

Two decades after Krompecher, Darier and Ferrand[32] introduced a classification of skin cancer in which they differentiated squamous cell carcinoma (épithélioma typique), basal cell carcinoma (épithélioma atypique), and a group of metatypical carcinomas which they subdivided into mixed (basosquamous) and intermediary types. Although the diagnosis basosquamous carcinoma continues to be made (according to Borel,[33] about 3.5 percent), we now are convinced that most of Darier's mixed carcinomas are nothing but keratotic basaliomas (see above), morphealike epitheliomas (see below), or basaliomas with attempts at organoid differentiation toward hair follicle (trichoepitheliomalike).

The fear of converting this type of lesion into squamous cell carcinoma by eradicating only the basal cell component with low doses of X-ray therapy is biologically absurd and not seen in practice. What may happen is development of new squamous cell cancer in an old X-ray dermatitis. Once in a while, one encounters pseudoepitheliomatous epidermal hyperplasia in connection with basal cell epithelioma, and in rare cases squamous cell carcinoma and basal cell epithelioma may develop in such close proximity that they are found side by side or intermingled in the same section. So-called intermediary cell carcinomas probably are now diagnosed as nodular hidradenomas or trichilemmomas in most cases.

At this point the *nevoid basalioma syndrome* (nevoid basal cell carcinoma syndrome[34,35]) may be mentioned because many authors speak in this connection of "basal cell nevi." According to the definition of the term "tissue nevus" (Sec. VII), it applies to a circumscribed malformation due to excess of one or several of the mature components of the skin. The skin lesions of the *Gorlin syndrome* (to use the eponymic term) are from the beginning basaliomas consisting of immature tumor cells. They are nevoid neoplasms, behave aggressively, and should be treated rigorously in the same way as other basaliomas.

Superficial Basal Cell Epithelioma

Some varieties of basalioma need special discussion. A biologically interesting variant (Fig. 39–9) is *superficial basal cell epithelioma*, to which the French apply the picturesque name "épithélioma pagetoide." It occurs most commonly on the trunk, more rarely on the extremities, but may be found on face and scalp just as well. Clinically, it is flat, rarely ulcerates, and may form plaques many centimeters in diameter. Histologically, it consists of a fibroepithelial plate replacing the papillary layer of the skin without invading the pars reticularis. Its epithelial portion is joined to the lower surface of the epidermis in numerous places and may replace short stretches of epidermis (Fig. 39–10). It forms a solid plate in early lesions. Later, the plate becomes fenestrated through local self-healing and may break up into multiple foci in the center. At the same time, it advances peripherally as a continuous ring.[36]

This description tries to do justice to the tumor as a biologic unit. In routine thin sections, cut vertically to the skin surface, one sees small epithelial nests attached to the lower surface of the epidermis and seemingly not connected to each other. The stroma may not be conspicuous in H&E sections unless one trains one's eye for it. Thus the desig-

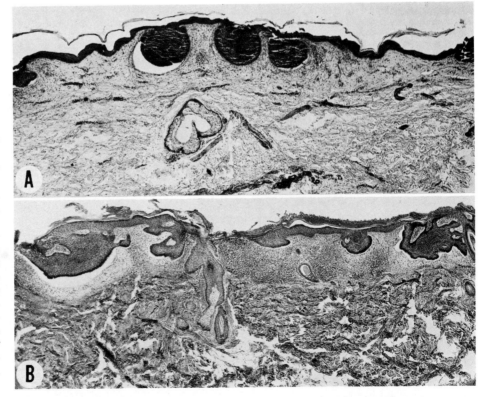

FIGURE 39–9.
Superficial basal cell epithelioma. Examination of serial sections probably would reveal that seemingly isolated epithelial nests are connected. In any case, the epithelial portion is embedded in vascularized stroma (more visible in **B***), which makes the entire tumor a solid plate occupying pars papillaris and riding on pars reticularis of the dermis. Note persistence of pilosebaceous complexes in and beneath tumor as indication of its relatively benign nature. Connections with epidermis and hair follicles are secondary contacts.* **A.** *H&E. X30.* **B.** *O&G. X45.*

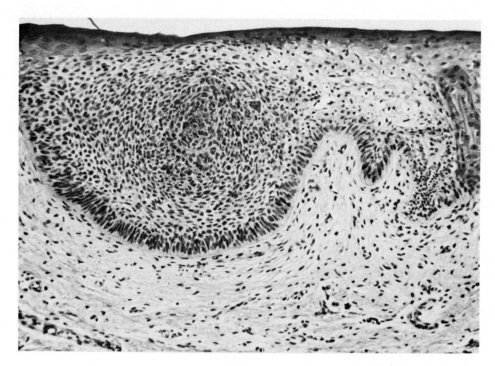

FIGURE 39–10.
Extremely superficial basal cell epithelioma, which becomes part of the surface epithelium. Keratinizing epidermis at far left is sharply delineated from tumor epithelium, which reaches the surface but does not keratinize. Note acrosyringium crossing the tumor at far right. H&E. X185.

nation "multicentric" epithelioma has taken a firm hold in American usage. Secondary multicentricity may indeed occur, as pointed out above, through partial self-healing in the center of larger lesions. However, the term "multicentric" implies the concept that there is a field of skin in which many new epitheliomas arise independently, and that is a misconception. Every superficial basalioma grows from one original neoplastic focus and spreads peripherally as a thin plate. Whether small or large, it can be cured by removal or destruction of the thin fibroepithelial plate to as little as 1 to 2 mm beyond the limit of the clinically visible lesion. This would not be possible if the peripheral skin had an innate tendency for neoplasia. No doubt patients affected with superficial epitheliomatosis may have several and even dozens of lesions. Each of their epitheliomas, however, is a unicentric neoplasm.

This is more evident if one pays attention to the mesodermal portion of the tumor, a task made easier by examination of O&G sections. Here it is evident (Fig. 39–9) that the stroma is a solid shield in which the epithelial nests are embedded. It replaces the pars papillaris, riding on the pars reticularis and lifting up the epidermis. It frequently extends laterally beyond the epithelial portion. The presence of this soft but solid mass, in which all epithelial nests are embedded, makes it possible to curette off the entire tumor without removing any of the reticular part of the dermis. It is not necessary to excise the entire thickness of the skin in order to cure superficial basalioma.

Premalignant Fibroepithelial Tumor

On the lower part of the trunk or in the groin or thigh region are sometimes found elevated or sessile lesions clinically resembling fibromas but, on microscopic examination, presenting the peculiar picture (Fig. 39–11) of an epithelial meshwork with hyperplastic mesodermal contents.[37,38] In three-dimensional interpretation we are dealing with an epithelial sponge, the compartments of which are filled with stroma resembling that of benign adnexoid tumors. What look like epithelial cords in paraffin sections actually are cross sections of thin septa. The cells composing them are a little larger and lighter staining than those of basaliomas, rather resembling those of trichoepithelioma. In some lesions, solid buds of small dark-staining cells which look like embryonic hair germs or the smallest basalioma nests are found sprouting from the epithelial septa (Fig. 39–11B). These may grow and replace parts or all of the preexisting tumor, a clear case of progression from a benign and balanced fibroepithelial growth to invasive and destructive, yet still organoid basal cell epithelioma. It was for this reason that Pinkus chose the designation *premalignant fibroepithelial tumors* when he called attention to them in 1953.[39]

Morphealike Epithelioma

Firm, skin-colored or yellowish white plaques, often having their start at an early age and slowly

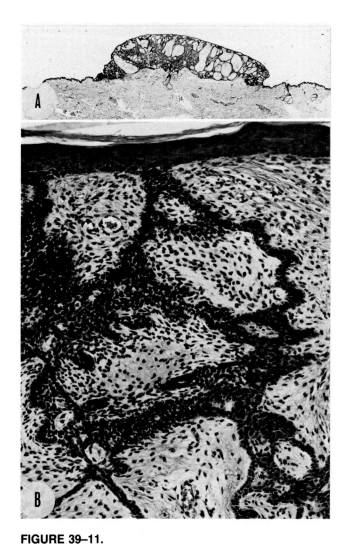

FIGURE 39–11.
*Premalignant fibroepithelial tumor. **A.** Low magnification of entire sessile and smooth-surfaced lesion. Note presence of pilosebaceous complex in contact with lower surface of tumor and presumably extending through it to surface since there is no evidence of obstruction. H&E. X8. **B.** Detail of spongelike pattern of epithelial septa between stromal compartments. H&E. X180.*

enlarging for many years before they ulcerate, constitute another variant of basalioma. They should not be confused with relatively superficial lesions on the face that act like brush fire, producing tiny ulcerations in their peripheral advance and leaving behind a somewhat atrophic scar in which residual epitheliomatous nests may be embedded. Morphealike epithelioma also is different from sclerotic basaliomas in which fibrous stroma seems to compress the epithelium into thin cords and which often grow fairly rapidly in circumference and depth (see above). On histologic examination, morphealike epitheliomas (Fig. 39–12) may be mistaken for squamous cell carcinoma, for desmoplas-

tic trichoepithelioma, or for syringoma, owing to the presence of epithelial cords that occasionally widen into tiny keratin-filled whorls or cysts. These are embedded in copious and fairly mature connective tissue without much inflammatory reaction. Tumors of this type[40] have been known to arise early in childhood. They may grow slowly for 10 to 20 years before attracting medical attention and, occasionally, may be mistaken for granuloma annulare even by experienced clinicians. Their clinical behavior is practically benign, but their eradication is difficult because it requires chemosurgery or generous excision, possibly with plastic repair.

In a sense, morphealike epithelioma may be classified tentatively as *basalioma* with *syringoid differentiation*. Otherwise, there are only two recent publications[41,42] relating basaliomas to sweat glands. The so-called adenoid basal cell epitheliomas certainly are not an expression of glandular differentiation (see above).

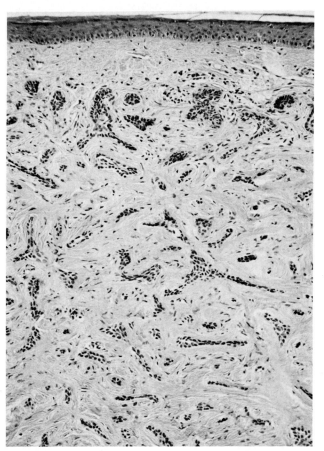

FIGURE 39–12.
Morphealike epithelioma. Epithelial cords and occasional lumenlike spaces produce a picture somewhat similar to syringoma and desmoplastic trichoepithelioma. Copious fibrous stroma completely replaces dermis. H&E. X135.

Intraepidermal Epithelioma

Jadassohn first proposed the concept that basal cell epithelioma may develop and grow within the epidermis without ever invading the dermis. He reported one case, the true nature of which can no longer be ascertained. It may well have been a seborrheic verruca with intraepidermal whorls (Chap. 33). The concept was perpetuated, modified, and sometimes confused with other phenomena of intraepidermal malignancy, and one must work with clear definitions in order to untangle the web.

The designation *intraepidermal tumor formation* should be restricted to the presence of sharply defined nests (or single cells) of neoplastic character surrounded completely by epidermal keratino-cytes. This is in contrast to *carcinoma in situ*, in which a sharply limited area of epidermis is completely replaced by neoplastic cells, which extend from the basement membrane to the surface. Examples of the latter are keratosis senilis and Bowen's dermatosis (Chap. 34).

Intraepidermal tumor nests[43] may represent three different biologic phenomena which may be designated by the names of Paget, Borst, and Jadassohn. The *Paget phenomenon* (Fig. 40–5) consists of adnexal or other nonkeratinocytic tumor cells intruding into the epidermis and forming colonies within it. Examples are Paget's disease and pagetoid malignant melanoma. The *Borst phenomenon* (Fig. 39–13) was described and clearly defined by that author as the invasion of epidermoid squamous can-

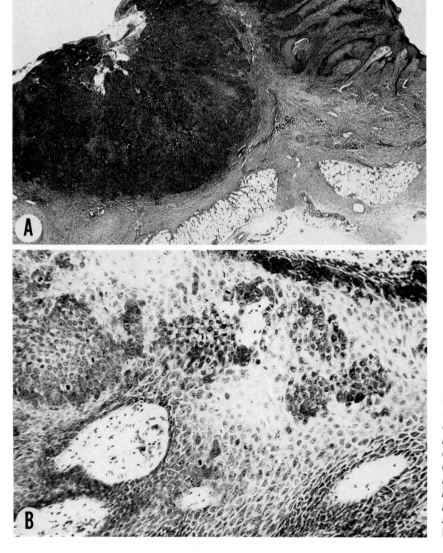

FIGURE 39–13.
*Squamous cell carcinoma of lower lip exhibiting Borst phenomenon. This tumor duplicates almost exactly Borst's original case and is a relatively small celled, nonkeratinizing carcinoma which has invaded deeply into the dermis and is ulcerated. Nests of squamous carcinoma cells also invade the hyperplastic surrounding epidermis. **A.** H&E. X45. **B.** H&E. X135.*

cer cells into the surrounding epidermis, where they form colonies. Borst observed this phenomenon in a carcinoma of the lip, which also invaded the dermis, and used it as a strong argument for the self-propagation of cancer, as contrasted with the concept of continual conversion of normal cells into cancer cells. The Borst phenomenon may also be found in some cases of Bowen's dermatosis (Fig. 34–13B), which then represent a combination of carcinoma in situ with intraepidermal carcinoma. The *Jadassohn phenomenon* indicates origin of neoplasia within the epidermis and colony formation of neoplastic cells which remain in the confines of the epidermis. Jadassohn's original observation actually may not have represented this phenomenon but may have been a seborrheic verruca with pseudonests of basaloid cells (Fig. 33–12). This is indeed the most common type of lesion suggesting intraepidermal neoplasia. Careful study of multiple sections shows that somewhere the border of each nest is not sharp and that the basaloid cells mature into prickle cells. These pseudonests are due to whorling and convolutions (basaloid eddies) within the substance of the seborrheic verruca.

There are, however, true instances of the Jadassohn phenomenon (Fig. 38–12). They were explained by Smith and Coburn[44] as arising from intraepidermal sweat duct material (*hidroacanthoma simplex*). While there is no proof of this concept, it has logical appeal and a sound biologic basis in the existence of the acrosyringium as a separate biologic unit. The concept can explain the absence of a demonstrable extraepidermal tumor in some cases of Paget's disease. The principal histologic difference between such cases and hidroacanthoma simplex is that the cells of the latter resemble the intraepidermal eccrine sweat duct unit and are closely connected to each other and surrounding epidermal keratinocytes by desmosomes. Just like the cells of eccrine poroma, they lack an organized system of tonofibrils and are generally incapable of keratinization. Malignant forms of hidroacanthoma[45] are porocarcinomas (Chap. 40).

We hope that this discussion will contribute to the discontinuation of the habit of hyphenating the names of Borst and Jadassohn in describing intraepidermal tumors.[46] It is true that Jadassohn quoted Borst's case as being similar to his, but he spoke at a time when the knowledge of epidermal biology was limited, and, moreover, he did not say the two cases were identical. On the basis of modern insight into the process of epidermal regeneration and symbiosis (Chap. 2), it has become evident that the two authors dealt with quite different phenomena and that there are no "Borst–Jadassohn tumors."[47,48]

REFERENCES

1. Pinkus H: Adnexal tumors, benign, not-so-benign, and malignant. In Montagna W, Dobson RL (eds): Carcinogenesis. Advances in Biology of Skin, vol 7. Oxford, New York, Pergamon, 1966, p 255
2. Lever WF: Pathogenesis of benign tumors of cutaneous appendages and of basal cell epithelioma II. Basal cell epithelioma. Arch Dermatol 57:709, 1948
3. Kint A, Piérard J: Ultrastructure de l'épithéliome basocellulaire. Arch Belg Dermatol 24:367, 1968
4. Brody I: Contributions to the histogenesis of basal cell carcinoma. J Ultrastruct Res 33:60, 1970
5. Raidbord HE, Wechsler HL, Fisher ER: Ultrastructural study of basal cell carcinoma and its variants with comments on histogenesis. Arch Dermatol 104:132, 1971
6. Kumakiri M, Hashimoto K: Ultrastructural resemblance of basal cell epithelioma to primary epithelial germ. J Cutan Pathol 5:53, 1978
7. Lerchin E, Rahbari H: Adamantinoid basal cell epithelioma: a histological variant. Arch Dermatol 111:586, 1975
8. Kerr JFR, Searle J: Suggested explanation for paradoxically slow growth rate of basal cell carcinomas that contain numerous mitotic figures. Cancer 29:1724, 1972
9. Malkinson FD, Pearson RW (eds): Year Book of Dermatology 1973. Chicago, Year Book, 1973, p 170
10. Rupec M, Vakilzadeh F: Über das Vorkommen von mehrkernigen Riesenzellen in Basaliomen. Arch Klin Exp Dermatol 235:198, 1969
11. Fellner MJ, Katz MJ: Pigmented basal cell cancer masquerading as superficial spreading malignant melanoma. Arch Dermatol 113:946, 1976
12. Deppe R, Pullmann H, Steigleder GK: Dopa-positive Zellen und Melanin im Basaliom. Arch Dermatol Res 256:79, 1976
13. Tezuka T, Ohkuma M, Hirose I: Melanosomes of pigmented basal cell epithelioma. Dermatologica 154:14, 1977
14. Weinstein GD, Frost P: Cell proliferation in human basal cell carcinoma. Cancer Res 30:724, 1970
15. Sloane JP: The value of typing basal cell carcinomas in predicting recurrence after surgical excision. Br J Dermatol 96:127, 1977
16. Massarelli G, Muzzetto P, Tanda F, et al.: Aspetti istochimici et significato istopatologico del connettivo mantellare nel carcinoma basocellulare. Ann Ital Derm Clin Sper 31:95, 1977
17. Steigleder GK: Besondere Aspekte des Basalioms (Pigmentierung, Stroma, Glucosaminoglycane, Kapillarmuster). Z Hautkr 53:55, 1978
18. McNutt NS: Ultrastructural comparison of the interface between epithelium and stroma in basal cell carcinoma and control human skin. Lab Invest 35:132, 1976
19. Mehregan AG, Staricco RG, Pinkus H: Elastic fibers in basal cell epithelioma. Arch Dermatol 89:33, 1964
20. Rudner EJ, Mehregan AH, Pinkus H: Elastic fibers in superficial basal cell epithelioma: occurrence on so-

lar protected areas. J Invest Dermatol 45:70, 1965

21. Berger H, Hübner S: Lichtmikroskopische Befunde zur Neubildung elastischer Fasern im Basaliomstroma. Arch Dermatol Forsch 252:119, 1975

22. Sümegi I: Elastase digestion of the amyloid-like substance surrounding mammary cancer and basal cell carcinoma of the skin. Acta Derm Venereol (Stockh) 53:99, 1973

23. Runne U, Orfanos CE: Amyloid production by dermal fibroblasts. Electron microscopic studies on the origin of amyloid in various dermatoses and skin tumors. Br J Dermatol 97:155, 1977

24. Pinkus H: The role of the mesoderm in basaliomas. In Proceedings, XIIIth International Congress of Dermatology. Berlin, Springer-Verlag, 1968, p 8

25. Wermuth BM, Fajardo LF: Metastatic basal cell carcinoma: a review. Arch Pathol 90:458, 1970

26. Jackson RT, Adams RH: Horrifying basal cell carcinoma: a study of 33 cases and a comparison with 435 non-horror cases and a report on four metastatic cases. J Surg Oncol 5:431, 1973

27. Hughes JN: Metastatic basal cell carcinoma: report of two cases and review of literature. Clin Radiol 24:392, 1973

28. Jager RM, Weiner LJ, Howell RS: Basal cell carcinoma with bony metastases producing myelofibrosis. Arch Dermatol 113:1288, 1977

29. Guillan RA, Johnson RP: Aspiration metastases from basal cell carcinoma. Arch Dermatol 114:589, 1978

30. Farmer ER, Helwig EB: Metastatic basal cell carcinoma. Arch Dermatol 114:1833, 1978

31. Belisario JC: Cancer of the Skin. London, Butterworth, 1959

32. Darier J, Ferrand M: L'épithélioma pavimenteux mixte et intermédiaire. Ann Dermatol Syphiligr 3:385, 1922

33. Borel DM: Cutaneous basosquamous carcinoma. Arch Pathol 95:293, 1973

34. Mason JK, Helwig EB, Graham JH: Pathology of the nevoid basal cell carcinoma syndrome. Arch Pathol 79:401, 1965

35. Howell JB: Genesis of the nevoid basal cell carcinoma syndrome. Dermatology 2(4):30, 1979

36. Madsen A: Histogenesis of superficial basal cell epitheliomas; unicentric or multicentric origin. Arch Dermatol 72:29, 1955

37. Pasternak F, Civatte J: Les tumeurs firboépitheliales de Pinkus a localisations extra-dorso-lombo-sacrées. A propos de 31 cas personnals. Ann Dermatol Syphiligr 103:275, 1976

38. Barr RJ, Herter RJ, Stone OJ: Multiple premalignant fibroepitheliomas of Pinkus. A case report and review of the literature. Cutis 21:335, 1978

39. Pinkus H: Premalignant fibroepithelial tumors of skin. Arch Dermatol 67:598, 1953

40. Botvinick I, Mehregan AH, Weissman F: Morphealike basal cell epithelioma in a child. Arch Dermatol 95:67, 1967

41. Freeman RG, Winkelmann RK: Basal cell tumor with eccrine differentiation (eccrine epithelioma). Arch Dermatol 100:234, 1969

42. Puente Duany N, Madden JJ, Golden GT: Multiple basal cell epithelioma of eccrine duct origin. Cutis 11:84, 1973

43. Mehregan AH, Pinkus H: Intraepidermal epithelioma: a critical study. Cancer 17:609, 1964

44. Smith JLS, Coburn JG: Hidroacanthoma simplex: assessment of selected group of intraepidermal basal cell epitheliomata and of their malignant homologues. Br J Dermatol 68:400, 1956

45. Ishikawa K: Malignant hidroacanthoma simplex. Arch Dermatol 104:529, 1971

46. Nicolis G, Capetanakis J, Panas E: Les épithéliomas intra-épidermiques de Borst et Jadassohn. Ann Dermatol Syphiligr 98:161, 1971

47. Holubar K: Das intraepidermale Epitheliom (sog. Borst-Jadassohn): verkörpert dieser Begriff eine Entität? Z Hautkr 44:391, 1969

48. Berger P, Baughman R: Intraepidermal epithelioma; report of case with invasion after many years. Br J Dermatol 90:343, 1974

Adenocarcinoma and Metastatic Carcinoma

Adenocarcinomas are rare tumors in the skin. They have the same grave prognosis as in other organs, and they must be separated sharply from benign adnexal tumors that have no potential for metastasis.

SEBACEOUS ADENOCARCINOMA

The clearest contrast is provided by sebaceous gland tumors. In Chapter 35, we discussed the spectrum ranging from sebaceous hyperplasia to sebaceous adenoma to sebaceous epithelioma to basal cell epithelioma with sebaceous maturation. All these are benign fibroepithelial tumors, and the distinction is mainly one of attained or not attained maturity of the cells until the telltale mark of inflammatory infiltrate sets apart the locally malignant but still rather innocuous tumor consisting almost entirely of basaloid cells interacting with supportive stroma.

A sebaceous adenocarcinoma, in contrast, may have many lipid-forming cells, but it has cytologic features of malignancy: large, irregular nuclei with large nucleoli; a jumbled arrangement of cells; and no palisading border (Fig. 40–1). It has the appearance of a carcinoma in the sense of general pathology, and it has the ability to metastasize.[1]

Meibomian Carcinoma

Adenocarcinomas of the meibomian glands of the eyelid are relatively more common than those of

sebaceous glands of the body surface[2,3] and are also more dangerous. They have a propensity to invade the conjunctival epithelium and to cause pagetoid lesions.[4]

ADENOCARCINOMA OF THE SWEAT APPARATUS

In carcinoma related to sweat glands, the distinction between eccrine and apocrine tumors may be even more insecure than in benign lesions.[5]

Eccrine Carcinoma

One personally observed eccrine adenocarcinoma arose in the palm of a middle-aged woman, imitated the configuration of the surrounding normal glands including the presence of diastase-resistant, PAS-positive material,[6] but differed in the absence of PAS-positive basement membranes. The tumor recurred after excision and metastasized to axillary lymph nodes. A similar tumor is illustrated in Figure 40–2.

Other tumors have been called clear cell carcinomas,[7] (Chap. 38), and tumors resembling adenoid basal epitheliomas[8] have been described. It is difficult to differentiate some sweat gland carcinomas from salivary gland tumors because salivary glands (being derived from ectodermal sources) also have two-layered epithelium. The possible occurrence of ectopic salivary gland tissue must be kept in mind

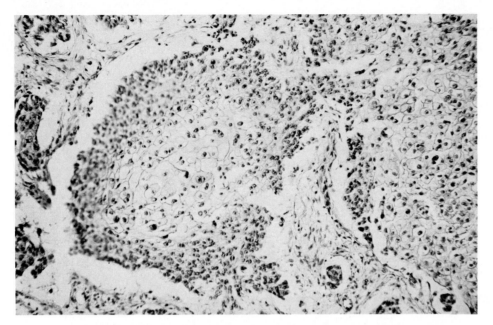

FIGURE 40–1.
Sebaceous adenocarcinoma. Compare and contrast with sebaceous epithelioma in Figure 35–7. Note cellular atypia and absence of basaloid outer layers. H&E. X135.

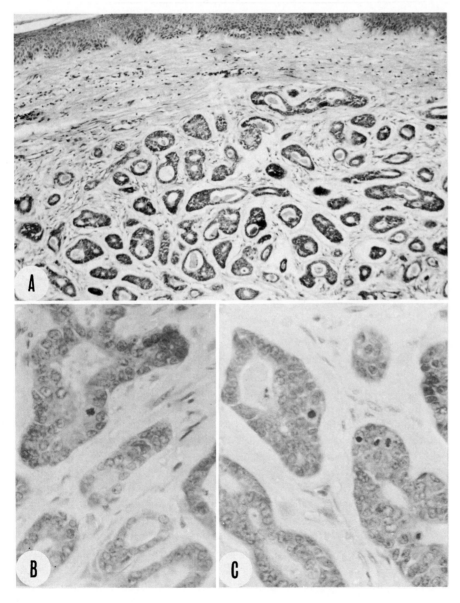

FIGURE 40–2.
Eccrine adenocarcinoma. **A.** *Tubular irregular configuration. H&E. X125.* **B** *and* **C.** *Many mitoses. H&E. X400.*

in the head and neck region, and agreement may not be reached among experts in individual cases.

Mucinous (Adenocystic) Carcinoma. Mendoza and Helwig's first publication[9] on primary mucinous carcinomas of sweat glands has been followed by several others. The observation[10] of tumors changing from a solid hidradenomatous pattern to one in which small islands of epithelial parenchyma are surrounded by lakes of mucinous stroma in recurrent lesions supports the eccrine nature of the cells and at the same time gives an interesting explanation for the very unusual picture (Fig. 40–3).

Porocarcinoma. A peculiar group of rare cases is biologically instructive in showing that malignant cells of the eccrine apparatus can maintain the ability of their normal progenitors to live within the epidermis and to form pagetoid nests. The first observation was an ulcerated tumor near the ankle of an elderly woman that metastasized and spread widely in the superficial lymphatics of the skin.[11] In hundreds of places, the tumor cells reentered the epidermis from below and produced nodules of intraepidermal nests (Fig. 40–4) along the lower extremity and on the abdomen. At least two similar cases[12,13] have since been described and document the morphologic similarity to benign eccrine poroacanthoma and to poroepithelioma.

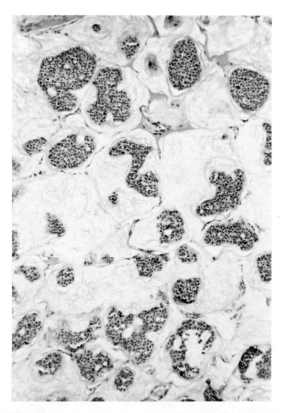

FIGURE 40–3.
Mucinous carcinoma of skin. A field of moderate expression of the great amount of mucinous stroma that can be associated with small nests of tumor cells. H&E. X250.

Apocrine Adenocarcinoma and Paget's Disease

Apocrine carcinomas are unusual, and in cases arising in the axilla, relation to aberrant mammary tissue rather than to sweat glands is the preferred interpretation. Special discussion is needed of those lesions known as *extramammary Paget's disease* because they are thought to be related to carcinoma of apocrine glands, even though this association has been established in only a few cases by demonstration of an underlying invasive carcinoma.

When Paget described the disease of the mammary areola which bears his name, he stressed the constant association with cancer of the breast, and his experience has been borne out over the years so regularly that the skin lesion is valid indication for amputation of the breast. There are, however, two diametrically opposed opinions concerning the mechanism of this association. One school of thought maintains that some as yet undefined carcinogenic stimulus induces cancerization of epidermal cells and milk apparatus cells. The histologi-

cally unmistakable *Paget cells* in the epidermis are supposed to be converted keratinocytes,[14] and their continued presence is thought to be due to continuous conversion of epidermal basal cells into Paget cells. The other school, to which we subscribe, feels that there is enough evidence to maintain[15] that Paget cells are mammary carcinoma cells which have migrated into and parasitized the epidermis, where they maintain themselves by mitotic division—in short, that Paget's disease is due to the presence of an *epidermotropic adnexal carcinoma.* A refinement of this concept[16] suggests that Paget's disease starts at the junction of the lactiferous duct with the epidermis as a neoplastic process that extends downward into the duct and laterally into the epidermis.

Electron microscopic studies supporting the conversion hypothesis cannot be considered conclusive as long as Paget cells have not been compared to normal intraepidermal lactiferous or apocrine duct cells and cognizance has not been taken of the facts that desmosomes may exist between epidermal and adnexal epithelial cells and that description of transitional cell forms has often proved fallacious in

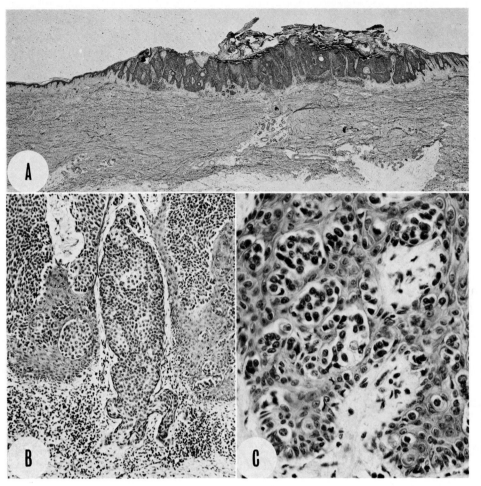

FIGURE 40–4.
Epidermotropic eccrine carcinoma. A. An entire metastatic lesion. H&E. X28. B. Tumor nest in a superficial dermal lymph vessel and multiple nests in epidermis. H&E. X90. C. Paget-like intraepidermal spread of carcinoma. H&E. X135. (From Pinkus and Mehregan. Arch Dermatol 88:597, 1963.)

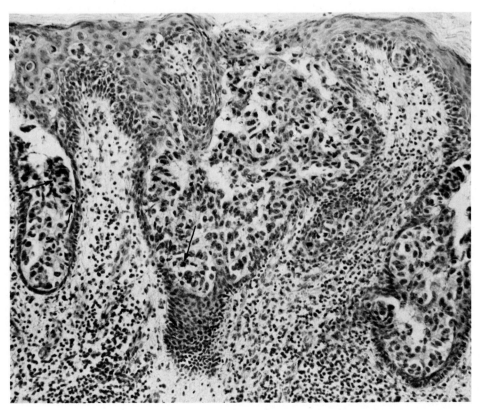

FIGURE 40–5.
Paget's disease of the nipple. Adenocarcinomatous cells are single or in small and large nests in epidermis. Three mitotic figures in Paget cells indicated by arrows. Epidermal basal layer is intact in most places. H&E. X185. (From Mehregan and Pinkus. Cancer 17:609, 1964.)

the last 100 years of anatomic investigation. We just state that the existence of epidermotropic carcinoma seems to have been established beyond a reasonable doubt (see above), and that the interpretation of Paget cells as epidermotropic cancer cells conforms with the concept of unicentric rather than multicentric origin of any single malignant neoplasm.

Extramammary Paget's disease[17-19] shares many clinical and histologic features with the classic areolar type. Its almost constant location in areas of apocrine gland prevalence, especially axilla and vulva, provides a good basis for the view that it represents *epidermotropic apocrine adenocarcinoma* in most instances. In some cases, it was found associated with carcinoma of the rectal mucosa, which is also biologically compatible with the adjoining epidermis. Such cases do not obligate one to

hypothesize the anatomically unsupported cloacogenic origin of much of the genital epidermis. There is histochemical support for the identity of the sialomucin of Paget cells and rectal mucosa.[20]

In Paget's disease of either areolar (Fig. 40–5) or extramammary (Fig. 40–6) type the epidermis may not be much thickened, but it usually is, and it is covered either by parakeratotic scale or crust. The specific cells are relatively large and light staining with H&E and are found singly or in smaller and larger groups within the epidermis. Occasionally, they form rosettes, suggesting adenomatous arrangement, and, in some cases, the epidermis seems to be a bag of keratinocytes filled with masses of the clear nonfibrillar cells. Mitoses are not infrequent and prove that the Paget cells multiply in situ. Paget cells are more prevalent in the lower part of the epidermis but are almost always

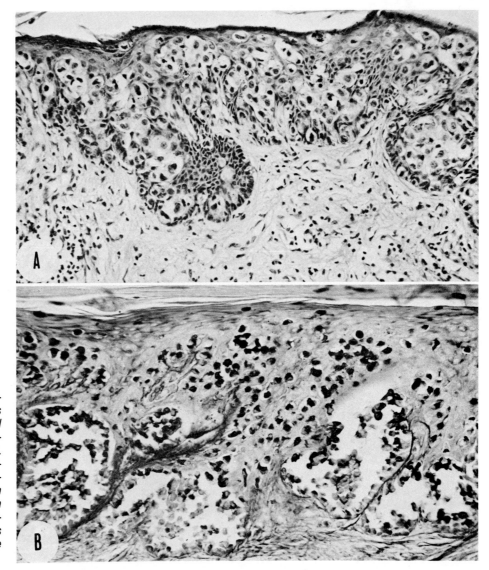

FIGURE 40–6.
Extramammary Paget's disease. In this case, some nests are not surrounded by basal cells but are confined by basement membrane. **A.** *H&E. X180.* **B.** *Alcian blue-PAS-picric acid stain shows sialomucin in Paget cells not only in living epidermis but also within horny layer. Very dark appearance of mucin is due to its having affinity for alcian blue as well as fuchsin. X180.*

separated from the dermis by a cohesive and fairly intact basal layer. However, they may invade the dermis (Fig. 40–6B). They may also be found in the higher epidermal layers, including the stratum corneum, but they do not keratinize themselves. In most cases, the cell is separated from surrounding keratinocytes by a narrow or broader space, not traversed by intercellular bridges. In a few cases, however, intercellular connections are present. This fact does not militate against the adnexal nature of Paget cells, since cells of the intraepidermal adnexal units (Chap. 2) normally are connected to their neighboring epidermal keratinocytes by bridges.

Paget cells of the areolar disease contain glycogen. Those of extramammary cases (Fig. 40–6B) regularly contain mucinous substances. Newer methods show these to be acid mucopolysaccharides and, in most instances, sialomucin, a substance found in hidradenomas. A dense inflammatory infiltrate consisting of small round cells and plasma cells in the upper dermis completes the histologic picture.

In areolar cases, a sufficiently large biopsy often shows the milk ducts affected by a so-called *comedo-type carcinoma*, but other forms of breast cancer may be present. In extramammary cases, Pa-

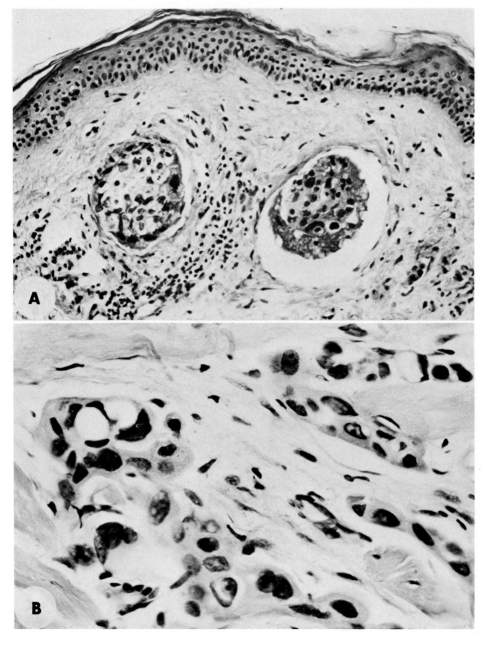

FIGURE 40–7.
Carcinoma metastatic to skin.
A. *Clinically erysipelaslike lesion produced by obstruction of lymphatics in carcinoma of breast. H&E. X225.* **B.** *Signet-ring cells in metastatic carcinoma of colon. H&E. X465.*

get cells often are present in the walls of eccrine and apocrine ducts and of hair follicles, presumably as a phenomenon of secondary migration. Careful serial sections enabled Cawley[21] to demonstrate a small apocrine gland carcinoma in an axillary case. Failure to find such a carcinoma in every case may have two reasons. Usually it proves impractical to examine all tissue in serial or step sections, especially if the superficial lesion is large. Second, the original focus may well be in the poral portion of a gland and may not lead to invasive carcinoma at all.

Beginners find it difficult to differentiate Paget cells from those of Bowen's disease on the one hand and from peculiar large cells of the normal areolar epithelium on the other. The last named are prickle cells with a large halo around the nucleus (intracellular edema). Thus, the empty space is between nucleus and cytoplasm, the cell adhering to surrounding cells with numerous desmosomes. In the Paget cell, on the other hand, nucleus and cytoplasm form a unit, and the empty space surrounds the entire cell. In Bowen's disease, some epidermal cells may undergo individual cell keratinization and become separated from their neighbors. However, this process is only one feature of the general dysplasia exhibited by the epidermis, while in Paget's disease, epidermal keratinocytes retain fairly normal morphology, although they may be compressed. Superficially spreading malignant melanoma has pagetoid features (Fig. 32–37) but may be differentiated in fresh material by the positive dopa reaction or in paraffin sections by the demonstration of melanin and premelanin (Fontana-Masson method) and also by the absence of acid mucopolysaccharides or glycogen in melanoma cells. Epidermotropic lymphomas (Chap. 44) may cause difficulties.

Trabecular Carcinoma

In 1972, Toker[22] described five cases of invasive carcinoma originating in the dermis or in the immediate subcutis and consisting of solid trabeculae that lack definite acini. Two of them metastasized. In a more recent publication[23] on three additional tumors using electron microscopy, the original thesis that the tumors are sweat gland carcinomas was corrected when dense-core membrane-bound granules were observed in the cells. The suggestion was offered that trabecular carcinoma originates from one of the neurocrest derivatives, most likely from Merkel cells (Chap. 2).

METASTATIC CARCINOMA

Cutaneous metastasis of internal cancer is relatively rare but is of diagnostic importance[24-26] because it may be the first manifestation of metastasis of a supposedly cured malignancy or even the first manifestation of an undiagnosed carcinoma.

With the exception of hypernephroma and a few other tumors,[24] the histologic features of cutaneous metastases do not permit identification of the primary site. The most common form of growth (Fig. 40–7A) is the formation of thin solid cords in the interfascicular spaces of the dermis. Presence of signet-ring cells, which contain mucin (Fig. 40–7B), suggests a primary focus in the gastrointestinal tract. There is rarely any inflammatory or fibrotic reaction, a fact that sets metastatic lesions apart from morphealike and sclerosing basaliomas. Rarely, carcinomatous cords approach and even invade the epidermis. This usually results in ulceration, but Paget-like pictures may be encountered.

The scalp is a site of predilection for metastatic cancer, especially of the breast. Any nodule arising on the scalp of an elderly person should be suspect. In rare cases, a patch of alopecia without tumor formation may be the site of a scirrhous carcinoma, with few nests of large cells within a fibrotic stroma that chokes off hair roots.

REFERENCES

1. Hernández-Pérez E, Baños E: Sebaceous carcinoma. Report of two cases with metastasis. Dermatologica 156:184, 1978
2. Bonink M, Zimmerman LE: Sebaceous carcinoma of the eyelid, eyebrow, caruncle and orbit. Trans Am Acad Ophthalmol Otolaryngol 72:619, 1968
3. Dixon RS, Mikhail GR, Slater HC: Sebaceous carcinoma of the eyelid. J Acad Dermatol 3:241, 1980
4. Lee SC, Roth LM: Sebaceous carcinoma of the eyelid with pagetoid involvement of the bulbar and palpebral conjunctiva. J Cutan Pathol 4:134, 1977
5. ElDomeiri AA, Brasfield RD, Huvos AG, et al.: Sweat gland carcinoma. A clinico-pathologic study of 83 patients. Ann Surg 173:270, 1971
6. Pinkus H: Adnexal tumors, benign, not-so-benign, and malignant. In Montagna W, Dobson RL (eds): Carcinogenesis. Advances in Biology of Skin, vol 7. New York, Pergamon, 1966, p 255
7. Hernández-Pérez E, Cruz TA: Clear cell hidradenocarcinoma. Report of an unusual case. Dermatologica 153:249, 1976
8. Piñol-Aguadé J, Pedragosa JR, Tomás JM, et al.: Falsos basaliomas y falsas metástasis cutáneos de carcinomas viscerales. A proposito de 7 observaciones de carcinoma ecrino. Med Cutan Iber Lat Am 4:23, 1976
9. Mendoza S, Helwig EB: Mucinous (adenocystic) carcinoma of the skin. Arch Dermatol 103:68, 1971

10. Santa-Cruz DJ, Meyers JH, Gnepp DR, et al.: Primary mucinous carcinoma of the skin. Br J Dermatol 98:645, 1978
11. Pinkus H, Mehregan AH: Epidermotropic eccrine carcinoma. A case combining features of eccrine poroma and Paget's dermatosis. Arch Dermatol 88:597, 1963
12. Mishima Y, Morioka S: Oncogenic differentiation of intraepidermal eccrine sweat duct: eccrine poroma, poroepithelioma, and porocarcinoma. Dermatologica 138:238, 1969
13. Hadida E, Sayag J, Sayag J, et al.: Poro-épithélioma avec metastases ganglionnaries. Bull Soc Fr Dermatol Syphiligr 79:271, 1972
14. Helwig EB, Graham JH: Anogenital (extramammary) Paget's disease: clinico-pathologic study. Cancer 16:387, 1963
15. Muir R: The pathogenesis of Paget's disease of the nipple and associated lesions. Br J Surg 22:728, 1935
16. Inglis K: Paget's Disease of the Nipple and Its Relation to Surface Cancers and Precancerous States in General. Oxford, Oxford Medical Publications, 1936
17. Pinkus H, Gould SE: Extramammary Paget's disease and intraepidermal carcinoma. Arch Dermatol 39:479, 1939
18. Pinkus H: In discussion of Murrell TW Jr, McMullan FH: Extramammary Paget's disease. Arch Dermatol 85:600, 1962
19. Jones RE, Austin C, Ackerman AB: Extramammary Paget's disease. A critical reexamination. Am J Dermatopathol 1:101, 1979
20. Woods WS, Culling CFA: Perianal Paget disease: histochemical differentiation utilizing borohydride-KOH-PAS reaction. Arch Pathol 99:442, 1975
21. Cawley LP: Extramammary Paget's disease. Am J Clin Pathol 27:559, 1957
22. Toker C: Trabecular carcinoma of the skin. Arch Dermatol 105:107, 1972
23. Tang C-K, Toker C: Trabecular carcinoma of the skin. An ultrastructural study. Cancer 42:2311, 1978
24. Mehregan AH: Metastatic carcinoma to the skin. Dermatologica 123:311, 1961
25. Brownstein MM, Helwig EB: Patterns of cutaneous metastasis. Arch Dermatol 105:862, 1972
26. Brownstein MM, Helwig EB: Spread of tumors to the skin. Arch Dermatol 107:80, 1973

Mesodermal Nevi and Tumors

Each of the mesodermal components of the skin can be the source of neoplasms, but their incidence and variability are much smaller than those of epithelial and fibroepithelial tumors. The number and variety of malignant mesodermal neoplasms are even smaller. The more important lesions are listed in Table 41-1, with the exception of vascular tumors, which are discussed in Chapter 42. Rather than giving systematic descriptions, we shall discuss differentiating features and points of biologic significance.

In addition to the usual task of identifying the specific cell or tissue of a tumor, we meet two peculiar difficulties in this field. All mesodermal tissues contain blood vessels, and sometimes it is not easy to decide whether a lesion is primarily or secondarily vascular. Furthermore, reactive proliferation of fibrous tissue must be differentiated from nevoid or neoplastic proliferation.

SCAR VERSUS KELOID VERSUS FIBROMA VERSUS CONNECTIVE TISSUE NEVUS

A good starting point with basic significance is the differentiation of the four conditions listed in the heading. As happens so often in dermatopathology, clinical data are important, and we must try to refine our histologic criteria to fit the clinical course. For instance, there has been much discussion on how to differentiate histologically a temporarily hypertrophic scar from a keloid at the time when the clinician is in doubt within the first few months after surgery, this being the most propitious time to institute treatment. Newer stains and more intensive investigation have clarified the differences to some degree.

Every young scar is a new growth of connective tissue and has some features of a neoplasm. However, just as atypical proliferation of epithelium in a healing wound or other tissue defect eventually subsides, so is the stage of proliferation of fibrocytes and blood vessels in a scar followed by a stage of maturation and return to relatively normal tissue homeostasis. *Keloid* tissue, on the other hand, remains immature for prolonged periods and has other peculiar characteristics.

Normal Scar

When scar tissue has replaced a defect in the skin, the area is characterized by three major features. Collagen bundles run a fairly straight course parallel to the skin surface. Small blood vessels extend perpendicularly between epidermis and subcutis, and elastic fibers either are absent or are thin and run parallel to the collagen bundles. Moreover, hair follicles and sweat glands are apt to be absent, and the papillae and rete ridges are either absent or poorly developed.

This picture comes about because the pars reti-

TABLE 41–1.
Mesodermal Nevi and Tumors

Fibrocytic
  Connective tissue nevi
    Collagenous
    Elastic
  Fibroma
    Nodulus cutaneus
    Keloid
    Fibroma molle (pendulum) and acrochordon
    Acquired fibrokeratoma
    Perifollicular fibroma
    Trichodiscoma
    Myxoma
    Osteoma
  Sarcoma
    Dermatofibrosarcoma protuberans
    Spindle cell sarcoma
    Pseudosarcomatous fasciitis
Histiocytic
  Benign lesions (Chap. 23)
  Langerhans cell granulomas (Chap. 24)
  Malignant histiocytomas
Lipocytic
  Nevus lipomatosus superficialis and nevus
    angiolipomatosus
  Lipoma and angiolipoma
  Liposarcoma
Muscular
  Leiomyoma
  Leiomyosarcoma
  Rhabdomyosarcoma

For a recent general review of mesodermal tumors, see Hajdu SI: *Pathology of Soft Tissue Tumors.* Philadelphia, Lea & Febiger, 1979.

cularis of the dermis is poorly vascularized, and granulation tissue, the first step in replacement of a tissue defect, arises primarily from the subcutaneous tissue, with some help from adnexal vascular tissue, and from the pars papillaris of the surrounding dermis. We emphasize that we are not dealing here with the healing of an incised and sutured wound but with the restitution of a sizable defect in the skin, such as an ulcer from whatever source. The components of *granulation tissue* (Fig. 41–1), vascular sprouts, and fibrocytes, coming from below, are at first directed vertical to the skin surface (Fig. 17–1). Fibroblastic cells containing myofilaments (myofibroblasts[1]) have been recognized recently in granulation tissue and contribute to its contraction. Blood vessels later become less numerous, but the persisting ones retain their telltale vertical arrangement. Fibrocytes and the collagen fibers and bundles formed by them are redeployed parallel to the skin surface but never achieve the resilient three-dimensional weave of normal dermis. Elastic fibers often are completely absent. They are regenerated more readily in young individuals but

always remain thin. While granulation tissue is rich in ground substance, this soon is reduced, and a maturing scar shows normal staining reactions with mucopolysaccharide and connective tissue stains.

Hypertrophic Scars and Keloids

Hypertrophic scars and keloids, on the other hand, grow in the dermis and produce curvilinear tracts and bundles, several of which form a whorl[2]. The interstitial tissue retains relatively large amounts of mucosaccharides for a longer time, giving H&E sections a bluish tinge. Abnormal cross-linking amino acids[3] have been described and the presence of myofibroblasts.[4] In the hypertrophic scar, there is gradual maturation, although the whorled arrangement may persist. In keloids, the process proceeds to the formation of tightly packed nodules of collagen with peripheral blood vessels. The tissue remains rich in cells and ground substance, and the collagen also is abnormal. This is best shown by Luxol fast blue, which stains normal collagen blue

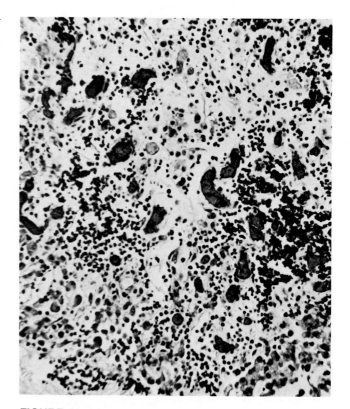

FIGURE 41–1.
Granulation tissue. Capillary blood vessels and a mixture of inflammatory cells embedded in immature connective tissue. H&E. X180.

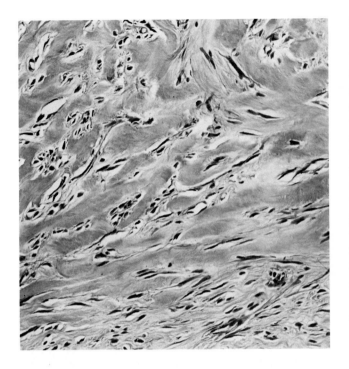

FIGURE 41–2.
Keloid, central portion exhibiting hyalinized collagen bundles and unusually large fibrocytes. (Compare with Fig. 15–9.) H&E. X225.

and that of keloid reddish. Later, in old keloids, collagen bundles may become very thick, hyaline, and eosinophilic (Fig. 41–2). There is no new formation of elastic fibers. Keloids that have developed in skin defects (burn keloids, scar keloids) have no normal pars papillaris. So-called *spontaneous keloids*, however, such as those that develop from minor trauma or acne lesions, are separated from the epidermis by fairly normal papillary dermis. Keloids are well circumscribed, often almost encapsulated, in contrast to histiocytomas (fibromas) and papular leiomyomas but similar to angioleiomyomas and neurofibromas.

Fibroma

What constitutes a dermal fibroma is not easy to define. It ought to be a continuing benign proliferation of less than mature connective tissue with deranged architecture. A keloid meets many of these criteria, but there remains some doubt as to its truly neoplastic nature. The tumor that bears the name *dermatofibroma (nodulus cutaneus, subepidermal nodular fibrosis)* also is in doubt because, in most cases, it is probably a fibrosed histiocytoma (Chap. 23). Another candidate is *fibrous papule of the nose,*[5,6] a common small lesion (Fig. 41–3) arising relatively late in life and consisting of fairly cellular fibrous tissue lacking elastic fibers. It is not known how often this may be fibrotic overgrowth in a subsiding dermal nevus. The tiny protrusions on the glans penis, known as *pearly penile papules,* also qualify as angiofibromas.[7]

Perifollicular Fibromas and Trichodiscomas

Other fibromatous lesions are related to the mesodermal portions of the pilar apparatus and have been described as *perifollicular fibromas*[8] and *trichodiscomas.*[9] Both are rare. Their existence, however, emphasizes what was said in Chapter 2—that the hair follicle has an integral mesodermal component which behaves independently from the interfollicular (skeletal) dermis. This follicle-related mesoderm forms the dermal papilla of the follicle, the perifollicular sheath, the arrector pili muscle, and the dermal pad of the hair disk.[10,11]

Perifollicular fibromas, which were mentioned in Chapter 36, may be present in three different forms,[12] as small single papules, as larger nodes, and as part of the tuberous sclerosis syndrome (Fig. 41–4). Cases described as multiple perifollicular fibromas of head and neck[13] seem to belong rather to

FIGURE 41–3.
Fibrous papule of nose. This lesion exhibits general, as well as perifollicular, overgrowth of fairly cellular collagenous tissue involving papillae and deeper dermal layers. H&E. X30. (For an instructive discussion of this and related lesions, see Ackerman AB (ed). Am J Dermatopathol 1:329–355, 1979.)

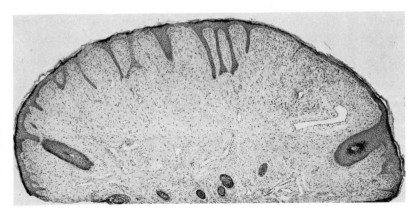

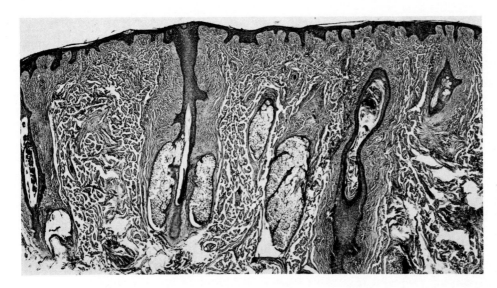

FIGURE 41–4.
Perifollicular fibromas (nevoid hyperplasia of follicular fibrous sheath) as a manifestation of Pringle's disease (tuberous sclerosis syndrome). H&E. X30.

a closely related entity, the *fibrofolliculoma* of Birt et al.[14] In a personal case (Fig. 36–17) of that type,[15] the substance of the papules was rich in reticulum fibers and stained prominently with PAS and alcian blue, an indication of neoplastic derangement of connective tissue maturation. The same patient also had a large connective tissue nevus of the interfollicular dermis, similar to those seen in tuberous sclerosis and offering a good example of the independence of the two components of the dermis. Moreover, he had unusually large dermal pads of haarscheibe associated with some of his fibrofolliculomas, while the patient of Birt et al.[14] had true *trichodiscomas* (Chap. 36, Fig. 36–18).

Connective Tissue Nevi

Under the term *connective tissue nevi* are grouped conditions that are congenital or arise later in life and have a relatively stable excess of mature vascularized connective tissue. It is understood that the sole cell capable of forming connective tissue is the fibroblast, although certain types of basement membrane-related collagens have recently been attributed to epithelial cells, and formation of elastin to smooth muscle cells. In lesions consisting of an excess of fibers, the fibroblasts usually are inconspicuous. The stimuli that prod them to lay down collagenous fibers, elastic fibers, and ground substance are unknown. We, therefore, can only describe the lesions we see and group them according to their clinical and histologic correlations, as has been done in Table 41–2, modified slightly from one presented by Hegedus and Schorr.[16] It appears preferable to give such an analysis of various forms

of nevoid conditions, rather than to use "connective tissue nevus" as a unifying term. One should remember that blood vessels are an essential part of any connective tissue and may be present in excess *(angiofibromas)*.

The *Pringle tumors* of the central face in tuberous sclerosis, for which "adenoma sebaceum" is an unfortunate misnomer (Chap. 1), are due to nevoid hyperplasia of vascular connective tissue either between or around hair follicles. *Shagreen plaques* of other regions are larger accumulations of mature connective tissue of the pars reticularis, and periungual fibromas are almost indistinguishable from acquired acral fibrokeratomas (see below). The *Buschke–Ollendorff syndrome*[17] consists of multiple skin papules of mature collagenous and elastic tissue in association with osteopoikilosos (Chap. 26), which also may be found associated with other types of *collagenoma*[18,19] and elastic tissue nevi. It seems likely that the histologically similar papules of *epidermolysis bullosa et albopapuloidea* of Pasini, which contain degraded chondroitin sulfate,[20] also belong here. Other connective tissue nevi have been described as *nevus elasticus* and *juvenile elastoma*. Nevus elasticus of the Lewandowsky type actually is a minus nevus as far as elastic fibers are concerned and rather is a collagenous nevus. Lesions described as juvenile elastoma (Fig. 26–16) do consist of circumscribed hyperplasia of elastic tissue (Chap. 26). Somewhat similar hyperplasia may be encountered in association with nevus cell nevi[21] and may overshadow the nevus cells. In other cases,[22] the fibromatous proliferation may be multiple, often involving muscle and only secondarily the subcutaneous tissue or the skin. Many of these cases defy exact classification, but although

TABLE 41–2.
Connective Tissue Nevi and Related Conditions

Clinical Diagnosis	Collagen	Elastic Fibers
Pringle tumors	Increased, vascular	Absent
Shagreen patch	Increased	Relatively decreased
Paving stone nevus (Lipschütz)	Hypertrophic, swollen homogeneous	Relatively decreased
Familiar cutaneous collagenoma	Increased	Relatively decreased
Dermatofibrosis lenticularis disseminata (Buschke-Ollendorff)	Increased	Decreased
Dermatofibrosis disseminata with microcysts (Verbov)	Increased perifollicular tissue	Decreased
Perifollicular fibroma	Increased perifollicular sheath	Absent
Fibrofolliculoma	Abnormal perifollicular sheath	Absent
Trichodiscoma	Decreased, edematous	Normal
Juvenile elastoma (Weidman, Mehregan, and Staricco)	No significant change	Increased, somewhat abnormal
Nevus elasticus (Lewandowsky)	No significant change	Spottily decreased and abnormal
Zosteriform connective tissue nevus	Abnormal, irregular, fine, short	Reduced, abnormal: shreds, granules
Epidermolysis bullosa et albopapuloidea (Pasini)	Degraded chondroitin sulfate	Absent

Adapted from Hegedus and Schorr.[16]

they may form tumor masses and may recur, they are not usually malignant. We shall refer to them later under juvenile digital fibromas.

Acrochordon, Fibroma Pendulum, Acquired Fibrokeratoma

In distinction from lesions that are located in the reticular dermis, there are those that project outward from the skin (papillomas). Most common is the *skin tag* or *acrochordon*. It consists of papillary dermis covered by thin epithelium and, in many cases, seems to be essentially one hyperplastic papilla. In other cases, however, there is more epidermal proliferation, and one wonders whether such a lesion is a papilloma in the sense of a combined new growth of epidermis and mesoderm (Chap. 33). This is particularly true in patients who have numerous lesions around the neck which are apt to vary clinically from skin tags to sessile and flat seborrheic warts.

Fibroma pendulum is the term used for larger lesions consisting purely of loose connective tissue of papillary type covered by epidermis. Some of these may be the end stage of a nevus cell nevus after the cells have atrophied. Some may contain fat tissue. Vascularity varies, and inflammation or torsion of the pedicle may lead to engorgement and hemorrhagic infarction. Fibroma pendulum does not contain hair follicles or sweat glands. If elastic fibers are present, they are of the thin papillary type.

Attention was called recently to not uncommon lesions (Fig. 41–5) on the acra under the name *acquired digital fibrokeratoma*.[23–25] Its differentiation from papillomas with hyperkeratotic acanthotic epidermal covering may seem to be a histologic nicety but actually has a biologic basis. The connective tissue core represents the pars reticularis as well as the pars papillaris and may include the two types of elastic fibers found in these layers. Some lesions also contain sweat ducts. Similar lesions occur on acral parts of the limbs other than the digits.

LESIONS WITH UNUSUAL DIFFERENTIATION OF CONNECTIVE TISSUE

Mucinous Lesions. True *myxomas* of the skin are rare, and the question arises in every case whether one is not dealing with a peculiar reaction to injury. The histologic picture resembles that of umbilical cord. *Mucinous papules* and so-called *synovial lesions* were discussed in Chapter 25. The so-called *giant cell tumor of tendon sheath* (Fig.

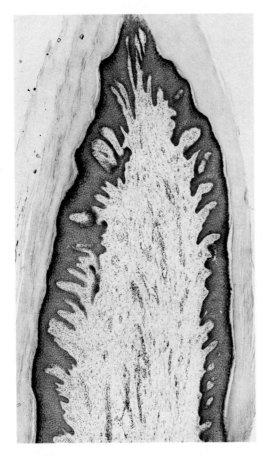

FIGURE 41–5.
Acquired digital fibrokeratoma. H&E. X30.

41–6), on the other hand, really is tenosynovitis with deposits of hemosiderin in a mixed foreign-body granuloma. It must not be mistaken for atypical fibroxanthoma (Fig. 41–12). In *mucinous carcinoma* (Chap. 40), epithelial nests may be so small and so widely separated by mucinous stroma that they may be overlooked in individual sections.

Juvenile Hyaline Fibromatosis. Several cases have been reported[26,27] in which large tumors appeared around the head, with small papules elsewhere and destructive lesions in long bones. The tumors consisted of large granular cells (Fig. 41–7) embedded in PAS-positive ground substance, giving the appearance of pseudocysts. This bizarre manifestation, possibly inherited in a recessive manner, ending fatally or improving, has been given the name juvenile hyaline fibromatosis.

Osteoma. Bone formation occurs in the skin and subcutaneous tissue under a variety of circumstances and was discussed in Chapter 27. Whether *osteoma* (Fig. 27–3) in the sense of primary neoplastic bone formation[28] exists in the skin is doubtful. Cases in which multiple tiny spheres of bone have been found on face and neck may well represent ossification of multiple epithelial milia. A few benign cartilaginous tumors have been found in the skin.[29]

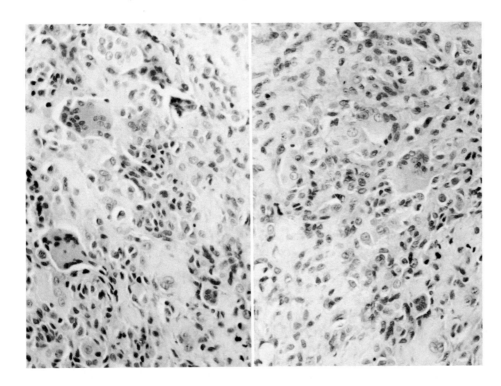

FIGURE 41–6.
Giant cell tumor of tendon sheath. These accumulations of histiocytes, macrophages, and multinucleated giant cells actually are foreign-body granulomas. They must be differentiated from pseudosarcomatous lesions, such as atypical fibroxanthoma (Fig. 41–12).

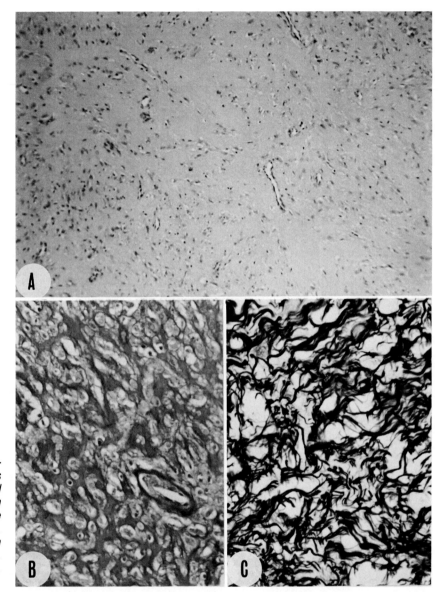

FIGURE 41–7.
Juvenile hyaline fibromatosis. **A.** *Fibroblasts and endothelial-lined capillaries embedded in a homogeneous ground substance. H&E. X100.* **B.** *PAS stain shows positive reaction of the hyaline material in the ground substance. X275.* **C.** *Reticulum stain demonstrates a rich network of reticulum fibers. X275. (Courtesy of Drs. J.K. Maniar and E. Wilson-Jones.)*

SARCOMA VERSUS HISTIOCYTOMA VERSUS PSEUDOSARCOMA

In the low-power histologic diagnosis of sarcoma, the classic division into round and spindle cell sarcomas retains its value. Round cell sarcomas will be discussed in Chapter 44, since practically all of them are malignant lymphomas in modern terminology. Tumors consisting predominantly of fusiform cells are more difficult to classify because a light microscopic differentiation of fibroblasts and histiocytes is very difficult. As pointed out in Chapters 2 and 5, histiocytes are identified by their ability to phagocytose. An inactive (resting) histiocyte is just a fixed-tissue-type cell, although the

electron microscope may reveal lysosomes and other differentiating features. It must be kept in mind, however, that fibrocytes and histiocytes most likely can transform one into the other. Benign histiocytomas can transform into fibromas and vice versa. The term *fibrous histiocytoma* expresses this ability[30] and injects considerable doubt into our ability for correct diagnosis. Recently, even greater doubt has been brought to our diagnostic efforts by well-trained investigators who reexamined spindle cell carcinomas and atypical fibroxanthomas under the electron microscope and had to reclassify considerable numbers of lesions (Chap. 34). Lesions consisting predominantly of fusiform cells are of three types: rare primary spindle cell sarcomas, dermatofibrosarcoma protuberans, and sarcomas originating in Kaposi's pigmented hemorrhagic sarcoma (Chap. 42). These must be differentiated from pseudosarcomatous lesions.

Spindle Cell Sarcoma

Spindle cell sarcoma consists of streams and bundles of large fusiform cells varying more or less in size of nuclei and cytoplasm and containing numerous mitoses. Interstitial tissue is minimal. The tumor as a rule arises in deeper tissues and invades subcutis and dermis. Kaposi's sarcoma may develop into a pure spindle cell sarcoma. An unusual tumor is the epithelioid sarcoma of Enzinger that consists of large, plump cells and may imitate a granuloma with central necrosis or a squamous cell carcinoma (Fig. 41–8). Heavy lymphocytic infiltrate is associated, and there are numerous mitoses.[31]

Histiocytoma

Infiltrative growth between dermal collagen bundles is not restricted to sarcomas. The nodulus cutaneus type of benign histiocytoma–fibroma has no

capsule and, at first glance, has an invading periphery. So does pseudosarcomatous fasciitis. For proper diagnosis of all these lesions, an ample biopsy, including central and peripheral portions, is essential. Closer analysis reveals the following differences. As discussed in Chapter 23, histiocytomas regularly have more or less prominent accumulations of round cells around small vessels outside the tumor periphery. Fat stains, if available, usually show lipid droplets in these inflammatory-looking cells and may show lipid in cells of the tumor itself, thus characterizing them as phagocytic histiocytes. Primary malignant fibrous histiocytomas (Fig. 41–9) of skin[32] are rare and are characterized, in addition to clinically progressive growth, by multinodularity and by invasion of blood vessels, subcutaneous tissue, and possibly bone. Electron microscopy reveals a mixture of fibrocytes, histiocytes, and intermediate cells, emphasizing the difficulties discussed above.

Dermatofibrosarcoma Protuberans

Dermatofibrosarcoma protuberans[33,34] exhibits extensive infiltration of fiber-forming spindle cells in the interfascicular spaces of the deeper dermis, a

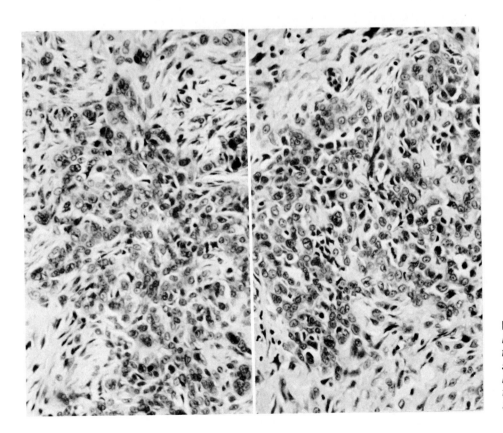

FIGURE 41–8.
Epithelioid sarcoma. Differentiation of these tumors from spindle cell squamous carcinomas and atypical fibroxanthomas may be difficult (Chap. 34). H&E. X225.

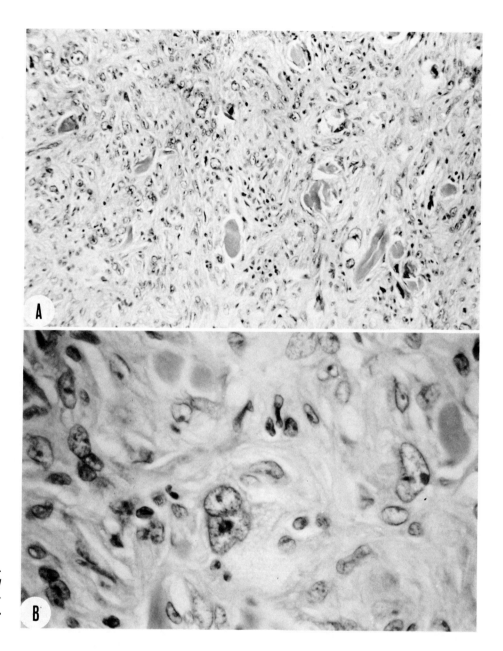

FIGURE 41–9.
*Malignant fibrous histiocytoma. Mixture of small and large atypical cells invading fibrous tissue. H&E. **A.** X125. **B.** X600.*

feature often discernible already in H&E sections (Fig. 41–10A). This shelf may extend not only for millimeters but for centimeters lateral to the nodular tumor and is the reason for recurrence if only the visible tumor is excised. The storiform cellular pattern inside the tumor was discussed for histiocytoma in Chapter 23. Some larger histiocytomas, which also extend into the subcutis, may imitate the peculiar cartwheel pattern (Fig. 41–10B) of the fibrosarcoma. On the other hand, the latter may become much more mature, with formation of much collagen and loss of the characteristic pattern, either in portions or throughout the lesion. In such cases, examination of the periphery is essential.

Attempts to consider dermatofibrosarcoma protuberans to be a histiocytoma on the basis of tissue culture and electron microscopy[35] cannot be considered successful for reasons mentioned repeatedly in our discussion. The possible relationship to perineural and endoneural cells seems better founded.[34]

Pseudosarcomas

Pseudosarcomas of the skin and subcutaneous tissue have been much discussed in recent years. There are two principal entities, both characterized clinically by rapid enlargement and benign behav-

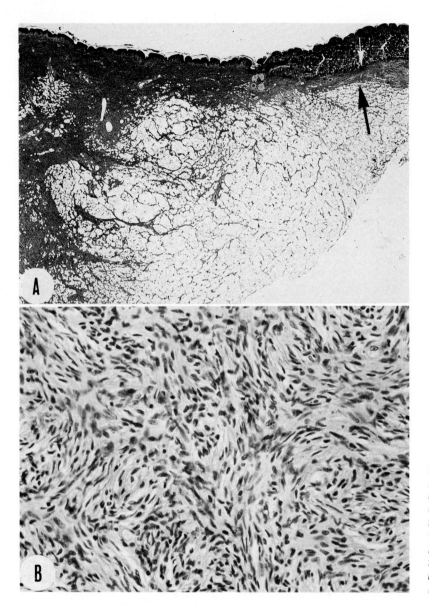

FIGURE 41–10.
Dermatofibrosarcoma protuberans. **A** *shows at left the edge of tumor which infiltrates dermis and subcutaneous tissue. While infiltration of subcutaneous tissue subsides toward right, there is a shelf of tumor tissue at border of dermis and hypoderm extending to edge of specimen at right. Upper and lower borders are indicated by arrows. H&E. X9.* **B.** *Cartwheel pattern. H&E. X225.*

ior, resulting in disappearance spontaneously or even after incomplete excision. One of them, nodular or *pseudosarcomatous fasciitis,*[36] is situated subcutaneously (Fig. 41–11). The other one, for which the name *atypical fibroxanthoma*[37] is commonly used, arises in the skin itself (Fig. 41–12). These lesions occur mainly in actinically damaged skin and consist either of dysplastic spindle cells forming poorly developed bundles or of bizarre polygonal and giant cells or of a mixture of these cell types. They infiltrate the surroundings in irregular fashion but usually do not recur after excision. Some well-documented cases of metastasis indicate, however, that some are true neoplasms. An electron microscopic study of two cases[38] revealed numerous Langerhans cells in one. It seems possible that a group of mesenchymal proliferative re-

actions occur in a similar clinical setting. Lipids are often demonstrable in frozen sections. There are fairly numerous mitoses, and the nuclei may be hyperchromatic but are not atypical. Pseudosarcomatous pictures may also be found years after radiotherapy and may be extremely difficult to tell from true sarcomas developing under similar circumstances.[39]

Recurrent Digital Fibrous Tumor of Childhood

Also to be mentioned here are fibrous tumors occurring on digits in children and having a strong tendency to recurrence but a relatively benign histologic picture, although they may extend from the

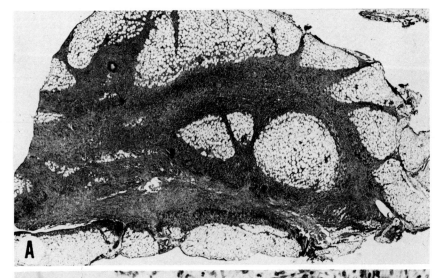

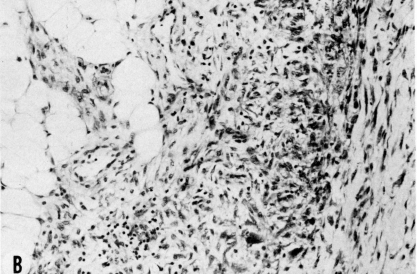

FIGURE 41–11.
Nodular (pseudosarcomatous) fasciitis.
A. *Subcutaneous nodule consists of densely cellular central area from which processes extend into surrounding fat tissue and suggest invasion. H&E. X14.*
B. *In the periphery of the lesion, there is a zone of granulomatous proliferation consisting of newly formed capillary blood vessels, histiocytes, giant cells, and scattered round cells. H&E. X135. (From Mehregan. Arch Dermatol 93:204, 1966.)*

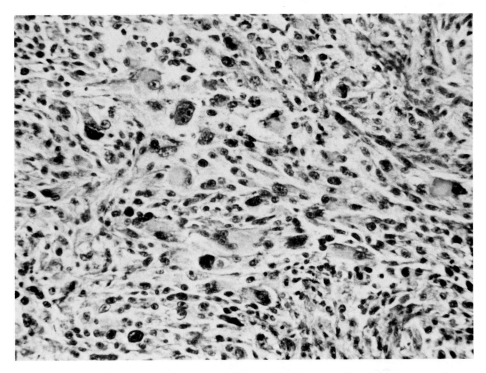

FIGURE 41–12.
Atypical fibroxanthoma. Greatly variable histiocytes, some multinucleated and foamy. Note resemblance to Sternberg–Reed cells (Fig. 44–4). H&E. X225.

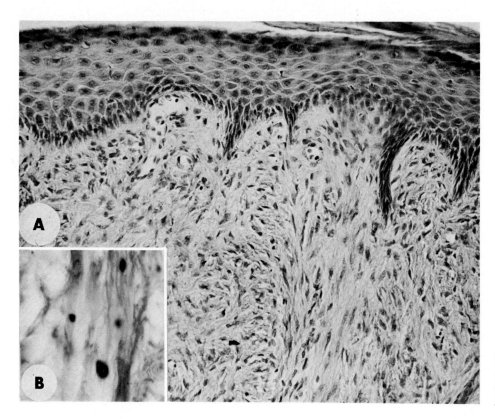

FIGURE 41–13.
Digital fibrous tumor of childhood. **A.** *H&E. X180.* **B.** *Cytoplasmic inclusions. H&E. X800.*

lower epidermal surface deep into the subcutaneous tissue. These recurring digital fibrous tumors of childhood[40,41] consist of whorls of spindle cells and fibrous tissue (Fig. 41–13A) and are identified by large cytoplasmic inclusions (Fig. 41–13B) which are visible in H&E sections but are much better demonstrated by phosphotungstic acid hematoxylin. They are not viral bodies. The spindle cells show the features of myofibroblasts on ultrastructural examination.[42]

LEIOMYOMA VERSUS HISTIOCYTOMA–FIBROMA

Many leiomyomas are so mature that the border between a smooth muscle nevus and a benign neoplasm is difficult to draw histologically. Most leiomyomas (Fig. 41–14) appear to be related to arrector pili muscle in localization and structure. Their frequent occurrence as multiple lesions becomes more plausible if we remember (Chap. 2)

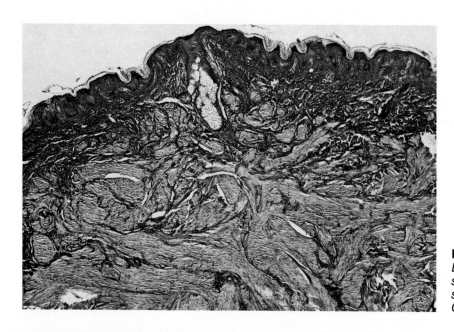

FIGURE 41–14.
Leiomyoma. Yellow-staining (light) masses of smooth muscle contrast with red-staining (dark) collagen bundles. Van Gieson. X45.

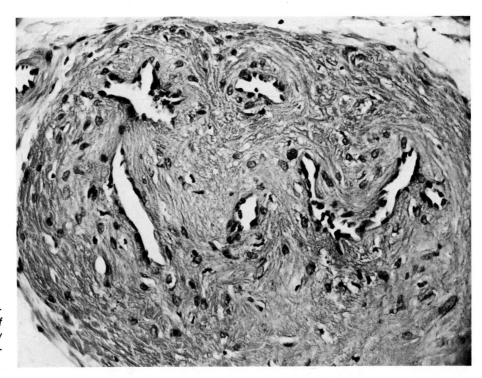

FIGURE 41–15.
Angioleiomyoma. Vascular channels embedded in a nodule of smooth muscle cells and strongly metachromatic ground substance. H&E. X135.

that in fetal life hair muscles originate in a diffuse metachromatic zone of the mesoderm, in spatial relation to, but not actually as part of, the fibroepithelial hair germ. Excessive production of muscle in these predisposed fields may lead to hamartomatous lesions, which may be stable, mature *muscle nevi* or less mature, progressively growing neoplasms.[43] Other much less common *angioleiomyomas* are related to vascular muscle.[44,45] These usually are solitary spherical lesions (Fig. 41–15) in the subcutaneous tissue of the legs, predominantly in women, and are easily diagnosed if one keeps in mind that not everything that looks pink and fibrous in H&E sections must be collagen. O&G or trichrome stains can be used for identification. O&G has three advantages in that it deemphasizes collagen, which may be present in any leiomyoma in considerable quantity, shows up elastic fibers, which frequently are newly formed as an accompaniment of smooth muscle formation,[46] and stains mucinous ground substance metachromatically, a feature common in tumors related to vascular wall.

Leiomyomas of a lesser degree of maturity have to be differentiated from histiocytomas and fibromas, and this may not be easy in H&E sections.[47] One should remember that smooth muscle usually forms fairly long and straight bundles, which intersect rather than whorl. Formation of much collagen may be disturbing, and in trichrome stains (Van Gieson or Masson-Mallory) the collagen may actually overshadow the cellular element. On the other hand, as mentioned in Chapter 23, histiocy-

tomas and fibromas contain only disjointed remnants of old elastic fibers, while leiomyomas frequently have newly formed fibers running parallel to the cell bundles. Demonstration of myofibrils with phosphotungstic acid hematoxylin may be attempted.

Leiomyosarcomas are rare and are characterized by the usual histologic attributes of malignancy: cellular atypia and more than 10 mitoses in 10 high-power fields. There may, however, be considerable spottiness in the distribution of mitoses, and treatment should be rather conservative.[48] Skeletal muscle occurs in the skin only on the face, and *rhabdomyosarcomas* are extremely rare.[49]

LIPOMA

Subcutaneous Lipoma

It is much more common to find normally constituted fat tissue in abnormal location or in abnormal amount than to find histologic aberrations truly classifiable as benign or malignant neoplasms. The histologic structure of the common subcutaneous lipoma is so much like normal fat tissue that it may be classified as a nevus of fat tissue on the basis of the maturity of its cells. Fat tissue (Chap. 2) develops in the embryo from small vascular foci (primitive fat organs), which by continuous accumulation of specific perivascular cells and their conversion into fat cells form individual

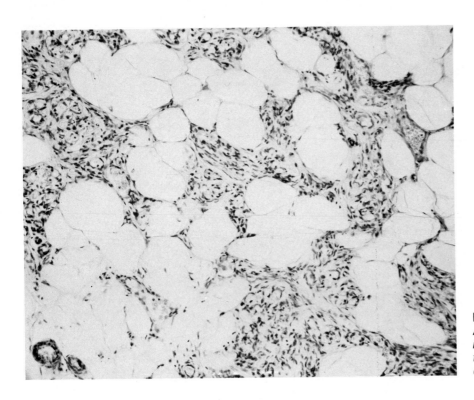

FIGURE 41–16.
Angiolipoma. Small portion of tumor is shown to demonstrate vascular tissue between normal-appearing fat cells. H&E. X135.

fat lobules. Thus, the development and extremely slow growth of unusually large, well-circumscribed nodes of fat tissue fit the definition of nevus also on the basis of tissue structure. *Angiolipoma* (Fig. 41–16) is a variant containing an unusual amount of vascular tissue.[50] Cases have been described in which encapsulated angiolipomas could be moved for considerable distances under the skin.[51] No explanation was given of how the blood supply of these tumors was maintained and how they were moved without disrupting surrounding tissue.

Fatty tumors may also project above the skin surface and may indicate, if in the sacral region, an underlying spina bifida with associated disturbances.[52]

Nevus Lipomatosus

Fat tissue, beyond the small amounts normally present around the deeper parts of hair follicles and sweat coils, is encountered within the skin in two conditions bearing the name nevus lipomatosus. One, the *nevus lipomatosus superficialis* of Hoffman and Zurhelle,[53,54] usually occurs as grouped lesions around the hip region, mainly of adolescent girls, and is of little practical importance. It consists of lobules of normal fat tissue which develop in the reticular portion of the dermis and partly replace the dermal connective tissue (Fig. 41–17). The other lesion, *nevus angiolipomatosus* of How-

ell[55] (Fig. 41–18), begins in early babyhood as accumulations of peculiar round cells and fat cells around small vessels of the pars papillaris, which are increased in number. The fat tissue may be sparse, and the lesion may resemble a superficial angioma, or fat tissue may crowd out the normal dermis until it practically disappears, and nevus fat lobes and subcutaneous fat lobes almost merge. There remains, however, a narrow layer of deep dermal collagenous tissue. This condition produces histologic pictures similar to the *focal dermal hypoplasia syndrome*, in which, according to Goltz et al.,[56] subcutaneous fat tissue replaces the hypoplastic dermis from below and extends upward close to the epidermis. This syndrome may cause pseudotumorous yellow protrusions above the level of the surrounding skin, and is associated with skeletal and other malformations.[57] Recent tissue culture studies[58] have shown that the fibroblasts of the upper dermis have abnormal metabolism.

Hibernoma

Yet another rare, and not really cutaneous, nevoid neoplasm has the structure of brown fat tissue, a type of vascular tissue with multivacuolar fat cells, which occurs mainly between the shoulder blades and probably is related to heat regulation in babies.[59] Because this tissue is prominently found in hibernating mammals, the tumor was given the

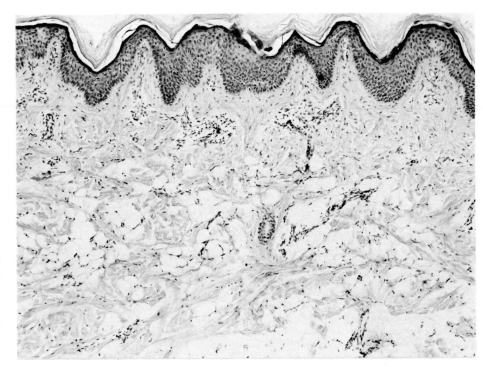

FIGURE 41–17.
Nevus lipomatosus superficialis. Fat cells of the nevus infiltrate and partly replace the reticular dermis. They remain below the superficial vascular plexus and also are not part of the subcutaneous tissue. H&E. X45. (From Mehregan, Tavafoghi, and Gandtchi. J Cutan Pathol 2:307, 1975. Copyright © 1975 Munksgaard International Publishers, Copenhagen.)

name *hibernoma*.[60] There is, however, the possibility[61] that this rare lesion truly represents neoplasia of fat tissue with retarded maturation.

Other Entities

Fat tissue may develop secondarily in other tumors. Cellular nevi often contain some fat cells and may be replaced by fat tissue (Fig. 32–28). A peculiar but characteristic feature is development of fat tissue in bone marrow-like fashion whenever bone develops in the skin (osteoma cutis and calcifying epithelioma).

Some subcutaneous lipomas contain a high proportion of spindle cells with evidence of transformation into lipocytes. No atypical cells are found, and the lesions are benign *spindle cell lipomas*.[62] *Liposarcomas* are very rare in dermatologic material. They must be differentiated from myxosarcomas and from lymphomatous round cell sarcomas. Even rarer is metastasis to the scalp of a retroperitoneal liposarcoma.[63]

REFERENCES

1. Majno G, Sabbiani G, Hirschel BJ, et al.: Contraction of granulation tissue in vitro: similarity to smooth muscle. Science 173:548, 1971
2. Linares HA, Kirscher CW, Dobrkonsky M, et al.: The histiocytic organization of the hypertrophic scar in humans. J Invest Dermatol 59, 323, 1972
3. Moriguchi T, Fujimoto D: Crosslink of collagen in

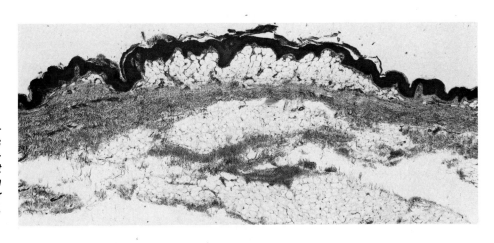

FIGURE 41–18.
Nevus angiolopomatosus. Nevoid fat tissue occupies pars papillaris of dermis and is separated from subcutaneous fat tissue by pars reticularis, which is being encroached on rather than being hypoplastic. H&E. X21.

hypertrophic scar. J Invest Dermatol 72:143, 1979

4. Baur PS, Larson DL, Stacey TR: The observation of myofibroblasts in hypertrophic scars. Surg Gynecol Obstet 141:22, 1975

5. Graham JH, Sanders JB, Johnson WC, et al.: Fibrous papule of the nose. A clinico-pathological study. J Invest Dermatol 45:194, 1965

6. Saylan T, Marks R, Wilson-Jones E: Fibrous papule of the nose. Br J Dermatol 85:111, 1971

7. Ackerman AB, Kornberg R: Pearly penile papules; acral angiofibromas. Arch Dermatol 108:673, 1973

8. Zackheim HS, Pinkus H: Perifollicular fibromas. Arch Dermatol 82:913, 1960

9. Pinkus H, Coskey RJ, Burgess GA: Trichodiscoma; a benign tumor related to haarscheibe (hair disk). J Invest Dermatol 63:212, 1974

10. Meigel WN, Ackerman AB: Fibrous papule of the face. Am J Dermatopathol 1:329, 1979

11. Pinkus H: Perifollicular fibromas: pure periadnexal adventitial tumors. Am J Dermatopathol 1:341, 1979

12. Mascaro JM, Galy-Mascaro C, Piñol Aguadé J: Fibroma perifolicular. Med Cutan 4:163, 1969

13. Belaïch S, Civatte J, Bonvalet D, et al.: Fibromes perifolliculaires multiples du visage et du cou posant le problème des adénomes sébacés symétriques blancs et fibreux. Ann Dermatol Venereol 105:959, 1978

14. Birt AS, Hogg GR, Dubé WJ: Hereditary multiple fibrofolliculomas with trichodiscomas and acrochordons. Arch Dermatol 113:1674, 1977

15. Weintraub R, Pinkus H: Multiple fibrofolliculomas (Birt-Hogg-Dubé) associated with a large connective tissue nevus. J Cutan Pathol 4:289, 1977

16. Hegedus SI, Schorr WF: Familial cutaneous collagenoma. Cutis 10:283, 1972

17. Schimpf A, Roth W, Kopper J: Dermatofibrosis lenticularis disseminata mit Osteopoikilie (Buschke–Ollendorff Syndrom). Dermatologica 141:409, 1970

18. Schorr WF, Optiz JM, Rayes CN: The connective tissue nevus-osteopoikilosis syndrome. Arch Dermatol 106:208, 1972

19. Smith LR, Bernstein BD: Eruptive collagenoma. Arch Dermatol 114:1710, 1978

20. Sasai Y, Saito N, Seiji M: Epidermolysis bullosa dystrophica et albopapuloidea; report of a case and histochemical study. Arch Dermatol 108:554, 1973

21. Mehregan AH, Staricco RG: Elastic fibers in pigmented nevi. J Invest Dermatol 38:271, 1962

22. Stevanovič D: Fibromatose multiple continué et progressive. Ann Dermatol Venereol 104:141, 1977

23. Bart RS, Andrade R, Kopf AW, et al.: Acquired digital fibrokeratomas. Arch Dermatol 97:120, 1968

24. Verallo VVM: Acquired digital fibrokeratomas. Br J Dermatol 80:730, 1968

25. Dupré A, Christol B, Bories M: Le fibro-kératome acquis. A propos de 8 observations. Ann Dermatol Venereol 104:611, 1978

26. Kitano Y: Juvenile hyaline fibromatosis. Arch Dermatol 112:86, 1976

27. Desmons F, Fontaine G, Farriaux J-P, et al.: Pseudokystes mucoides congenitaux multiples du cuir chevelu. Ann Dermatol Venereol 104:861, 1977

28. O'Donnell TF, Geller SA: Primary osteoma cutis. Arch Dermatol 104:325, 1971

29. Holmes HS, Boenmeyer JA: Cutaneous cartilaginous tumor. Arch Dermatol 112:839, 1976

30. Ronan SG, Tso MOM: Multiple periorbital fibrous histiocytomas. A light and electron microscopic study. Arch Dermatol 114:1345, 1978

31. Saxe N, Botha JBC: Epithelioid sarcoma. A distinctive clinical presentation. Arch Dermatol 113:1106, 1977

32. Headington JT, Niederhuber JE, Repola DA: Primary malignant fibrous histiocytoma of skin. J Cutan Pathol 5:329, 1978

33. Mopper C: Primary fibrosarcoma of the skin. JAMA 152:570, 1953

34. Hashimoto K, Brownstein MH, Jacobiec FA: Dermatofibrosarcoma protuberans. A tumor with perineural and endoneural cell features. Arch Dermatol 110:874, 1974

35. Ozzello L, Hamels J: The histiocytic nature of dermatofibrosarcoma protuberans. Am J Clin Pathol 65:136, 1976

36. Konwaler BE, Keasbey L, Kaplan L: Subcutaneous pseudosarcomatous fibromatosis (fasciitis). Am J Clin Pathol 25:241, 1955

37. Fretzin DF, Helwig EB: Atypical fibroxanthoma of skin; clinicopathologic study of 140 cases. Cancer 31:1541, 1973

38. Alguacil-Garcia A, Unni KK, Goellner JR, et al.: Atypical fibroxanthoma of the skin. An ultrastructural study of two cases. Cancer 40:1471, 1977

39. Kint A, Geerts ML: Pseudosarkome der Haut. Fortschr Dermatol Venerol 7:59, 1973

40. Mehregan AH, Nabai H, Matthews JE: Recurring digital fibrous tumor of childhood. Arch Dermatol 106:375, 1972

41. Fleischmajer R, Nedwich A, Reeves J: Juvenile fibromatosis. Arch Dermatol 107:574, 1973

42. Bhawan J, Bacchotts C, Joris I, et al.: Infantile digital myofibroblastoma (recurrent digital fibrous tumors of childhood). J Cutan Pathol 5:286, 1978

43. Montgomery H, Winkelmann RK: Smooth-muscle tumors of the skin. Arch Dermatol 79:32, 1959

44. MacDonald DM, Sanderson KV: Angioleiomyoma of the skin. Br J Dermatol 91:161, 1974

45. Bardach H, Ebner H: Das Angioleiomyom der Haut. Hautarzt 26:638, 1974

46. Ross R: The smooth muscle cell. II. Growth of smooth muscle in culture and formation of elastic fibers. J Cell Biol 50:172, 1971

47. Pinkus H: In discussion of Montgomery H, Winkelmann RK: Smooth-muscle tumors of the skin. Arch Dermatol 79:32, 1959

48. Headington JT, Beals TF, Niederhuber JE: Primary leiomyosarcoma of skin: a report and critical appraisal. J Cutan Pathol 4:308, 1977

49. Staindl O, Zelger J: Rhabdomyosarkom der Haut. Hautarzt 28:574, 1977

50. Howard WR, Helwig EB: Angiolipoma. Arch Dermatol 82:924, 1960

51. Sahl WJ Jr: Mobile encapsulated lipomas. Formerly called encapsulated angiolipomas. Arch Dermatol 114:1684, 1978

52. Tavafoghi V, Ghandchi A, Hambrick GW Jr, et al.: Cutaneous signs of spinal dysraphism. Report of a patient with a tail-like lipoma and review of 200 cases in the literature. Arch Dermatol 114:573, 1978

53. Mehregan AH, Tavafoghi V, Ghandchi A: Nevus lipomatosus cutaneus superficialis (Hoffman-Zurhelle). J Cutan Pathol 2:307, 1975

54. Wilson-Jones E, Marks R, Pongsehirun, D: Nevus superficialis lipomatosus. A clinicopathological report of twenty cases. Br J Dermatol 93:121, 1975

55. Howell JB: Nevus angiolipomatosus vs focal dermal hypoplasia. Arch Dermatol 92:238, 1965

56. Goltz RW, Henderson RR, Hitch JM, et al.: Focal dermal hypoplasia syndrome; a review of the literature and report of two cases. Arch Dermatol 101:1, 1970

57. Gottlieb SK, Fisher BK, Violin GA: Focal dermal hypoplasia; a nine year follow-up study. Arch Dermatol 108:551, 1973

58. Uitto J Bauer EA, Santa-Cruz DJ, et al: Focal dermal hypoplasia: Abnormal growth characteristics of skin fibroblasts in culture. J Invest Dermatol 75:170, 1980

59. Aherne W, Hull D: The site of heat production in the newborn infant. Proc R Soc Med 57:1172, 1964

60. Bonarandi JJ, Privat Y: Hibernoma. Bull Soc Fr Dermatol Syphiligr 80:72, 1973

61. Angervall L, Nilsson L, Stener B: Microangiographic and histological studies in two cases of hibernoma. Cancer 17:685, 1964

62. Brody HJ, Meltzer HD, Someren A: Spindle cell lipoma. An unusual dermatologic presentation. Arch Dermatol 114:1065, 1978

63. Peison B, Benisch B, Williams MC: Retroperitoneal liposarcoma metastatic to scalp. Arch Dermatol 114:1358, 1978

CHAPTER

42

Vascular Nevi and Tumors

Mesodermal neoplasms related to blood and lymph vessels are listed in Table 42–1. A broad practical classification of vascular lesions for clinical purposes might separate lesions that are present at birth or that appear early in childhood from lesions arising later in life. Histologic classification for diagnostic and prognostic purposes might best be based on whether we are dealing with an excess of fully formed vessels, usually blood vessels, or with an excess of vessel-associated cells with or without the formation of vessels. Lesions of the first type are easily recognized and are, with few exceptions, benign. Lesions of the second type may be benign but usually carry implications of malignancy. Their histologic identification may be difficult.

LESIONS CONSISTING OF VESSELS

Objective examination under the microscope without clinical data does not always permit us to say whether an excess of blood vessels in a section is either reactive or nevoid and stable or proliferative in the sense of a benign *hemangioma*. Hemangiomas[1,2] generally are subdivided into *capillary* types with relatively small lumina and thin walls and *cavernous* types with large spaces and thin or thick fibrous walls. Rare *angiosarcomas*, of course, show atypicality of vessels and the cells lining them. Of the congenital vascular lesions, *nevus flammeus* (port-wine stain) is counted among the

telangiectasias (see below), the *strawberry mark*[3] among the capillary hemangiomas, and deep-seated lesions are more commonly cavernous.

Usually, the pathologist is charged by the clinician to distinguish between a vascular tumor and a tumor of different type, melanoma being the most frequent differential diagnosis. Clinical uncertainty may arise from a deep-seated angioma, causing dark color of the skin surface. Another common occasion for recognizing a benign vascular lesion where malignant melanoma was suspected is thrombosis of a small superficial *hemangioma*, which may have been a tiny birthmark, a *senile angioma*, or a *venous lake* (Fig. 42–1) or *varix*. In these cases, all or much of the preexisting lesion may be in the process of transepidermal elimination, and, in some cases, nothing is visible but a hemorrhagic crust. In other cases, enough viable tissue is left in the dermis to permit definite diagnosis.

Bartonellosis *(verruga peruana)* may have so much vascular proliferation that a hemangioma is simulated. The organisms are found in the endothelial cells.[4]

Some predominantly epithelial tumors may be so vascular as to cause confusion. Thus, eccrine spiradenomas may be misdiagnosed as hemangiomas or as glomangiomas. The latter (see below) are particularly confusing because the diagnostic cuboidal glomus cells strongly resemble epithelial cells and may be mistaken for sweat epithelium

TABLE 42–1.
Vascular Nevi and Tumors

Vascular nevi
  Telangiectatic
  Cavernous
Proliferation of vessels
  Arterial hemangiomas (spiders)
  Acquired hemangiomas, venous lakes, and cirsoid
    aneurysms
  Angiokeratomas
  Lymphangioma circumscriptum
  Angiosarcoma
Proliferation of cellular elements related to vessels
  Hemangioendothelioma
  Granuloma pyogenicum
  Hemangiopericytoma
  Glomangioma
  Malignant angioendothelioma
  Kaposi sarcoma and Stewart–Treves syndrome

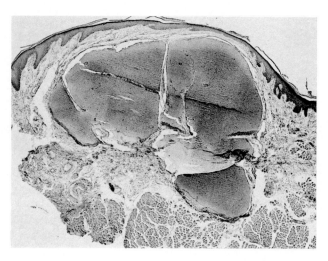

FIGURE 42–1.
Venous lake (varix) of lip. This is an almost physiologic phenomenon. In many elderly people, the vein near the lateral border of the lower lip between epidermis and skeletal muscle enlarges. It may become thrombosed or cause discomfort due solely to its size, as in the case illustrated. H&E. X45.

and vice versa. Another hidradenoma, eccrine poroma, often has a highly vascular stroma and may be suspected to be granuloma pyogenicum on clinical and cursory histologic examination. Once in a while, the pathologist may have to decide whether a nodule arising later in life in a port-wine mark is benign or malignant.

Telangiectasias

A number of vascular lesions are neither congenital (nevoid) and stable nor truly neoplastic. They are usually classified as telangiectasias, although ves-

sels larger than capillaries may be affected and some vascular proliferation may be involved. One example is *essential telangiectasia* (Fig. 42–2), appearing as spidery red spots in adult life. Another is *angioma serpiginosum* that must be separated from pigmented purpuric eruptions (Chap. 13).[5] Similar telangiectasias are found in the *CRST syndrome* (systemic sclerosis), in thyroid disease,[6] and in Osler's *familial hemorrhagic telangiectasia*. Von Lo-

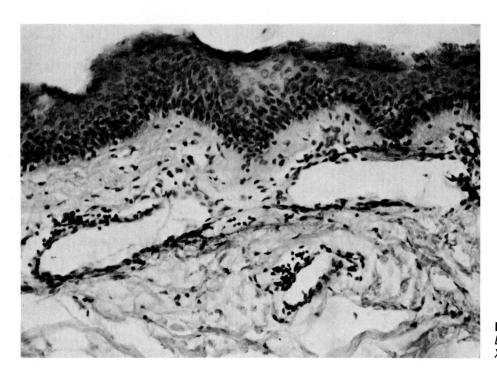

FIGURE 42–2.
Essential telangiectasia. H&E. X225.

huizen's cutis marmorata telangiectatica[7] is another example of widespread livedolike involvement of the skin in which telangiectatic capillaries and anomalies of larger vessels[8] are combined. Somewhat different are *arterial spiders*,[9] less appropriately called nevus araneus or spider nevus. They possess a central arteriole with muscular wall which widens into a subepidermal ampulla and splits up into radiating thin-walled vessels. Yet another eruption bearing the name telangiectasia is related to urticaria pigmentosa (Chap. 44): *telangiectasia macularis eruptiva perstans*[10] presents a combination of more numerous and dilated small vessels in the upper dermis with mild round cell infiltrate and some increase of mast cells. Diagnosis requires staining with toluidine blue or Giemsa solution.

Cirsoid Aneurysm

A peculiar lesion, most commonly encountered as a skin-colored papule on the face and not usually diagnosed clinically, consists of coiled thick-walled vessels embedded in fibrous stroma. The walls lack normal muscle and elastic fibers, and consist mainly of fibrocytes, collagen, and ground substance (Fig. 42–3). Biberstein and Jessner, the first describers,[11] pointed out that these not uncommon lesions are probably not true hemangiomas but *cirsoid aneurysms*, due to coiling of an abnormal vessel. They have been redescribed as arteriovenous shunts[12] or acral arteriovenous tumors.[13] The preferred name is *arteriovenous hemangioma*.[2]

Angiokeratoma

Angiokeratoma is the name given to a superficial hemangioma or telangiectasia associated with reactive hyperkeratosis of the epidermis. The Mibelli[14] and Fordyce (scrotal) types are defined clinically rather than histologically. The Fabry type[15,16] has now been recognized as the expression of metabolic aberration. There is inherited deficiency of alpha-galactosidase leading to the deposition of ceramid trihexosidase. Electron microscopic examination shows dense, laminated inclusions in lysosomes.[17] Under the light microscope (Fig. 42–4), demonstration of lipid droplets in smooth muscle is the diagnostic feature, and these must be looked for in larger vessels and arrector pili muscles. Very similar cutaneous manifestations may be found in *fucosidosis*, an autosomal recessive deficiency of the lysosomal enzyme alpha-L-fucosidase causing accumulation of fucose.[18,19]

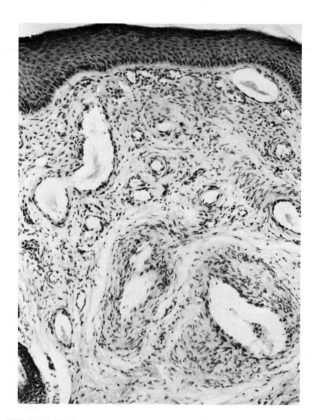

FIGURE 42–3.
Cirsoid aneurysm, also called arteriovenous hemangioma. Thick walled coiled-up blood vessels form a papule in facial skin. H&E. X125.

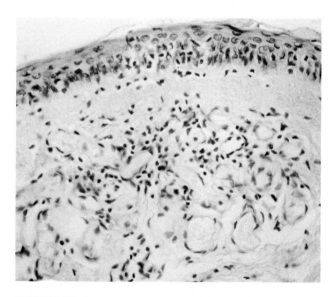

FIGURE 42–4.
Angiokeratoma of Fabry. Cluster of capillary vessels in the upper dermis. Mild thickening and hyperkeratosis of overlying epidermis. Minimal round cell infiltrate. H&E. X250.

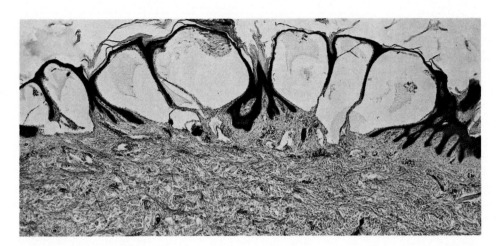

FIGURE 42–5.
Lymphangioma circumscriptum corporis. H&E. X30.

Lymphangioma

Lymphangioma, usually encountered in the form of *lymphangioma circumscriptum*,[20] expresses itself in a routine biopsy specimen as endothelium-lined spaces which may be so closely applied to the lower surface of the epidermis as to simulate intraepidermal vesicles (Fig. 42–5). It is, however, essential to realize[21] that the small superficial angiectasias are in communication with large subcutaneous cisterns consisting of muscle-coated lymphatic vessels and that these must be excised in order to effect cure.

LESIONS DUE TO PROLIFERATION OF VESSEL-ASSOCIATED CELLS

Of the lesions mentioned so far, all consist of well-formed, almost normal vessels in excess. Although the endothelial cells of hemangiomas may be more prominent than those of normal vessels, they are not atypical, and they are not more numerous than needed to line the vascular lumen. If their number exceeds that requirement and if, therefore, they project in papilliferous form into the lumen or form vascular buds and incompletely canalized structures, we are dealing with a tumor consisting of vessel-associated cells, and the differential diagnosis requires much more analysis.

Hemangioendothelioma and Hemangiopericytoma

These terms include benign as well as malignant tumors, and the differentiation depends often more on clinical behavior than on histologic criteria. *Angioendotheliomas* consist of cells within the basement membrane as demonstrated by reticulum stain or PAS. *Pericytomas* of Stout,[22] in contrast, show plain endothelial lining of vessels and tumor cells outside the basement membrane, a distinction very difficult to make in routine sections.

A rare disease, *proliferating systematized angioendotheliomatosis*, in which benign-appearing endothelial cells proliferate profusely in dermal and systemic capillaries,[23] resulting often in a fatal outcome, may be due to a circulating angiogenic factor.[24]

Intravascular Papillary Endothelial Hyperplasia (IPEH)

How difficult it is to differentiate benign proliferations of vessel-associated cells from neoplasia is exemplified by the considerable literature that has recently been devoted[25] to a lesion first described by Masson in 1923 as vegetating intravascular hemangioendothelioma. One must remember that in the organization of an intravascular thrombus, there is considerable temporary proliferation of endothelia, perithelia, and other cells. It is generally held now that these processes, if they become excessive, and especially if they take place in preexisting hemangiomas, may mimic *angiosarcoma*, another term that has been applied to various malignant forms of vascular proliferation (see Kaposi sarcoma, below). It is important in making the diagnosis of IPEH to ascertain the intravascular location of the tumor and to find fibrin which offers the basis for the florid papillary endothelial proliferation.

Malignant Angioendothelioma

Lesions of IPEH have to be differentiated from aggressive neoplasms that are clinically ill-defined, almost inflammatory appearing plaques on the

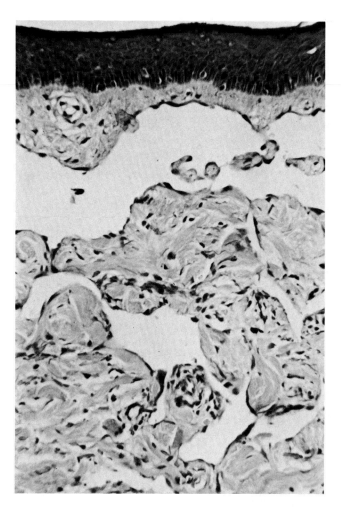

FIGURE 42–6.
Malignant hemangioendothelioma. Atypical hyperchromatic cells seem to line interfascicular spaces of the dermis rather than form complete blood vessels. H&E. X180.

scalps of elderly people. In this malignant angioendothelioma,[26] which German authors considered an angioplastic reticulosarcoma,[27,28] one finds wide capillaries in the papillary layer and massive accumulations of endothelial cells between the collagen bundles of the deep dermis,[29] but especially prominent are atypical endothelial cells coating collagen bundles of the reticular dermis rather than forming closed vessels (Fig. 42–6).

Granuloma Pyogenicum

Another lesion mimicking a neoplasm but probably exemplifying inflammatory reactive proliferation is granuloma pyogenicum. It is composed of lobes of incompletely formed vessels (Fig. 42–7) with considerable excess of endothelial and interstitial cells. Characteristically, it is sessile *(granuloma pediculatum)* and is fed by a large arterial vessel entering

its base. Therefore, it will recur if this vessel is not excised or destroyed by cauterization. The surface of a granuloma pyogenicum usually is covered by a purulent crust, but that is not essential and is a complication due to mechanical trauma or secondary infection. Protection and mildly antibacterial treatment will cause reepithelization, and many lesions are always covered by thin, smooth epithelium *(granuloma telangiectaticum)*. A frightening but, in fact, harmless experience is the formation of multiple satellites after surgical removal of a granuloma pyogenicum,[30,31] especially when these secondary lesions develop deep in the skin and thus are histologically indistinguishable from hemangioendothelioma. So-called atypical granuloma pyogenicum will be discussed in Chapter 44.

Glomangioma

The neuromyoarterial glomus of Masson (Chap. 2) gives rise to a tumor called *glomangioma* or *glomus tumor.*[32] It may consist of a variable combination of vascular, muscular, and neural components. The most common and most characteristic element is the glomus cell (Fig. 42–8),[33,34] a cuboidal cell with round nucleus and light-staining cytoplasm, which may form solid epitheliumlike masses

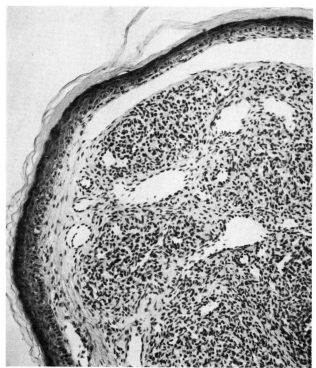

FIGURE 42–7.
Granuloma pyogenicum. Portion of a well-epithelized sessile lesion is shown. H&E. X135.

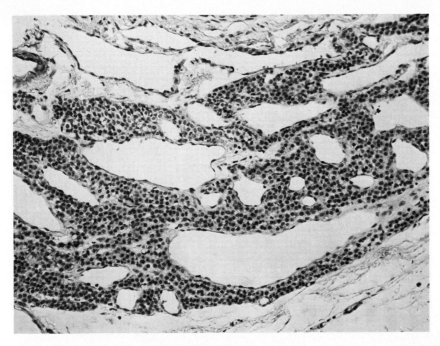

FIGURE 42–8.
Glomangioma. Cuboidal glomus cells fill spaces between endothelium-lined capillaries. H&E. X180.

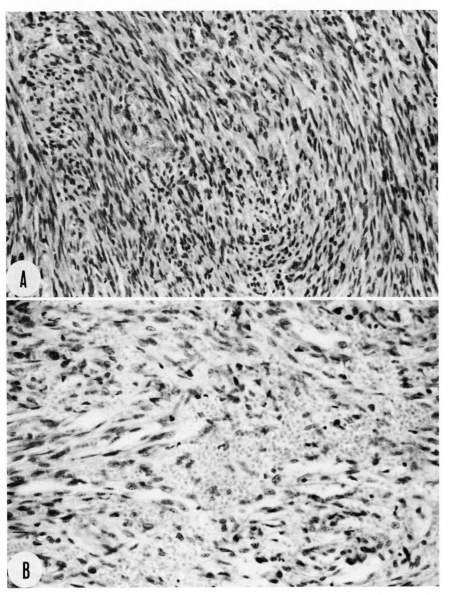

FIGURE 42–9.
*Kaposi's pigmented hemorrhagic sarcoma. **A.** Late stage consisting almost entirely of spindle cells. Many nuclei appear round because they are cross sectioned where the cell streams bend. H&E. X400. **B.** Early phase shows vessels and vascular slits lined by endothelial cells. Some round cells, many red blood cells inside and outside of vascular channels. The picture does not show hemosiderin deposits, which are often present. H&E. X400.*

or may be associated with vascular spaces. In the latter case, glomus cells lie outside a lining of flat endothelial cells. While most glomangiomas are single and occur in general on the acral parts of the extremities, a fair number of cases with multiple lesions have been described.[35,36]

Blue Rubber Bleb Nevus

Bean described multiple lesions under this picturesque name. Their relationship to glomangioma was discussed because they also have multiple perivascular layers of epithelioid cells. However, it seems assured now that blue rubber bleb nevus is clinically and histologically a separate entity. It is clinically associated with systemic cavernous hemangiomas, and fatalities have been reported. Under the electron microscope, the peripheral cells resemble smooth muscle cells.[37]

Kaposi's Sarcoma

Early lesions of the *multiple hemorrhagic* and *pigmented sarcoma* of Kaposi (Fig. 42–9) require considerable experience for differential diagnosis from benign reactive conditions. Among the latter are pigmented purpuric eruptions of the Schamberg–Majocchi type, peculiar hypertrophic plaques of the legs, related either to venous stasis (Chap. 15) or other vascular anomalies, especially arteriovenous fistulas,[38,39] papular tumors on face and neck, now usually classified as angiolymphoid hyperplasia (Chap. 44), and even exuberant granulomatous lesions in diaper dermatitis (granuloma glutaeale infantum, Chap. 21).

One must keep in mind that even though the name includes "multiple," every lesion of the Kaposi sarcoma[40] is solitary and nodular and arises in the reticular dermis or deeper tissues through the atypical proliferation of one vessel. Hypertrophic stasis dermatitis, on the other hand, is diffuse and involves proliferation of small vessels of the pars papillaris. The proliferative process of Kaposi's lesion produces incomplete vessels, often mere vascular slits between a mixture of round cells and fixed-tissue-type cells. Red cells leaking from the vascular spaces are engulfed by histiocytes with the formation of hemosiderin. Lesions of the early stage of the disease may show considerable fibrosis, and the entire process may be obliterated by scar tissue containing some pigmented macrophages. In later stages, fusiform cells often prevail over round cells and vessels, and eventually pure spindle cell sarcomas may be found.[41]

The histologically similar process arising in lymphedematous arms after mastectomy (Stewart–Treves syndrome[42]) is thought to be due to proliferation of lymph vessels.

REFERENCES

1. Schnyder UW: Hämangioma (einschliesslich Teleangiektasien und verwandte Hauterscheinungen). In Jadassohn (ed): Handbuch der Haut- und Geschlechtskrankheiten, Ergänzungswerk, vol 3. Berlin, Springer-Verlag, 1963, p 494
2. Johnson WC: Pathology of cutaneous vascular tumors. Int J Dermatol 15:239, 1976
3. Masuda M: A histological and electron microscopical study on strawberry nevus (strawberry mark). Jpn J Dermatol [B] 81:104, 1971
4. Arona G, Small O: Verruga peruana o enfermedad de Carrión. Dermatologia, Revista Mexicana 18:20, 1974
5. Marriott PJ, Munro DD, Ryan T: Angioma serpiginosum—familial incidence. Br J Dermatol 93:701, 1975
6. Thomson JA, Mackie RM: Localized secondary telangiectasia in patients with thyroid disease. Br J Dermatol 89:561, 1973
7. Dupont C: Cutis marmorata telangiectatica congenita (Von Lohuizen's syndrome). Br J Dermatol 97:437, 1977
8. Way BH, Herrmann J, Gilbert EF, et al.: Cutis marmorata telangiectatica congenita. J Cutan Pathol 1:10, 1974
9. Bean WB: The arterial spider and similar lesions of the skin and mucous membranes. Circulation 8:117, 1953
10. Klotz L: Telangiectasia macularis eruptiva perstans; Beitrag zur Kenntnis einer Sonderform der Urticaria pigmentosa. Hautarzt 21:372, 1970
11. Biberstein HH, Jessner M: A cirsoid aneurysm in the skin. Dermatologica 113:129, 1956
12. Girard C, Graham JH, Johnson WC: Arteriovenous hemangioma (arteriovenous shunt). A clinicopathological and histochemical study. J Cutan Pathol 1:73, 1974
13. Carapeto FJ, Armijo M: Tumeur acrale arterio-veineuse. Ann Dermatol Venereol 105:977, 1978
14. Dave VK, Main RA: Angiokeratoma of Mibelli with necrosis of the finger tips. Arch Dermatol 106:726, 1972
15. Van Mullem PJ, Ruiter M: Fine structure of the skin in angiokeratoma corporis diffusum (Fabry's disease). J Pathol 101:221, 1970
16. Wallace HJ: Anderson-Fabry disease. Br J Dermatol 88:1, 1973
17. Hashimoto K, Lieberman P, Lamkin N Jr: Angiokeratoma corporis diffusum (Fabry disease). Arch Dermatol 112:1416, 1976
18. Smith EB, Graham JL, Ledman JA, et al.: Fucosidosis. Cutis 19:195, 1977
19. Dvoretzky I, Fisher BK: Fucosidosis. Int J Dermatol 18:213, 1979
20. Flanagan BP, Helwig EB: Cutaneous lymphangioma. Arch Dermatol 113:24, 1977

21. Whimster IW: The pathology of lymphangioma circumscriptum. Br J Dermatol 94:473, 1976
22. Metz J, Barabasch R: Das Hämangiopericytom. Z Hautkr 46:95, 1971
23. Kauh YC, MacFarland JP, Camabuci GG, et al.: Malignant proliferating angioendotheliomatosis. Arch Dermatol 116:803, 1980
24. Person JR: Systemic angioendotheliomatosis: a possible disorder of a circulating angiogenic factor. Br J Dermatol 96:329, 1977
25. Barr RJ, Graham JH, Sherwin LA: Intravascular papillary endothelial hyperplasia. A benign lesion mimicking angiosarcoma. Arch Dermatol 114:723, 1978
26. Wilson-Jones E: Malignant angioendothelioma of the skin. Br J Dermatol 76:21, 1964
27. Weidner F, Braun-Falco O: Über das angioplastische Reticulosarkom der Kopfhaut bei älteren Menschen. Hautarzt 21:60, 1970
28. Ehlers G, Herbstreit A, Kampffmeyer U: Klinische, histologische und cytophotometrische Untersuchungen über primärcutane metastasierende angioblastische Reticulosarcome. Hautarzt 22:245, 1971
29. Mehregan AH, Usndek HE: Malignant angioendothelioma. Arch Dermatol 112:1565, 1976
30. De Graciansky P, Leclerq R, Timsit E, et al.: Granulome pyogénique récidivant avec multiples satellites. Ann Dermatol Syphilgr 98:408, 1971
31. Zala L: Satellitenförmige Rezidive bei telangiektatischem Granulom. Dermatologica 147:18, 1973
32. Schnyder UW: Über Glomustumoren. Dermatologica 131:83, 1964
33. Goodman TF, Abele DC: Multiple glomus tumors. A clinical and electron microscopic study. Arch Dermatol 103:11, 1971
34. Reinhard M, Sasse D, Lüders G: Zur Histochemie der Epitheloidzellen in Glomustumoren. Arch Dermatol Forsch 242:165, 1972
35. Conant MA, Wiesenfeld SL: Multiple glomus tumors of the skin. Arch Dermatol 103:481, 1971
36. McEvoy BF, Waldman PM, Tye MJ: Multiple hamartomatous glomus tumors of the skin. Arch Dermatol 104:188, 1971
37. Chandon J-P, De Micco C, Lebreuil G, et al.: Blue rubber bleb naevus et glomangiomatose: unicité ou dualité? A propos de 2 cas. Ann Dermatol Venereol 105:123, 1978
38. Rusin LJ, Harrall R: Arteriovenous fistula. Cutaneous manifestations. Arch Dermatol 112:1135, 1976
39. Stewart W-M: Pseudo-angiosarcomatose de Kaposi par fistules arterio-veineuses. Ann Dermatol Venereol 104:391, 1977
40. Ackerman LV (ed): Symposium on Kaposi Sarcoma. Unio Internat Contra Cancrum 18:322, 1962
41. O'Connell KM: Kaposi's sarcoma: histopathological study of 159 cases from Malawi. J Clin Pathol 30:687, 1977
42. Wolff K: Das Stewart-Treves-Syndrom. Arch Klin Exp Dermatol 216:468, 1963

CHAPTER

43

Neural Tumors

Although nerve tissue is ectodermal rather than mesodermal, its nevoid and neoplastic manifestations are put here for convenience, while melanogenic lesions, also of neuroectodermal origin, were discussed in Chapter 32.

NEUROMA

Simple hyperplasia of cutaneous nerves was described in prurigo nodularis (Chap. 7) as an essential feature. Proliferation of myelinated nerves (Fig. 43–1) similar to that seen in *amputation neuromas* may ocur in the skin and, more commonly, in oral mucosa (Chap. 45), probably secondary to minor trauma. Nontraumatic solitary tumors may occur on the face,[1] and cases of multiple cutaneous and muscosal neuromas have been described.[2,3] The stubs remaining after amputation of *supernumerary digits* in infancy contain large nerve trunks and many Meissner's corpuscles (Fig. 43–2). This picture, which had been assumed to be pathognomonic, was recently found in an undoubtedly traumatic neuroma on the hand by Shapiro et al.,[4] who, therefore, reinterpreted the rudimentary digit as an amputation neuroma. Their argument sounds convincing. Tumors consisting almost entirely of immature pacinian corpuscles have been described.[5,6]

NEUROFIBROMA

The most common cutaneous tumor related to nerves is neurofibroma (Fig. 43–3), which may be solitary or a manifestation of *Von Recklinghausen's disease.*[7] It is differentiated from fibromas and other cutaneous nodules by three features. The cells are relatively small, with short ovoid nuclei, and frequently are not arranged in definite bundles. They often point in all directions. Finely fibrillar interstitial substance does not stain like collagen in trichrome stains and appears light blue rather than pink in O&G sections. The latter also bring out the presence of numerous large mast cells, which are usually roundish rather than ameboid and are scattered throughout the tumor. Large nerve bundles may be encountered in the tumor. The neoplasm usually has a sharp border but no capsule. Old lesions may become secondarily fibrotic. Malignant transformation of cutaneous neurofibromas is extremely rare.[8]

NEURILEMOMA

Neurilemoma (Fig. 43–4) is a benign tumor of Schwann cells, rare in the skin. The characteristic regimentation of nuclei, sometimes in the form of *Verocay bodies*, makes it easy to diagnose if this feature is present. Otherwise, neurilemoma may be suspected if one sees wavy streams of elongated cells resembling the course of nerve bundles. Nerve fibers, however, are usually not demonstrated in routine sections.

OTHER FORMS

Extremely rare are *cutaneous meningiomas*, also called *psammomas*[9,10] (Fig. 43–5), *gliomas*, usually

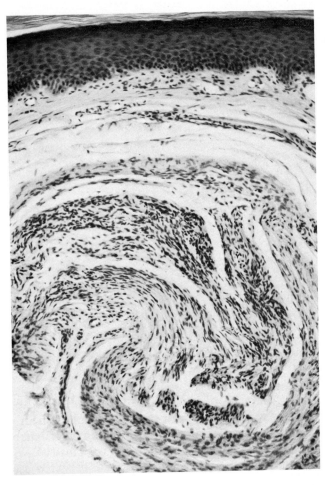

FIGURE 43–1.
Neuroma in finger skin, probably posttraumatic. H&E. X135.

developing subcutaneously in the noses of young children[11,12] and having sometimes intracranial connections, and infantile *neuroblastomas*,[13] which may mature into *ganglioneuromas*.[14]

Morton's neuroma is sometimes suspected in painful lesions of the sole, which in many cases are nothing but painful scars resulting from repeated surgical treatment of plantar verrucae or calluses. The true Morton's lesion is local degeneration of an interdigital nerve due to pressure or trauma, and on microscopic examination, it presents degenerating nerve fibers with proliferation of Schwann cells and fibrocytes. Fibrosis may involve the adjacent fat tissue and even adjacent arteries.[15]

Granular Cell Myoblastoma

Although the histogenesis of granular cell myoblastoma (Fig. 43–6) remains debated, it is discussed here because schwannian origin is one of the prominent hypotheses. Diagnosis is relatively easy once one realizes that the cytoplasm of the large pale cells is granular rather than foamy.[16] In some lesions, the smallest peripheral groups of cells are seen around nerves. However, while this feature speaks for affinity of the tumor cells for nerves, it cannot be used as an argument for origin from nerves, as we discussed in the introduction to the section on neoplasms (Sec. VII). Ultrastructural observation[17] has not helped to clarify histogenesis except to rule out myoblastic and schwannian origin. The granules are probably related to lysosomes, but there is no other evidence for histiocytic origin.

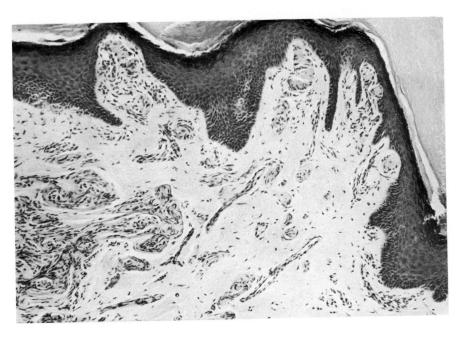

FIGURE 43–2.
Supernumerary digit. Part of a stub-like protrusion in the typical location at the base of the small finger. History was not clear whether a longer digit had been amputated in infancy or whether this was the original condition. Large coiled nerve trunks and several deformed Meissner's corpuscles in the subepidermal papillae. H&E. X45.

Neural Tumors / 505

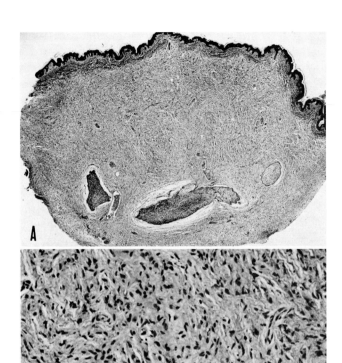

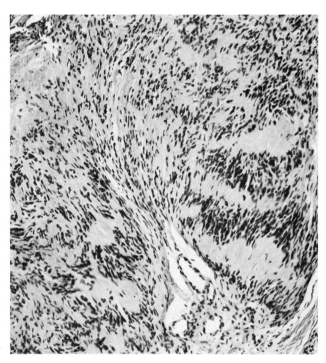

FIGURE 43–3 (left).
Neurofibroma: Von Recklinghausen type. **A.** *Low power shows sharp delineation of tumor without capsule and relative lack of fasciculation. Hypertrophied nerves deep in tumor. H&E. X28.* **B.** *At higher power, cells are short spindle cells with short nuclei forming convoluted bundles. One deformed nerve near lower border. H&E. X400.*

FIGURE 43–4.
Neurilemoma. H&E. X185.

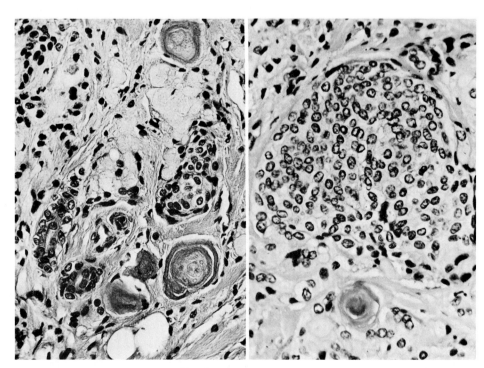

FIGURE 43–5.
Cutaneous meningioma (psammoma). Nests of meningothelial cells, some of which undergo hyaline degeneration. Lamellated and partly calcified psammoma bodies. H&E. (From Bain and Shnitka. Arch Dermatol 74:590, 1956.)

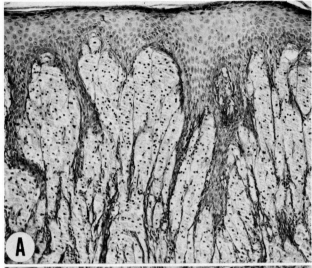

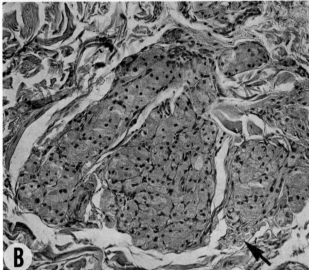

FIGURE 43–6.
*Granular cell myoblastoma. **A.** Superficial portion of a lesion exhibiting epidermal hyperplasia, although not of pseudoepitheliomatous pattern. H&E. X90. **B.** Small outlying nest of large granular cells in dermis. (Compare with Fig. 23–2, xanthelasma.) Several cells have multiple nuclei. Cross sections of myelinated nerve fibers indicated by arrow. H&E. X135.*

An intriguing feature of practical importance is the tendency of the overlying epithelium, especially that of mucous membranes, to react with pseudoepitheliomatous proliferation. It may resemble squamous cell carcinoma so much that a superficial biopsy may lead to mistaken diagnosis. In a case of our experience, laryngectomy was barely avoided when a small biopsy from the vocal cord region was first interpreted as carcinoma until a few large granular cells at the lower border of the section led to the correct diagnosis, which was confirmed by conservative surgery. Malignant granular cell tumors occur but rarely.[18] They have the cytologic features of dysplasia and mitotic activity.

REFERENCES

1. Reed RJ, Fine RM, Meltzer HD: Palisaded, encapsulated neuromas of the skin. Arch Dermatol 106:865, 1972
2. Holm TW, Prawer SE, Sahl W, et al.: Multiple cutaneous neuromas. Arch Dermatol 107:608, 1973
3. Schnitzler L, Simard C, Bandoux C, et al.: Neuromes cutanés et muqueux avec étude histopathologique et ultrastructurale. Ann Dermatol Venereol 100:241, 1973
4. Shapiro L, Juhlin EA, Brownstein MH: "Rudimentary polydactyly." Arch Dermatol 108:223, 1973
5. Bennin B, Barsky B, Salgia K: Pacinian neurofibroma. Arch Dermatol 112:1558, 1976
6. Owen DA: Pacinian neurofibroma. Arch Pathol Lab Med 103:99, 1979
7. Heine H, Schaega P, Nasemann T: Licht-und elektronenmikroskopische Untersuchungen zur Pathogenese der Neurofibromatose. Arch Dermatol Res 256:85, 1976
8. Knight WA, Murphy WK, Gottlieb JA: Neurofibromatosis associated with malignant neurofibromas. Arch Dermatol 107:747, 1973
9. Bain GO, Shnitka TK: Cutaneous meningioma (psammoma). Arch Dermatol 74:590, 1956
10. Lopez DA, Silvers DN, Helwig EB: Cutaneous meningiomas: clinico-pathologic study. Cancer 34:728, 1974
11. Baran R, Kopf A, Schnitzler L: Le gliome nasal. A propos de quatre cas, avec étude d'un cas au microscope électronique. Ann Dermatol Syphiligr 100:395, 1973
12. Krebs A, Zala L, Meyer A, et al.: Nasales Gliom. Dermatologica 153:136, 1976
13. Shapiro L: Neuroblastoma with maturation to ganglioneuroma. Arch Dermatol 105:613, 1972
14. Collins JP, Johnson WC, Burgoon CF Jr: Ganglioneuroma of the skin. Arch Dermatol 105:256, 1972
15. Asbury AK, Johnson PC (eds): Pathology of Peripheral Nerve. Philadelphia, Saunders, 1978
16. Caputo R, Bellone AG, Tagliavini R: Ultrastructure of the granular cell myoblastoma, so-called Abrikossof's tumor. Arch Dermatol Forsch 242:127, 1972
17. Chrestian MA, Gambarelli D, Hassoun J, et al.: Granular cell myoblastoma. J Cutan Pathol 4:80, 1977
18. Al-Sarraf M, Loud A, Vaitkevicius V: Malignant granular cell tumor. Arch Pathol 91:550, 1971

CHAPTER

44

Lymphoreticular Neoplasms

In approaching histologic diagnosis and differential diagnosis of neoplastic lesions of the lymphoreticular system in the skin, one must be aware of several difficulties which make absolute diagnosis hazardous in many cases and impossible in some. The principal difficulties are differentiation between inflammatory and neoplastic infiltrates and identification of cell types. Both difficulties are due in great part to technical factors and to the fact that pathologic classification and diagnostic features described for lymphomas[1] are based on their morphology in lymph nodes. Such criteria as destruction of normal architecture, invasion of capsule, and involvement of peripheral sinuses are not applicable to the skin, where there is no preexisting lymphatic tissue. Cytologic diagnosis is hazardous in H&E-stained paraffin sections, and even O&G stain often is not very informative in routinely fixed skin specimens. The method of tissue imprints which has been so helpful in hematopathology encounters great difficulty in the skin, where infiltrates often are not massive and cells are held firmly in tough connective tissue. Modern methods have made it possible to identify T cells and other types in tissue sections, but special techniques are required.

Another difficulty is introduced by the great mobility of many of the cells seen. We discussed the origin of cells in granulomatous inflammation in Section IV. We must remember that many of the cells we encounter in lymphoreticular neoplasia come to the skin from other sites, mainly from lymph nodes or bone marrow. This "lymphocyte traffic"[2] is, however, not reserved to malignancy but is a normal phenomenon of body function and of immunologic processes. It is likely that certain cells have learned to consider the skin their home base to which they return preferentially.[3] Thus, the formation of lymph follicles with germinal centers is encountered in malignant and in benign conditions and is even found occasionally without any special significance in chronic inflammatory disease.

To some degree, then, dermatopathologists must develop their own rules and should use restraint in their reports. We should, without a feeling of inferiority, recommend other diagnostic procedures, including lymph-node biopsy and blood and bone marrow examination and, in general, should seek the assistance of the hematopathologist. On the other hand, since we have the advantage of familiarity with clinical differential diagnosis of dermatoses and with the multiple histologic reaction patterns of the skin, we also have the duty of moderating either overdiagnosis or underdiagnosis by pathologists who may try to transfer their rules too rigidly from lymph nodes and bone marrow to the skin.

CYTOLOGIC INTERPRETATION

While features of some normal and abnormal cells were mentioned in Chapters 2 and 5, more must be said here about those elements apt to be encountered in lesions of the lymphoreticular system. A primitive approach to cellular interpretation is this: Cells that are round or roundish without cytoplasmic projections or intercellular connections may be normal or abnormal cells of the lymphoid series, any type of primitive blast form, plasma cells, monocytes, or macrophages, depending on the characteristics of their nuclei and cytoplasm. Cells that are fusiform, stellate, or have obvious intercellular connections are fixed-tissue-type cells (Chap. 5) and may be fibrocytes, histiocytes, endothelial cells, or undifferentiated mesenchymal (reticular) cells. Specialized cells, such as muscle cells, Schwann cells, or mast cells, are left out of consideration.

Round Cells

Although the term *lymphocyte* has been used in this book freely, as is done by all but the most scrupulous pathologists, it is actually very difficult to know with certainty that a small round cell with a dark-staining round nucleus is a lymphocyte unless one encounters it in a lymph node. Considerable progress has been made in the identification and differentiation of cells in tissue sections by modern immunochemical methods.[4,5] T cells, B cells, and other types can be told apart by special procedures.[6] Whether the small round cell is part of an inflammatory or neoplastic process in the skin must be determined by other factors than its morphology. Even the nature of somewhat larger mononuclear cells remains doubtful, and one should remember that fixation, dehydration, and processing of the sections after embedding may influence the appearance of cells considerably. The individual examiner should be particularly cautious in the interpretation of material prepared by different techniques in other laboratories. The beginner must also learn that not every round image of membrane-limited chromatin in a section represents a spherical nucleus but may be the cross section of an ovoid or rod-shaped nucleus.

Cells having a fair amount of light-staining cytoplasm and an indented nucleus have been called *monocytes* but may be stimulated lymphocytes. If the nucleus is ovoid or round, they may be monocytes or histiocytes. It is safest to describe such cells as "larger mononuclears." One should never forget that mast cells may be indistinguishable in H&E stains, although their cytoplasm may have somewhat greater affinity to hematoxylin. Giemsa or toluidine blue stain is needed for identification. Plasma cells (Figs. 5–14, 44–1, and 45–1) have strongly basophilic cytoplasm, an eccentric coarsely granular nucleus, and a paranuclear light spot in typical instances.

Certain types of macrophages which are not obviously foamy furnish the largest cells in the round cell category. They usually have small vesicular

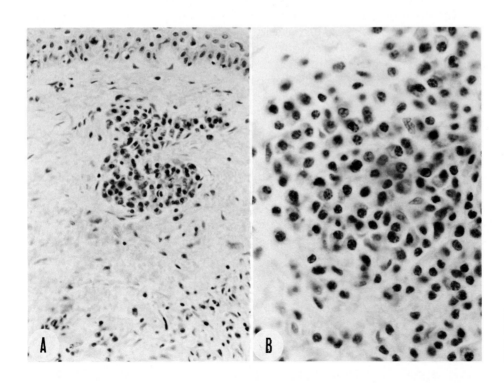

FIGURE 44–1.
Plasma cell leukemia. Plasma cells in dermal blood vessels. H&E. A. X250. B. X800.

nuclei and are designated as *epithelioid cells* if closely aggregated. Primitive blast cells of all phyla also are in this category and may be identified by their large, immature nuclei.

The nuclei of all these cell types are normochromatic. Based on the rule that most normal and many abnormal tissue cells have similar (diploid) amounts of chromatin, a small nucleus will stain darker than a larger one in which the same amount of DNA is distributed in a greater volume. If a cell has a large and dark-staining nucleus, we say it is "hyperchromatic," a feature most commonly found in malignant cells (Fig. 44–6B). The feature of a convoluted nucleus (Lutzner cell, Fig. 44–8B) is best recognized in electron micrographs. Very large and bizarre nuclei may occur but are not necessarily malignant (Fig. 44–9).

Fixed-Tissue-Type Cells

Normal skin contains four types of cells in this category: endothelial cells, fibrocytes, histiocytes, and undifferentiated mesenchymal cells. Endothelia are identified by their location in the walls of blood vessels or lymph vessels. Resting fibrocytes and histiocytes are practically indistinguishable. Fibrocytes are more easily recognized under pathologic conditions, e.g., the giant forms of chronic X-ray dermatitis (Fig. 15–9) and cells in keloids (Fig. 41–2) or other situations where fibers are produced. Histiocytes become recognizable only when they begin to phagocytize unless ultrastructural methods are used. Mast cells may have almost any shape and are not easily identified in H&E sections.

The undifferentiated mesenchymal cell is mentioned here for theoretical reasons. We presume that it exists in the skin as in most other tissues and that it plays a part in various reactive and neoplastic processes. No claim, however, is made that it can be identified in normal skin. We said at this point in the first edition that "reticulum cell" is one of the most abused terms in pathology. Meanwhile, terminology has been modified, especially through the work of Rappaport as codified in his fascicle.[1] His nomenclature, which has been accepted by many authors, eliminates "reticulum cell." It is pointed out that the potential for hematic or stromal differentiation is retained in the adult tissues by inconspicuous fixed cells. These *undifferentiated mesenchymal (primitive reticular) cells* preferentially are located in the vascular adventitia. They are considered the precursors of all types of blood and connective tissue cells and, in stained sections, are characterized by oval pale nuclei, which have delicate chromatin structure

and small, often indistinct nucleoli and pale-staining cytoplasm. According to Rappaport, there are strong similarities between the primitive reticular cell and one of its derivatives, the histiocyte, in their general distribution, association with fibrillar reticulum, and morphology. The histiocyte is said to have a more abundant cytoplasm. It is capable of phagocytosis, especially erythrophagocytosis, under appropriate stimulation and can store vital dyes. These latter abilities, one must add, are overt only under pathologic or experimental conditions. More recently, many of the cells called histiocytes by Rappaport have been classified as T lymphocytes on a functional basis. This will be discussed later.

Cells corresponding to primitive reticular cells and histiocytes in Rappaport's sense are encountered in the skin mainly in two situations. They are encountered if there is an infiltrate of fairly small cells with fairly small, round, or ovoid nuclei and closer inspection reveals that the cells are not round cells but have cytoplasmic projections which appear to connect them with neighboring cells. Such pictures usually signify parapsoriasis of premycotic type. The other situation concerns lesions which have the architectural characteristics of lymphosarcoma but consist of larger cells with larger ovoid nuclei and polyhedral or elongated bodies (reticulum cell sarcomas).

Multinucleated Cells

Multinucleated giant cells are usually found in granulomatous disease (Sec. IV), and it is a general rule that the presence of multinucleated cells excludes sarcoma (Fig. 41–6). There are, however, exceptions. Best known is the relatively small multinucleated cell (Fig. 44–4) of Hodgkin's disease, the Sternberg–Reed cell, which may also be found in mycosis fungoides. It must be distinguished from solid vascular endothelial buds, which may occur in any granulation tissue.

STRUCTURAL INTERPRETATION

Cytologic identification being uncertain,[7] histologic diagnosis of cutaneous reticulosis and lymphoma of non-Hodgkin type must seek help from the distribution, arrangement, and other structural features of the infiltrate. The important criteria are quantity, polymorphism versus monomorphism, involvement of the various dermal layers, involvement of the epidermis and adnexal structures, and destructiveness.

Quantity of Infiltrate

Heavy cellular infiltrate makes one suspect neoplasia, while a minimal number of cells tends to rule it out. This, however, is not an infallible criterion because many granulomas may have just as heavy or heavier infiltrate, and cellularity may be surprisingly small in some lymphomas, especially of the epidermotropic type.

Polymorphism Versus Monomorphism

With the exception of mycosis fungoides and Hodgkin's disease, malignant lymphomas are monomorphous, or at least one cell type predominates heavily. However, since mycosis fungoides is the prototype of cutaneous lymphoblastoma, the rule of monomorphism is generally not applicable in our field.

Involvement of Dermal Strata

We pointed out in Section III that sparing of the pars reticularis separates most simple inflammatory dermatoses from the lupus erythematosus group and granulomatous inflammation. We now add that involvement of the reticular dermis should make one suspicious also of lymphoreticular disease. Again, this rule applies only with reservations to mycosis fungoides, which may be quite superficial in early stages (Fig. 44–5) and, in its epidermotropic form, may remain so for many years. For all other neoplastic diseases of the lymphoreticular system, whether they take the form of leukemia or of sarcomatous proliferation, deep involvement of skin and subcutaneous tissue is characteristic. Figure 44–3A illustrates the most typical distribution, which outlines the entire vasculature of the skin, including superficial and deep plexus and the perforating vessels which usually accompany the adnexa. In leukemia cutis, the cells usually form sharply defined nodular infiltrates around the vessels, while they infiltrate the interfascicular spaces in aggressively growing sarcomas. In sarcomas the Indian-file arrangement of columns of single cells (Fig. 44–2B) is often seen. A rule of considerable value in differentiating lymphocytic lymphomas from inflammatory diseases, and especially from chronic lupus erythematosus, is that in the latter the cells are spaced by edema so that they can easily be scrutinized individually. In a lymphoma, the cells are so tightly packed (Fig. 44–2) that their features are obscured except in very thin sections.

Involvement of Epidermis and Adnexa

Leukemic infiltrates do not usually invade the epidermis. They are separated from it by a grenz zone of compressed connective tissue. Sarcomatous tumors, on the other hand, may destroy the epidermis and lead to ulceration. It was mentioned in Chapter 24 that Langerhans cell granuloma, which often comes into differential diagnosis, has a strong tendency to invade and even destroy the epidermis. In mycosis fungoides we meet the paradoxical situation that the infiltrate often involves the subpapillary zone more than the papillae, while on the other hand, epidermal invasion in the form of Pautrier abscesses (Fig. 44–5) is a diagnostic feature. Both phenomena may be found in the same section.

The condition of hair follicles and sweat glands may serve as an indication of the relative benignity or destructiveness of the process. The adnexa may be fairly normal in benign lymphoplasia, although they are embarrassed by massive infiltrate. They become atrophic in leukemia and are invaded and destroyed by sarcomas. Sebaceous glands usually suffer first, hair follicles next, but eccrine glands are surprisingly resistant.

TERMINOLOGY AND CLASSIFICATION

Concepts and nomenclature of cutaneous lymphoreticular proliferation have grown and changed over the years, just as in other fields of dermatology, but have been influenced much more by parallel developments in general pathology and immunology. Rappaport's classification was morphologic and had to be changed when modern immunologic methods brought new views of histogenesis and function. Five new classifications have been proposed by Lukes and Collins,[8] Dorfman,[9] a British group,[10] the World Health Organization,[11] and a group of German authors (the so-called Kiel classification).[12,13] These have been subjected to a critical comparative analysis very recently,[14] which proposes a compromise classification and ends with the hope that it will stimulate others to offer modifications and bring about a final solution to the classification of non-Hodgkin's lymphomas. In this status of transition and partial disagreement, our present third edition can only try to give guidelines for the dermatologic lymphomas. Leukemic infiltrates and other disorders affecting the skin secondarily will not be discussed in detail. Those histiocytic lesions that we consider to be granulomatous rather than neoplastic were the subject of Chapter 23. It is to be admitted that the differentiation between reactive and neoplastic lesions is less secure than in any other field of dermatohistopathology because we are dealing here with the same tissue elements that are the substrate of inflammation. Presence of some mitoses cannot decide the issue, unless they are numerous and atypical. Cellular atypy must be evaluated with great caution. The old rule still holds true that presence of multinucleated cells and evidence of considerable phagocytosis of lipid and iron pigment proves that the tumor cells are reactive histiocytes and, therefore, not malignant. It is confusing that the name "histiocyte" has been used with an entirely new meaning. We, therefore, continue to use "reticulum cell" where it seems appropriate. Table 44–1 lists the conditions discussed in this chapter.

SPECIFIC DISORDERS

Leukemia Cutis

Any of the recognized forms of leukemia may produce specific infiltrates in the skin, but *chronic lymphatic leukemia* (Fig. 44–2) is the most common cause,[15] even in aleukemic cases.[16] *Monocytic leukemia* is next, while *myeloid leukemia cutis* is very rare. In monocytic leukemia, local proliferation of abnormal cells may take place in the skin,

TABLE 44–1.
Proliferative Lymphoreticular Affections of the Skin

Benign (Possibly Premalignant) Proliferations
    Parapsoriasis en plaques
    Benign lymphoplasia (lymphocytoma, lymphadenosis
      benigna)
    Lymphomatoid papulosis
    Woringer–Kolopp disease
    Crosti's reticulohistiocytoma of the back
Malignant Proliferations
    Mycosis fungoides
    Sézary's syndrome
    Primary Hodgkin's disease of skin
    Primary lymphosarcomas and reticulum cell sarcomas
      (including Spiegler–Fendt sarcoid)
    Secondary involvement by leukemias, Hodgkin's
      disease, and lymphosarcoma
Pseudolymphoma
    Arthropod bites
    Actinic reticuloid
    Angiolymphoid hyperplasia

simulating malignant reticulosis.[17] Even in subacute lymphatic leukemia, trauma leading to hemorrhage can cause leukemic cells to be deposited in the skin, where they then may multiply, producing a specific focus due to a nonspecific cause. There are, however, pruritic and unexplainable nonspecific inflammatory skin lesions in patients having leukemia, and to these the diagnosis *leukemid* may be applied.

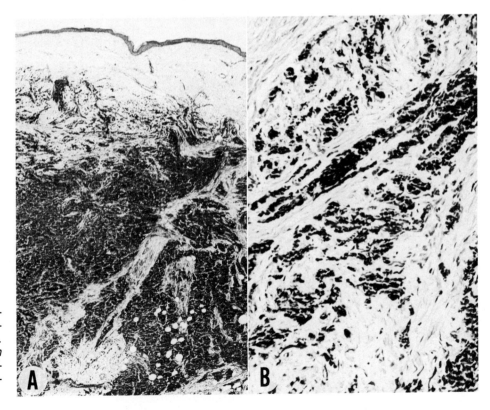

FIGURE 44–2.
Lymphatic leukemia. **A.** *Massive infiltrate does not approach epidermis. H&E. X21.* **B.** *Monomorphic cells in clumps and Indian-file columns between collagen bundles. H&E. X185.*

Sarcomas and Hodgkin's Disease

We continue to use the diagnoses *lymphosarcoma* and *reticulum cell sarcoma* because "malignant lymphoma" has often been used in a much wider sense for all lymphoproliferative diseases.

By definition, sarcomatous lesions should be locally destructive in contrast to simply space-occupying leukemic deposits or benign lesions (Sec. VII). Histologically, one finds interfascicular spread of specific cells in the pars reticularis (Fig. 44–3), in addition to more or less massive perivascular accumulations. Epithelium of adnexa and epidermis may be invaded. Cytologic differential diagnosis should be made with caution in paraffin sections and should be confirmed by touch imprints or other hematologic and immunologic methods. Occasionally, lesions of this type may originate in the skin and spread to lymph nodes and other organs later. Thorough systemic examination of the patient is essential in every case.

Reticulum Cell Sarcoma. Reticulum cell sarcomas (Fig. 44–3B) are composed of smaller or larger

stellate or fusiform cells with atypical nuclei. If there is evidence of phagocytic activity of the tumor cells, especially of erythrophagia, the lesion is properly called *malignant histiocytosis*[18] or histiocytic medullary reticulosis.[19] Large tumors may show considerable variation of histologic pattern from place to place. Tumors containing a mixture of reticular cells and round cells may occur.

Lymphosarcoma. Lymphosarcomas consist either of relatively large cells of lymphoblastic type or of small elements resembling mature lymphocytes.[20] Differential diagnosis of lymphosarcomas from clinically benign lymphoplasias can be most difficult in a biopsy specimen, and diagnosis often must be deferred.

Hodgkin's Disease. Hodgkin's disease manifests itself in the skin but rarely, and primary cutaneous localization is highly exceptional.[21] The histologic picture does not differ from that in other organs, and the *Sternberg-Reed cell* (Fig. 44–4) is essential in diagnosis. Hodgkin's disease may supervene in a patient with mycosis fungoides as a

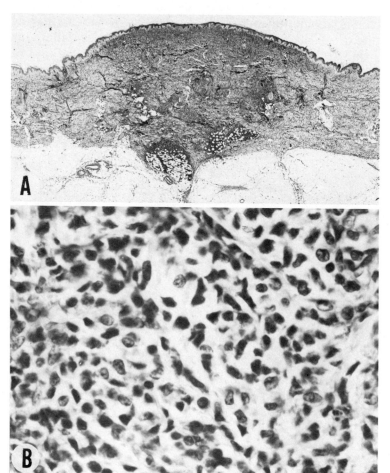

FIGURE 44–3.
Reticulum cell sarcoma. **A.** *Characteristic distribution of many lymphomatous infiltrates, which outline entire vasculature of skin. Pattern is somewhat obscured in this case because sarcomatous cells also infiltrate interfascicular spaces. H&E. X14.* **B.** *Polygonal and interconnected cells permit tentative cytologic diagnosis of reticulum cells rather than lymphoid cells. Diagnosis should be checked by hematologic methods. H&E. X400.*

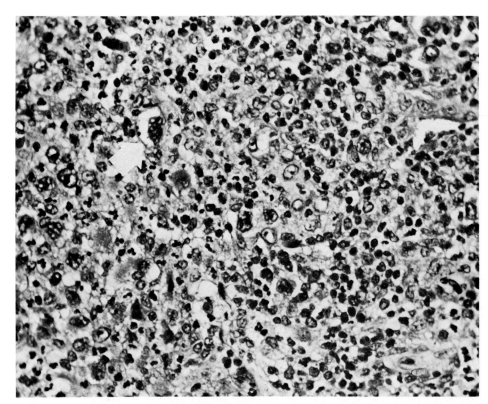

FIGURE 44–4.
Hodgkin's disease. Mixed infiltrate of atypical mononuclear cells interspersed with a few eosinophils. Sternberg–Reed cells (arrow) have one nucleus or, more commonly, several nuclei containing very large nucleoli. H&E. X370.

terminal event and may remain distinct in localization and histologic expression (personal observation).

Mycosis Fungoides

Definition. Mycosis fungoides is the principal lymphoreticular neoplasm originating in the skin, and it often remains confined to the skin for many years and even to the end of life. Since the clinicopathologic concept of mycosis fungoides is not the same everywhere, we have to define our own. We believe that it is a neoplastic, or at least proliferative, process from the very beginning rather than an inflammatory or granulomatous one. This statement includes *parapsoriasis en plaques* and *parapsoriasis lichenoides* (Chap. 13) as obligatory precursor lesions. On the other hand, mycosis fungoides may superimpose itself on inflammatory diseases which are facultative precursors, such as *psoriasis* or *alopecia mucinosa*. The histologic picture of mycosis fungoides has been identified recently as a *T cell lymphoma*,[22] and one may consider the possibility that it is an immunologically induced lymphoma.[23]

We include under mycosis fungoides any case exhibiting the characteristic clinical progression from the eczematoid or parapsoriatic stage through the plaque stage to the tumor stage, regardless of the histologic substrate, which may be the classic mixed one or a monomorphous one of round cells or fixed-tissue-type cells. On the other hand, we do not rule out *erythrodermatous* or *d'emblée* cases if they do show a mixed infiltrate.[24] The reasons for this broad definition are several. The course of the disease is variable, and the stages may occur in reversed order. The histologic picture may show progression from a mixed infiltrate to a monomorphous infiltrate, and this may occur early or late. The most reasonable explanation for the histologic picture seems to be that given by Van Scott et al.[25] that the neoplastic cells may be relatively few in earlier stages and are overshadowed by inflammatory infiltrate, a situation similar to that in Hodgkin's disease.[1] It is assumed that the infiltrate is a reaction to the malignant cells and keeps them in check until, in later stages, the immunologic status of the patient deteriorates. In addition, as in other neoplasms, the neoplastic cell may show progression and change in character. Leukemia, reticulum cell sarcoma, lymphosarcoma, or Hodgkin's disease may develop secondarily in mycosis fungoides. That is the reason that the old term *lymphoblastoma*[26] should not be forgotten. It is broader and more comfortably applicable to the spectrum of cutaneous disease than the term *malignant lymphoma*, which implies disease of lymph nodes. *Cu-*

taneous *lymphoblastoma*, of which mycosis fungoides is the outstanding example, has as its implied and most important characteristic that it originates in the skin and usually remains confined to the skin for prolonged periods, regardless of the exact nature of clinical or histologic manifestations.

Histologic Features. In attempting the histologic diagnosis of mycosis fungoides (Fig. 44–5), one must pay attention to the epidermis as well as the dermis. For reasons to be detailed later, the epidermis often is acanthotic in a peculiar manner

which attracts attention once one has learned to recognize it. The rete ridges are long and rounded and often bulbous in cross section. Papillae are correspondingly prominent and often bulbous, the combination producing a festoonlike contour of the dermoepidermal junction in a single section. The epidermis usually shows some intracellular and intercellular edema and also parakeratosis. It often is invaded by mononuclear cells, which may lie singly or in groups within small cavities called *Pautrier abscesses* (Figs. 44–5 and 44–8). The cells may be simply small round cells but often are larger mononuclears, sometimes possessing atypical nuclei. Cells are apt to invade the epidermis singly[27] in parapsoriasis en plaques. Well-developed Pautrier abscesses are almost pathognomonic for mycosis fungoides, but their absence does not rule out the diagnosis. The number of cells invading the epidermis varies greatly from case to case. In some cases, it becomes so great that the epidermis appears honeycombed, and Paget's disease is simulated if the invading cells are large and hyperchromatic (Fig. 44–6A). One then speaks of *epidermotropic lymphoblastoma*[28,29] (Fig. 44–7).

The epidermal involvement has been clarified or at least rationalized in the last several years. We

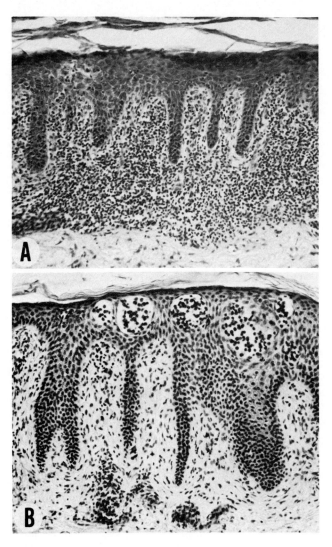

FIGURE 44–5.
Mycosis fungoides, plaque stage. **A.** *Rather diffuse and fairly monomorphous infiltrate, which is heavier in subpapillary layer than in some papillae and does not involve pars reticularis. Acanthotic epidermis is invaded in only a few places. H&E. X135.* **B.** *Higher degree of acanthosis and crowded Pautrier abscesses in lesion which exhibits relatively mild dermal infiltrate. Many of epidermotropic cells, and some in dermis, are hyperchromatic. H&E. X135.*

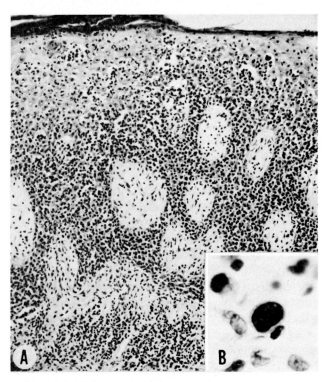

FIGURE 44–6.
Epidermotropic form of mycosis fungoides. **A.** *Acanthotic and papillomatous epidermis is diffusely invaded by hyperchromatic mononuclear round cells. H&E. X135.* **B.** *Mycosis fungoides cell in the dermal infiltrate. H&E. X800.*

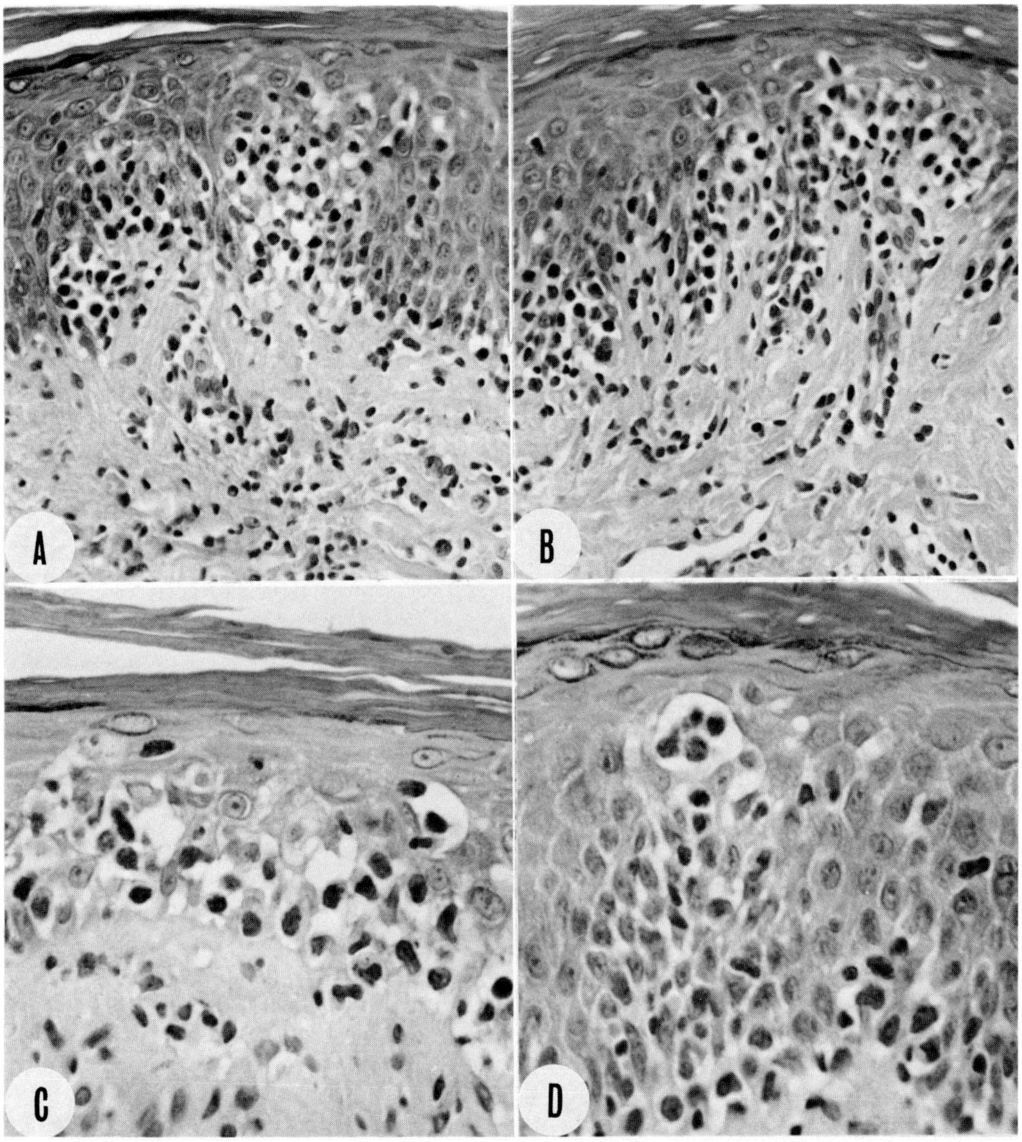

FIGURE 44–7.
Epidermotropic lymphoma. Hyperchromatic cells invade the epidermis diffusely, forming Pautrier abscesses occasionally. Relatively few of these cells are present in the dermis. H&E. **A** *and* **B**. *X400.* **C** *and* **D**. *X600.*

mentioned that mycosis fungoides has been identified as a T cell lymphoma (Fig. 44–8). The hypothesis[3] of homing of T cells to epithelial tissues other than the thymus has been invoked to explain intraepidermal occurrence of the atypical cells (ecotaxis). Very recently, Rowden et al.[30] have investigated the role of Langerhans cells in this process, basing their work on the role of Langerhans cells in contact dermatitis (Chap. 7) as intermediaries in antigen recognition and presentation. They found apposition of lymphocytes to Langerhans cells and suggest that subsequent destruction of L cells acts as the focus for the development of Pautrier mi-

croabscesses. Schuppli[23] had found that patients with mycosis fungoides tend to be exquisitely sensitive to metals, and Langerhans cells have been found to recognize and bind metals preferentially. It seems possible that these findings may lead to further identification of antigen persistence as a cause of mycosis fungoides. Long-continued stimulation may in the end lead to neoplastic transformation.

In its classic expression, the dermal infiltrate of mycosis fungoides spares the papillae in spite of its epidermotropism. In the earlier, pretumor stages, infiltrate may form a relatively dense and broad

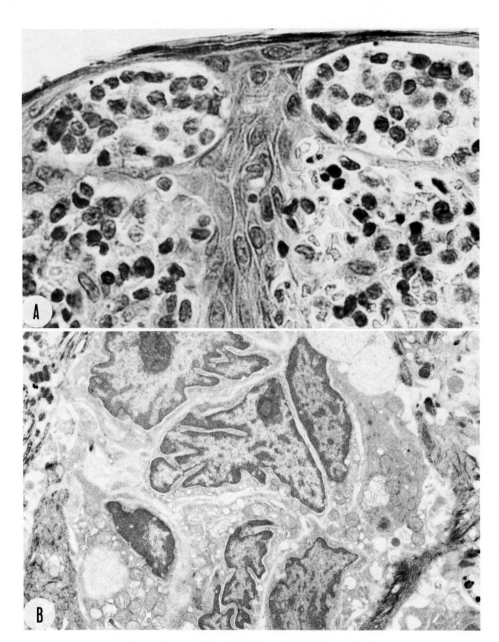

FIGURE 44–8.
Pautrier abscesses and Lutzner cells. **A.** *Accumulations of large mononuclear cells, presumably T lymphocytes, in epidermis. H&E. X800.* **B.** *Electron micrograph of Lutzner cells with indented nuclei in a Pautrier abscess. (Courtesy of Dr. M. Taylor.)*

zone in the subpapillary layer and may involve the pars reticularis in variable depth. It consists of a mixture of cells in which mononuclear cells of various sizes predominate. Plasma cells, eosinophils, and neutrophilic polymorphonuclear cells may be present in descending order of frequency. Mast cells play no significant role. Fixed-tissue-type cells usually are increased in number, and there may be a diffuse increase of fibrocytes and/or histiocytes throughout the dermis. The characteristic mycosis cell is a fairly large cell (Fig. 44–6B) with a single, large, and hyperchromatic nucleus. It has attracted renewed attention because of attempts of electron microscopists to identify it *(Lutzner cell)* (Fig. 44–8B). It soon became apparent, however, that similar atypical cells with highly convoluted nuclei

are present also in other lymphoreticular diseases, not all of them neoplastic.[31,32] They have been identified in the bloodstream of patients suffering from dermatitis and psoriasis.[33] Lutzner cells are of diagnostic importance in histologic sections only if present in appreciable numbers. An occasional hyperchromatic cell may be identified in various other dermatoses, especially in parapsoriasis en plaques, where it supports the view that this disease is a premycotic affection but has no prognostic significance. Destruction of elastic fibers is a helpful, but not infallible, criterion. In the tumor stage, infiltrate becomes so massive that diagnosis is easy.

Edelson[34] has pointed out that cutaneous T cell lymphoma (CTCL) progresses often from the epidermotropic form to a nonepidermotropic form and that this transition carries a poor prognosis, especially if it is associated with lymph node involvement.

Differential Diagnosis. Commonly, the pathologist is asked to rule out or confirm the diagnosis of lymphoblastoma in a patient who has long-standing and stubborn eczema, parapsoriasis en plaques, or other ill-defined skin disease. The decision is among the most difficult in dermatopathology, and one should proceed with cautious reserve. The mental attitude should be "Must I diagnose MF?" rather than "Can I diagnose MF?" Mycosis fungoides, while eventually fatal, has a long course extending often over many years[24,35] and not infrequently punctuated by spontaneous remissions. In contrast to Hodgkin's disease, in which some patients are encountered at a stage when only one group of lymph nodes is involved and eradication of the neoplasm by vigorous treatment is feasible, mycosis fungoides practically always involves large areas of skin by the time diagnosis is made. Although some hopeful voices have been heard recently, in general there is only palliative treatment, no cure. Experienced dermatologists know that the best therapeutic measures are the mildest ones that give the patient relief. Even ultraviolet rays may be effective for relatively long times. Precocious diagnosis may induce the less experienced therapist to rush in with heavy guns that exhaust the patient's immunologic and general resistance prematurely and may enhance the fatal outcome rather than retard it. Thus, if the diagnosis of mycosis fungoides is delayed several months or even a few years in a questionable case, little is lost, and much may be gained by avoiding diagnostic error.

The list of confusing differential diagnoses includes parapsoriasis, eczematous dermatitis, especially of the dermal contact sensitivity type, alopecia mucinosa, psoriasis, and less common ones, some of which will be mentioned in the discussion of pseudolymphoma.

As mentioned repeatedly and discussed in Chapter 13, the histologic differences between parapsoriasis of the plaque, lichenoid, and reticulated types and early plaques of mycosis fungoides are ill defined. In some cases, one can diagnose parapsoriasis with assurance on the basis of mild and superficial infiltrate and little epidermal involvement. In other cases, heavy and deep infiltrate and some Pautrier abscesses fairly prove mycosis fungoides. In many cases, the turning point is judged more accurately by the clinical features of thickening of the plaques and onset of severe pruritus.

Dermal contact sensitivity reaction (Chap. 7)

was recognized only recently and is easily confused with early mycosis fungoides, since the epidermis shows acanthosis, parakeratosis, and round cell invasion but no spongiosis or vesiculation, while the dermal infiltrate is heavy and mixed and extends into the pars reticularis. There may be destruction of elastic fibers. This little-known type of contact dermatitis should be mentioned in every applicable case, and the clinician should be asked to rule it out, if necessary, by intradermal testing.

Alopecia mucinosa was discussed in Chapter 18. In some cases, the mixed infiltrate may become so heavy as to suggest mycosis fungoides. In other cases follicular mucinosis has been found associated with true mycosis fungoides, and in still others the transition from benign alopecia mucinosa to lymphoblastoma has been observed clinically as well as histologically. That event is recognizable by the appearance of atypical cells in the infiltrate, and by the infiltrate's becoming dissociated from the altered follicles and occurring independently, usually in perivascular distribution.

There are documented cases in which psoriasis eventuated into mycosis fungoides. Histologically, this event is indicated by much heavier infiltrate than one usually sees in psoriasis, by its mixed character, and by the presence of Pautrier abscesses rather than of Munro abscesses.

Clinical Variants. Cases of *general exfoliative dermatitis* and of *generalized erythroderma* without exfoliation may be diagnosed as mycosis fungoides if they present the classic histologic picture. Other cases may represent leukemia cutis, lymphosarcoma, or the Sézary syndrome. Sometimes a rather nonspecific and often relatively mild inflammatory infiltrate characterizes the skin disease as an –id in cases of otherwise proved lymphoma. Rarely, epidermal invasion by mononuclear cells and edema become so severe in mycosis fungoides that clinical *bullae* are seen, and the histologic picture may include acantholysis.[36] More common is the clinical picture of *poikiloderma* (Chap. 9). Here, the histologic features of mycosis fungoides are to be looked for, with the exception of epidermal hyperplasia. On the contrary, the epidermis may be severely atrophic and exhibit basal cell degeneration in connection with invasion by atypical mononuclear cells.[37] In other cases, truly verrucoid hyperplasia of the epidermis may be found.[38]

Erythroderma and Sézary's Syndrome

Generalized redness of the skin accompanied by clinical infiltration and more or less prominent scaliness, often to the point of exfoliation, is always suspected to be a manifestation of lymphoreticular neoplastic proliferation. The diagnosis, however, must be carefully evaluated by clinicopathologic correlation and often by repeated biopsies and prolonged observation. *Generalized erythroderma* was mentioned as the most severe manifestation of eczematous dermatitis and especially of the dermal contact sensitivity reaction in Chapter 7, as psoriatic erythroderma in Chapter 8, and as the chronic form of pityriasis rubra pilaris in Chapter 18. It may develop as a rare manifestation of histoplasmosis[39] and was misdiagnosed as mycosis fungoides for many months in a personally observed case until it cleared up completely under antibiotic therapy for the oral histoplasmic ulcers, which had developed as a supposed complication.[40]

Considered a variant of mycosis fungoides by some, *Sézary's syndrome* seems to emerge as a universal erythroderma characterized by atypical T lymphocytes in skin and circulating blood.[41,42] The circulating cells originate in the skin. Electron microscopically, the Lutzner cells of mycosis fungoides may be found also in Sézary's syndrome.[43,44] In tissue sections, the skin contains a not very heavy and quite superficial infiltrate of mononuclear cells, some of which seem to be lymphocytes, others fixed-tissue-type cells resembling reticulum cells. The atypical cells often invade the epidermis and show mitotic activity in the epidermis.[45] Diagnosis often requires several biopsies at intervals of a few months and correlation with the clinical picture of intractable pruritic erythroderma, which involves palms and soles and is associated with thick and deformed nails.

Lymphomatoid Papulosis

Since Macaulay[46] first insisted that a patient with a case of so-called atypical Mucha-Habermann's disease actually had repeated periodic accumulations of malignant lymphoma cells in epidermis and dermis and, therefore, applied the name *lymphomatoid papulosis* (Figs. 44–9 and 44–10) to this continuing self-healing eruption that is clinically benign in spite of the paradoxical histologic appearance of malignancy, quite a number of similar observations have been published.[47] Macaulay's disease is now recognized as a T cell affection, in which apparently clones of grossly abnormal cells proliferate in the uppermost dermis and the epidermis and are reacted to and probably destroyed by an inflammatory infiltrate. While each individual lesion heals, an unpredictable number of new foci will arise. Recently, a possible role has been assigned to immunoglobulin A in the causation of lymphomatoid papulosis on the basis of one case.[48] There are patients in whom the benign condition after many years ended as a malignant lymphoma.[49,50] There are other cases in which nodules, plaques, and tumors rather than papules underwent similar paradoxical rhythmic evolution and involution. We have placed this discussion behind mycosis fungoides and Sézary syndrome as a third manifestation of T cell lymphoma in the skin instead of putting it under the benign lymphoplasias, as in the second edition of our book, because we believe that much more investigation and follow-up of individual cases will be needed before we can consider the condition as truly benign.

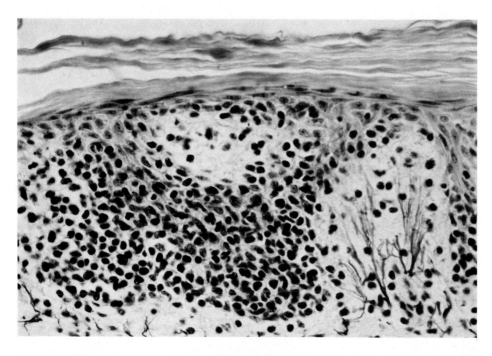

FIGURE 44–9.
Lymphomatoid papulosis. Early lesion of Macaulay's case. Bizarre hyperchromatic cells have invaded epidermis, which shows no evidence of acanthotic reaction (compare Fig. 44–7). O&G. X225. (From Macaulay. Arch Dermatol 97:23, 1968.)

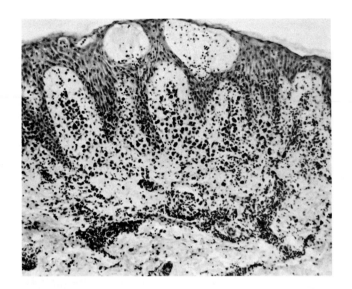

FIGURE 44–10.
Lymphomatoid papulosis. Fully developed lesion shows large T cells in upper dermis, associated with inflammatory infiltrate. Epidermis is acanthotic and exhibits inflammatory and degenerating cells in vesicles. H&E. X125.

Mastocytosis and Plasmacytoma

Mast cells are a normal component of the dermis and are found in small numbers, mainly in the surroundings of blood vessels and adnexa. Larger num-

bers occur without pathologic significance in the stroma of benign tumors and basal cell epitheliomas. Some unusual cases of acral dermatitis, possibly associated with atopy, were found to have a striking increase of mast cells in the papillary dermis.[51] Otherwise, large numbers of these cells are almost pathognomonic of *urticaria pigmentosa*. Papules and nodules composed of mast cells usually are benign and often self-healing skin lesions. However, in some cases, they are part of systemic mastocytosis.[52] The histologic picture of urticaria pigmentosa (Fig. 44–11) varies from massive accumulations of mast cells in the entire dermis to moderate increase of these cells in perivascular arrangement. The former is more often found in children, the latter in adults. Because the granules do not stain specifically in H&E sections, mast cells may be overlooked or mistaken for histiocytes unless special stains (toluidine blue, PAS, alcian blue) are done. Routine use of O&G staining obviates this difficulty. Mast cell granules are stained purple by this method. A variant called *telangiectasia macularis eruptiva perstans* was mentioned in Chapter 42. Bullous and pseudoxanthomatous lesions may be found.

Multiple myeloma, the proliferation of neoplastic plasma cells in the bone marrow, rarely causes skin manifestations, although the related dyspro-

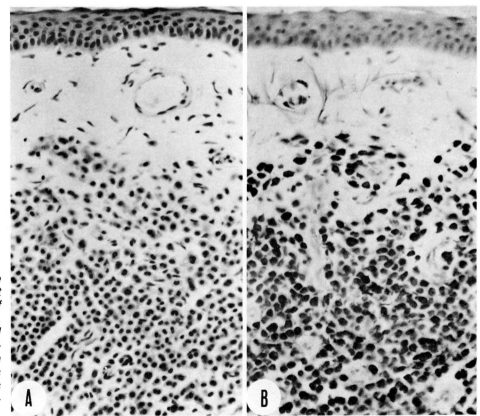

FIGURE 44–11.
Urticaria pigmentosa. **A.** *Dense dermal infiltrate of cells that have a moderate amount of stainable cytoplasm. H&E. X250.* **B.** *Similar section stained with O&G shows dense granulation of these cells, which cannot be resolved at this magnification. The granules stain purple with Giemsa solution (Chap. 3).*

teinemias of Waldenström and other types may produce vascular disturbances, which were mentioned in Chapter 15. Occasionally, primary cutaneous plasmacytomas are encountered,[53,54] which consist of more or less atypical elements (Fig. 5–14), in contrast to heavy plasma cell infiltrates of a reactive nature (Fig. 38–6). The rare picture of plasma cell leukemia in the skin is illustrated in Figure 44–1.

Rare Localized Forms

Woringer–Kolopp Disease. A peculiarly localized and chronic form of epidermotropic lymphoma was described in a 13-year-old girl by Woringer and Kolopp[55] in 1939. Since its rediscovery in 1970,[56,57] several cases have been reported, some of them generalized. The frame of the term, Woringer–Kolopp disease, has been stretched on the basis of histologic resemblance to include forms which we mentioned as epidermotropic types of mycosis fungoides (see above).

We prefer to restrict the concept of *pagetoid reticulosis* to localized cases which have been found to be curable by total excision.[58] The few generalized cases were in old people, while the typical localized lesions were found mainly in young patients preceding the common age of onset of mycosis fungoides (which ordinarily is not curable by surgery). A new thought has been introduced by

Reonz and Touraine,[59] who found dense granules characteristic of Merkel cells in the pagetoid cells and favor the Merkel cell as the tumor cell. This concept awaits confirmation, but it is interesting to note that the Merkel cell has been implied recently as the proliferating cell of the invasive trabecular carcinoma of the skin (Chap. 40).

The histologic picture (Fig. 44–12) of Woringer–Kolopp disease is very characteristic. There is tremendous verrucous hyperplasia of the epidermis, in which are localized in pagetoid fashion large pale cells that do not react with any of the reagents used for melanoma or for Paget cells (Fig. 44–13). There is some inflammatory infiltrate in the dermis.

Crosti's Reticulohistiocytoma of the Back. Cerutti and Santoianni[60] described four cases in which lesions were localized to the back. The histologic picture was dominated by histiocytic cells of fibrocytic type and by lymphocytic and monocytic cells, all situated in the mid-dermis. Other cases have been reported.[61,62] Ultrastructurally, the cells resemble histiocytes. The tumors are radiosensitive but may recur.

The reason we mention these puzzling rarities is to point out that the field of cutaneous lymphoreticular proliferation is far from exhausted and that, in certain cases, one does not know whether the clinically benign course or the atypical histologic pictures should be used for classification. This is even more true for the two groups to be discussed next.

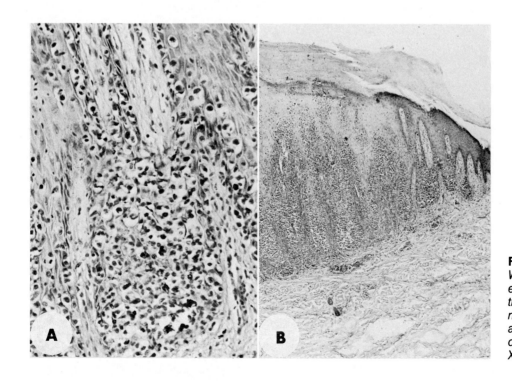

FIGURE 44–12.
Woringer–Kolopp disease. Pagetoid picture is produced by the presence of large mononuclear cells in the highly acanthotic and verrucous epidermis. **A.** *H&E. X180.* **B.** *H&E. X30.*

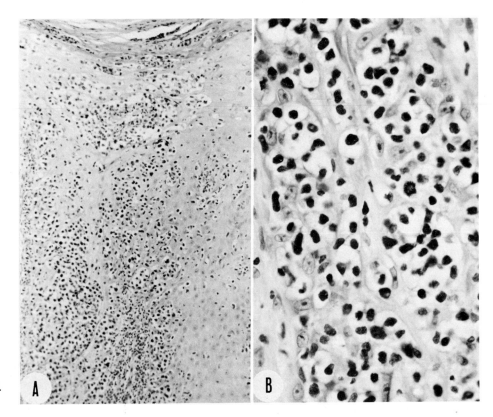

FIGURE 44–13.
Woringer–Kolopp disease. H&E.
A. *X135.* **B.** *X600.*

Benign Lymphoplasia

The manifestations of presumably benign cutaneous infiltrates of lymphoid cells are many. One of the easiest to diagnose is typical *lymphocytoma cutis* (Fig. 44–14), in which sharply defined nodules of small round cells surround germinal centers. If the latter are absent, one may still deal with benign lymphocytoma but must consider *Jessner's lymphocytic infiltration* on one hand and the old *Spiegler–Fendt sarcoid* on the other. Jessner's disease was discussed in Chapter 14. Its overall

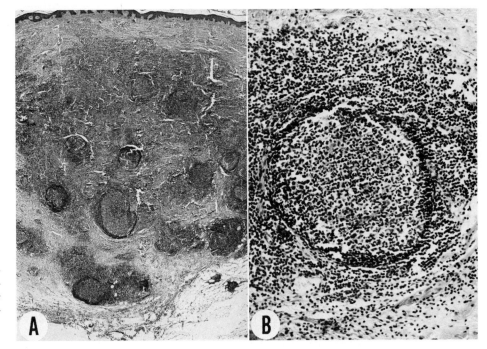

FIGURE 44–14.
Lymphocytoma cutis (lymphadenosis cutis benigna). Well-delineated germinal centers surrounded by small lymphocytes in lymphadenoid pattern.
A. *H&E. X30.* **B.** *H&E. X135.*

features are those of an inflammatory perivascular infiltrate rather than those of neoplastic nodularity. Spiegler-Fendt sarcoid is considered by some a low-grade lymphosarcoma, by others a manifestation of Baefverstedt's *lymphadenosis cutis benigna*.[63] The old-fashioned designation comes in handy when massive nodes of small or somewhat larger round cells occupy dermis and subcutaneous tissue. Only the clinical course or associated findings can bring a decision in such cases. A case in point was described[64] after the injection of antigenic material. The skin lesions consisted of large pleomorphic cells and showed many germinal centers. The case was described as pseudolymphoma, and we shall encounter on the next pages various lesions in which a faulty immune reaction mimics lymphomatous lesions.

Pseudolymphoma

This term is fairly new and is applicable to any lesion that simulates malignant lymphoreticular proliferation histologically. However, it is more specifically used for certain lesions which are different from the benign lymphoplasias discussed in the preceding paragraph and have features of destructiveness or cytologic atypicality.

An unusually aggravating syndrome has been encountered with the use of anticonvulsant drugs related to hydantoin. The illness is of a systemic nature and often involves the skin with a papular pruritic eruption that histologically may mimic mycosis fungoides with Pautrier microabscesses.[65] Lymph node involvement shows destruction of architecture, as in lymphoma. These immune reactions usually subside rather quickly but may run a prolonged course.[66]

Arthropod Bites. It has long been known that solitary lesions resembling various lymphomas, but especially mycosis fungoides, may be unusual chronic reactions to *arthropod bite* (Fig. 44–15). They may persist for many months and, on biopsy, present massive mixed infiltrate, usually containing eosinophils and sometimes atypical mononuclear cells. However, the infiltrate may be monomorphous. This diagnosis should always be considered when a solitary nodule or tumor resembles lymphoblastoma. With the recent recrudescence of *scabies*, nodular-persistent reactions to this infestation are being seen more frequently.[67]

Actinic Reticuloid. So far observed only in elderly men, actinic reticuloid is a highly unusual tissue reaction to sun exposure.[68] It may have been

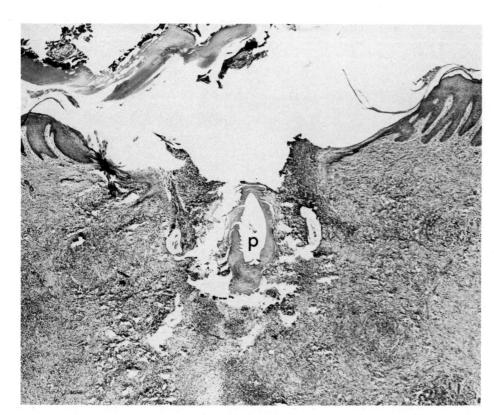

FIGURE 44–15.
Arthropod bite reaction. Proboscis of tick (p) is embedded in heavy granulomatous infiltrate in dermis which contains many eosinophils, while parts of chitinous shell of engorged body are visible near upper rim of picture. H&E. X30.

included in the frame of polymorphic light eruptions by earlier authors. There is deep-reaching and often pleomorphic infiltrate, which may also invade the epidermis and strongly simulate mycosis fungoides. The clinical restriction to light-exposed areas and proof of hypersensitivity to ultraviolet and visible light will lead to the correct diagnosis.

Angiolymphoid Hyperplasia. Through the work of several authors,[69,70] a variable but fairly well defined picture has emerged that probably is best designated as *angiolymphoid hyperplasia with eosinophils.* It is related to and possibly identical with *Kimura's disease*[71] and also has similarities to vascular papules around the head and neck described as *papular angioplasia*[72] and as *atypical granuloma pyogenicum.*[73] The lesions (Figs. 44–16 and 44–17) usually occur on the head and neck but may develop on the hand.[74] They may involve dermis or subcutaneous tissue, or both, and are characterized by two components in variable combination. There is new formation of vessels, partly thick-walled, partly immature, and there is a cellular infiltrate of small and larger mononuclear cells mixed with eosinophils and some mast cells. Multiple lymph follicles may be formed. Differential diagnosis includes malignant hemangioendothelioma, malignant and benign lymphoreticular processes, and chronic reaction to arthropod bite.

Angioimmunoblastic Lymphadenopathy. Recognized since 1975, and until then often mistaken for Hodgkin's disease, a disease of lymph nodes has been described as angioimmunoblastic lymphadenopathy.[75,76] It is considered to be a benign lymphoproliferative process, possibly due to faulty stimulation of the immune system by medication, and presents a characteristic triad of vascular neogenesis, polymorphous cellular proliferation, and deposits of acidophilic intercellular substances in the affected lymph nodes. In more than half of the cases, it is accompanied by a maculopapular skin rash that may occasionally produce tumors. Histologically, the skin lesion may not present more than focal lymphohistiocytic perivasculitis, but in other cases, it may simulate a tuberculoid granuloma or may resemble the more specific picture found in the lymph nodes. In any case, the clinician confronted with a maculopapular eruption accompanied by lymphadenopathy should take this unusual disease, which may terminate as a true lymphoma, into consideration.[77,78]

Sinus Histiocytosis with Massive Lymphadenopathy. This affection is a generally self-limited disease that typically affects cervical lymph nodes of children, most commonly in Africa and the West Indies. It tends to resolve spontaneously but may last for years. It is unknown whether there is a spe-

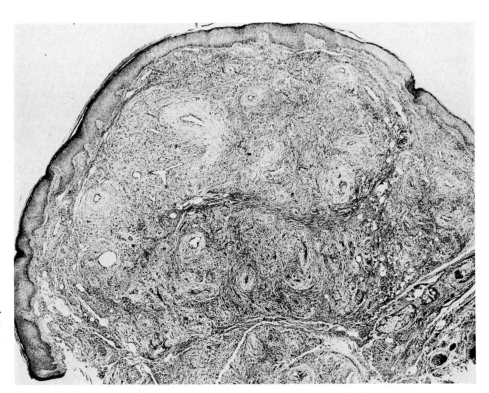

FIGURE 44–16.
Angiolymphoid hyperplasia with eosinophils. Nodular lesion consists of unusual blood vessels accompanied by cellular infiltrate rich in lymphocytes and interspersed with eosinophils (Fig. 44–17). H&E, X14. (From Mehregan and Shapiro. Arch Dermatol 103:50, 1971.)

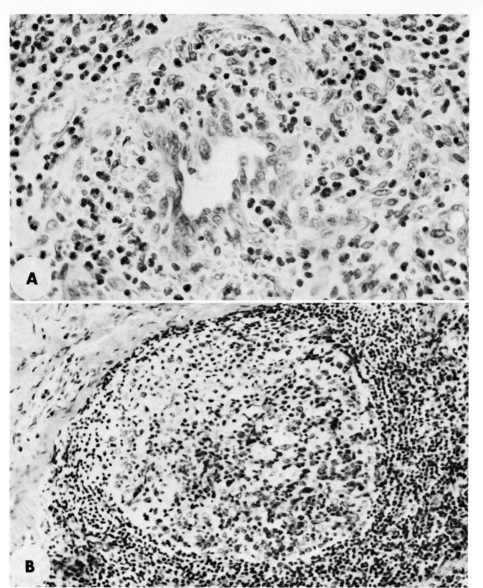

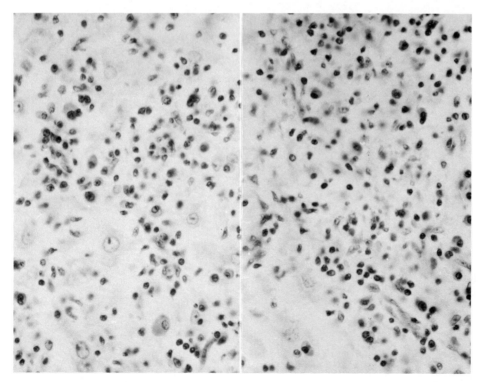

FIGURE 44–17.
Angiolymphoid hyperplasia with eosinophils. **A.** *Small blood vessel surrounded by lymphocytes and fixed-tissue-type cells. Polymorph nuclei belong to eosinophils. H&E. X250.* **B.** *Lymphoid follicle in deeper portion of lesion. H&E. X250. (From Mehregan and Shapiro. Arch Dermatol 103:50, 1971.)*

FIGURE 44–18.
Sinus histiocytosis (with massive lymphadenopathy). Large, lipid-laden histiocytes, embedded in an infiltrate consisting of lymphoid cells and clusters of plasma cells, in the wall of a central necrosis. H&E. X400.

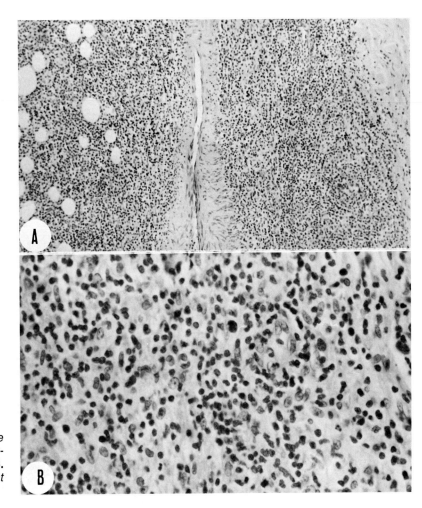

FIGURE 44–19.
Lymphomatoid granulomatosis. **A.** *Dense granulomatous infiltrate surrounds a thick-walled artery in fat tissue. H&E. X125.* **B.** *Details of mixed granulomatous infiltrate at higher power. H&E. X400.*

cific infection or an immunologic disturbance involved in the causation. About 10 percent of patients have skin manifestations,[79] and one young man we encountered had skin manifestations only (Fig. 44–18). He had traveled widely and had developed six separate deep cutaneous nodes that did not recur after excision. The histologic picture was characterized by a sharply limited granuloma with central necrosis. The infiltrate consisted of lymphoid mononuclear cells in the periphery and of large, lipid-laden histiocytes near the center. Numerous plasma cells were scattered and formed small accumulations between the histiocytes.

Lymphomatoid Granulomatosis. Lymphomatoid granulomatosis, described by Liebow et al. in 1972, is an angiocentric and angiodestructive infiltrative process, primarily of the lung. It affects the skin in more than one in three cases.[80] A similar or possibly identical affection has been described in the upper respiratory tract as *polymorphic reticulosis*,[81] where it may involve the mucous membranes of nose and mouth. Wegener's granulomatosis has to

be considered in differential diagnosis. A relation to immunosuppression has been suggested.[82]

Skin lesions are erythematous, macular, sometimes plaquelike, and may improve spontaneously[83] while the systemic disease progresses. There is a perivascular infiltrate consisting of lymphocytes, lymphoblasts, plasma cells, and histiocytes (Fig. 44–19).

REFERENCES

1. Rappaport H: Tumors of the Hematopoietic System. Atlas of Tumor Pathology, Sec. 3, Fascicle 8. Washington, DC, Armed Forces Institute of Pathology, 1966
2. Streilein JW: Lymphocyte traffic, T-cell malignancies and the skin. J Invest Dermatol 71:167, 1978
3. Goudie RB, MacFarlane PS, Lindsay MK: Homing of lymphocytes to nonlymphoid tissues. Lancet 1:292, 1974
4. Edelson RL, Smith RW, Frank MM, et al.: Identification of subpopulations of mononuclear cells in cutaneous infiltrates. I. Differentiation between B cells, T cells, and histiocytes. J Invest Dermatol 61:82, 1973

5. Burg G, Braun-Falco O: Classification and differentiation of cutaneous lymphomas. Enzyme-cytochemical and immunocytochemical studies. Br J Dermatol 93:597, 1975

6. Stingl G, Wolff K, Diem E: In situ identification of lymphoreticular cells in benign and malignant infiltrates by membrane receptor sites. J Invest Dermatol 69:231, 1977

7. Nair KG, Han T, Minowada J: T-cell chronic lymphocytic leukemia. Report of a case and review of the literature. Cancer 44:1652, 1979

8. Lukes RJ, Collins RD: Immunologic characterization of human malignant lymphomas. Cancer 34:1488, 1974

9. Dorfman RF: Pathology of the non-Hodgkin's lymphomas: new classifications. Cancer Treat Rep 61:945, 1977

10. Henry K, Bennett MH, Farrer-Brown G: Morphological classification on non-Hodgkin's lymphomas. Recent results. Cancer Res 64:38, 1978

11. Mathé G, Rappaport H, O'Conor GT, et al.: Histological and cytological typing of neoplastic diseases of hematopoietic and lymphoid tissues. In WHO International Histological Classification of Tumors, No. 14. Geneva, World Health Organization, 1976

12. Gerard-Marchant R, Hamlin I, Lennert K, et al.: Classification of non-Hodgkin's lymphomas. Lancet 2:406, 1974

13. Lennert K, Mohri N: Histopathology and diagnosis of non-Hodgkin's lymphomas. In Uehlinger E (ed): Malignant Lymphomas Other than Hodgkin's Disease. New York, Springer-Verlag, 1978, pp 111–469

14. Nathwani BN: A critical analysis of the classifications of non-Hodgkin's lymphomas. Cancer 44:347, 1979

15. Fayolle J, Coeur P, Bryon PA, et al.: Les manifestations cutanées des leucémies lymphoides chroniques. Ann Dermatol Syphiligr 100:5, 1973

16. Yoder FW, Schuen RL: Aleukemic leukemia cutis. Arch Dermatol 112:367, 1976

17. Burg G, Schmoeckel C, Braun-Falco O, et al.: Monocytic leukemia clinically appearing as "malignant reticulosis of the skin." Arch Dermatol 114:418, 1978

18. Liao KT, Rosai J, Daneshbad K: Malignant histiocytosis with cutaneous involvement and eosinophilia. Am J Clin Pathol 57:438, 1972

19. Rabinowitz BN, Naguchi S, Bergfeld WF: Tumor cell characterization of histiocytic medullary reticulosis. Arch Dermatol 113:927, 1977

20. Goldberg J, Davey FR, Lowenstein F, et al.: Lymphoma cutis of apparent B-cell origin. Arch Pathol Lab Med 102:15, 1978

21. Rubins J: Cutaneous Hodgkin's disease. Indolent course and control with chemotherapy. Cancer 42:1219, 1978

22. Edelson RL: Cutaneous T-cell lymphomas: clues of a skin-thymus interaction. J Invest Dermatol 67:419, 1976

23. Schuppli R: Is mycosis fungoides an "immunoma?" Dermatologica 153:1, 1976

24. Puissant A, Durepaire R-M, Tousch MA, et al.: Mycosis fungoides—le practicien devant les problèmes nosologiques, diagnostiques, pronostiques des lymphomes épidermotropes. Dermatologica 157:365, 1978

25. Van Scott EJ, Clendenning WE, Brecher G: Mycosis fungoides. Relationship to malignant cutaneous reti-

culosis and the Sézary syndrome. Arch Dermatol 89:785, 1964

26. Keim HL: The lymphoblastomas, their interrelationship. Arch Dermatol 19:533, 1929

27. Sanchez JL, Ackerman AB: Early diagnosis of mycosis fungoides: criteria for the histologic diagnosis of the patch stage of the disease. Arch Dermatol 114:1831, 1978

28. Ketron LW, Goodman MH: Multiple lesions of the skin apparently of epithelial origin resembling clinically mycosis fungoides. Report of a case. Arch Dermatol 24:758, 1931

29. Brier RL, Steele CH: Mycosis fungoides. A prolonged course and association with adenocarcinoma of the breast. South Med J 51:919, 1958

30. Rowden G, Phillips TM, Lewis MG, et al.: Target role of Langerhans cells in mycosis fungoides: transmission and immune-electron microscopic studies. J Cutan Pathol 6:364, 1979

31. Petrozzi JW, Reque CJ, Goldschmidt H: Malignant lymphoma, reticulum cell type: demonstration of Lutzner cell. Arch Dermatol 104:38, 1971

32. Flaxman BA, Zelasny G, Van Scott EJ: Nonspecificity of characteristic cells in mycosis fungoides. Arch Dermatol 104:141, 1971

33. Duncan SC, Winkelman RK: Circulating Sézary cells in hospitalized dermatology patients. Br J Dermatol 99:171, 1978

34. Edelson RL: Cutaneous T-cell lymphoma: Mycosis fungoides, Sézary syndrome, and other variants. J Am Acad Dermatol 2:89, 1980

35. Redmond WJ, Rahbari H: Mycosis fungoides: a retrospective study. J Am Acad Dermatol 1:431, 1979

36. Roenigk HH, Castrovicki AJ: Mycosis fungoides bullosa. Arch Dermatol 104:402, 1971

37. Pinkus H: Lichenoid tissue reactions. Arch Dermatol 107:840, 1973

38. Price NM, Fuks ZY, Hoffman TE: Hyperkeratotic and verrucous features of mycosis fungoides. Arch Dermatol 113:57, 1977

39. Cramer HJ: Erythrodermatische Hauthistoplasmose. Dermatologica 146:249, 1973

40. Samovitz M, Dillon TK: Disseminated histoplasmosis presenting as exfoliative erythroderma. Arch Dermatol 101:216, 1970

41. Winkelmann RK: T-cell erythroderma (Sézary syndrome). Arch Dermatol 108:205, 1973

42. Zucker-Franklin D: Thymus-dependent lymphocytes in lymphoproliferative disorders of the skin (Sézary syndrome and mycosis fungoides). J Invest Dermatol 67:412, 1976

43. Lutzner MA, Hobbs JW, Horvath P: Ultrastructure of abnormal cells in Sézary syndrome, mycosis fungoides, and parapsoriasis en plaques. Arch Dermatol 103:375, 1971

44. Whang-Peng J, Lutzner M, Edelson R, et al.: Cytogenetic studies and clinical implications in patients with Sézary's syndrome. Cancer 38:861, 1976

45. Saghier-Guedon I, Pruniéras M, Durepaire R, et al.: Preferential replication of Sézary cells in the epidermis. Bull Cancer (Paris) 64:259, 1977

46. Macaulay WL: Lymphomatoid papulosis. A continuing self-healing eruption, clinically benign—histologically malignant. Arch Dermatol 97:23, 1968

47. Macaulay WL: Lymphomatoid papulosis. J Int Dermatol 17:204, 1978

48. Praudi G, Alessi E, Stefani B, et al.: La papulose lymphomatoide. Rôle possible des IgA dans sa pathogenèse. Ann Dermatol Venereol 104:165, 1977

49. Black MM, Wilson-Jones E: "Lymphomatoid" pityriasis lichenoides, a variant with histological features simulating a lymphoma. A clinical and histopathological study of 15 cases with details of long-term follow-up. Br J Dermatol 86:329, 1972

50. Dupont A: Transformation maligne très tardive d'une réticulose papuleuse à évolution prolongée (lymphomatoid papulosis). Ann Dermatol Syphiligr 100:141, 1973

51. Winkelmann RK, Gleich GJ: Chronic acral dermatitis: association with extreme elevations of IgE. JAMA 225:378, 1973

52. Bazex A, Dupré A, Christol B, et al.: Les mastocytoses familiales. Présentation des deux observations, revue générale, interêt nosologique. Ann Dermatol Syphiligr 98:241, 1971

53. Bork K, Weigand U: Multiple Plasmocytome der Haut mit IgA—Vermehrung im Serum ohne Knochenmarksbeteiligung. Arch Dermatol Res 254:245, 1976

54. Klein M, Grishman E: Single cutaneous plasmacytoma with crystalloid inclusions. Arch Dermatol 113:64, 1977

55. Woringer F, Kolopp P: Lésion érythémato-squameuse polycyclique de l'avant-bras évoluant depuis 6 ans chez un garçonet de 13 ans. Histologiquement infiltrat intraépidermique d'apparence tumorale. Ann Dermatol Syphiligr 10:945, 1939

56. Gisiger O: Zur Differentialdiagnose der von Woringer und Kolopp beschriebenen Retikulose. Dermatologica 140 [Suppl 2]:19, 1970

57. Braun-Falco O, Marghescu S, Wolff HH: Pagetoide Retikulose, Morbus Woringer-Kolopp. Hautarzt 24:11, 1973

58. Lever WF: Localized mycosis fungoides with prominent epidermotropism, Woringer-Kolopp disease. Arch Dermatol 113:1254, 1977

59. Reonz J, Touraine R: Maladie de Woringer et Kolopp. Dermatologica 157:377, 1978

60. Cerutti P, Santoianni P: A relatively benign reticulosis: Crosti's "reticulohistiocytoma of the back." Int J Dermatol 12:35, 1973

61. Laugier P, Hunziker N, Olmos L: Réticulo-histiocytome du dos de l'adulte. Réticulose cutanée circonscrite à évolution lente. Dermatologica 149:350, 1974

62. Gamby T, Chaudon J-P, Dor J-F, et al.: La réticulose de Crosti. A propos de 3 cas dont un avec étude ultrastructurale. Ann Dermatol Venereol 105:821, 1978

63. Schmoeckel C, Burg G, Wolff HH, et al.: The ultrastructure of lymphadenosis benigna cutis (pseudolymphoma cutis). Arch Dermatol Res 258:161, 1977

64. Bernstein H, Shupack J, Ackerman AB: Cutaneous pseudolymphoma resulting from antigen injections. Arch Dermatol 110:756, 1974

65. Schreiber MM, McGregor JG: Pseudolymphoma syndrome. A sensitivity to anticonvulsant drugs. Arch Dermatol 97:297, 1968

66. Halevy S, Feuerman EJ: Pseudolymphoma syndrome. Dermatologica 155:321, 1977

67. Konstantinov D, Stanoeva L: Persistent scabious nodules. Dermatologica 147:321, 1973

68. Ive FA, Magnus IA, Warin RP, et al.: "Actinic reticuloid." A chronic dermatosis associated with severe photosensitivity and the histological resemblance to lymphoma. Br J Dermatol 81:469, 1969

69. Wells GC, Whimster IW: Subcutaneous angiolymphoid hyperplasia with eosinophilia. Br J Dermatol 81:1, 1969

70. Mehregan AH, Shapiro L: Angiolymphoid hyperplasia with eosinophilia. Arch Dermatol 103:50, 1971

71. Reed RJ, Terazakis N: Subcutaneous angioblastic lymphoid hyperplasia with eosinophilia (Kimura's disease). Cancer 29:489, 1972

72. Wilson-Jones E, Marks R: Papular angioplasia: vascular papules of the face and scalp simulating malignant vascular tumors. Arch Dermatol 102:422, 1970

73. Wilson-Jones E, Bleehen SS: Inflammatory angiomatous nodules with abnormal blood vessels occurring about the ears and scalp (pseudo or atypical pyogenic granuloma). Br J Dermatol 81:804, 1969

74. Grimwood R, Swinehart JM, Aeling JL: Angiolymphoid hyperplasia with eosinophilia. Arch Dermatol 115:205, 1979

75. Frizzera G, Moran EM, Rappaport H: Angioimmunoblastic lymphadenopathy: diagnosis and clinical course. Am J Med 59:803, 1975

76. Lukes RJ, Tindle BH: Immunoblastic lymphadenopathy: a hyperimmune entity resembling Hodgkin's disease. N Engl J Med 292:1, 1975

77. Lessana-Leibowitch M, Mignot L, Bloch C, et al.: Manifestations cutanées des lymphoadénopathies angioimmunoblastiques. Ann Dermatol Venereol 104:603, 1977

78. Matloff RB, Neiman RS: Angioimmunoblastic lymphadenopathy. A generalized lymphoproliferative disorder with cutaneous manifestations. Arch Dermatol 114:92, 1978

79. Thawerani H, Sanchez RL, Rosai J, et al.: The cutaneous manifestations of sinus histiocytosis with massive lymphadenopathy. Arch Dermatol 114:191, 1978

80. Katzenstein A-L A, Carrington CB, Liebow AA: Lymphomatoid granulomatosis. A clinicopathologic study of 152 cases. Cancer 43:360, 1979

81. DeRemee RA, Weiland LH, McDonald TJ: Polymorphic reticulosis, lymphomatoid granulomatosis. Two diseases or one? Mayo Clin Proc 53:634, 1978

82. Jauregin HO: Lymphomatoid granulomatosis after immunosuppression for pemphigus. Arch Dermatol 114:1052, 1978

83. Bender BL, Kapadia SB, Synkowski DR, et al.: Lymphomatoid granulomatosis preceded by chronic granulomatous dermatitis. Arch Dermatol 114:1547, 1978

VIII

MUCOUS MEMBRANES, HAIR, AND NAIL

After discussing histopathology of the skin, we feel there are three portions of the body surface left that have their peculiarities and need special techniques and knowledge for adequate examination. The plan of the *Guide* brings together changes that enter differential diagnosis in the examination of a tissue section or other microscopic material. The accessible mucous membranes of mouth, nose, eye, and anogenital area have features that do not lend themselves to exact comparison with those of the diseases of the skin proper but have similarities to each other. The hair and nail are tissues that require special handling and special knowledge of their structure under normal and pathologic circumstances. Thus, we decided to unite mucous membranes, hair, and nail in one section.

Details of the histology of oral mucosa were surveyed in a recent symposium[1] and a small text,[2] and there are several recent textbooks and atlases on oral pathology,[3,4] but they take in much more than dermatologic conditions, while we shall restrict discussion to dermatoses and some neoplastic lesions of the mucosa. There is a recent text on diseases of the vulva[5] which also includes discussion of development and normal structure. Again, we shall confine ourselves to conditions apt to come to the attention of dermatologists.[6]

The hair has attracted considerable attention in the last few years. Two symposiums[7,8] in this country and an international meeting[9] dealt with many aspects of normal and pathologic hair, and there is a comprehensive book[10] just published. The nail

also was treated in several books.[11-13] Our discussion will be somewhat short and will pay attention only to some features of special interest.

REFERENCES

1. Squier CA, Meyer J (eds): Current Concepts of the Histology of Oral Mucosa. Springfield Ill, Thomas, 1971
2. Squier CA, Johnson NW, Hopps, RM: Human oral mucosa. Development, Structure and Function. Oxford, London, Blackwell, 1976
3. Gorlin RJ, Goldman HM: Thoma's Oral Pathology, 6th ed. St. Louis, Mosby, 1970, Vol 2
4. Rushton MA, Cooke BED, Duckworth R: Oral Histopathology, 2nd ed. Edinburgh, Churchill-Livingstone, 1970
5. Gardner HL, Kaufman RH: Benign Diseases of the Vulva and Vagina. St. Louis, Mosby, 1969
6. Ridley CM: A review of the recent literature on diseases of the vulva. Parts I, II, III. Br J Dermatol 86:641, 87:58, 87:163, 1972
7. Brown AC (ed): The First Human Hair Symposium. New York, Medcom, 1974
8. Brown AC, Crounse RG (eds): Hair, Trace Elements and Human Illness. New York, Praeger, 1980
9. First International Congress of Hair Research. Hamburg, 1979
10. Orfanos CE (ed): Haar und Haarkrankheiten. Stuttgart, New York, Gustav Fischer Verlag, 1979
11. Pardo-Castello V, Pardo OA: Diseases of the Nails, 3rd ed. Springfield Ill, Thomas, 1960
12. Samman PD: The Nails in Disease, 2nd ed. Springfield Ill, Thomas, 1972
13. Alkiewicz J, Pfister R: Nagelpathologie. Stuttgart, Schattauer Verlag, 1975

Lesions of Mucous Membranes

In this chapter, affections of the vermilion of the lips, the oral mucosa, the glans penis, and the non-hair-bearing portions of the vulva will be considered. Conjunctiva and anus will be mentioned as occasion arises. Although some of these tissues are not true mucous membranes, they have the common features of weak or parakeratotic keratinization above a stratified epidermislike epithelium and absence of the cutaneous adnexa, except free sebaceous glands (Fig. 2–37).[1] They are frequently involved in some dermatoses, rarely in others, and they have some diseases of their own. They also are subject to neoplasia of various types. The following discussion will be divided broadly into inflammatory, bullous, ulcerative, and neoplastic conditions. White- or dark-appearing lesions will be grouped together.

INFLAMMATORY LESIONS

Just as the skin, mucous membranes can become inflamed as the result of physical or chemical trauma or contact allergic mechanisms. They then present a histologic picture of noncharacteristic, acute, subacute, or chronic inflammatory infiltrate in the membrana propria, while the epithelium may become hyperplastic and edematous but more often becomes necrotic or separated from its base, with the formation of fleeting bullae followed by erosion. It is the frequent and far from easy task of

the pathologist to discern such nonspecific *stomatitis, balanitis,* or *vulvitis* from the changes of specific dermatoses, which we shall now enumerate. It must be kept in mind that, with the exception of the hard palate and the tongue, a granular layer is normally absent or very thin on mucosal surfaces, that a nucleated horny layer usually represents the normal condition, and that a thick granular layer with compressed keratin is, in fact, abnormal. It is also true, especially in the mouth, that inflammatory infiltrate may contain many plasma cells without special significance.

Plasmocytosis Mucosae

An exception is *plasma cell balanitis* (Chap. 34), a benign lesion of unknown origin,[2,3] in which plasma cell-rich dermal infiltrate is covered by a thin epidermis (Fig. 45–1). In the latter, cells may be distorted but are not dysplastic. Similar lesions have been observed on the female genitalia, oral mucosa, and conjunctiva *(plasmocytosis mucosae).*[4,5]

Psoriasis, Geographic Tongue, Balanitis Circinata

Psoriasis of the oral mucosa does exist but is extremely rare.[6,7] The mucosa being normally parakeratotic and having fairly high mitotic counts,

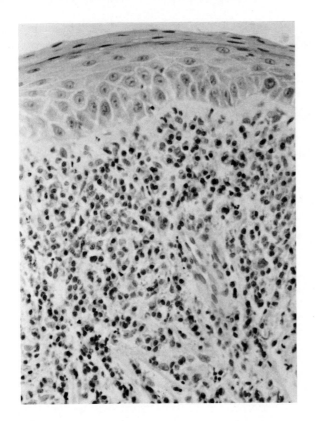

FIGURE 45–1.
Plasma cell balanitis. The epidermis is parakeratotic but not as thin and atrophic as it sometimes is. There is almost pure plasma cell infiltrate in the dermis. H&E. X400.

leukocytic invasion of the epithelium (from whatever cause) produces a psoriasiform histologic picture, and the diagnosis must be supported by continuity of oral and cutaneous plaques and response to therapy. The histologic picture of *geographic tongue* or *migrating glossitis* (Fig. 45–2) is indistinguishable from that of psoriasis,[8,9] but nosologic relation of these two common affections is highly questionable. The histologic picture of psoriasis of the vulva and the glans penis does not differ in principle from that on other parts of the skin, although pronounced acanthosis is uncommon. The changes are very similar to *balanitis circinata* and related lesions on the vulva,[10] which are manifestations of *Reiter's disease* (Chap. 8) in the group of psoriasiform tissue reactions.

Lichen Planus and Lupus Erythematosus

The oral mucosa is much more commonly involved by *lichen planus* than by *lupus erythematosus*. Either may produce whitish streaks or, less frequently, ulceration, and the histologic picture may be even more convergent than that of skin lesions (Chap. 14). The epithelium consists of large cells (hypertrophy) and develops multiple granular and orthokeratotic horny layers. Basal cells show

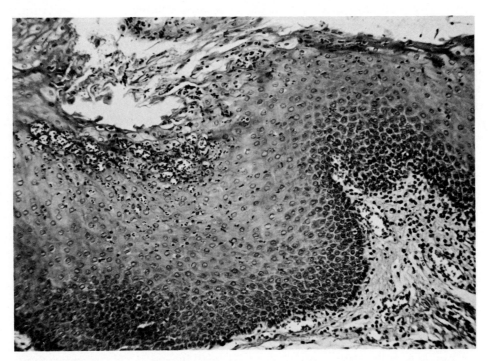

FIGURE 45–2.
Benign migratory glossitis (geographic tongue). Note remarkable similarity to a psoriasiform lesion (Figs. 8–9 and 8–16). H&E. X135.

degenerative changes,[11,12] and the lower strata are invaded by round cells from the dense lymphocytic-plasmacytic infiltrate[13] that is present subepithelially. The picture must be differentiated from precancerous leukoplakia by paying attention to cytologic details (see under leukoplakia). In *erosive lichen planus* and similar lesions due to lupus erythematous, one must try to find diagnostic features in the edge of the ulcer. Histologic diagnosis of lichen planus on the glans and other genital areas offers no special difficulties.

Lichen Sclerosus et Atrophicus

Lichen sclerosus et atrophicus (LSA) (Chap. 25) deserves special mention here because this benign dermatosis has a predilection for the female genitoanal region and has been confused with *leukoplakic vulvitis* and *kraurosis vulvae*. Without entering into clinical differential diagnosis, we state that the combination of epithelial atrophy with hyperkeratosis and edematous homogeneous connective tissue characterizes LSA[14] and that "atrophic stage of leukoplakic vulvitis" and "kraurosis" are antiquated misnomers[15] which have led to radical surgical procedures in many cases amenable to dermatologic therapy and cure. It is only when LSA persists for many years and the pruritic atrophic tissues are injured by long-continued excoriation that secondarily leukoplakic changes and cancer may supervene as uncommon and usually preventable complications.[16] Their presence should be verified by expert histopathologic examination. When LSA affects the glans penis, it has been called *balanitis xerotica obliterans*, another name that may be eliminated without loss. Occurrence of LSA on the vulva of small girls is not uncommon, and it has been reported on the glans penis of young boys.[17,18]

Syphilis

Syphilis has a preference for mucous membranes in all of its stages, but biopsy material will come to the pathologist's attention more often by mistake than by intent. Such instances have become more frequent through a combination of unusual sexual habits of patients and lack of suspicion on the part of clinicians. Chancres of tonsil and rectum have been biopsied on the suspicion of carcinoma. Mucous plaques of the secondary stages may be mistaken for leukoplakia. Late *gummatous syphilis* and especially *interstitial syphilitic glossitis*, with

its great tendency to malignant transformation, are genuine objects of biopsy. The syphilitic hallmarks (Chap. 20 and below) of endovasculitis and plasma cell infiltrate or fibrosis following tuberculoid granulomatous infiltration should rouse the pathologist's attention.

BULLOUS LESIONS

The greater fragility of mucous membrane epithelium makes it more difficult to obtain specimens of unbroken blisters. The patient should be watched carefully, and biopsy should be done at the earliest possible moment, preferably by an oral surgeon who is more apt to have the proper instruments and skill for this task. Proper procedures, which should include immunofluorescent and ultrastructural studies, are particularly important in cases in which no skin lesions are present.[19,20]

Pemphigus, Pemphigoid, Erythema Multiforme

The acantholytic process of *pemphigus vulgaris* can still be recognized in a deroofed lesion if the basal layer remains adherent to the membrana propria (Fig. 45–3). The bulla of *mucous membrane pemphigoid* (Fig. 45–4)[21,22] is subepithelial, and the stratified epithelium is well preserved in the roof, in contrast to the situation with *erythema multiforme*, where it is apt to be more or less necrotic. Late lesions of mucous membrane pemphigoid show adhesions and scarring, which as such are noncharacteristic but do not occur in other bullous diseases. Scarring does take place in Behçet's syndrome (aphthosis, see below). *Desquamative gingivitis*[23] often develops into cicatricial pemphigoid. An extensive review of the entire field of erosive, ulcerative, and bullous lesions of the oral mucosa was given by Rogers.[24]

Darier's and Hailey–Hailey's Diseases

Rare but well-documented occurrence of Darier's disease and warty dyskeratoma on the oral mucosa[25] and other mucous membranes[26] shows that the name "keratosis follicularis" is a misnomer. The disease of Hailey–Hailey also has been observed in mucosal localization.[27] The expression of these disorders is similar to that on the skin (Chap. 28) but is even more difficult to differentiate from pemphigus vulgaris. Presence of corps ronds and

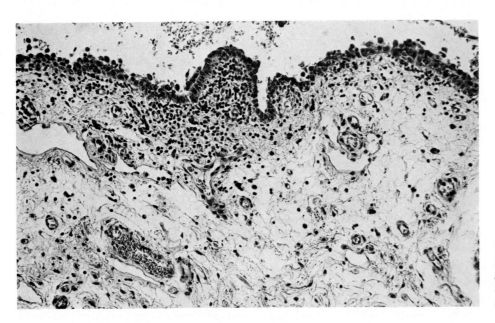

FIGURE 45–3.
Pemphigus vulgaris of buccal mucosa. Acantholytic cells above the adherent layer of basal cells. H&E. X185.

absence of degenerating acantholytic cells are to be looked for. In addition, proliferative epithelial budding often is found in the diseases of Darier and Hailey–Hailey and does not occur in pemphigus vulgaris. Tzanck smears may be helpful.[28]

ULCERATIVE LESIONS

Any of the bullous lesions just mentioned may lead to denudation and superficial ulceration. Erosive lichen planus and lupus erythematosus may cause painful ulcers. There are, in addition, several diseases which are primarily ulcerative, ranging from tiny aphthae to large granulomatous defects. We can give only some directions for their histologic differentiation (Chap. 17).

Aphthae and Aphthosis

Corresponding to the clinical picture, simple aphthae[29] show loss of epithelium, superficial mesodermal necrosis, and a more or less severe sub-

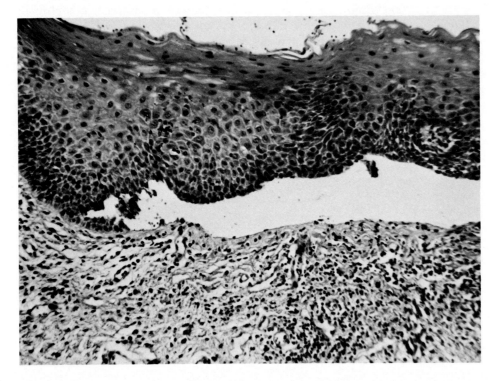

FIGURE 45–4.
Benign mucous membrane pemphigoid. Complete separation of viable epithelium from membrana propria. Oral lesion. H&E. X180.

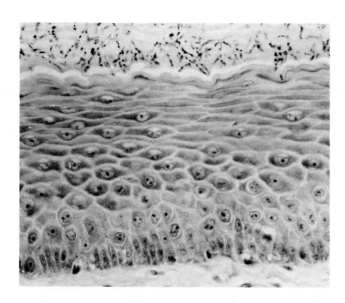

FIGURE 45–5.
Candidiasis of oral mucosa. Epithelium preserved and regular. Hyphae and spores in horny layer but not penetrating living tissue. O&G. X400.

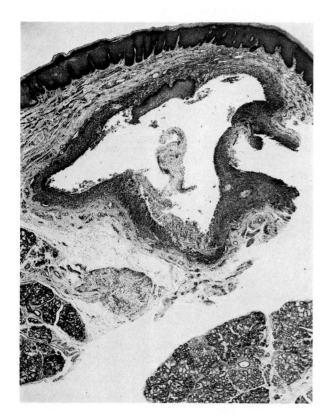

FIGURE 45–6.
Mucocele. Oral epithelium above, mucous glands below cystic lesion which is only partly lined with stratified epithelium. Most of wall consists of granulomatous membrane. H&E. X14.

acute inflammatory infiltrate with no specific features. When herpes simplex affects the mucous membranes, it produces lesions indistinguishable from aphthae, unless one can demonstrate the specific cytologic changes (Chap. 12). *Behçet's syndrome (aphthosis)* produces painful lesions on oral, ocular, and genital membranes, very similar to aphthae, but possibly leading to synechiae.[30] Favorable sections may reveal vascular changes in the form of hyalinization and endarteritis,[31] and mast cells have been reported to be increased.[32]

Perlèche

We mention here perlèche (angulus infectiosus), an erosive lesion of the commissure of the lips that may be due to maceration in edentulous or excessively salivating patients with or without infection with streptococci or *Candida*. In the latter case,[33] numerous hyphae (Fig. 45–5) are easily seen in the keratin layer by O&G or PAS stain. Otherwise, there is subacute inflammatory infiltrate and edema or loss of epithelium without characteristic features.

GRANULOMATOUS DISEASES

Cheilitis Glandularis and Mucocele

A rare affection of the small mucosalivary glands[34] produces recurrent ulcers in which granulomatous destruction of gland tissue is the outstanding feature. Quite common, on the other hand, is a lesion, probably of traumatic origin, which is known as *mucous retention cyst* or *mucocele*.[35,36] It probably results from the rupture of a duct which lets mucous secretion enter the tissue. Although remnants of an epithelial lining are sometimes found, the cyst usually has a thick wall of granulation tissue (Fig. 45–6) that may be mistaken for an infectious granuloma of gummatous type. The lesion is benign, although it may recur. In other cases, secondary atypical metaplasia may take place in surviving remnants of the gland and may simulate squamous cell carcinoma *(necrotizing sialometaplasia)*.[37]

Infectious Granulomas

Tuberculosis orificialis of the oral and anal mucosa was discussed in Chapter 20 as a now rare affection of marasmic individuals with waning immune response. It is due to implantation of mycobacteria stemming from an open lesion in lung or bowel. Syphilitic chancre, secondary mucous plaques, and late interstitial glossitis were mentioned. *Tertiary syphilis* may also produce severely destructive gummatous lesions (Chap. 20) of bone and soft tissues around the nose and mouth, and on the genitalia the so-called *chancre redux*, which has the histologic characteristics of a gumma. *South American leishmaniasis* and *histoplasmosis* commonly produce stubborn ulceration at mucocutaneous junctions or in the mouth and must be diagnosed by the demonstration of the respective organisms in a predominantly mononuclear granuloma (Chap. 21). One should not forget that *granuloma inguinale* may occur in the oral mucosa.[38,39]

Noninfectious Granulomas

Langerhans cell granuloma (Chap. 24), in manifestations of the Hand–Schüller–Christian type, may produce severely destructive lesions in the genitoanal area and in the mouths of children as well as adults.[40] The presence of large and often foamy histiocytes and variable numbers of eosinophils leads to histologic diagnosis. *Wegener's granulomatosis* (Chap. 15) may present as gingivitis[41] and frequently produces oral ulcers. The histologic picture shows a combination of necrotizing vasculitis, which may involve small and larger vessels, and a mixed granulomatous infiltrate usually including multinucleated giant cells of the foreign-body type. The *lethal midline granuloma* of the face sooner or later causes destruction of the palate. It presents a mixed infiltrate without specific characteristics. Finally, it should be mentioned that manifestations of *Crohn's disease* of the gut may be found in the mouth,[42] where they present a sarcoid type of tissue reaction.

WHITE LESIONS

The term *leukoplakia* is another of the old descriptive names that have changed in interpretation from clinical to histologic and have become either meaningless as a diagnosis or fraught with undesirable overtones. While the word means nothing but white plaque, many clinicians consider it as synonymous with precancer, and the pathologist should use it only in this connotation. It must be understood that leukoplakia can be used only for lesions of mucous or semimucous membranes not normally possessing a layer of keratohyaline granules (Chap. 2) which reflect and diffuse incident light and modify the red color of vascularized tissue. Inasmuch as the skin normally has a granular layer,

any excessive whiteness due to its thickening is attributable to specific cutaneous disease, such as lichen simplex, lichen planus, or lichen sclerosus et atrophicus. It never is leukoplakia.

Leukoplakia

In proper use, pathologists refer to leukoplakia as a lesion of oral or genital mucous or semimucous membrane that exhibits abnormal keratinization in the form of a more or less prominent granular layer in association with cellular evidence of dysplasia or carcinoma in situ. If the living epithelium is not dysplastic, other terms should be employed. Cytologic expression of precancerous change in the oral mucosa can vary from the relatively mild derangement of the basal layer shown in Figure 45–7B, with occasional dyskeratotic cells, to pronounced bowenoid pictures. The granular layer may be thick or may be represented by only a few cells, but the keratin layer always is dense and different from the normal appearance of swollen bulky cells.[32] Presence of reactive inflammatory infiltrate below the epithelium is essential[43] but is not pathognomonic because it is shared with lichen planus and other inflammatory lesions. If the lower epithelial surface shows atypical budding, this is a danger signal, and the presence of horny pearls usually signifies beginning invasion. Precancerous leukoplakia may occur as the result of chronic irritation, especially in smokers, in the course of late syphilis, and in the rare familial condition *dyskeratosis congenita*.[44]

Benign White Plaques

Lichen planus, lupus erythematosus, secondary syphilis, and lichen sclerosus et atrophicus were already mentioned as causes of white discoloration. In children and debilitated persons, infection with *Candida* may produce adherent white plaques *(thrush)*. Histologic examination reveals a pseudomembrane consisting of desquamating epithelium, debris, and possibly necrotic tissue matted together by numerous fungal hyphae.[33] Other circumscribed white plaques on oral mucosa result from chronic trauma of ill-fitted dentures, ragged teeth, and so on. Their histologic expression is *epidermization* (Fig. 45–7A) of the oral epithelium, and either this term or *benign leukokeratosis* may be used for diagnosis.

A special form is the condition described as *stomatitis nicotina* and also known as smoker's palate. Small or larger white papules usually have a

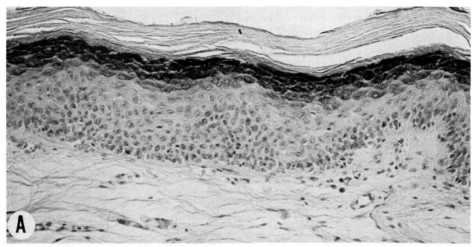

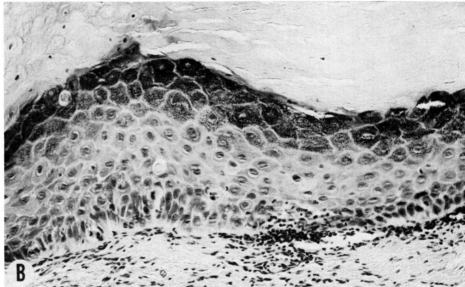

FIGURE 45–7.
A. *Benign leukokeratosis (epidermization) of buccal mucosa. Note regular basal layer and orderly configuration of upper strata. Absence of inflammatory infiltrate. H&E. X135.*
B. *Leukoplakia of buccal mucosa. This is a minimal lesion but exhibits a disturbed basal layer with hyperchromatic nuclei and increased mitotic activity, individually keratinizing cells, and some inflammatory infiltrate. Note also larger size of all cells. H&E. X135.*

red center, which corresponds to a keratinized mucous gland duct[45] associated with glandular hyperplasia.[46] The epithelium is orthokeratotic and not dysplastic, and the condition is usually benign. A peculiar diffuse bluish whiteness of pigmented buccal mucosa is not infrequently seen in blacks and has been given the name *leukoedema*.[47] The clinician should not confuse it with the opalescent mucous plaques of secondary syphilis or with leukoplakia. Histologically, it exhibits only thickened epithelium without inflammation or dysplasia.

Nevoid and Verrucous White Lesions

Occasionally, a *viral wart* (Fig. 45–8) may cause a small white plaque on the oral mucosa. It is remarkable and unexplained why wart virus does not usually produce condyloma acuminatum in the mouth as it does on the genitals but rather gives

rise to hard keratinizing lesions. The phenomenon may be an indication that the virus of condyloma acuminatum is not truly identical with that of verruca vulgaris.

Heck's Disease. *Familial focal epithelial hyperplasia* was first described in American Indians[48] but has now been found in various parts of the world. The search for a virus was futile except in Van Wyck's cases[49] in South Africa, in which papova-like intranuclear bodies were found. The crowding of cases in families and schools makes an infectious etiology likely. The slightly elevated whitish papules consist of acanthotic epithelium without cellular atypicalities.

Fordyce's Condition. It was mentioned in Chapter 2 that free sebaceous glands occur on mucous membranes (Fig. 2–37). They were described in the mouth by Fordyce as a "disease" in the nineteenth

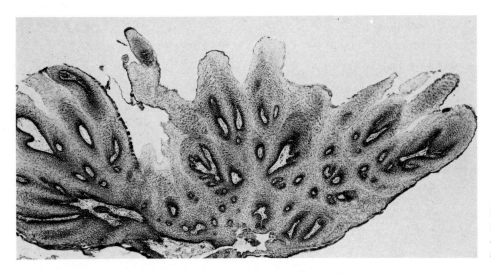

FIGURE 45–8.
Verruca vulgaris of tongue. Small amount of connective tissue in relation to bulky epithelium differentiates this lesion from condyloma acuminatum (Fig. 31–9). H&E. X29.

century but are an almost normal feature and have a slightly yellow tinge. Sebaceous glands also occur on the labia minora, sometimes in great numbers, and rarely on the glans and inner prepuce.

White Sponge Nevus. A familial condition, Cannon's white sponge nevus (Fig. 45–9)[50,51] may produce small wartlike lesions or large soggy protuberances. It causes white color without keratohyalin through the piling up of swollen parakera-

totic cells. Similar lesions occur in *pachyonychia congenita* (Chap. 46). These are benign affections[52] but may simulate in their clinical and pathologic features florid oral papillomatosis.

Uremia. In uremic patients, parakeratotic thickening of the oral epithelium may produce white lesions without inflammatory infiltrate (erythematopultaceous form), which regress when the patient's condition improves.[53]

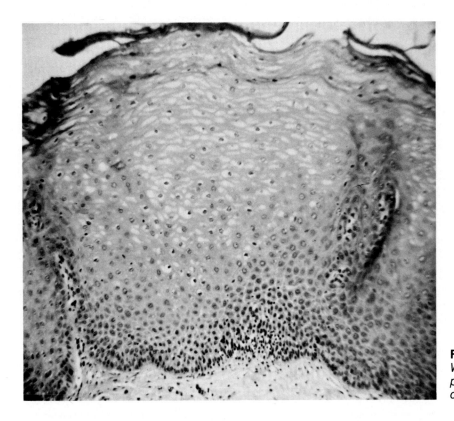

FIGURE 45–9.
White sponge nevus. Exaggeration of physiologic parakeratosis of buccal mucosa with cellular atypy. H&E. X135.

Florid Oral Papillomatosis

Protruding whitish lesions, also known as *papillomatosis mucosae oris carcinoides*,[54] have been described[55] as florid oral papillomatosis and have a serious prognosis. They probably are variants of Ackerman's *verrucous carcinoma* (see below), usually recur after treatment, and may end up as highly immature squamous carcinomas. Their histologic picture (Fig. 45–10) presents soggy and bulky parakeratotic cells, which are similar to those of the white sponge nevus, overlying more highly cellular and somewhat dysplastic living epithelium.

DARK LESIONS

Melanin Pigmentation

We group together several disparate lesions because they may be submitted for microscopic exclusion of malignant melanoma. Benign pigmented nevi and malignant melanomas do occur on conjunctiva, oral mucosa, and the other membranes occasionally and do not offer any special diagnostic difficulty. Epidermal melanin pigmentation is very rarely encountered in normal Caucasian buccal or gingival mucosa but is common in more pigmented races. A Swedish study[56] revealed a considerable incidence of pigmentation of the attached gingiva in heavy smokers *(smoker's melanosis)*. Pigmentation of the tongue is much rarer and is said to be diagnostic of Addison's disease in Orientals.[57] In blacks, subepidermal bluish pigmentation of the tongue occurs in large plaques, but epithelial melanin is uncommon and usually is restricted to individual fungiform papillae.[58]

Vascular Lesions

Varicose widening of veins is not uncommon in elderly people near the lateral ends of the lower lips, and thrombosis may occur.[59] Similar processes may be found on the female genitalia, and scrotal angiokeratomas (Chap. 43) also may look so dark that histologic examination is requested.

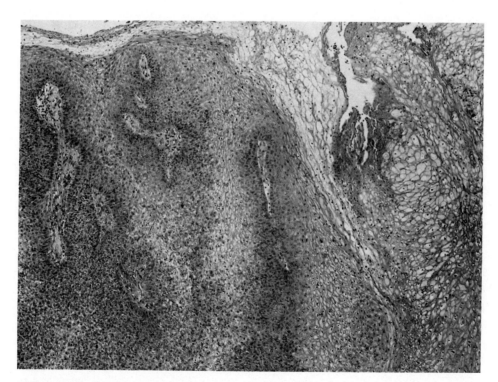

FIGURE 45–10.
Florid oral papillomatosis exhibiting physiologic type of oral keratinization in exaggerated degree. Extremely bulky acanthosis and retarded maturation of the epithelial cells. Specimens of this type must be carefully examined for evidence of epithelial downgrowth in the manner seen in verrucous carcinoma (Fig. 45–11). H&E. X70.

Tattoos

Very dark macules may be produced in the mouth by the slip of a dentist's drill that carries silver or mercury into the mucosa. These metals are preferentially deposited on elastic fibers (Fig. 30–2A) and can be tentatively identified by darkfield examination (Chap. 3).

NEOPLASMS

Epithelial Neoplasms

Viral warts and some congenital conditions (white sponge nevus, dyskeratosis congenita) were already mentioned. Extramammary Paget's disease was treated in Chapter 40. We shall not deal with tumors of salivary, mucous, or other glands of the mucous membranes because they are in the field of general pathology. It remains to discuss here epidermoid neoplasia.

Squamous Cell Carcinoma. By far the most common epithelial tumor in the mouth, as well as on the lips and on male and female genitalia, is squamous cell carcinoma. It has a much higher tendency to early metastasis and is relatively immature more often than tumors on the skin proper. It is, therefore, more important to note and report even minor evidence of invasion in a precancerous leukoplakia than it would be in an actinic keratosis.

Verrucous Carcinoma. A peculiarly deceptive variant (Fig. 45–11) is verrucous carcinoma,[60] which is most common in the mouth but may be found on the genitalia. It shows little evidence of dysplasia, often has an intact basement membrane, and invades deeper tissue by pushing solid masses of epithelium downward rather than by growing in an infiltrating manner. Attempts to differentiate it from florid papillomatosis in the mouth and from the Buschke–Loewenstein variant of giant condyloma acuminatum on the genitals (Chap. 31) have led to the conclusion that all these are variants of verrucous carcinoma and that carcinoma cuniculatum of the sole of the foot (Chap. 34) should be included in this grouping. All these lesions do not metastasize readily, but complete excision may meet great technical difficulties.

Carcinoma in Situ. Of precancerous conditions, leukoplakia was discussed earlier in this chapter. It is to be stressed that the superficial epidermal layers need not show atypical cells and that high-power examination of the basal layer is essential. In contrast to lichen planus and lupus erythematosus, there is no liquefaction or other loss of basal cells. On the contrary, the lowest epithelial layers consist of somewhat irregular cells with large nuclei and nucleoli in spite of inflammatory cells being present among them (Fig. 45–7B). This feature also differentiates precancerous leukoplakia and the invasive verrucous carcinoma from benign papillomas in which one basal row of cells under-

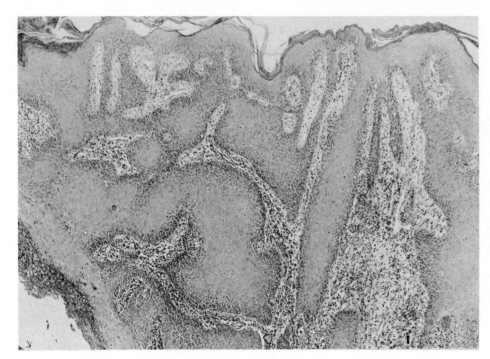

FIGURE 45–11.
Verrucous carcinoma of oral mucosa. Portion of a large tumor, which protruded above the surface and extended down to striated muscle. The picture illustrates the deceptively benign histologic structure. H&E. X70. (Specimen supplied by Dr. T.C. Knechtges, V.A. Hospital, Allen Park, Michigan.)

lies the prickle cell layers (Fig. 45–7A). Marked atypicality of cells and dyskeratosis is the expression of Bowen's disease, a name that dermatologists are not apt to abandon in favor of carcinoma in situ.[61] The reason for this statement is that epithelium exhibiting the characteristic bowenoid changes (Chap. 34) may at low power have all kinds of configurations, from a thin atrophic epidermis to acanthosis to papillomatosis. The horny layer may be orthokeratotic or parakeratotic.

"Bowenoid Papules" of the Genitalia. The overriding importance of cytologic abnormalities over structural benignity of a lesion has been brought to the foreground of differential diagnosis by widespread observations over the last several years that lesions considered to be condylomata acuminata or lichen planus on the penis and vulva of young people were found on histologic examination (Fig. 45–12) to have all the features of a premalignant bow-

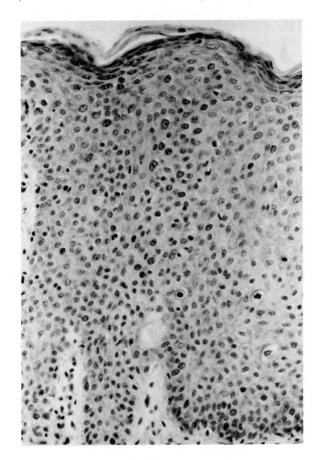

FIGURE 45–12.
Bowenoid appearance of a lesion diagnosed as condyloma acuminatum clinically. The general unrest of the epidermis and the presence of several mitoses in the right half of the picture sets this epithelium apart from the regular large prickle cells of condyloma acuminatum (Fig. 31–8). H&E. X250.

enlike epithelium.[62] The unusual features were the young age of the patients and the widespread appearance of this precancerous picture in many parts of the country. A few cases of invasive carcinoma have been seen. On the other hand, spontaneous involution of some lesions also has been seen.[63] What such lesions actually are is impossible to say at this time. Papova virus has been found in some cases.[64] Bowen's disease is well known to involve the anogenital area of older people.[65] It is not apt to become invasive for many years. One has to consider, however, that this histologic picture is a new finding, one that has not been reported by the careful observers of years past but that has been seen often in recent years.[66] The advice to the pathologist would be to report Bowen's disease and advise watchfulness but no radical procedures. It seems better not to minimize the involved weighty questions by using a euphemistic term like "bowenoid papules."[67]

Actinic Cheilitis. Another important lesion is actinic cheilitis, which shares many features with keratosis senilis of the skin (Chap. 34) but usually has a much heavier inflammatory infiltrate, consisting of lymphocytes and plasma cells, and often has a rather inconspicuous and even fragmentary, parakeratotic, and uneven epithelium. The absence of adnexal structures on the lip vermilion probably is responsible for the fragility of the epithelial cover. Multiple sections should be examined with care in order to identify any invasive cords or nests of epithelial cells, which usually are nonkeratinizing.

Keratoacanthoma. A number of solitary keratoacanthomas of the oral cavity[68,69] and one on the inner surface of the prepuce[70] have been reported. These instances make the relationship of keratoacanthoma to the hair follicle (Chap. 34) questionable.

Basaloid Carcinoma of the Anus. True basal cell epitheliomas are extremely rare in oral mucosa[71] and are uncommon in the genitoanal area. The anal mucosa, however, gives rise to a specific malignant tumor called either *basaloid carcinoma*[72] or *cloacogenic carcinoma*.[73] These nonkeratinizing neoplasms are apt to metastasize and have a cure rate of less than 50 percent in spite of a deceptive histologic appearance simulating that of basal cell epithelioma. The epithelial cells have little cytoplasm and dark-staining nuclei. There may be peripheral palisading and central necrosis with the formation of pseudocysts. Mitotic activity is fairly high.

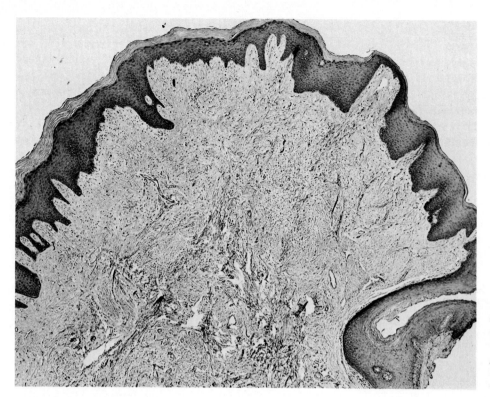

FIGURE 45–13.
Angiofibroma of buccal mucosa. Epidermization of buccal epithelium above a protruding papule consisting of fairly mature vascular connective tissue. H&E. X14.

Mesodermal and Neural Neoplasms

Of very common occurrence are small, often sessile, papular lesions of the tongue or labial mucosa, which may be reactions to trauma rather than true neoplasms. These *angiofibromas* (Fig. 45–13) are usually covered with keratinizing epidermoid epithelium and have a core of vascular collagenous tissue. They are benign. Much rarer are *granular cell myoblastomas* (Chap. 43), which may have pseudocarcinomatous epithelial covering.[74] *Neuromas* are encountered as solitary reaction to trauma and as multiple lesions in the *oral mucosal neuroma–medullary thyroid carcinoma syndrome.*[75] *Verruciform xanthomas* of oral mucosa[76–78] and the vulva[79] have been described in which the xanthomatous cells are overlaid by a papillomatous epidermis.

REFERENCES

1. Sewerin I: The sebaceous glands in the vermilion border of the lips and in the oral mucosa of man. Acta Odontol Scand 33[Suppl 68]:1, 1975
2. Brodin MB: Balanitis circumscripta plasmacellularis. J Am Acad Dermatol 2:33, 1980
3. Stern JK, Rosen T: Balanitis plasmacellularis circumscripta (Zoon's balanitis plasmacellularis). Cutis 25:57, 1980
4. Lüders G: Plasmocytosis mucosae; ein oft verkanntes neues Krankheitsbild. Munch Med Wochenschr 114:8, 1972
5. Baughman RD, Berger P, Pringle WM: Plasma cell cheilitis. Arch Dermatol 110:725, 1974
6. Doty CA, Hasley CK, Blumenthal F, et al.: Psoriasis of skin and oral mucosa. Arch Dermatol 38:808, 1938
7. White DK, Leis HJ, Miller AS: Intraoral psoriasis associated with widespread dermal psoriasis. Oral Surg 41:174, 1976
8. O'Keefe E, Braverman IM, Cohen I: Annulus migrans. Arch Dermatol 107:240, 1973
9. Banóczy J, Szabo L, Csiba A: Migratory glossitis: a clinical-histologic review of seventy cases. Oral Surg 39:113, 1975
10. Thamba IV, Dunlap R, Thin RN, et al.: Circinate vulvitis in Reiter's syndrome. Br J Vener Dis 53:260, 1977
11. Shklar G, Flynn E, Szabo G: Basement membrane alterations in oral lichen planus. J Invest Dermatol 70:45, 1978
12. Shklar G, McCarthy PL: Histopathology of oral lesions of discoid lupus erythematosus. Review of 25 cases. Arch Dermatol 114:1031, 1978
13. Regezi JA, Deegan MJ, Heyward JR: Lichen planus: immunologic and morphologic identification of the submucosal infiltrate. Oral Surg 46:44, 1978
14. Oberfield RA: Lichen sclerosus et atrophicus and kraurosis vulvae; are they the same disease? Arch Dermatol 83:806, 1961
15. Friedrich EG Jr (ed): New nomenclature for vulvar diseases. Int J Dermatol 15:126, 1976 [also in gynecologic journals]
16. Hart WR, Norris HJ, Helwig EB: Relation of lichen

sclerosus et atrophicus of the vulva to development of carcinoma. Obstet Gynecol 45:369, 1975

17. Mikat DM, Ackerman HR Jr, Mikat KW: Balanitis xerotica obliterans; report of case in an 11-year-old and review of literature. Pediatrics 52:25, 1973

18. Götz H, Zabel M, Patiri C: Lichen sclerosus et atrophicus. Erstmalige Beobachtung am Genitale eines Knaben. Hautarzt 28:235, 1977

19. Meurer M, Millus JL, Rogers RS III, et al.: Oral pemphigus vulgaris. A report of ten cases. Arch Dermatol 113:1520, 1977

20. Braun-Falco O, Wolff HH: Elektronenmikroskopie von Mundschleimhautläsionen des Pemphigus vulgaris. Hautarzt 26:483, 1975

21. Susi FR, Shklar G: Histochemistry and fine structure of oral lesions of mucous membrane pemphigoid. Arch Dermatol 104:244, 1971

22. Brauner GJ, Jimbow K: Benign mucous membrane pemphigoid; an unusual case with electron microscopic findings. Arch Dermatol 106:535, 1972

23. Rogers RS III, Sheridan PJ, Jordan RE: Desquamative gingivitis: clinical, histopathologic, and immunopathologic investigations. Oral Surg 42:316, 1976

24. Rogers RS III: Recent advances in erosive, ulcerative, and bullous diseases of the oral mucosa. I and II. Prog Dermatol 12 (1,2), 1978

25. Tomich CE, Burkes EJ: Warty dyskeratoma (isolated keratosis follicularis) of the oral mucosa. Oral Surg 31:798, 1971

26. Brünauer SR: Morbus Darier: Schleimhautveränderungen. In Jadassohn J: Handbuch der Haut- und Geschlechtskrankheiten, vol 8, pt 2. Berlin, Springer-Verlag, 1931, pp 230–34

27. Botvinick I: Familial benign pemphigus with oral mucous membrane lesions. Cutis 12:371, 1973

28. Medak H, Burlakow P, McGrew EA, et al.: Cytopathologic study as an aid to the diagnosis of vesicular dermatoses. Oral Surg 32:204, 1971

29. Dolby AE: Mikulicz's recurrent oral aphthae: histopathological comparison with two experimentally induced immunological reactions. Br J Dermatol 83:674, 1970

30. Curth HO: L'aphthose. Ann Dermatol Syphiligr 83:130, 1956

31. Haensch R: Behçet's disease (aphthosis). Cutis 14:353, 1974

32. Haim S: The pathogenesis of lesions in Behçet's disease. Dermatologica 158:31, 1979

33. Winner JI: Candidosis. In Baker RD (ed): The Pathologic Anatomy of Mycoses. Handbuch der speziellen pathologischen Anatomie und Histologie, vol 3, pt 5. Berlin, New York, Springer-Verlag, 1971, pp 731–61

34. Weir TW, Johnson WC: Cheilitis glandularis. Arch Dermatol 103:433, 1971

35. Cataldo E, Mosadomi A: Mucoceles of oral mucous membrane. Arch Otolaryngol 91:360, 1970

36. Lattanand A, Johnson WC, Graham JH: Mucous cyst (mucocele). Arch Dermatol 101:673, 1970

37. Rangi GJ, Kessler S: Necrotizing sialometaplasia. A condition simulating malignancy. Arch Dermatol 115:329, 1979

38. Garg BR, Lal S, Bedi BMS, et al.: Donovanosis (granuloma inguinale) of the oral cavity. Br J Vener Dis 51:136, 1975

39. Rao MS, Kameswari VR, Ramulu C, et al.: Oral lesions of granuloma inguinale. J Oral Surg 34:1112, 1976

40. Winther JE, Fejerskov O, Philipsen HP: Oral manifestations of histiocytosis X. Acta Derm Venereol (Stockh) 52:75, 1972

41. Scott J, Finch LD: Wegener's granulomatosis presenting as gingivitis. Review of the clinical and pathologic features and report of a case. Oral Surg 34:920, 1972

42. Stankler L, Ewen SWB, Kerr NW: Crohn's disease of the mouth. Br J Dermatol 87:501, 1972

43. Boncinelli U, Fornieri C, Muscatello U: Relationship between leukocytes and tumor cells in precancerous and cancerous lesions of the lip: a possible expression of immune reaction. J Invest Dermatol 71:407, 1978

44. Sirihavin C, Trowbridge AA: Dyskeratosis congenita: Clinical features and genetic aspects: Report of a family and review of the literature. J Med Genet 12:339, 1975

45. Forsey RR, Sullivan TJ: Stomatitis nicotina. Arch Dermatol 83:945, 1961

46. Laugier P, Extermann J-C, Michau C, et al.: L'ouranite glandulaire. Dermatologica 142:344, 1971

47. Martin JL, Crump EP: Leukoedema of the buccal mucosa in Negro children and youth. Oral Surg 34:49, 1972

48. Schock RK: Familial focal epithelial hyperplasia; report of a case. Oral Surg 28:598, 1969

49. Van Wyck CW: Focal epithelial hyperplasia of the mouth: recently discovered in South Africa. Br J Dermatol 96:381, 1977

50. Whitten JB: The electron microscopic examination of congenital keratoses of the oral mucous membranes. I. White sponge nevus. Oral Surg 29:69, 1970

51. Frithiof L, Bánóczy J: White sponge nevus (leukoedema exfoliativum mucosae oris): ultrastructural observations. Oral Surg 41:607, 1976

52. Witkop CJ Jr, Gorlin RJ: Four hereditary mucosal syndromes. Comparative histology and exfoliative cytology of Darier-White's disease, hereditary benign intraepithelial dyskeratosis, white sponge nevus, and pachyonychia congenita. Arch Dermatol 84:762, 1961

53. Jaspers MT: Unusual oral lesions in a uremic patient: review of the literature and report of a case. Oral Surg 39:934, 1975

54. Richter G, Engel S, Jacobi H: Zum Krankheitsbild der sogenannten "oral florid papillomatosis" (papillomatosis mucosae oris carcinoides). Dermatologica 144:75, 1972

55. Wolff K, Tappeiner J: Floride orale Papillomatose (papillomatosis mucosae carcinoides). In Braun-Falco O, Petzoldt D (eds): Fortschritte der Praktischen Dermatologie und Venerologie, vol 7. Berlin, Springer-Verlag, 1973, pp 40–51

56. Hedin CA: Smoker's melanosis. Occurrence and localization in the attached gingiva. Arch Dermatol 113:1533, 1977

57. Kitamura K, Mishima Y: Zur Frage der Zungenpigmentierung bei Morbus Addison. Hautarzt 8:484, 1957

58. Pinkus H: Die Makroskopische Anatomie der Haut. In Marchiorini A (ed): Jadassohn: Handbuch der Haut- und Geschlechtskrankheiten, Ergänzungswerk, vol 1, pt 2. Berlin, Springer-Verlag, 1965, p 17

59. Weathers DR, Fine RM: Thrombosed varix of oral cavity. Arch Dermatol 104:427, 1971

60. Ackerman LV: Verrucous carcinoma of the oral cavity. Surgery 23:670, 1947

61. Bender ME, Katz HI, Posalaky Z: Carcinoma in situ of the genitalia. JAMA 243:145, 1980

62. Lupulescu A, Mehregan AH, Rahbari H, et al.: Venereal warts vs Bowen's disease. A histologic and ultrastructural study of five cases. JAMA 237:2520, 1977

63. Berger BW, Hori Y: Multicentric Bowen's disease of the genitalia. Spontaneous regression of lesions. Arch Dermatol 114:1698, 1978

64. Kimura S, Hirai A, Harada R, et al.: So-called multicentric pigmented Bowen's disease. Report of a case and a possible etiologic role of human papilloma virus. Dermatologica 157:229, 1978

65. Grussendorf EI, Gahlen W: Morbus Bowen bei Condylomata acuminata. (Zur Frage der Möglichkeit virusbedingter Tumorinduktion). Hautarzt 25:443, 1974

66. Katz HI, Posalaky Z, McGinley D: Pigmented penile papules with carcinoma in situ changes. Br J Dermatol 99:155, 1978

67. Wade TR, Kopf AW, Ackerman AB: Bowenoid papules of the genitalia. Arch Dermatol 115:306, 1979

68. Scofield HA, Werning JT, Shakes RC: Solitary intraoral keratoacanthoma. Oral Surg 37:889, 1974

69. Svirsky JA, Freedman PD, Lumerman H: Solitary intraoral keratoacanthoma. Oral Surg 43:116, 1977

70. Lejman K, Starzycki Z: Giant keratoacanthoma on the inner surface of the prepuce. Br J Vener Dis 53:65, 1977

71. Peters RA, Gingrass RP, Teyes CN, et al.: Basal cell carcinoma of the oral cavity: report of case. J Oral Surg 30:73, 1972

72. Pang LSC, Morson BC: Basaloid carcinoma of the anus. J Clin Pathol 20:128, 1967

73. Kheir S, Hickey RC, Martin RG, et al.: Cloacogenic carcinoma of the anal canal. Arch Surg 104:407, 1972

74. Dixter CT, Konstat MS, Ginnta JL, et al.: Congenital granular cell tumor of alveolar ridge and tongue; report of two cases. Oral Surg 40:270, 1976

75. Walker DM: Oral mucosal neuroma-medullary thyroid carcinoma syndrome. Br J Dermatol 88:599, 1973

76. Shafer WG: Verruciform xanthoma. Oral Surg 31:784, 1971

77. Zegarelli DJ, Zegarelli-Schmidt E, Zegarelli EV: Verruciform xanthoma; further light and electron microscopic studies with the addition of a third case. Oral Surg 40:246, 1976

78. Cobb CM, Holt R, Denys FR: Ultrastructural features of the verruciform xanthoma. J Oral Pathol 5:42, 1976

79. Santa Cruz DJ, Martin SA: Verruciform xanthoma of the vulva. Am J Clin Pathol 71:224, 1979

In the formation of the epidermis, every basal germinative cell appears to be equivalent to its neighbors, and the horny layer seems to be a diffuse mass of cells the origin of which is of no great significance. That there is order in epidermal keratinization was shown only some years ago.[1] That individual basal cells are distinctly different from their neighbors becomes obvious only in precancerous keratoses and some benign tumors, where sharp boundaries separate normal and abnormal cells and their progeny (Sec. VII and Chap. 34).

In the formation of hair and nail (the *phanera* of the skin to use a French and German term), sharp boundaries between adjoining basal cells are the obvious rule which gives rise to these phaneric structures.

In the nail, the limits of proximal matrix, nailbed, anterior matrix, and nailfold are absolutely sharp (Fig. 46–1), and each type of basal cell (although it is practically indistinguishable from its neighbor across the line of division) forms its predetermined end product—nail, horn of the sole, cuticle—and will continue to do so even after surgical or incidental trauma and disruption.

In the hair, the boundaries are even more defined in the formation of three layers of internal root sheath and three layers of hair out of an immature and indistinguishable mass of pilar matrix cells. They are surrounded by the trichilemma (outer root sheath) with its specific and peculiar type of keratinization. In tumors of pilar nature, the specificity of individual cells becomes even more obvious.

It is, therefore, not surprising that hair and nail exhibit a variety of pathologic changes closely related to minor and major disturbances of their matrix cells, and a detailed knowledge of their normal anatomic structure is essential to interpret these changes correctly (Chap. 2). Knowledge of the normal and abnormal chemistry and metabolism of the tissues of hair and nail is just beginning to develop. It has already contribted to our understanding and can be expected to do much more.[2]

DISTURBANCES OF HAIR

It may seem arbitrary to separate inflammatory and keratotic lesions of the hair follicle (Chap. 18) from lesions of hair itself, and a strict separation, admittedly, is not feasible. We shall, however, describe in this chapter mainly those changes seen if one puts an entire hair or portions of one under the microscope and will refer to pictures seen in embedded tissue sections only secondarily.

Microscopic Examination of Hair

Elaborate methods have been devised for examination of hair,[2-4] but we will outline here only a relatively simple routine that does not use special

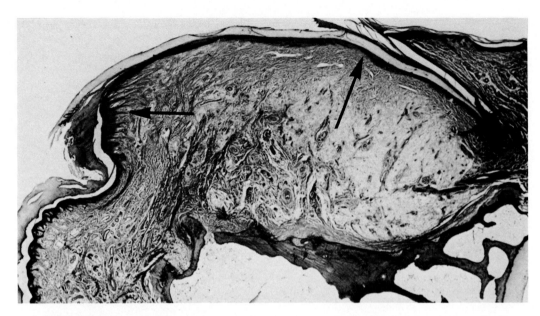

FIGURE 46–1.
Longitudinal section of toe illustrating the anatomy of the nail. Terminal phalanx with cartilage of interphalangeal joint at bottom of picture. The distance between phalanx and nail is increased, and the tissue shows hypervascularity and edema as evidence of a mild case of pulmonary osteoarthropathy. The nailplate emerges from the posterior nailfold at right and increases in thickness while moving over the matrix, the anterior border of which is indicated by an arrow. The nail then moves over the nailbed, which does not add appreciable substance to it, and emerges free on the left. Beneath the free end of the nail is thick keratin furnished by epidermis with long rete ridges (second arrow). This part is the horn of the sole, and corresponds to the main portion of the horse's hoof. It is the distal matrix of the nail that adds considerable material and binds the distal end of the nail firmly to the underlying tissues. At the lower end of the distal matrix is a shallow anterior groove and below this the epidermis of the tip of the phalanx which carries eccrine glands (not illustrated). The posterior nailfold is covered with keratin which projects beyond its anterior end (eponychium) and produces on its lower surface a thin layer of keratin, which is bound to the surface of the nail and lifts up a short distance anterior to the nailfold. This is the cuticle of the nail, which can be pushed back except in some persons where it is tightly bound to the nail as pterygium unguis. H&E. X8. (From Pinkus. In Andrade et al. (eds). Cancer of the Skin, 1976. Courtesy of W.B. Saunders Co.)

equipment. A single hair or a few hairs may be put lengthwise on a glass slide if they are relatively short. For a quick preliminary orientation, we find it convenient to put a number of hairs into one of the plastic holders for name cards that are given out at every scientific meeting and put the holder under the microscope. After that, individual hairs can be selected. Longer hairs should be cut into convenient pieces. For some purposes, e.g., examination of pili torti, it is preferable to cut the hair into 1 to 1.5 cm lengths. A long coverglass or, if high-power examination is not necessary, a second glass slide is put on top and, preferably, held in place with a piece of tape. The hair should first be examined in air and then in immersion oil, which can be added drop by drop between the two glass surfaces. For some purposes, one may want to use water first instead of oil but should permit the hair

to dry out again before changing from water to oil. After bright-light examination, one should use polarizing equipment. For most purposes, two pieces of Polaroid film, one below and one above the preparation, are adequate (Chap. 3).

Examination should take into account diameter of the shaft and possible local variations, condition of the cuticle, pigment content of cortex, pigment or gas content of medulla, condition of the hair root (anagen, catagen, telogen—Chap. 2), twists and other abnormalities of the shaft, and condition of the free end (natural tip, cut, broken, or frayed). One should examine many normal hairs in order to be able to differentiate truly abnormal states from artifacts or insignificant variations.

Individual variations of hair diameter are great. In order to assess decreased diameter, one should compare hairs from the balding area with those from the patient's occiput, which may be assumed to be normal. Two other types of examination are recommended. According to the method of F. Pinkus,[5] one asks the patient to collect assiduously all combed-out hair, even short pieces, for 24 hours into a dated envelope and to repeat the procedure every day for one week. No shampooing is permitted during this time. By counting the hairs in each envelope, one can get a good idea of the severity of hair loss. Up to 100 hairs are lost daily from a healthy scalp. While counting, one separates hairs representing less than one year's growth (approximately 12 cm) from longer ones, or if the hair has been trimmed to less than 12 cm into those with cut ends and those with natural tips. If more than about 20 percent of short hairs (or hairs with natural tips) are present, it is an indication of severe chronic weakening of hair growth and most likely of pattern alopecia, if other diseases of the scalp can be ruled out. The newer method, pioneered by Van Scott et al.,[6] is somewhat traumatic but less complicated. One grasps approximately 50 hairs in a padded hemostat and pulls them out with a quick jerk. The roots are then trimmed off for examination. If more than about 20 percent are telogen hairs, this speaks for increased hair loss *(telogen effluvium[7])* but does not differentiate between acute and chronic loss.

Pattern Alopecia

We discussed various types of hair loss associated with more or less inflammation in Chapter 18. The gradual thinning and disappearance of hair in male and female pattern alopecia[8] is expressed in decrease of diameter of hair follicle and hair and shortening of the hair root.[9] Simultaneously, there is hyperplasia of sebaceous glands. Inflammation may be minor or absent. It takes a good knowledge of size and length of normal hair follicles to appraise early stages of the process. Looking at a biopsy from the scalp of a woman who shows appreciable clinical thinning of hair, one may be surprised to find a practically normal histologic picture until one realizes that every follicle and its hair are reduced in size and do not penetrate any more into the subcutis. In a really bald male pate, the hair roots are mere appendages to the large sebaceous glands, but they do persist (Fig. 46–2). Examination of shed or plucked hairs under the microscope reveals no conspicuous abnormalities.

There is one specific change in biopsy sections that was recognized only lately.[10] It was mentioned in Chapter 2 that many growing hairs form a small

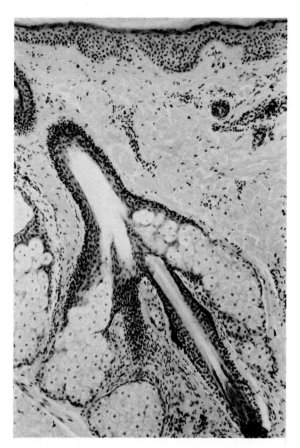

FIGURE 46–2.
Short, small anagen hair root among large sebaceous glands in advanced male pattern alopecia. H&E. X125.

cluster of elastic tissue in the neck of the papilla (the Arao-Perkins body) and that these fibers are clumped in catagen and stay behind at the lowest point to which the papilla extended in anagen (Fig. 46–3). In male pattern baldness, the next anagen hair is a little shorter than the previous one, and its Arao-Perkins body will be left behind a distance above the first one. Eventually, in scalps that form good elastic fibers, there will be a row of elastic clumps stacked within the remnants of collapsed fibrous root sheath like the rungs of a ladder. This picture is absolute proof of male or female pattern alopecia.

Acute Hair Loss

Although much less frequent than in times past, acute loss of hair *(telogen effluvium)* continues to be observed after febrile illness, surgical procedures, complicated childbirth, and other sudden systemic impairment of health. In these cases, the mortally affected hair will go into telogen and will fall out 60 to 90 days later, while less severely af-

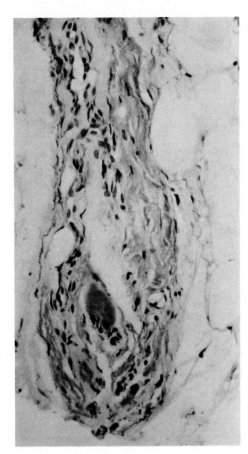

FIGURE 46–3.
Collapsed fibrous root sheath forms a persistent streamer in the subcutis, indicating the extent of the previous hair growth. Near its lower end, a clumped Arao-Perkins elastinlike body (Chap. 2). O&G. X250.

special features consisting of dyskeratotic and necrolytic changes with parakeratosis and spongiform abscesses in the hair follicles and induction of telogen.

Hypertrichosis

The most spectacular form of generalized hypertrichosis is congenital *hypertrichosis lanuginosa*, which

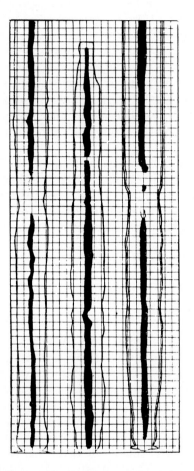

FIGURE 46–4.
Shown are graphs of three hairs obtained by measuring diameter of cortex and medulla from mm to mm along their length and entering values on a scale exaggerated 1000X for width. Hairs had been plucked from a patient's head 98 days after he fell ill with pneumonia and show Pohl-Pincus' mark. Young hair in center was least affected and grew faster than two older hairs, only bottom halves of which are shown. While older hairs show constriction and loss of medulla (black) beginning 37 and 39 mm from the base and extending for 5 to 7 mm, the vigorous young hair has only a slight constriction and loss of medulla at 41 mm. At average growth rate of 0.4 mm a day, 98 days correspond to 39.2 mm, a value confirming connection of Pohl's mark with febrile illness. (From Pinkus. Die Einwirkung von Krankheiten auf das Kopfhaar des Menschen, 2nd ed, 1928. Courtesy of S. Karger.)

fected hairs will show a temporary local constriction and loss of medulla. Plucked anagen hairs (preferentially white ones because their medulla is more conspicuous) should be examined either by simple microscopic inspection or by the more accurate methods developed by F. Pinkus (Fig. 46–4). The transient decrease in diameter can also be found following the administration of antimitotic drugs,[6] immunosuppressive drugs,[11] and other drugs,[12] and following X-ray therapy.[13] The common denominator is decrease or cessation of mitotic activity in the hair root. If the hair matrix recovers, temporary thinning of shaft and disappearance of the medulla in a circumscribed zone will result, and this is pushed outward as *Pohl–Pincus's mark*. If the insult was too severe, the hair undergoes precipitous catagen and exhibits a fusiform end instead of a club (Fig. 46–5A).

The effect of oral administration of thallium salts,[14] which leads to diffuse hair loss, has some

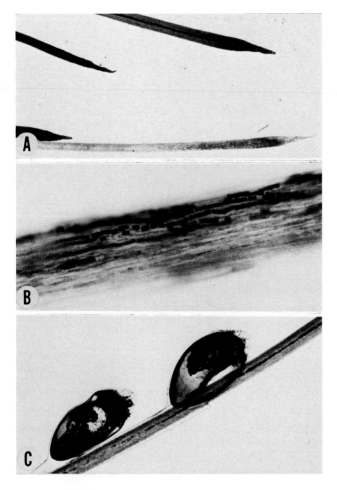

FIGURE 46–5.
Abnormal hairs. **A.** *Filiform roots in X-ray defluvium. X30.*
B. *Endothrix. X225.* **C.** *Nits in pediculosis capitis. X25.*

in fact represents an arrest of hair differentiation so that silky hair resembling fetal lanugo grows to great length, but the specific forms of scalp and terminal hair are not developed. On the other hand, *acquired hypertrichosis lanuginosa* (or *vellosa*), a rare skin manifestation of internal malignancy,[14] results from the conversion of preexisting vellus follicles on face and other areas. Their roots grow longer, often bending sideways (Fig. 46–6), and they form long, soft, and usually colorless hairs (malignant down[15]). A relation to carcinoembryonic antigen was suggested[16] inasmuch as this substance is found in fetuses between the second and sixth months and was elevated in several patients. Other forms of hypertrichosis, whether in porphyria or in virilizing syndromes *(hirsutism)*, are due to conversion of small hair follicles into stronger ones. No new hair roots are formed.

Rhythmic and Discontinuous Disturbances

A detailed and amply illustrated chapter on structural abnormalities of the hair shaft has been written by Price.[17] It testifies to the value of scanning electron microscopy. The use of polarized light also furnishes beautiful and instructive pictures, as shown by Dupré and Bonafé.[18] *Trichorrhexis nodosa* (Fig. 46–7A), *monilethrix*[19] (Fig. 46–7B), *pili torti* (Fig. 46–7C), and *bamboo hairs*[20,21] (Fig. 46–8A) must be due to rhythmic or discontinuous disturbances of hair formation. Little is known concerning the pathomechanisms causing these

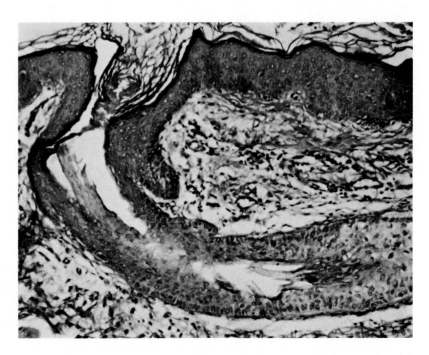

FIGURE 46–6.
Hypertrichosis vellosa (acquired hypertrichosis lanuginosa) in a case of internal cancer. Lateral deviation of hyperplastic root of a vellus hair. H&E. X100. (From Hegedus and Schorr. Arch Dermatol 106:84, 1972.)

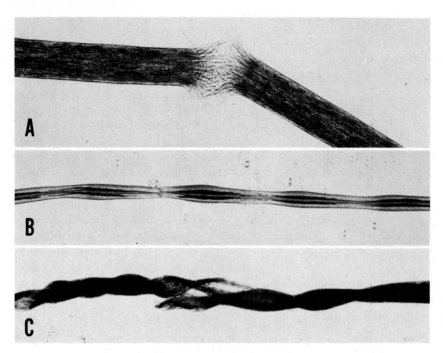

FIGURE 46–7.
*Abnormal hairs. **A.** Trichorrhexis nodosa. **B.** Monilethrix. **C.** Pilus tortus also exhibiting trichorrhexis.*

disturbances, but their manifestations are easily identified. *Pili anulati* require closer examination[22] because they are characterized by groups of tiny gas bubbles in the cortex, while *pili pseudoanulati*[23,24] are due to partial twists of hairs having elliptical cross section.

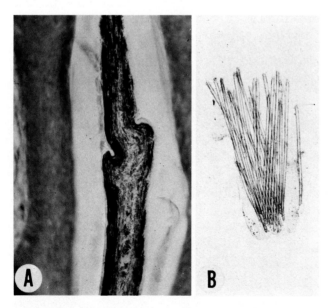

FIGURE 46–8.
*Abnormal hairs. **A.** Trichorrhexis invaginata (bamboo hair), longitudinal section of hair in follicle. O&G. X180. **B.** Trichostasis spinulosa, bundle of hairs (tysanothrix) expressed from a small hair follicle. X30.*

Unmanageable Hair

Several other abnormalities have been described in recent years and accounts may be found in review articles,[17,25] abstracts in the Year Books of Dermatology, and the books quoted earlier.

One of these abnormalities has attracted considerable attention. It was first described as "spun glass" hair[26] because of the refractoriness of the surface of the hairs, each one of which protrudes from the scalp in its own direction and does not lie down. This has led to the appellation "cheveux incoiffables" *(unmanageable hair)*. Biopsies and electron microscopy have shown that the hair shafts are triangular or fluted and are surrounded in the follicle by inner root sheath of the same configuration. The papilla and matrix appear normal.[27] Unmanageable hair is a purely cosmetic defect which seems to regress[28] as the children get older. It occurs in siblings, but nothing is known about inheritance.

Hair in Congenital Disorders

Hair is a good genetic marker,[29] and many peculiarities of hair growth and color are visible to the naked eye and do not require microscopic examination. Hair dysplasia often is associated with dysplasia of other cutaneous adnexa.[30] In some of these long-known disorders, microscopic examination of scalp biopsies and hair can add interesting new findings.

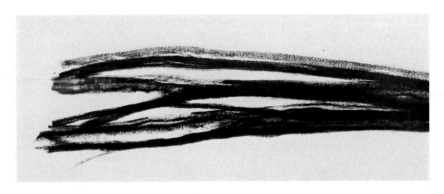

FIGURE 46–9.
Pili multigemini. Upper end of multiple hair formation consisting of several branching and reuniting asymmetrical shafts (pagothrix). Formations of this type can be differentiated from trichoptilosis (longitudinal splitting of a single hair) by the much greater combined volume of the several hairs, each of which has its own cuticle.

We mention the Marie Unna type of hereditary hypotrichosis,[31,32] in which fluting and twisting of hair shafts and unusual epithelial outgrowths on hair follicles may be seen, and Menkes' disease[33] in which copper metabolism is deranged and kinky hairs are a prominent manifestation. Such experiences should encourage dermatologists to take biopsies in cases of macroscopic abnormality of hair more often. It can be expected that missing links in the spectrum of follicular malformation may be thus discovered. A case in point is the discovery of generalized follicular hamartomas where alopecia totalis had been diagnosed on clinical examination.[34]

Circumscribed Abnormalities

Occurrence of abnormal hairs in circumscribed areas was mentioned in Chapter 36. They are often described as woolly hair nevi. The term *woolly* in connection with human hair is confusing. Many authors refer to negroid curly hair as woolly, but the wool of sheep has quite different structural and histochemical characteristics, which are not found in any human hair.[35] The negroid hair follicle has a regular semicircular curve (Figs. 2–24 and 18–10), and the hair continues the curl imposed on it during its keratinizing phase after it leaves the skin. Most authors do not define exactly what they mean by woolly hair,[36] and it is likely that measurements of hair and biopsy of scalp would reveal different anomalies in different cases. It would be better to refer to localized abnormalities of hair as *curly* or *kinky hair nevi* than as woolly hair nevi.

Pili Multigemini

Scattered abnormal hairs may be found on close examination, especially in the beard, and rarely cause symptoms. These abnormalities vary from fluted hairshafts to hair with double medulla, bifurcate,[37] and other monstrous hairs (pagothrix), and in the fullest expression *multiple hairs* (pili multigemini[8,38,39]), in which up to seven asymmetric hairs (Fig. 46–9) each with its own inner root sheath, arise from a single multiheaded papilla (Fig. 46–10).

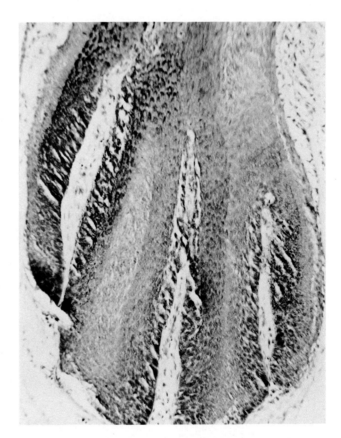

FIGURE 46–10.
Pili multigemini. Hair bulb showing subdivision of dermal papilla into several lobes, each surrounded by matrix and keratinizing cells which partly unite higher up into a very thick shaft that will break up into multiple hairs (Fig. 46–9). H&E. X135. (From Mehregan and Thompson. Br J Dermatol 100:315, 1979.)

The papilla is unusually large, and the total diameter of the divided hair is much thicker than normal,[40] causing difficulties in shaving.

Trichostasis Spinulosa

The occurrences described above must be sharply differentiated from the condition trichostasis spinulosa, in which several to dozens of dead vellus hairs are retained in a follicle (Fig. 46–8B), each formed successively from the normal matrix.

Disturbances of Hair Due to External Causes: Traction Alopecia and Trichotillomania

The alterations of hair due to common cosmetic procedures cannot be discussed here. Definitely pathologic changes, however, are produced by those manipulations leading to traction alopecia. These include tight braiding and attachments of nurse's caps.[41] Affected follicles enter telogen and become surrounded by fibrosis and may even undergo irreversible atrophy. The histologic picture may imitate pseudopelade (Chap. 18). A different picture, so-called *trichomalacia* (Fig. 46–11), is produced by compulsive pulling at hair, trichotillomania.[42–44] Here, the number of hair follicles does not decrease, but many are found in catagen, a stage rarely seen in other conditions because of its short duration. Strong follicles may contain peculiar deformed hairs or just keratinous and pigmented debris. Perifollicular hemorrhage and some inflammation may be present.

Trichosporosis and Trichomycosis

Changes of the hair due to dermatophytic infection were mentioned in Chapter 18. Spores and mycelia

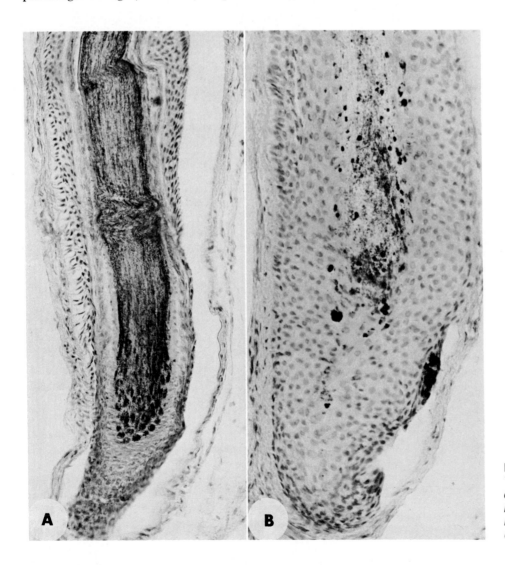

FIGURE 46–11.
Trichomalacia in a case of trichotillomania. **A.** *Deformed hair in fairly normal follicle.* **B.** *Pigmented debris in another follicle.* H&E. X135.

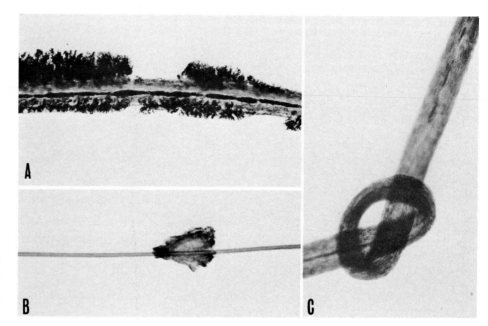

FIGURE 46–12.
*Abnormalities of hairs. **A.** Trichomycosis axillaris (black piedra). Hair shaft densely surrounded by organisms. X250. **B.** Hair cast. X125. **C.** Trichonodosis. X250.*

around and in the shaft can be seen in plucked hairs suspended in oil, crushed in xylene,[45] or cautiously treated with 10 percent potassium hydroxide. PAS stain, as illustrated in Figure 46–5B, is rarely necessary. Other organisms, such as *Trichosporon cutaneum* causing *white piedra*,[46,47] and *Corynebacterium tenue* causing *trichomycosis axillaris*,[48,49] (Fig. 46–12) also attack hair of axillae and pubic region. In these and other disturbances of the hair shaft, scanning electron microscopy has provided beautiful and instructive pictures, the discussion of which, however, is beyond the scope of the present volume.

Trichonodosis

Trichonodosis, the formation of true knots (Fig. 46–12C) is easily recognized under the microscope and is more common than generally believed,[50] especially in kinky scalp hair.

Extraneous Material on Hair

In the microscopic examination of shed or plucked hair, extraneous matter is often seen. Commonly, adherent dirt or hair dye is of no consequence except in forensic medicine.[51] The growing anagen hair, when plucked, usually is enveloped in the soft portions of inner and outer root sheath, forming a semitransparent coat around the lower end. This is absent in catagen and telogen hairs.

Hair Casts

Keratinized remnants of inner root sheath, on the other hand, may be found as sliding whitish rings (Fig. 46–12B) around hair shafts.[52] They sometimes are mistaken for nits (Fig. 46–5C) on naked-eye examination but are movable and can easily be distinguished under the microscope, where they resemble napkin rings.

DISTURBANCES OF NAIL

Punch biopsy specimens of nail and nailbed can be obtained without permanent deformity, if the matrix region is avoided.[53] If the matrix must be biopsied, two longitudinal incisions should be made about 2 mm apart and the gap sutured in order to obtain a strip of tissue with minimal scarring.[54] Small punch biopsies can also be taken of the matrix after it is exposed by incising and reverting the posterior fold. Skillful surgery is a prerequisite. Otherwise specimens are of little value, and the nail may remain deformed.

Various Dermatoses

Pathologic changes of the soft tissues under the nailplate do not differ materially from those of other regions in many inflammatory and neoplastic conditions and need little specific discussion.

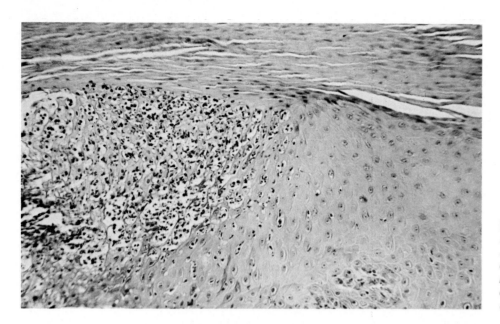

FIGURE 46–13.
Pustular psoriasis of nailbed. Spongiform pustule and excess formation of parakeratotic material are similar to the processes seen in other areas (Figs. 8–11 and 8–12).

Nailbed changes in pustular psoriasis[55] are shown in Figure 46–13, those of lichen planus[56] in Figure 46–14. Zaias and Ackerman[57] described characteristic dyskeratotic changes of the soft tissues around the nail in Darier's disease and multinucleated giant cells in the cornified portions of nailplate and nailbed. Scabies mites may occasionally affect the nail and surrounding keratinized tissue.[58]

Bowen's disease and keratoacanthoma may affect the nail matrix and nailbed and may require differential diagnosis from squamous cell carcinoma and from verruca vulgaris. The latter can involve the nailbed for a considerable distance from the distal or lateral margins. These diagnoses require resolute measures for adequate biopsy. The nailplate must be avulsed in order to inspect the underlying tissues and to obtain a sufficiently large and deep specimen. Another indication for radical exploration is pigmentation of the nail. A longitudinal pigmented streak in the nail of a Caucasian (darker skinned persons are excepted from this rule) means the presence of a melanin-forming lesion in the nail matrix. A decision whether this lesion is a benign nevus, a malignant nevocytoma, or a lentigo maligna can only be made by adequate incisional biopsy after removal of the nailplate.

The nail itself is rarely submitted for histopathologic analysis, and its examination is often unsatisfactory. Silver,[59] melanin, and mycelia can be demonstrated in sections of nail, if that is indicated.

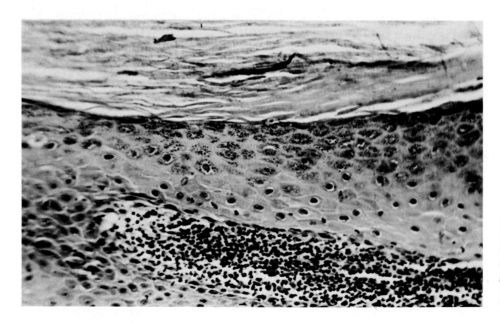

FIGURE 46–14.
Lichen planus of nailbed. Loss of basal layer and formation of a granular layer, not normally present in the bed of the nail. Dense lymphocytic infiltrate. H&E. X180.

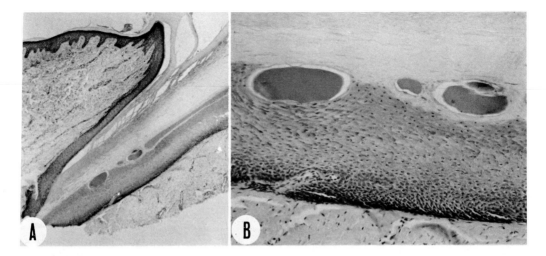

FIGURE 46–15.
*Subungual hemorrhage. **A.** The blood is deposited as several coagulated masses between the nail matrix and the forming nail plate. H&E. X125. **B.** At higher power, it is seen that the clot at the left indents the nail matrix, while the clot at the right has been incorporated into the nail (a form of transepithelial elimination). H&E. X250. Note also in **A** the obvious division of the keratin of the posterior nailfold into eponychium and cuticle (see Fig. 46–1).*

Hemorrhage

Hemorrhages involving the nail matrix (Fig. 46–15) will be incorporated into the nailplate as it forms and keratinizes and will either make it so abnormal that it disintegrates or will appear on the surface as the nail moves forward. On the other hand, hemorrhages into the nailbed distal to the lunula will remain below the nailplate but will be moved forward with it.

Pachyonychia Congenita

In pachyonychia congenita (Fig. 46–16), in spite of its name, the nailplate and the proximal nail matrix from which it arises are quite normal.[60,61] The normally semisterile nailbed epithelium, however, and the distal matrix, which normally forms only a small amount of keratin (horn of the sole, hyponychium), are hyperplastic and papillomatous and produce large quantities of abnormal horny mate-

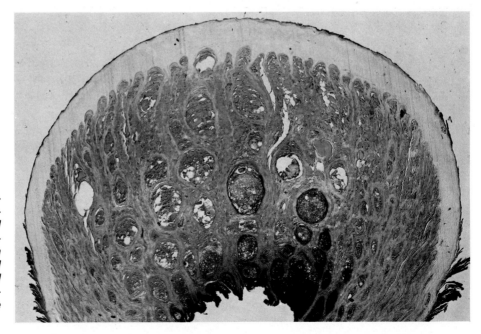

FIGURE 46–16.
Cross section of nail in pachyonychia congenita shows well-formed sturdy nailplate and papillomatous distal matrix tissue producing abnormal keratin honeycombed with coagulated PAS-positive material (colloid keratosis). Configuration resembles a horse's hoof. Compare Figure 46–1. H&E. X21.

rial mixed with hyaline masses (*colloid keratosis*[62]). Each of the deformed nails resembles a miniature horse's hoof histologically as well as clinically.

Pterygium Inversum Unguis

A minor deformity of the distal matrix which may occur as a congenital or acquired phenomenon is pterygium inversum unguis.[63,64] Here, the keratin formed by the distal matrix adheres tightly to the lower surface of the nail and is pulled forward.

The monographs on diseases of the nails mentioned in the introduction to Section VIII should be consulted for more detailed discussion.

REFERENCES

1. Christophers E: Cellular architecture of the stratum corneum. J Invest Dermatol 56:165, 1971
2. Jarrett A (ed): The Hair Follicle. The Physiology and Pathophysiology of the Skin, vol 4. London, New York, Academic, 1977
3. Kobori T, Montagna W (consulting eds): Biology and Disease of the Hair. University of Tokyo Press, 1976
4. Orfanos CE (ed): Haar und Haarkrankheiten. Stuttgart, New York, Gustav Fischer, 1979
5. Pinkus F: Die Einwirkung von Krankheiten auf das Kopfhaar des Menschen, 2nd ed. Berlin, Karger, 1928
6. Van Scott EJ, Reinertson RP, Steinmuller R: The growing hair roots of the human scalp and morphologic changes therein following amethopterin therapy. J Invest Dermatol 29:197, 1957
7. Kligman AM: Pathologic dynamics of human hair loss. I. Telogen effluvium. Arch Dermatol 83:175, 1961
8. Baccaredda-Boy A, Moretti G, Fry JR (eds): Biopathology of Pattern Alopecia. Basel, Karger, 1968
9. Lattanand A, Johnson WC: Male pattern alopecia. A histopathologic and histochemical study. J Cutan Pathol 2:58, 1975
10. Pinkus H: Differential patterns of elastic fibers in scarring and non-scarring alopecias. J Cutan Pathol 5:93, 1978
11. Kostanecki W, Mazurkiewicz W, Górkiewicz A, et al.: Haarveränderungen bei immunsuppressiver Therapie. Z Hautkr 46:704, 1971
12. Levantine A, Almeyda J: Drug-induced alopecia. Br J Dermatol 89:549, 1973
13. Van Scott EJ, Reinertson RP: Detection of radiation effects on hair roots of the human scalp. J Invest Dermatol 29:205, 1957
14. Hegedus SI, Schorr WF: Acquired hypertrichosis lanuginosa and malignancy: clinical review and histopathologic evaluation with special attention to "mantle" hair of Pinkus. Arch Dermatol 106:84, 1972
15. Fretzin DF: Malignant down. Arch Dermatol 95:294, 1967
16. Ikeya T, Izumi A, Suzuki M: Acquired hypertrichosis lanuginosa. Dermatologica 156:274, 1978
17. Price VH: Strukturanomalien des Haarschaftes. In Orfanos CE (ed): Haar und Haarkrankheiten. Stuttgart, New York, Gustav Fischer, 1979
18. Dupré A, Bonafé J-L: Étude en lumière polarisée des dysplasies pilaires. Essai d'actualisation de la nomenclature. Ann Dermatol Venereol 105:921, 1978
19. Comaish S: Autoradiographic studies of hair growth and rhythm in monilethrix. Br J Dermatol 81:443, 1969
20. Netherton EW: A unique case of trichorrhexis nodosa—"bamboo hairs." Arch Dermatol 78:483, 1958
21. Nikulin A, Šalamon T: Über die Entstehung der Nodositäten der Haare beim Netherton-Syndrom. Polarisations-mikroskopische Untersuchungen. Z Hautkr 44:1015, 1969
22. Dawber R: Investigations of a family with pili annulati associated with blue nevi. Trans St Johns Hosp Dermatol Soc 58:51, 1972
23. Price VH, Thomas RS, Jones FT: Pseudopili annulati. Arch Dermatol 102:354, 1970
24. Arnold HA: Pili pseudoannulati. Arch Dermatol 103:104, 1971
25. Porter PS: Genetic disorders of hair growth. J Invest Dermatol 60:493, 1973
26. Stroud JD, Mehregan AH: "Spun glass" hair. A clinicopathologic study of an unusual hair defect. In Brown AC (ed): The First Human Hair Symposium. New York, Medcom, 1974
27. Dupré A, Bonafé J-L, Litoux F, et al.: Le syndrome des cheveux incoiffables. Pili trianguli et canaliculi. Ann Dermatol Venereol 105:627, 1978
28. Laurent R, Yulzari M, Makki S, et al.: Syndrome des cheveux incoiffables. Deux nouveaux cas familiaux avec étude au microscope électronique à balayage. Ann Dermatol Venereol 105:633, 1978
29. Muller SA: Alopecia: syndromes of genetic significance. J Invest Dermatol 60:475, 1973
30. Freire-Maio N: Ectodermal dysplasias. Hum Hered 21:309, 1971
31. Solomon LM, Esterly NB, Modenica M: Hereditary trichodysplasia: Marie Unna's hypotrichosis. J Invest Dermatol 57:389, 1971
32. Hutchinson PE, Wells RS: Hereditary hypotrichosis (Marie-Unna type). Two cases. Proc R Soc Med 68:534, 1975
33. Enjolras O, Lessana-Leibowitch M, Hewitt J, et al.: Maladie de Menkes. Anomalies ultrastructurales cutanéophanériennes nouvelles. Ann Dermatol Venereol 105:493, 1978
34. Brown AC, Crounse RG, Winkelmann RK: Generalized hair follicle hamartoma. Arch Dermatol 99:478, 1969
35. Histology of wool and hair and of the wool follicle. In Proceedings of the International Wool Textile Research Conference, Australia 1955, Vol F. Melbourne, Commonwealth Scientific and Industrial Research Organization, 1956
36. Verbov J: Woolly hair: Study of a family. Dermatologica 157:42, 1978
37. Weary PE, Hendricks AA, Wawner F, et al.: Pili bifurcati; a new anomaly of hair growth. Arch Dermatol 108:403, 1973
38. Pinkus H: Multiple hairs (Flemming-Giovannini). J Invest Dermatol 17:291, 1951

39. Mehregan AH, Thompson WS: Pili multigemini. Report of a case in association with cleidocranial dysostosis. Brit J Dermatol 100:315, 1979

40. Pierard G-E: Structure et interprétation pathogénique. Dystrophies acquises du cheveu. Ann Dermatol Syphiligr 102:137, 1975

41. Renna FS, Freedberg IM: Traction alopecia in nurses. Arch Dermatol 108:694, 1973

42. Mehregan AH: Trichotillomania; a clinicopathologic study. Arch Dermatol 102:129, 1970

43. Muller SA, Winkelmann RK: Trichotillomania; a clinicopathologic study of 24 cases. Arch Dermatol 105:535, 1972

44. LaChapelle JM, Pierard SE: Traumatic alopecia in trichotillomania: a pathogenetic interpretation of histologic lesions in the pilosebaceous unit. J Cutan Pathol 4:51, 1977

45. Shelley WB, Wood MG: New technic for instant visualization of fungi in hair. J Am Acad Dermatol 2:69, 1980

46. Smith JD, Murtishaw DA, McBride ME: White piedra (trichosporosis). Arch Dermatol 107:439, 1973

47. Krempl-Lamprecht L: Ein Fall von weisser Piedra in München. Castellania 3:1, 1975

48. Orfanos CE, Schloesser E, Mahrle G: Hair-destroying growth of *Corynebacterium tenuis* in the so-called trichomycosis axillaris. Arch Dermatol 103:632, 1971

49. White SW, Smith J: Trichomycosis pubis. Arch Dermatol 115:444, 1979

50. English DT, Jones HE: Trichonodosis. Arch Dermatol 107:77, 1973

51. Berg S: Der Identifizierungswert des menschlichen Haares. Arch Kriminologie 159:65, 1977

52. Dawber RPR: Hair casts. Br J Dermatol 100:417, 1979

53. Scher RK: Punch biopsies of nails: a simple, valuable procedure. J Dermatol Surg Oncol 4:528, 1978

54. Fosnaugh RP: Surgery of the nail. In Epstein E, Epstein E Jr (eds): Skin Surgery. Springfield Ill, Thomas, 1977

55. Lewin K, DeWit S, Ferrington RA: Pathology of the fingernail in psoriasis; a clinicopathologic study. Br J Dermatol 86:555, 1972

56. Alkiewicz J, Nowak Z: Zur Klinik und Histologie des Lichen ruber planus ungium. Arch Klin Exp Dermatol 238:346, 1970

57. Zaias N, Ackerman AB: The nail in Darier-White disease. Arch Dermatol 107:193, 1973

58. Saruta T, Nakamizo Y: Usual scabies with nail infestation. Arch Dermatol 114:956, 1978

59. Plewig G, Lincke H, Wolff HH: Silver-blue nails. Acta Dermatol Venereol (Stockh) 57:413, 1977

60. Kelly EW Jr, Pinkus H: Report of a case of pachyonychia congenita. Arch Dermatol 77:724, 1958

61. Achten G, Wanet-Ronard J: Pachyonychia. Br J Dermatol 83:56, 1970

62. Alkiewicz J, Lebioda J, Rokita Z: Über Kolloidkeratose. Dermatol Monatsschr 158:329, 1972

63. Odom RB, Stein KM, Maibach HI: Congenital, painful, aberrant hyponychium. Arch Dermatol 110:89, 1974

64. Catteral MD, White JE: Pterygium inversum unguis. Clin Exp Dermatol 3:437, 1978

Index

Boldface indicates figures.